Spectral, Photon Counting Computed Tomography

Devices, Circuits, and Systems
Series Editor - Krzysztof Iniewski

Low Power Semiconductor Devices and Processes for Emerging Applications in Communications, Computing, and Sensing
Sumeet Walia and Krzysztof Iniewski

Sensors for Diagnostics and Monitoring
Kevin Yallup and Laura Basiricò

Biomaterials and Immune Response
Complications, Mechanisms and Immunomodulation
Nihal Engin Vrana

High-Speed and Lower Power Technologies
Electronics and Photonics
Jung Han Choi and Krzysztof Iniewski

X-Ray Diffraction Imaging
Technology and Applications
Joel Greenberg and Krzysztof Iniewski

Compressed Sensing for Engineers
Angshul Majumdar

Low Power Circuits for Emerging Applications in Communications, Computing, and Sensing
Krzysztof Iniewski and Fei Yuan

Labs on Chip
Principles, Design, and Technology
Eugenio Iannone

Energy Efficient Computing & Electronics
Devices to Systems
Santosh K. Kurinec and Sumeet Walia

Spectral, Photon Counting Computed Tomography
Technology and Applications
Katsuyuki Taguchi, Ira Blevis and Krzysztof Iniewski

For more information about this series, please visit: https://www.crcpress.com/Devices-Circuits-and-Systems/book-series/CRCDEVCIRSYS

Spectral, Photon Counting Computed Tomography

Technology and Applications

Edited by

Katsuyuki Taguchi
Ira Blevis
Krzysztof Iniewski

CRC Press
Taylor & Francis Group
Boca Raton London New York

CRC Press is an imprint of the
Taylor & Francis Group, an **informa** business

First edition published 2020
by CRC Press
6000 Broken Sound Parkway NW, Suite 300, Boca Raton, FL 33487-2742
and by CRC Press
2 Park Square, Milton Park, Abingdon, Oxon, OX14 4RN

Library of Congress Cataloging-in-Publication Data

Names: Taguchi, Katsuyuki, editor.
Title: Spectral, photon counting computed tomography : technology and applications / edited by Katsuyuki Taguchi, Ira Blevis, Krzysztof Iniewski.
Description: First edition. | Boca Raton : CRC Press, 2020. | Series: Devices, circuits, & systems | Includes bibliographical references and index.
Identifiers: LCCN 2020011034 (print) | LCCN 2020011035 (ebook) | ISBN 9781138598126 (hbk) | ISBN 9780429486111 (ebk)
Subjects: LCSH: Tomography--Methodology.
Classification: LCC RC78.7.T6 S63 2020 (print) | LCC RC78.7.T6 (ebook) | DDC 616.07/57--dc23
LC record available at https://lccn.loc.gov/2020011034
LC ebook record available at https://lccn.loc.gov/2020011035

ISBN: 978-1-138-59812-6 (hbk)

ISBN: 978-0-429-48611-1 (ebk)

Contents

PART IV Image Reconstruction for Spectral CT

Preface

X-ray computed tomography (CT) provides enormous and by now essential diagnostic benefits as the first cross-sectional imaging modality used in most hospitals; however, the performance of the current x-ray CT has not reached its full potential because current CT detectors measure the intensity of x-rays and ignore fingerprints of soft tissues or contrast agents in the x-ray spectrum. Transmitted x-ray spectra contain information about different tissue types such as muscle, fat, bone, contrast agents, etc. Spectral dual-energy (DE-)CT was the first step toward acquiring such spectral information; various system concepts and designs have been introduced and dedicated clinical applications developed. They have made significant contributions to the accuracy of clinical CT-based diagnosis. Recently developed, energy-sensitive photon counting detectors (PCDs) work on a different principle, counting photons individually, and capturing energy-dependent information within 2–8 energy windows. As a result, photon counting (PC-)CT has the potential not only to further improve the current CT images, but also to enable new class of clinical applications, such as higher spatial resolution, better soft tissue contrast, stronger contrast agent enhancement, radiation dose reduction, quantitative CT imaging and biomarkers, accurate soft tissue material characterization, K-edge imaging, and simultaneous multi-contrast agent imaging. PC-CT is expected to be the next generation of x-ray CT after DE-CT.

This book is the first one that covers the latest developments of spectral DE-CT and spectral PC-CT comprehensively and we believe this is the right timing for such a book. One of the editors authored a Vision 20/20 paper on PCDs for medical imaging for the journal *Medical Physics* in 2013 [1], which covered detectors, imaging algorithms, system designs, and clinical applications. Since then, a few prototype whole-body research PC-CT systems have been developed by CT manufactures and installed and field-tested at their luminary sites worldwide. Clinical assessments provided realistic views of PC-CT and due to the increasing levels of clinical activities, a much larger number of researchers with different backgrounds are coming to this field. This book will serve as a great textbook for such new investigators as well as for experts to understand emerging areas outside of their expertise.

In this book, leading world experts on each subject review detectors and electronics, detector and system modeling, image reconstruction methods, a simulation tool, nanoparticle contrast agents, and clinical applications for spectral CT. Spectral CT is an emerging area of clinical and technical research; and therefore, it is natural that there exist different opinions. It was our intention to provide readers such different views on related topics. Readers are encouraged to read all of the closely related chapters. If there is an agreement on some topic among a few chapters, it means that it has become or is becoming a consensus in the community. If there are differences among authors' opinions, it may indicate that it remains a topic of debate. In the near future, the differences may be resolved and a consensus may be formed, or it may still remain an open discussion.

The book consists of four parts: Part I on spectral DE-CT and its clinical perspective and applications; Part II on spectral PC-CT and its clinical perspective and applications; Part III on detector systems; and Part IV on image reconstruction methods. Overview of all the four parts is provided here.

Part I consists of three chapters (Chapters 1–3) and is devoted to clinical perspective and application of DE-CT. Chapter 1 provides a theoretical background on the principles of DE-CT, outlines different techniques in use, and includes some discussion of the advantages and disadvantages of different methods and design choices. Chapter 2 presents different DE-CT designs with a clinician's perspective, image processing techniques, and reviews various clinical applications for neuroimaging comprehensively. Chapter 3 outlines clinical perspective on DE-CT for various radiology and oncology applications, as well as artifacts and safety issues.

Part II consists of six chapters (Chapters 4–9) and is devoted to clinical perspective and application of PC-CT. Chapter 4 focuses on the use of PC-CT for breast imaging and provides a brief overview of the current breast CT imaging systems, the benefits of PC-breast-CT, different design requirements and their trade-offs, and promising applications. Chapters 5–7 are authored by top researchers with invaluable experiences with prototype whole-body research PC-CT systems developed by Siemens, Philips, and MARS imaging, respectively. The three CT systems use very different PCDs, and therefore, understanding the agreements and disagreements between their views may be of interest to the readership.

Chapters 8 and 9 discuss contrast agents, which are the key element for very unique clinical applications for PC-CT such as K-edge imaging and molecular imaging. Chapter 8 provides technical aspects of contrast agents, including the necessary considerations of potential atomic elements for PC-CT-specific contrast agent development and their development into nanoparticle-based contrast agents. Chapter 9 outlines clinical aspects of contrast agents, including the clinical requirements, potential clinical merits, and various design and targeting issues.

Part III consists of nine chapters (Chapters 10–18) and covers detectors and imaging systems analyses. Chapters 10, 11, and 13 discuss PCDs. Chapter 10 describes the PCDs including the basics of signal formation and the primary failure modes at the very high flux employed for x-ray CT and the impact of detector design trade-offs such as pixel size. Chapter 11 dissects detector response functions and details various factors including noise, charge sharing, fluorescence x-rays, pulse pileup, Compton scattering, recombination of electron-hole pairs, etc. Chapter 13 presents theories and modeling focusing on the detector signal formation.

Chapters 14 and 15 cover application specific integrated circuit (ASIC) and electronics. Chapter 14 discusses requirements to readout detector signals and minimizes systematic errors passed onto data processing reconstruction schemes. Chapter 15 presents an ASIC design and performance evaluation results for an electronics configuration in use in one of spectral photon counting CT prototypes.

Chapters 12, 16–18 cover detector and system modeling for imaging science. Chapter 12 starts with nonlinear shift-variant imaging systems model and outlines how charge summing mode restores shift-invariance. Chapter 16 presents beautiful new detector modeling effort for PCDs using cascaded systems approaches. Energy thresholding in PCDs forces a substantial departure from the traditional cascaded systems approaches, including joint probabilities of pre-thresholding signals at neighboring pixels. Chapter 17 outlines how several PCD parameters control trade-offs in systems level performance such as PCD pixel sizes, the number of energy windows, and pulse shaping time. New technologies, such as charge summing and dynamic filters, which can improve the performance of PCDs in the future, are discussed. Chapter 18 presents a simulation tool, Photon Counting Toolkit (PcTK), which are made available to academic researchers at pctk.jhu.edu to help the community. PcTK can compute energy responses of PCDs with given design parameters and generate noisy PC-CT projection data of user-defined objects.

Part IV consists of three chapters (Chapters 19–21) and covers image reconstruction for spectral CT. Chapter 19 provides an overview of image reconstruction algorithms. Various aspects, such as material decomposition and image prior information, are discussed. Chapter 20 presents an algorithm that integrates a detector model and compensates for severe spectral distortions induced by charge sharing. A nonlinear CT systems model is broken into two linear steps and one correction step with the use of "x-ray transmittance" that models the attenuation of x-ray spectra. It is computationally very efficient and bias and noise are comparable or better than maximum-likelihood approaches. Chapter 21 outlines an innovative algorithm that takes advantage of the rich information that PC-CT provides. The algorithm is based on a new concept and jointly estimates tissue/material types and densities of basis functions (or CT images) for each image voxel. The estimated tissue type maps are used to regularize CT images effectively and accurately, while improved CT images make tissue type maps more accurate.

Overall, the hope is that this book will provide readers comprehensive views of the state of the art of the emerging spectral, DE-CT and PC-CT, as well as a future perspective of spectral PC-CT.

Note: [1] Taguchi, K and Iwanczyk, JS. Vision 20/20: Single photon counting x-ray detectors in medical imaging, *Medical Physics*, 2013;40(10):100901.

Editors

Katsuyuki (Ken) Taguchi (ktaguchi@jhmi.edu) is professor in The Russell H. Morgan Department of Radiology and Radiological Science, The Johns Hopkins University School of Medicine. Dr. Taguchi received his M.Sc. degree in mechanical engineering science from Tokyo Institute of Technology (Tokyo, Japan) in 1991 and his Ph.D. degree in information science and electrical engineering from University of Tsukuba (Tsukuba, Japan) in 2002. He has worked for Toshiba Medial Systems (Otawara, Japan and Lincolnshire, IL, USA) between 1991–2005 and served as a senior imaging scientist toward the end. He has pioneered and implemented algorithms for prototypes and commercial scanners such as multislice CT in 1998, cardiac CT in 2000, and 256-slice CT in 2002. Due to those seminal works and his significant contribution, Dr. Taguchi has received IEEE Nuclear and Plasma Sciences Society 2008 Young Investigator Medical Imaging Science Award. Working on PC-CT since 2006, Dr. Taguchi has quickly become one of the world's leading experts of PCDs and the systems modeling and image reconstruction for PC-CT. He has organized two international spectral imaging workshops (with SPIE MI in 2008 and IEEE NSS/MIC in 2013), and given four keynote speeches on PC-CT (at AAPM meeting in 2008, at RSNA in 2011, at CERN Workshop in 2011, and at a joint symposium in Japan in 2012) as well as numerous invited departmental talks. Dr. Taguchi published a Vision 20/20 paper on PC-CT in *Medical Physics* journal and authored a section on the PCD technology for a statement-type article on radiation dose management in *Radiology* journal.

Ira Blevis (Ira.Blevis@philips.com) is principal scientist in Philips Healthcare developing semiconductor radiation detectors and Photon Counting CT based on them. Recent progress with the detectors led to a prototype PC scanner based on CZT, which served as a basis for an EU H2020 grant awarded to develop a full-size prototype for clinical use. Ira served a term as director of the Philips Project and serves as Philips PI on the grant. Prior to Philips, Ira was principal engineer at General Electric Medical Systems, leading R&D of CZT for Nuclear Medicine and attenuation correction CT (1999–2012), leading to first imaging prototypes and to commercial products. Ira also worked with the team building the first active matrix a-Se panels at University of Toronto. Ira received his Ph.D. in Particle Physics from the Weizmann Institute (Rehovot, Israel) for work at CERN (Geneva, Switzerland) and then participated in the Nobel Prize winning SNO collaboration (Ottawa, Canada) to measure neutrino oscillations, also sharing in the 2016 Breakthrough Prize in Physics. Ira has an extensive bibliography in Physics, Medical Detectors, and Medical Imaging, and holds numerous international patents in imaging and detectors; he is a repeated invited speaker and has contributed to published books in the field.

Krzysztof (Kris) Iniewski (kris.iniewski@gmail.com) is managing R&D development activities at Redlen Technologies Inc., a compound semiconductor detector company based in British Columbia, Canada. During his 12 years at Redlen, he managed development of highly integrated CZT detector products in medical imaging and security applications. Prior to Redlen, Kris held various management and academic positions at PMC-Sierra, University of Alberta, SFU, UBC, and University of Toronto. Dr. Iniewski has published over 250 research papers in international journals and conferences. He holds 18 international patents granted in USA, Canada, France, Germany, and Japan. He wrote and edited several books for Wiley, Cambridge University Press, McGraw-Hill, CRC Press, and Springer. He is frequent invited speaker and has consulted for multiple organizations internationally. He received his Ph.D. degree in electronics (honors) from the Warsaw University of Technology (Warsaw, Poland) in 1988.

Contributors

Sikiru A. Adebileje
University of Otago
Christchurch, New Zealand
Human Interface Technology Laboratory New Zealand, University of Canterbury
Christchurch, New Zealand

Steven D. Alexander
University of Canterbury
Christchurch, New Zealand

Ami Altman
Philips Healthcare
CT/AMI
Haifa, Israel

Kenji Amaya
Tokyo Institute of Technology
Tokyo, Japan

Maya R. Amma
University of Otago
Christchurch, New Zealand

Fatemeh Asghariomabad
University of Otago
Christchurch, New Zealand

Ali Atharifard
MARS Bioimaging Limited
Christchurch, New Zealand

Benjamin Bamford
University of Otago
Christchurch, New Zealand

Stephen T. Bell
MARS Bioimaging Limited
Christchurch, New Zealand

Rick Bergmans
Technical Medicine
University of Twente
Enschede, Netherlands

Srinidhi Bheesette
University of Otago
Christchurch, New Zealand
European Organisation for Nuclear Research (CERN)
Geneva, Switzerland

Ira Blevis
Philips Healthcare
Haifa, Israel

Loic Boussel
Radiology Department of Cardiothoracic and Vascular Imaging, Louis Pradel Hospital, Hospices Civils de Lyon
and
CREATIS Laboratory, Claude Bernard Lyon 1 University
Lyon, France

Christian Broennimann
Dectris Ltd., Taefernweg
Baden-Daettwil, Switzerland

Anthony P. H. Butler
MARS Bioimaging Limited, Christchurch
and
University of Canterbury
and
University of Otago
and
Human Interface Technology Laboratory New Zealand, University of Canterbury
Christchurch, New Zealand
European Organisation for Nuclear Research (CERN)
Geneva, Switzerland

Philip H. Butler
MARS Bioimaging Limited
and
University of Canterbury
and
University of Otago
and
Human Interface Technology Laboratory New Zealand, University of Canterbury
Christchurch, New Zealand
European Organisation for Nuclear Research (CERN)
Geneva, Switzerland

Liang Cai
Canon Medical Research Inc.
Vernon Hills, Illinois, USA

Pierre Carbonez
University of Otago
Christchurch, New Zealand
European Organisation for Nuclear Research (CERN)
Geneva, Switzerland

Alexander I. Chernoglazov
MARS Bioimaging Limited
and
Human Interface Technology Laboratory New Zealand, University of Canterbury
Christchurch, New Zealand

David P. Cormode
Department of Radiology, Department of Bioengineering, and Department of Cardiology
University of Pennsylvania
Philadelphia, Pennsylvania, USA

Ian Cunningham
Imaging Research Laboratories
and
Robarts Research Institute
and
Department of Medical Biophysics
The University of Western Ontario
London, Ontario, Canada

Shishir Dahal
University of Otago
Christchurch, New Zealand
and
Ministry of Health, Nepal
National Academy of Medical Sciences
Kathmandu, Nepal

Jérôme Damet
University of Otago
Christchurch, New Zealand
and
European Organisation for Nuclear Research (CERN)
Geneva, Switzerland
and
Institute of Radiation Physics, Lausanne University Hospital
Lausanne, Switzerland

Niels J. A. de Ruiter
MARS Bioimaging Limited
and
University of Canterbury
and
University of Otago
and
Human Interface Technology Laboratory New Zealand, University of Canterbury
Christchurch, New Zealand

Robert M. N. Doesburg
MARS Bioimaging Limited
Christchurch, New Zealand

Philippe Douek
Radiology Department of Cardiothoracic and Vascular Imaging, Louis Pradel Hospital, Hospices Civils de Lyon
and
CREATIS Laboratory, Claude Bernard Lyon 1 University
Lyon, France

Thorsten Fleiter
Department of Diagnostic Imaging
University of Maryland School of Medicine
Shock Trauma Center
Baltimore, Maryland, USA

Bahaa Ghammraoui
Office of Science and Engineering Laboratories, CDRH
U.S. Food and Drug Administration
Silver Spring, Maryland, USA

Steven P. Gieseg
University of Canterbury
and
University of Otago
Christchurch, New Zealand

Stephen J. Glick
Office of Science and Engineering Laboratories, CDRH
U.S. Food and Drug Administration
Silver Spring, Maryland, USA

Brian P. Goulter
MARS Bioimaging Limited
Christchurch, New Zealand

Rajiv Gupta
Department of Radiology
Massachusetts General Hospital and Harvard Medical School
Boston, Massachusetts, USA

Conny Hansson
Redlen Technologies
Saanichton, British Columbia, Canada

Joseph L. Healy
MARS Bioimaging Limited
Christchurch, New Zealand

Christoph Herrmann
Philips Research Europe
High Tech Campus
Eindhoven, Netherlands

Scott S. Hsieh
Department of Radiology
Mayo Clinic
Rochester, Minnesota, USA

Krzysztof Iniewski
Redlen Technologies
Saanichton, British Columbia, Canada

Praveen K. Kanithi
University of Canterbury
and
Human Interface Technology Laboratory New Zealand, University of Canterbury
Christchurch, New Zealand

Johoon Kim
Department of Radiology and
Department of Bioengineering
University of Pennsylvania
Philadelphia, Pennsylvania, USA

Thomas Koenig
Ziehm Imaging GmbH
Nuremberg, Germany

Mayo Clinic Graduate School of Biomedical Sciences
Rochester, Minnesota, USA

Xiaochun Lai
Canon Medical Research Inc.
Vernon Hills, Illinois, USA

Stuart P. Lansley
MARS Bioimaging Limited
Christchurch, New Zealand

Okkyun Lee
Department of Robotics Engineering
Daegu Gyeongbuk Institute of Science and Technology
Daegu, Republic of Korea

Shuai Leng
Department of Radiology
Mayo Clinic
Rochester, Minnesota, USA

Amir Livne
Philips Healthcare
Haifa, Israel

Chiara Lowe
University of Otago
Christchurch, New Zealand

V. B. H. Mandalika
MARS Bioimaging Limited
and
University of Canterbury
and
Human Interface Technology Laboratory New Zealand, University of Canterbury
Christchurch, New Zealand

Emmanuel Marfo
University of Otago
Christchurch, New Zealand

Aysouda Matanaghi
University of Otago
Christchurch, New Zealand

Cynthia H. McCollough
Department of Radiology
Mayo Clinic
Rochester, Minnesota, USA

Charis McNabney
Department of Radiology
St. Paul's Hospital
Vancouver, British Columbia, Canada

Mahdieh Moghiseh
MARS Bioimaging Limited
and
University of Otago
Christchurch, New Zealand

Cyril Mory
Univ Lyon, INSA-Lyon
Université Claude Bernard Lyon 1
UJM-Saint Etienne, CNRS
INSERM, CREATIS, Centre Léon Bérard
Lyon, France

Darra T. Murphy
Department of Radiology
St. Paul's Hospital
Vancouver, British Columbia, Canada

Pratap C. Naha
Department of Radiology
University of Pennsylvania
Philadelphia, Pennsylvania, USA

Peter B. Noël
Department of Radiology
Perelman School of Medicine
University of Pennsylvania
Philadelphia, Pennsylvania, USA

Raj K. Panta
MARS Bioimaging Limited
and
University of Otago
Christchurch, New Zealand

Maarten Poirot
Technical Medicine
University of Twente
Enschede, Netherlands

Hannah M. Prebble
MARS Bioimaging Limited
Christchurch, New Zealand

Shamir Rai
Department of Radiology
St. Paul's Hospital
Vancouver, British Columbia, Canada

Aamir Y. Raja
MARS Bioimaging Limited
and
University of Otago
Christchurch, New Zealand

Kishore Rajendran
Department of Radiology
Mayo Clinic
Rochester, Minnesota, USA

Simon Rit
Univ Lyon, INSA-Lyon
Université Claude Bernard Lyon 1
UJM-Saint Etienne, CNRS
INSERM, CREATIS, Centre Léon Bérard
Lyon, France

Nanette Schleich
University of Otago
Wellington, New Zealand

Emily Searle
University of Canterbury
Christchurch, New Zealand

Nadav Shapira
Philips Healthcare
CT/AMI
Haifa, Israel

Jereena S. Sheeja
University of Otago
Christchurch, New Zealand

Salim Si-Mohamed
Radiology Department of Cardiothoracic and Vascular Imaging, Louis Pradel Hospital, Hospices Civils de Lyon
and
CREATIS Laboratory, Claude Bernard Lyon 1 University
Lyon, France

Chris Siu
BCIT
Burnaby, British Columbia, Canada

Roger Steadman
Philips Research Europe
High Tech Campus
Eindhoven, Netherlands

Katsuyuki Taguchi
Radiological Physics Division
The Russell H. Morgan Department of Radiology and Radiological Science
Johns Hopkins University School of Medicine
Baltimore, Maryland, USA

Jesse Tanguay
Department of Physics
Ryerson University
Toronto, Ontario, Canada

Shengzhen Tao
Department of Radiology
Mayo Clinic
Rochester, Minnesota, USA

Richard Thompson
Canon Medical Research Inc.
Vernon Hills, Illinois, USA

Peter Trueb
Dectris Ltd., Taefernweg
Baden-Daettwil, Switzerland

Rayhan Uddin
University of Canterbury
Christchurch, New Zealand

Lieza Vanden Broeke
University of Canterbury
Christchurch, New Zealand

Vivek V. S.
MARS Bioimaging Limited
Christchurch, New Zealand

Naor Wainer
Philips Healthcare, CT/AMI
Haifa, Israel

E. Peter Walker
University of Otago
Christchurch, New Zealand

Michael F. Walsh
MARS Bioimaging Limited
Christchurch, New Zealand

Manoj Wijesooriya
University of Canterbury
Christchurch, New Zealand

Yoad Yagil
Philips Healthcare, CT/AMI
Haifa, Israel

Pietro Zambon
Dectris Ltd., Taefernweg
Baden-Daettwil, Switzerland

Kevin Zimmerman
Canon Medical Research Inc.
Vernon Hills, Illinois, USA

Part I

Spectral, Dual-Energy CT: Clinical Perspective and Applications

1 Spectral Imaging Technologies and Apps and Dual-Layer Detector Solution

Nadav Shapira, Yoad Yagil, Naor Wainer, and Ami Altman
Philips Healthcare, CT/AMI, Haifa, Israel

CONTENTS

1.1 INTRODUCTION

Dual-energy computed tomography (DECT) is already an established clinical tool, which possesses diagnostic advantages over conventional CT systems. These advantages enable improvements in tissue characterization and material separation and pave the way for the quantitative imaging in CT. While conventional CT utilizes measurements of the total energy difference that was absorbed in a detector for an x-ray beam traversing an object verses that for an x-ray beam of the same characteristics traversing air, DECT is based on acquiring this difference for two different photon energy spectra. There are different technologies in use utilizing different approaches to create the two different photon energy spectra. A comparison between the different approaches will be discussed later in this chapter.

Taking advantage of information from two different photon energy spectra is actually not a new concept, but rather one that is known from color vision in the animal kingdom [1]. There is an analogy between DECT and animal color vision that can provide some intuition for the main concept behind the spectral theory of DECT.

In vision, the main source of light is the sun. The sun emits photons in a range of energies, or wavelengths ($\lambda_\gamma = hc / E_\gamma$), where the amount of emitted power per unit volume per wavelength comprises the spectrum of the sun. See Figure 1.1.

Photons which are reflected from various objects have been the sole evolutionary input for vision. In an earlier phase of evolution, animals had no capability to distinguish between colors. The total amount of detected light was absorbed by photoreceptor cells containing light-sensitive proteins which evolved in the retina. Each photoreceptor cell responded only to the total energy it absorbed, i.e., $Signal = \sum E \times n(E)$, where E is the energy of the photon and $n(E)$ is the number of photons of energy E that compose the reflected light and were successfully absorbed by the photoreceptor cell. This scheme allowed for a one-dimensional, i.e., gray-scale, intensity map of the reflected light

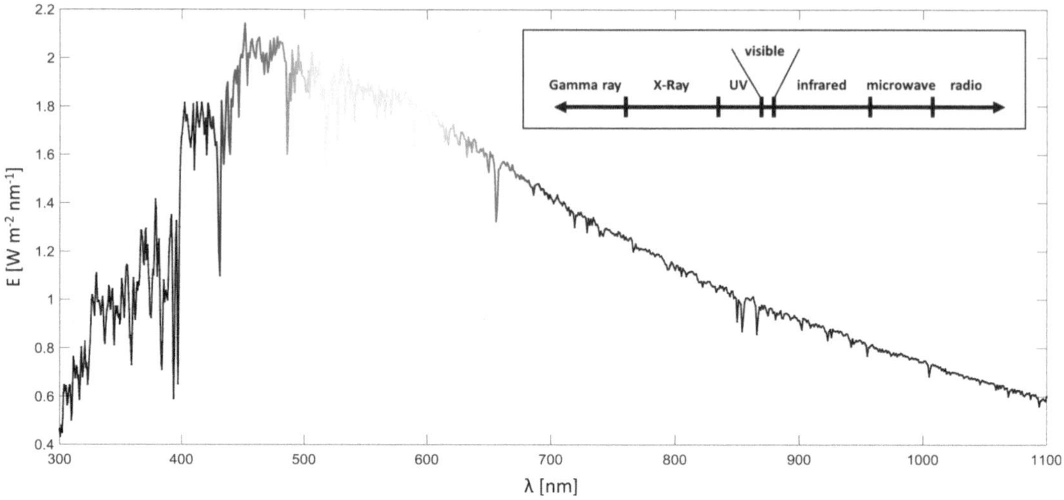

FIGURE 1.1 The electromagnetic spectrum of the sun, with visible light wavelengths shown in gray-scale, and a schematic of the range of classes of electromagnetic radiation. Based on data from Ref [2].

from the scene and later detected by the eye. However, since different objects may reflect the same amount of combined energy despite being composed of different wavelengths, e.g., a large number of yellow (low-energy) photons versus a small number of blue (high-energy) photons, detecting objects in the scene by the energy reflected from their surfaces can fail when objects reflect a similar amount of energy as each other or the background.

Following the principle of natural selection, two kinds of photoreceptor cell evolved with different energy response. While these new types of photoreceptor cells still maintain the basic mechanism of response that is dependent on the total amount of absorbed energy, each type exhibits a different spectral sensitivity, i.e., different detection efficiencies for the same light spectrum. That is, not to say that there is a complete energy separation between the two spectral responses, but that, despite the partial overlap between the two response spectra, a different detection signal is produced by each type of photoreceptor cell. This new scheme allowed for the differentiation between objects or surfaces that presented little or no signal difference in the one-dimensional scheme and provided an evolutionary advantage in various situations. The interpretation of the signals by the brain is now referred to as color vision, which combines information of both the integrated energy and the wavelength contrasts to detect objects for signals from cells, or channels, in the same areas of visual space. When the integrated energy contrast between different objects is absent or insufficient, "wavelength contrast" [1] may still be available to differentiate between them – it may be that two objects reflect the same amount of energy; however, it is unlikely that they reflect the same wavelength composition.

Exactly the same as in vision, the signal that is produced by conventional CT detectors depends on the total (integrated) amount of x-ray energy that is absorbed in the detector and does not contain information regarding the x-ray spectrum. Thus, the same as in animal kingdom vision, while detection by total energy absorption might fail when different objects absorb a similar amount of energy, spectral imaging allows detection when single energy contrast is absent or minimal.

1.2 SPECTRAL THEORY

Figure 1.2(a) shows the attenuation curves of various clinically relevant materials in the energy range relevant for the photon spectrum that is emitted from a typical CT tube. The attenuation is measured in units of HU, which is attenuation normalized to water in the sense that it is defined

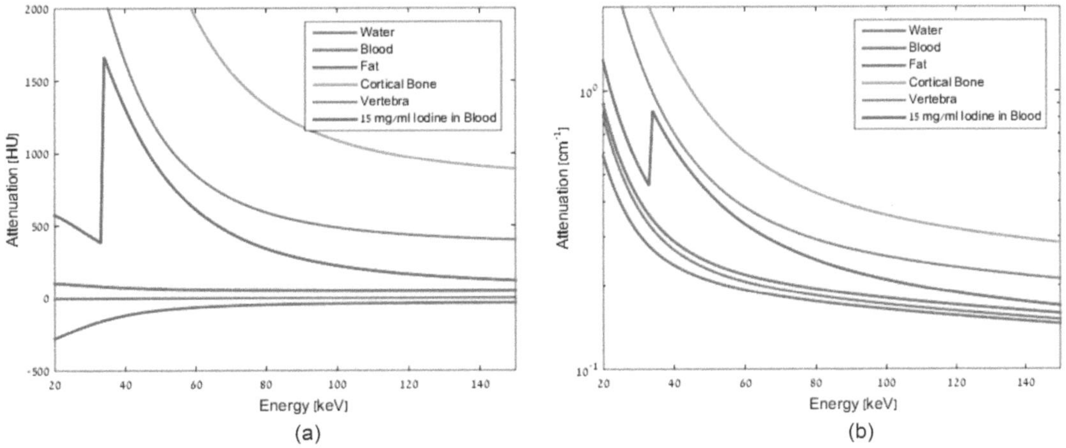

FIGURE 1.2 (a) HU attenuation curves and (b) physical attenuation curves of clinically relevant materials in a typical CT tube energy range. HU attenuation curves are related to the physical attenuation curves according the Eq. (1.1) and by definition results in 0 HU for water over the entire energy range.

as 1000 times the difference between the physical attenuation of the material, in units of cm^{-1}, to the physical attenuation of water and scaled by the physical attenuation of water. This definition is prescribed for each energy, i.e.,

$$HU(keV) = 1000 \times \frac{\mu(E) - \mu_{water}(E)}{\mu_{water}(E)} \tag{1.1}$$

Although the physical attenuation coefficient of the material is linked to the physical process of the attenuation, i.e., Beer-Lambert's law of $I = I_0 e^{-\mu\Delta x}$, it is less useful for clinicians who are accustomed to evaluating tissues on a scale where 0 HU describes water, −1000 describes air, and all other materials are quantified based on their relative difference from water.

The HU attenuation curves in Figure 1.2(a) were converted from the physical attenuation curves shown in Figure 1.2(b) by use of Eq. (1.1). The physical attenuation curves themselves were derived using well-accepted published data [3] of the elemental compositions and physical densities of tissues and by using the following formula:

$$\mu_{compound}(E) = \rho_{compound} \sum_i f_i \tilde{\mu}_i(E) \tag{1.2}$$

where $\mu_{compound}(E)$ is the physical attenuation of a specific compound at energy E, $\rho_{compound}$ is the physical density of the material, in units of g/cm^3, f_i is the fraction by mass of each element in the compound, and $\tilde{\mu}_i(E)$ is the mass-attenuation coefficient of each element at the given energy. The summation is over all the different elements composing the compound. Values of $\tilde{\mu}_i(E)$ can be found in various databases; here we have used the NIST-XCOM database [4].

In conventional CT, the measured HU results from the integrated energy that was absorbed in the detector from photons of all energies. Thus, the conventional HU value depends not only on the tube spectrum, which includes the user selected kVp, the pre-patient filtration including the selected bowtie filter material and shape utilized by each CT vendor for each scanning mode, as well as the spectral sensitivity of the detectors, but also on the entire variety of materials and material densities that the beam traverses before reaching the detector. This dependence is primarily due to the fact that the imaged materials themselves attenuate a different amount of x-ray photons at different energies, as can be seen in Figure 1.2(b), which consequently implies that for each projection angle the spectrum of the beam changes as it traverses the patient or object leading to different values of total attenuation for that specific region of space at that specific projection angle.

To a first order approximation, and neglecting the beam-hardening effect, the conventional HU attenuation value corresponds to the attenuation value at some effective energy, E_{eff}, which can be calculated as the single energy value at which the HU is equal to the same as the mean attenuation over averaged all energies.

The equation that relates the spectrum of the absorbed x-rays to a single attenuation value can be written as:

$$HU^{conv} = \frac{\mu(E_{eff}) - \mu^0_{water}}{\mu^0_{water}} \times 1000 \tag{1.3}$$

where $\mu^0_{water} = \mu_{water}(E_0)$ is a predefined water attenuation value used for the definition of HU^{conv} calculation and $E_{eff} \equiv \int s(E)EdE$.

The definition of the effective energy at which the attenuation matches the measurement holds, to a first order approximation, also for DECT technologies. In DECT technologies, two different x-ray photon spectra serve as the fundamental signals for a process which is referred to as spectral decomposition, and both result in detected attenuation values that can be noted by two different effective energies, E_{low} and E_{high}. Next, we will discuss the spectral decomposition process.

All existing spectral technologies are based on measurements of the same object with the two different photon energy spectra: kVp-switching DECT technology measures x-ray-paths from two photon energy spectra using the same detection system, dual-source DECT technology measures each image voxel using two photon energy spectra sources and two detection systems, "spectral detector" DECT technology measures two photon energy spectra of each x-ray-path using energy sensitive detector layers (where the upper detection layer absorbs most of the low-energy photons and the bottom absorbs most of the high-energy photons) and "spin-spin" DECT technology measures x-ray-paths from two photon energy spectra using the same detection system. As in color vision, there exists some level of overlap between the two photon energy spectra in all these existing spectral technologies.

In addition, all existing spectral technologies are based on the decomposition theory (1976) that was first described in a seminal paper by Alvarez and Macovski [5]. The theory prescribes a method to convert the two measurements at the two different photon energy spectra into two universal energy-dependent physical phenomena. These two universal energy-dependent physical phenomena, referred to as basis functions or the two-base model, are in fact any energy-dependent functions that are chosen beforehand and are kept consistently during the entire process. Alvarez and Macovski themselves prescribed that the optimal selection of basis functions would be empirical. We will further discuss the selection of the optimal basis functions later in this chapter. The decomposition process should be perceived as a non-linear transformation from the pair of measurements at the two different photon energy spectra into two coefficients. These coefficients serve as the factors of a linear combination built from the two basis functions that best describes the attenuating material:

$$\mu_{comp}(E) = \alpha \times \mu^{base1}(E) + \beta \times \mu^{base2}(E) \tag{1.4}$$

The advantages of describing the attenuation of a material as a linear combination of two basis functions rises from the fact that such a description unveils additional information about the material that can be further used for better quantification and visualization. In addition, such a description can be utilized to take into account and properly address various effects that may otherwise lead to image and quantification artifacts including the interference between the detection layers of a detection-based dual energy detector or beam-hardening effects.

As discussed above, the goal of the decomposition process is to find the best linear combination of the two-base functions that describe the attenuation of a material. To better understand this goal, let us look at an example of a specific two-base model selection and the method used to describe with it a third material. Suppose that we are interested in describing the attenuation of vertebrae (see Figure 1.2(b) and in Figure 1.3(a)) as a linear combination of the attenuation curves of 15 mg/mL iodine and of 1000 mg/mL water (Figure 1.3(a)). In order to define the goodness of this linear combination or another, one must define an error function that will serve as a quantity that shall be minimized. A simple, and perhaps naïve, example of such an error function that can serve as input to a specific choice of a decomposition process is the sum of absolute differences squared of attenuations at any number of given energies, or, as in this simple example, just at two selected energies – 60 and 80 keV, i.e.,

$$Err = \sum_{E=\{60,80\}kev} \left| \mu_{vertebra}(E) - \left(\alpha \times \mu^{Base1}(E) + \beta \times \mu^{Base2}(E)\right) \right|^2 \quad (1.5)$$

For this specific choice of error function and selected two-base model, the best linear combination to represent the attenuation of vertebra is given in Figure 1.3. The uniqueness of this solution can be visualized in Figure 1.3(b), which show the values of the error function *Err* for different linear combinations of the selected two-base model in log scale. Please note that this naïve error function was selected arbitrarily for the sake of explanation; however, all decomposition methods require not only the two-basis functions as an input, but also a consistent definition of an error function that will be used throughout the process.

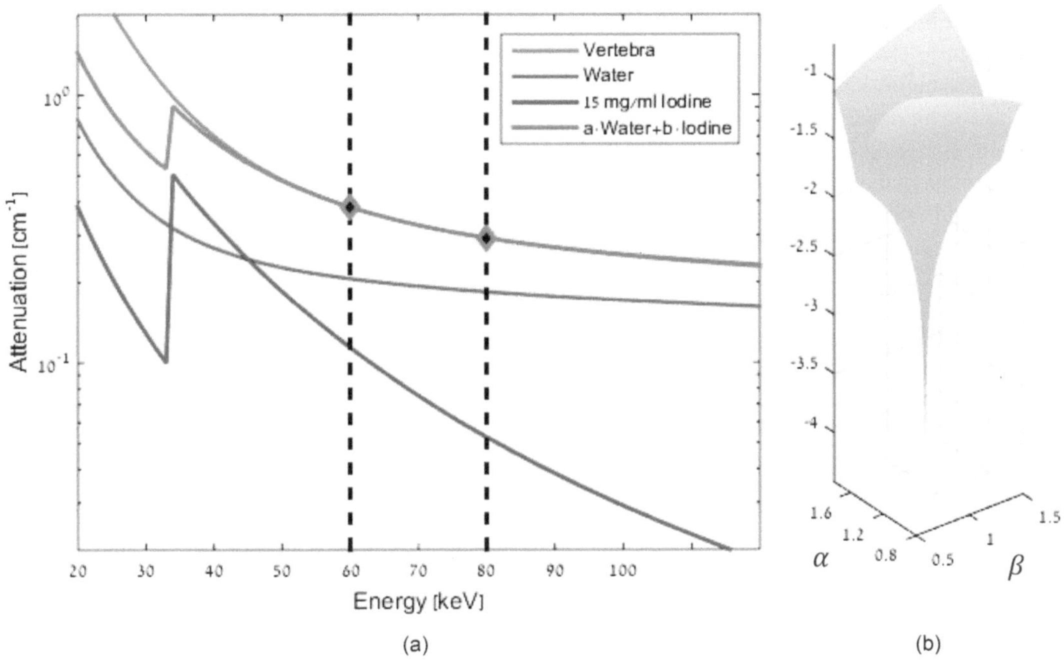

FIGURE 1.3 (a) Example of a two-base model selection of 15 mg/mL iodine and 1 g/mL water and their best linear combination that describes a third material – vertebra. The best linear combination was obtained by minimizing the error function defined in Eq. (1.5). (b) A visualization of the value of the error function for different linear combinations of the selected two-base model in log scale.

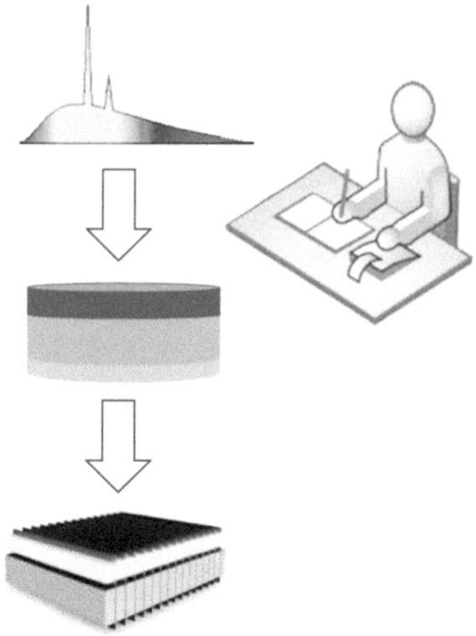

FIGURE 1.4 Thought experiment as a means of calculating the decomposition transformation: a beam of a known energy spectrum traverses an object composed of a stack of known materials and material densities and is detected by a spectral detector of a known energy response where the upper detection layer absorbs most of the low-energy photons and the bottom absorbs most of the high-energy photons.

In practice, the calculation of the non-linear transformation between the low-energy and high-energy signals obtained by the scanner to the coefficients that best describe the line integral or voxel can be computed beforehand. This is easier to understand for the projection-based decomposition technologies, which perform the decomposition process prior to the transformation to image space via Filtered Back Projection (FBP) or any other solution of the inverse problem. Consider the following thought experiment, depicted in Figure 1.4. An x-ray beam of a known spectrum is traversing an object composed of a stack of known materials and material densities. A detector of a known energy response then detects the beam. For a spectral detector-based DECT, the difference in DECT signals arises from the difference in energy response of the detectors, where the upper detection layer is mostly sensitive to low-energy photons and acts as a filter for the bottom layer, which detects almost all of the remaining high-energy x-rays. For fast-kVp switching-based DECT and spin-spin-based DECT, differences in DECT signals arise from the difference of the two tube spectrums, such as the differences in DECT signals for dual-source DECT, but these are obtained only in the image domain. A comparison between projection-based decomposition and image-based decomposition has been performed by Maass et al. [6]. It was found that the best results with respect to material quantification and beam-hardening artifact reduction are obtained by decomposition in the projection domain, not the image domain. Since this method requires that the acquired projection signals would be completely aligned, both in time and space, this method is naturally applicable to a spectral detector-based DECT and can be achieved through the technique of interpolation in fast-kVp switching DECT.

Returning to the thought experiment, the following two independent calculations can be performed:

1. A detailed simulation of the resulting signal for each of the energy spectrums and due to the stack's attenuation including physical effects such as beam hardening or the interference between layers for the case of the spectral detector technology.
2. A calculation aimed to find the optimal representation of the (already known) physical attenuation of the stack as a linear combination of the chosen two-base model. Note that this step requires an additional definition of the error function as an input.

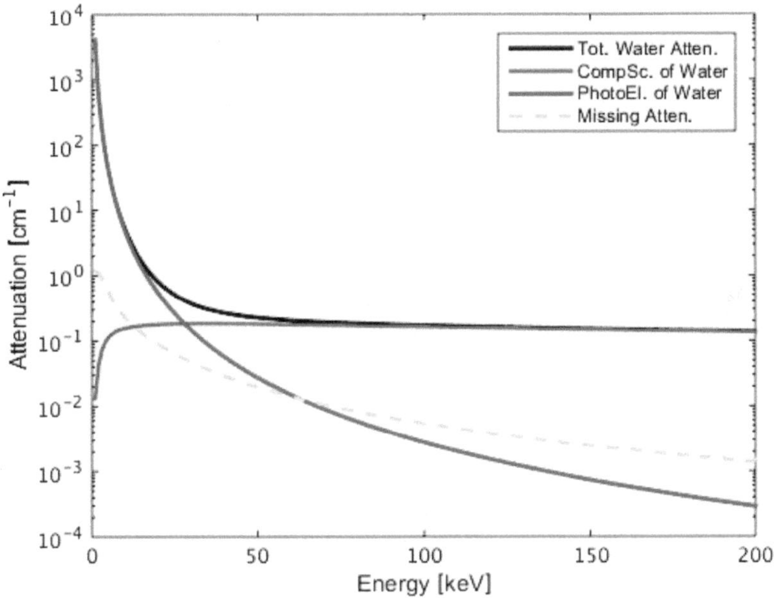

FIGURE 1.5 Log scale of the total attenuation of water separated into the two most important forms of light-matter interaction contribution to the attenuation – Compton scattering and the photoelectric effect. The missing attenuation is due to an additional physical process, Rayleigh scattering, which is distinct from the interactions above.

Once these two calculations have been completed, we have in fact mapped one of the transformation paths that take a specific pair of low-energy and high-energy signals and map them into their corresponding coefficients of the selected two-base model. This exercise can then be repeated over and over until the entire space of possible low-energy and high-energy signal pairs has been entirely mapped. The obtained mapping between any low-energy and high-energy pair into their corresponding two-base model coefficients can be computed before any acquisition process and stored in the system.

Concluding the description of the method used to obtain the decomposition mapping function, let us now return to the subject of the two-base model selection. Any physical material can have different representations depending on different selections of a two-base model. To understand the implications of this choice, let us begin by examining another set of basis functions that are also universal energy-dependent physical phenomena, to describe the vertebra attenuation in Figure 1.2. Instead of describing a tissue or material as a linear combination of iodine and water, one could describe it as a linear combination of the attenuation of water due to Compton scattering and the attenuation of water due to the photoelectric effect (Figure 1.5).

These two physical phenomena are the most important forms of x-ray-matter interaction in the relevant energy range of x-rays (Figure 1.6). They are distinct in their underlying physical mechanisms. While in Compton scattering a photon can be perceived as being rerouted from its path, in the photoelectric effect the photon energy is completely absorbed. The two different interaction forms have different dependencies on the transmitted photon energies. Different materials exhibit different portions of each of the physical processes, Compton scatter and photoelectric absorption; however, the dependence of each of these two phenomena on photon energy and atomic number is common for the different materials. Note that this universal dependence is still an approximation which has residual deviations.

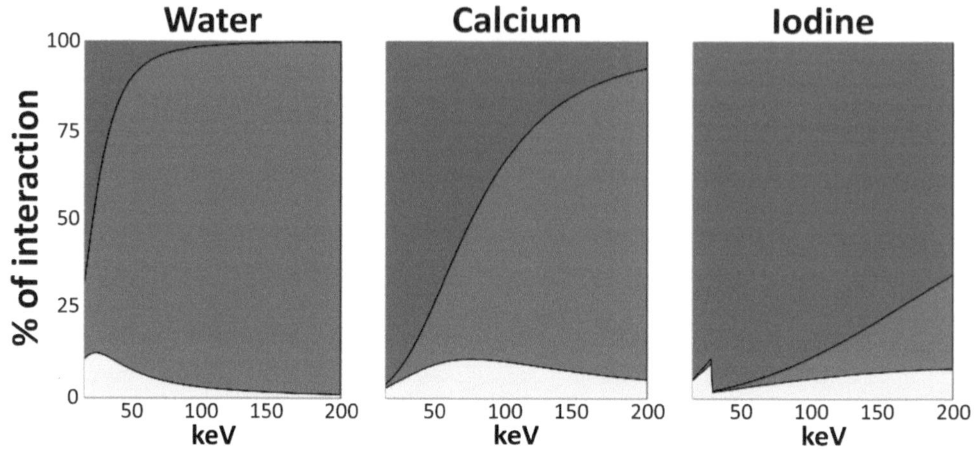

FIGURE 1.6 The relative amount of interaction due to the different x-ray-matter interaction processes, Compton scattering (light gray), photoelectric effect (dark gray), and Rayleigh scattering (white) for three different clinically relevant materials – water, calcium, and iodine. It can be seen that Rayleigh scattering composes less than 10% of the interaction for most of the energy range in each of the three materials. Data taken from the NIST-XCOM database [4].

Returning to the comparison with the second two-base model representation, the same process of finding the best linear combination of the two-base functions that described the attenuation of a material can be applied again by using the same error function that was described in the previous example Eq. (1.5). For the water Compton scatter and photoelectric effect-based two-base model selection, the optimal linear combination found is shown in Figure 1.7(a). Comparing the deviations of the attenuation curve, which describes the vertebra in each of the example two-base models, we find that for both two-base models, the tissue description deviates from the true attenuation of the tissue. Moreover, we find that these deviations are different in their magnitude and sign for each of the models and at different energy values. Such residual deviations, non-zero and different in magnitude and sign, would be found for any two-base model selection and would present themselves differently for different materials.

As mentioned above, it was understood from the very first days of spectral CT [5] that there is freedom in the selection of the model and that some empirical effort is still required. Let us elaborate on that. The definition of the optimal two-base model could be as follows: the selected two-base model shall provide minimal errors, as defined by a predefined error function, for a specific variety of materials at a specific energy range. In addition, not all materials need to have an equal standing – the contribution of each material may be tuned based on its clinical abundance and clinical significance with the use of a weighting function. Taking all this into account, in order to achieve the optimal choice of the two-base model, one must perform theoretical and experimental work to achieve a pair of basis functions, which reduces quantification errors as much as possible, based on the intended (clinical) use of the system and the expected materials that it would encounter. One must do so bearing in mind that, even theoretically, there exists no perfect basis such that it can eliminate all quantification errors for all the materials that the system will encounter. Through the research and development of the spectral-detector DECT solution (IQon, Philips Healthcare), the optimal basis for materials that are of clinical relevance (including, e.g., contrast agents) was implemented as a basis that is a slightly modified version of the pure Compton scatter and photoelectric effect components of pure water. This modification accounts for other materials, which slightly deviate from the universal assumption for the behavior of the two basic physical interactions.

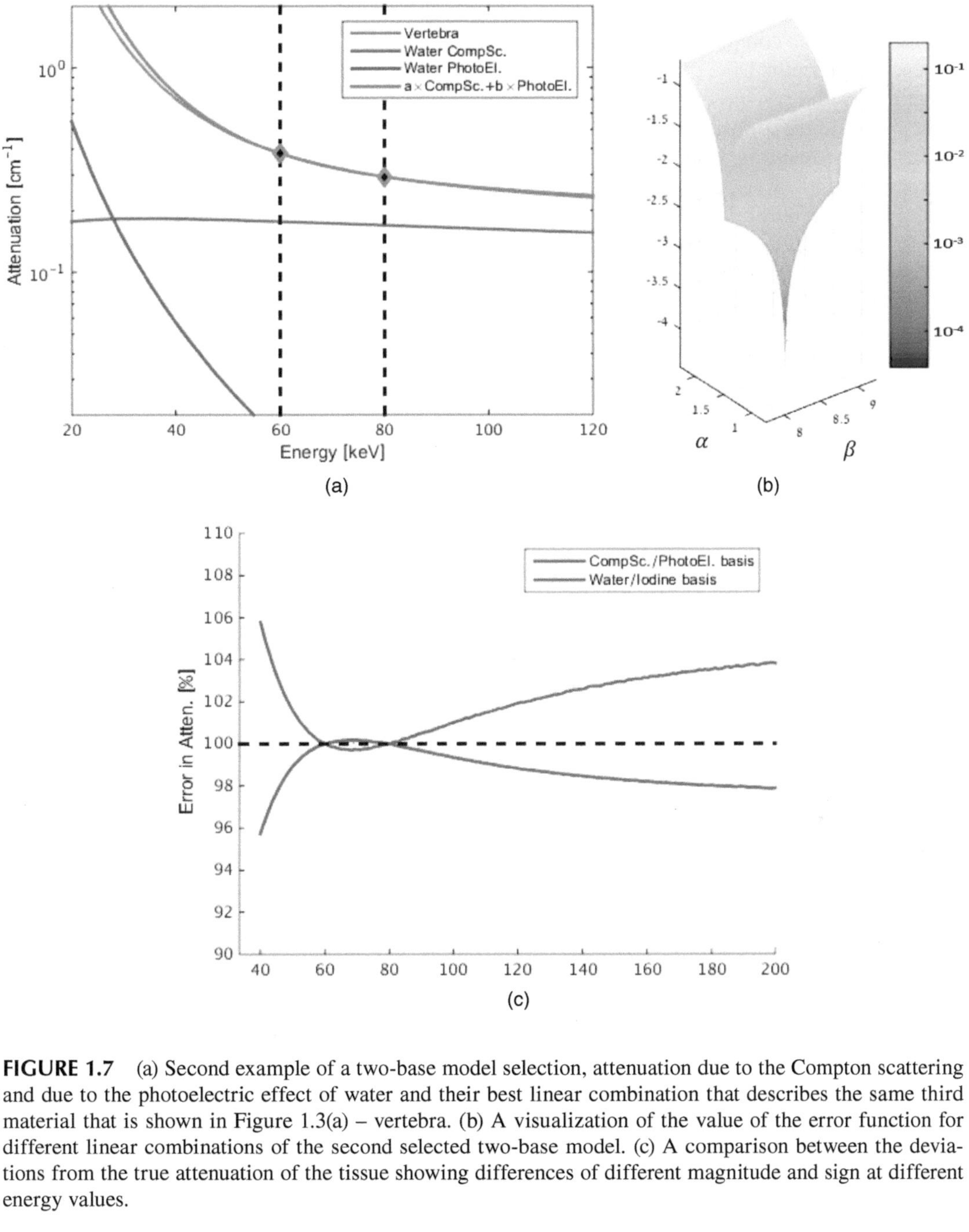

FIGURE 1.7 (a) Second example of a two-base model selection, attenuation due to the Compton scattering and due to the photoelectric effect of water and their best linear combination that describes the same third material that is shown in Figure 1.3(a) – vertebra. (b) A visualization of the value of the error function for different linear combinations of the second selected two-base model. (c) A comparison between the deviations from the true attenuation of the tissue showing differences of different magnitude and sign at different energy values.

1.3 DIFFERENCES BETWEEN DIFFERENT DECT TECHNOLOGIES

For all different DECT technologies, the input for the decomposition process includes the high- and low-energy integrated signals. It is useful to redefine these inputs as the sum of the two signals and the difference between the two signals. The sum of the signals has a relatively low noise and is an indication of the amount of material that the beam traversed. The difference of the signals, i.e., the low-energy signal minus the high-energy signal, contains most of the information regarding the kind of material that the beam traversed; however, this difference is more susceptible to noise.

Thus, it is this low-high (to be read low minus high) signal for a given object or tissue that should be considered when comparing one technology with the other. While it is true that as the energy difference of a specific DECT system, i.e., the difference between the effective energies of the low- and high-detected x-ray spectra for a given tissue, grows, so does that the low-high signal (Figure 1.8); however, one must always compare a signal to its noise when performing such evaluations. To better understand this, assume a comparison between a DECT system, which exhibits an effective energy separation, i.e., of 20 keV (Figure 1.8(a)), and a DECT system, which exhibits an effective energy separation of 30 keV (Figure 1.8(b)) for the same scanned object/tissue. If there was no noise in either of the systems and both low-high signals were of the same accuracy, there would be no advantage for the DECT technology of higher energy separation – both systems would provide the same representation when using the same two-base model and error function. However, noise is also present in the detected signal due to various sources. These sources include any geometric inconsistencies between both spectra, any temporal inconsistencies (motion) between both spectra, cross-scatter between dual tube-detection systems (when present), beam-hardening effect residuals,

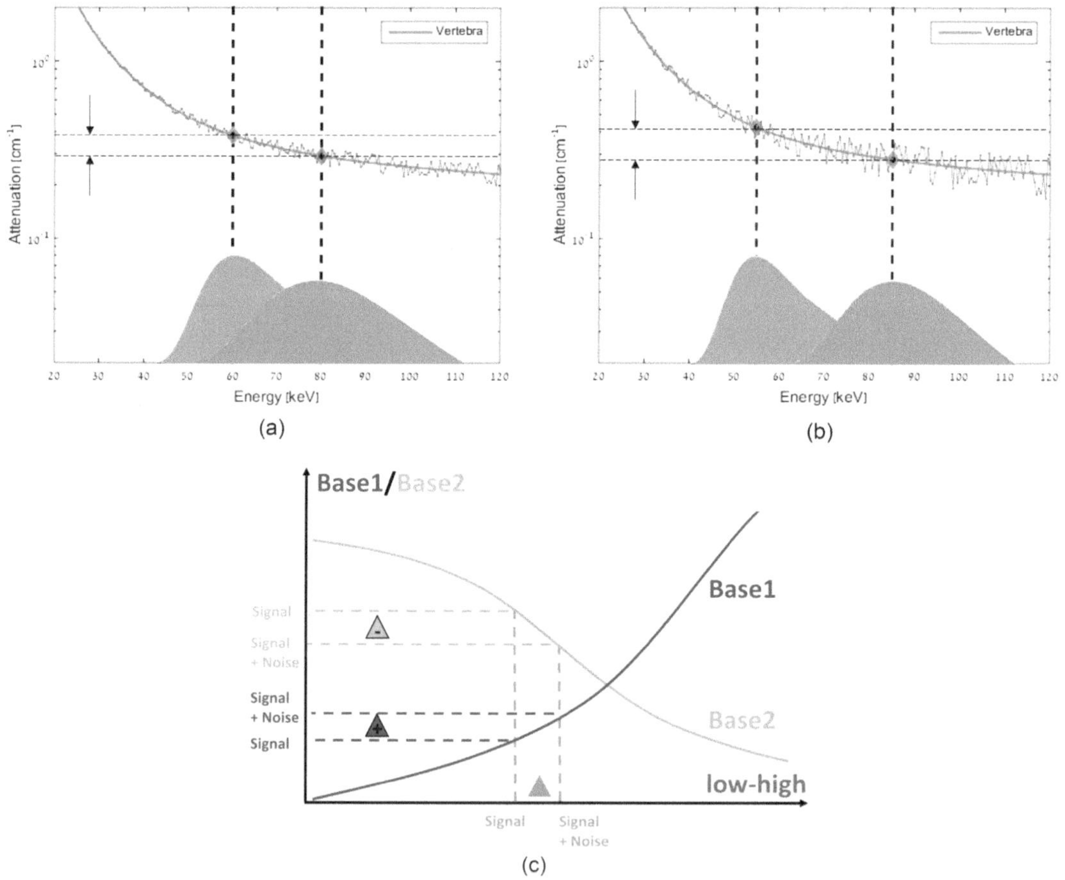

FIGURE 1.8 (a-b) Spectral signal and its sensitivity to noise versus energy separation: while the spectral signal (black arrows) increases with energy separation, as in many other measurement systems, it is the signal-to-noise ratio (SNR), which determines the spectral accuracy and spectral separation capabilities of each technology. Noise sources that influence the spectral signal include geometric inconsistencies between both spectra, temporal inconsistencies (motion) between both spectra, cross-scatter between both spectra, beam-hardening effect residuals, and the signal noise for each spectrum signal. (c) Schematic plot describing the source of anti-correlated noise between the two signals of the basis functions: a signal increase in one of the basis functions due to noise in the difference between the high- and low-energy signals is accompanied by a signal decrease of the other basis function.

and the signal noise for each spectrum, which itself contains a contribution from quantum (Poisson) noise and electronic noise. Note that in the spectral detector-based DECT technology, there is complete registration and consistency between both spectra, both in space and in time, by the nature of the system. In addition, since the total noise of a system σ_{tot} is due to contributions from different noise sources $\sigma_a, \sigma_b, \ldots$ that are summed quadratically, i.e., $\sigma_{tot} = \sqrt{\sigma_a^2 + \sigma_b^2 + \ldots}$, it is the higher noise source of a system that dominates the total noise of the signal. The consequence of the additional unavoidable noise of the signal is loss in accuracy of the decomposition process (see more below) and implies that the energy difference is not sufficient for comparing DECT technologies and that an alternative figure of merit is required. One proposed quantity that is more adequate to describe the spectral capabilities of a DECT system is the *spectral signal-to-noise ratio (SNR)*, which is calculated as the ratio between the low-high signal, for a specific material or stack of materials, divided by the noise of the signal due to all the contributing noise sources mentioned above, i.e.,

$$Spectral\ SNR = \frac{Low\text{-}energy\ signal - High\text{-}energy\ signal}{Total\ noise\ of\ the\ signals} \tag{1.6}$$

Despite providing a better representation of the spectral capabilities of a DECT system, i.e., accurate attenuation quantification and/or classification into different materials, spectral SNR is a difficult quantity to calculate or measure and the authors are unaware of any publication quantifying this figure of merit for different DECT systems.

The decomposition process is extremely sensitive to the noise in the low-energy and high-energy signals. This sensitivity arises from the fact that the function itself is sensitive to the difference between the low signal and the high signal and consequently lead to that all decomposition methods amplify noise [7]. This noise has the property of being anti-correlated between the two basis signals, which means that when there is a deviation in one point of a basis image, there is a statistical tendency for the deviation to be opposite in the other basis image. The source of this anti-correlation can be explained by the fact that, for any reasonable choice of basis functions, the slopes of the resulting two-base coefficients are opposite to each other (see Figure 1.8(c)). In a sense, using the prior knowledge of this unique statistical property of the post-decomposition noise turns the noise into a signal with additional information from its unique signature. It enables the design of dedicated algorithms that target noise in both images by searching for such anti-correlated deviations between both two-base signals, either in the projection domain or in the image domain or in both. Such is the case for the IQon spectral detector-based scanner in which the spectral reconstruction algorithms apply anti-correlated noise denoising of the two-base signals both in the projection domain and in the image domain.

1.4 SPECTRAL RESULTS

There is a large variety of spectral results that can be produced from a DECT scanner, each result with its own clinical usage. In most of the DECT technologies, i.e., in the kVp switching, dual-kVp, and spin-spin technologies, producing spectral results require selection of a dual-energy type acquisition beforehand; however, in the spectral detector-based technology, these results are available from any acquisition (currently for kVp values of 120 and above). This is due to the fact that in the spectral detector-based technology the tube is operated in the same fashion as it would be for a conventional scanner, i.e., constant kVp; the separation between the two energy spectra is inherent in the detectors enabling a dual conventional and spectral-always mode of operation where the spectral results are either requested prospectively or produced retrospectively in addition to the HU results. Next, we will describe a selected subset of the various spectral results that are available on a commercial DECT scanner, explain their physical interpretation and provide examples for a selection of their clinical use. Please note that the spectral results can be separated into two main types of results – HU based (or "HU modified") and non-HU based results. The HU based (or HU modified) results have the units of attenuation, converted to HU, that may or may not been modified based on some specific material properties. An example of such a result, which we will further discuss later, is the Virtual Non-Contrast result which is aimed to mimic a non-contrast-CT HU image even though it was reconstructed from a contrast-CT acquisition. The second type of results, the non-HU type, are composed of voxel-values that represent physical quantities that differ from the material attenuation, such as the amount of iodine density (units of mg/mL) in a voxel or the electron density in the same voxel.

1.4.1 Conventional Result

The aim of this result is to mimic a CT image that is produced from a conventional, i.e., non-DECT, scanner. Although this is not a spectral result per se, we should mention the different approaches taken to create such a result when it is produced from a preselected DECT protocol on the kVp-based technologies or for any protocol in the spectral detector-based technology. While in the kVp-based technologies the conventional result is produced by mixing or blending signals which originated from the two different kVp values, and thus not accurately representative of any single kVp value, the spectral detector-based technology works differently. The spectral detector-based technology is able to use the pre-reconstructed sum of the signals from both detector layers, which accounts for the total amount of absorbed energy in the detector per the single selected kVp value, in exactly the same way as a true conventional CT.

1.4.2 MonoE XX keV

MonoE XX keV, also known as a virtual mono-energetic image (VMI), is a family of results distinguished by their keV values that aim to represent the quantified attenuation that would have been obtained from a pure monochromatic beam at a specific keV value. To illustrate this, if one would be able to integrate an (monoenergetic) x-ray laser [11] into a CT system and in addition filter out any scattered photons by applying an energy filter before the detector, the amount of missing energy that did not reach the detector would be directly related to the attenuation of the object at the specific energy value.

The different MonoE results have been shown to reduce beam-hardening artifacts [8], improve iodine conspicuity at low keV values [9], and improve metal artifact reduction at mid-high keV values [10]. The implication of the greatly reduced beam-hardening artifacts is the near-elimination of size dependency in the attenuation representation that is found in conventional CT, which in due time may enable the potential adoption of quantitative CT techniques.

Theoretically, since the total attenuation of the material is linearly dependent on the physical density, as are the attenuations of the selected two-base model, it is expected that the different MonoE images would be comprised of a linear sum of the two-base model. In this sum the values of the coefficients are proportional to the attenuation value of each basis at the selected keV and are independent on the voxel attenuation or value, i.e.,

$$MonoE(x,y,z,keV) = C_1(keV) \times Base1(x,y,z) + C_2(keV) \times Base2(x,y,z) \quad (1.7)$$

Since the behavior of the chosen universal energy-dependent basis is known at high energies, MonoE results can be synthesized also for keV values higher than the used kVp value or values of the acquisition. In fact, in their paper Alvarez and Macovski themselves presented data for 200 keV attenuation values with errors only up to 1% [5]. In the existing DECT technologies, different vendors allow different maximal keV values. Currently the Philips IQon provides the highest value of 200 keV, the same value that was suggested by Alvarez and Macovski in their paper in 1976.

1.4.3 Effective Z

A result that aims to quantify the effective atomic number of different materials. While the atomic number is a quantity that describes, if not defines, pure elements, when dealing with materials composed of more than one element, the effective atomic number is the number of most interest in terms of the dependencies of x-ray-matter interactions on the atomic number. In many scientific publications and textbooks, the following proposed formula for the effective atomic number, Z_{eff} for x-ray attenuation, is employed [11]:

$$Z_{eff} = \sqrt[2.94]{\sum_i f_i \, Z_i^{2.94}} \tag{1.8}$$

where f_i is the fraction of the total number of electrons associated with each element and Z_i is the atomic number of each element. The power varies in different publications; the value of 2.94 given here is accordance with the Mayneord formula [12] and other publications [11, 13]. The values of Z_{eff} are independent on the density of the imaged object or tissue and are thus especially useful for differentiating between isoattenuating tissues [14] and for classification of different material compositions such as different stone types [15]. For the spectral-detector DECT solution (IQon, Philips Healthcare), a phantom study [16] concluded that the median deviation of Z_{eff} ranged from −2.3% to 1.7% for soft tissue and bone inserts.

1.4.4 Iodine Density

A result that aims to quantify the amount of iodine, in mg/mL, in different tissues. Diagnosis based on attenuation of iodinated contrast enhancement is commonly used in routine CT practice for various applications. Accurate quantification is required to differentiate between isoattenuating structures and for quantitative CT evaluations of iodinated regions.

In the spectral-detector DECT solution, iodine densities are derived through a simple linear basis transformation from the Compton-scatter/photoelectric-like basis into a NIST-based iodine and water basis. In this new basis representation, the iodine density of each image voxel is quantified by a scaling of the corresponding iodine projection. Using this implementation, a phantom study [16] concluded that the median absolute iodine deviations were up to 0.3 mg/mL from the nominal values for iodine concentrations of 2–20 mg/mL where the overall median deviation is 0.1 mg/mL.

1.4.5 Virtual Non-Contrast (VNC)

A result that provides the attenuation values of a non-contrast-CT acquisition from the data obtained in a contrast-CT acquisition. In common practice there are a large number of two-phase CT studies in which two CT acquisitions are performed, one before injection of a contrast agent and one after the injection. The VNC results aim to replace the non-contrast scan by using the spectral information obtained in the contrast-CT scan with the valuable effects of reducing radiation dose and patient discomfort. In addition, incidental findings in a single-phase contrast-CT exam may require the non-contrast information for evaluation of the finding. For such cases, a retrospectively requested VNC result importantly removes the need to schedule the patient for an additional CT study.

The VNC result is based on the iodine quantification values obtained as described above. The attenuation contribution of a unit of iodine, i.e., 1 mg/mL iodine, on each of the two-base model components is computed beforehand and can thus be proportionately subtracted for each quantified iodine value in each of the voxels. The results of the subtraction are in fact "VNCed" Basel and Base2 basis images that can then be used to create a variety of spectral results such as any of the MonoEs. For Philips IQon, for example, the VNC image is computed as a MonoE 70 keV image calculated according to Eq. (1.7) where Basel and Base2 are replaced by a VNCed Basel and VNCed Base2, respectively.

REFERENCES

1. Gouras P. Color Vision, *Progress in Retinal Research.* 1984;3:227–261.
2. Gueymard CA. The sun's total and spectral irradiance for solar energy applications and solar radiation models, *Solar Energy.* 2004;76(4):423–453.
3. International Commission on Radiation Units and Measurements (ICRU). Tissue substitutes in radiation dosimetry and measurement. ICRU Report Vol. 44. Bethesda, MD: ICRU; 1989.
4. Berger MJ, Hubbell JH, Seltzer SM, Chang J, Coursey JS, Sukumar R, Zucker DS, and Olsen, K. (2010), XCOM: Photon Cross Section Database (version 1.5). [Online] Available: http://physics.nist.gov/xcom [2019, June 4]. National Institute of Standards and Technology, Gaithersburg, MD.
5. Alvarez RE and Macovski A. Energy-selective reconstructions in x-ray computerized tomography, *Physics in Medicine and Biology.* 1976;21(5):733–744.
6. Maass C et al. Image-based dual energy CT using optimized precorrection functions: A practical new approach of material decomposition in image domain, *Medical Physics.* 2009;36(8):3818–3829.
7. Kalender WA et al. An algorithm for noise suppression in dual energy CT material density images, *IEEE Transactions on Medical Imagining.* 1988;7(3):218–224.
8. Fahmi R et al. Effect of beam hardening on transmural myocardial perfusion quantification in myocardial CT imaging, Proc. SPIE 9788, Medical Imaging 2016: Biomedical Applications in Molecular, Structural, and Functional Imaging, 97882I (29 March 2016).
9. Neuhaus V et al. Comparison of virtual monoenergetic and polyenergetic images reconstructed from dual-layer detector CT angiography of the head and neck, *European Radiology.* 2018;28(3):1102–1110.
10. Wellenberg RH et al. Quantifying metal artefact reduction using virtual monochromatic dual-layer detector spectral CT imaging in unilateral and bilateral total hip prostheses, *European Journal of Radiology.* 2017;88:61–70.
11. Murty RC. Effective atomic numbers of heterogeneous materials, *Nature.* 1965;207:398–399.
12. Mayneord WV. The significance of the roentgen, *Acta International Union Against Cancer.* 1937;2:271–282.
13. Goodsitt MM, Christodoulou EG, and Larson SC. Accuracies of the synthesized monochromatic CT numbers and effective atomic numbers obtained with a rapid kVp switching dual energy CT scanner, *Medical Physics.* 2011;38:2222–2232.
14. Punjabi GV. Multi-energy spectral CT: Adding value in emergency body imaging, *Emergency Radiology.* 2018;25:197–204.
15. Joshi M et al. Effective atomic number accuracy for kidney stone characterization using spectral CT, Proc. SPIE 7622, Medical Imaging 2010: Physics of Medical Imaging, 76223K (22 March 2010)
16. Hua CH et al. Accuracy of electron density, effective atomic number, and iodine concentration determination with a dual-layer dual-energy computed tomography system, *Medical Physics.* 2018;45(6):2486–2497.

2 Clinical Applications of Dual Energy CT in Neuroradiology

Rajiv Gupta,[1] Maarten Poirot,[2] and Rick Bergmans[2]
[1]Department of Radiology, Massachusetts General Hospital and Harvard Medical School, Boston, Massachusetts, USA
[2]Technical Medicine, University of Twente, Enschede, Netherlands

CONTENTS

2.1 INTRODUCTION

This chapter provides an overview of the applications of dual energy computed tomography (DECT) in neuroimaging. We briefly describe six different implementations of the DECT technology. Irrespective of the technological implementation; however, the fundamental capabilities provided by DECT remain the same and include: (1) material decomposition to separate different tissue types, (2) material quantification to predict presence or concentration of a specific material, and (3) generation of the so-called virtual monochromatic images. These capabilities, which are offered by both dual and multispectral CT scanners, have several useful and promising applications in neuroimaging and the most of the chapters are devoted to describing these different applications. Specifically, we describe the following applications of DECT: (1) differentiation of intracranial hemorrhage from iodinated contrast extravasation, (2) differentiation of hemorrhage from dystrophic calcifications in the brain, (3) accentuation of contrast enhancement when only a small volume of contrast material can be used due to renal insufficiency, (4) metal artifact reduction, (5) atherosclerotic plaque characterization, (6) tumor characterization, and (7) predicting risk of intracranial hematoma expansion. The chapter will discuss the pertinent literature and describes the above application with examples from routine clinical care of patients. As we will show, multispectral imaging is an integral part of the routine clinical care of patients today because it improves image quality, reduces radiation dose by eliminating multiphasic examinations (e.g., by eliminating the need for both a non-contrast and contrast-enhanced CT), and provides more specific diagnostic information for certain pathologies in head and neck imaging.

2.2 FUNDAMENTAL PRINCIPLES

As an x-ray beam travels through the body it is attenuated by the various tissues it encounters in its path. A map of this attenuation forms the basis of both projection radiography and cross-sectional CT. The degree of attenuation imparted by any tissue is dependent on the energy of the x-ray beam and the elements comprising that tissue. At the x-ray energies used for medical imaging, the overall attenuation is predominantly determined by two main phenomena: photoelectric effect and Compton scattering. In a single-energy scanner, one observes the net effect of the overall photoelectric effect and Compton scattering.

Dual energy CT (DECT) – and, in general, multispectral CT – leverages the fact that for each material, the overall attenuation is composed of a unique combination of photoelectric and Compton components. Further, these components are dependent on the energy of the incident x-rays. For example, a polychromatic beam generated by a tube voltage setting of 80 kVp has a higher proportion of photons near the k-edge of iodine than a beam coming from 140 kVp.[1] As a result, the photoelectric effect has a larger contribution to the total attenuation of the lower energy beam than to the higher energy beam. By acquiring the data at two or more energies, one can compute the relative contribution of photoelectric and Compton components to the overall attenuation. Since the energy dependence of both these effects is known a priori, one can make simulated or virtual monochromatic images for any x-ray energy level. One could also use such decomposition to estimate the proportion of different materials in a voxel, assuming that the tissue consists of only two types of materials.

2.3 DECT TECHNOLOGY IMPLEMENTATIONS

A simple way to acquire CT projection data at two different energies is to do two separate scans, one at a low-tube voltage and a second at a high-tube voltage. Such sequential acquisition using two separate scans – though technically simple – is not optimal because the two scans are quite far apart in time and any patient motion will interfere with voxel by voxel registration between the two scans. The field has seen multiple advances in the design of x-ray sources, detectors, filters, and gantry that overcome this problem. There are six different implementations of Dual and Multispectral CT technologies. In the following paragraphs, we briefly describe them.

2.3.1 SEQUENTIAL SCANNING

As the name implies, sequential scanning approaches to DECT entails two separate scans of the same anatomy. It is one of the earliest approaches because technologically it is a straightforward way to obtain data at two energies. One can acquire the two scans at the same patient table position, or move the table back and forth, changing the tube voltage at the end of each excursion. As mentioned earlier, the main limitation of this approach is the delay between the high- and low-energy scan. This delay can be minimized by using the first approach; nonetheless, a full rotation of the CT gantry that may take up to 1 second is too slow for accurate voxel level registration between the acquired volumes (Figure 2.1).

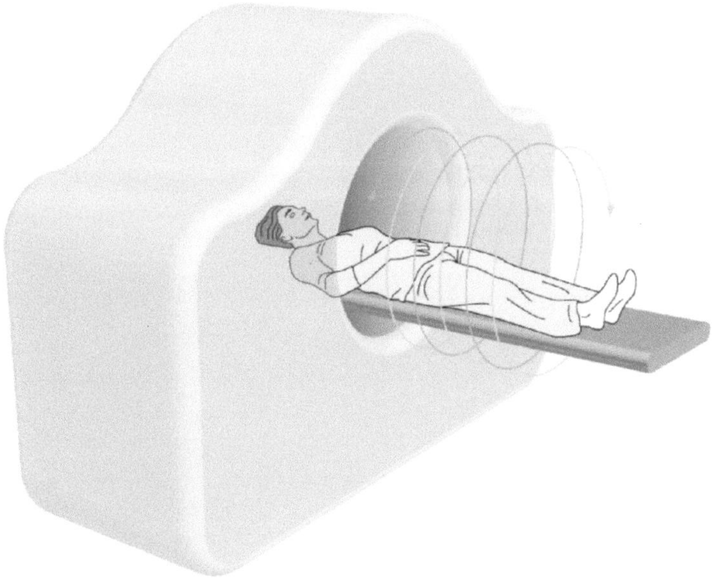

FIGURE 2.1 Sequential scanning for DECT.

2.3.2 Beam Filtration DECT

This implementation of DECT modifies a standard, single source CT scanner with a special x-ray beam filtration to enable dual energy CT. TwinBeam DECT (Siemens AG, Forchheim, Germany), as it is sometimes called, is schematically shown in Figure 2.2. Schematic illustration of this type of a single source-detector combination system in which a split filter consisting of gold and tin is placed at the output of the tube, results in separation of the beam into low- and high-energy spectra. The corresponding halves of the detector are then used for detection of the low- and high-energy spectra.

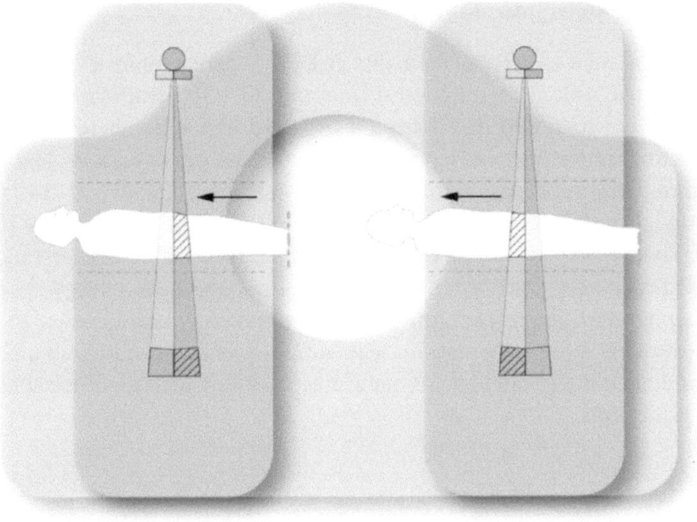

FIGURE 2.2 Beam filtration for DECT.

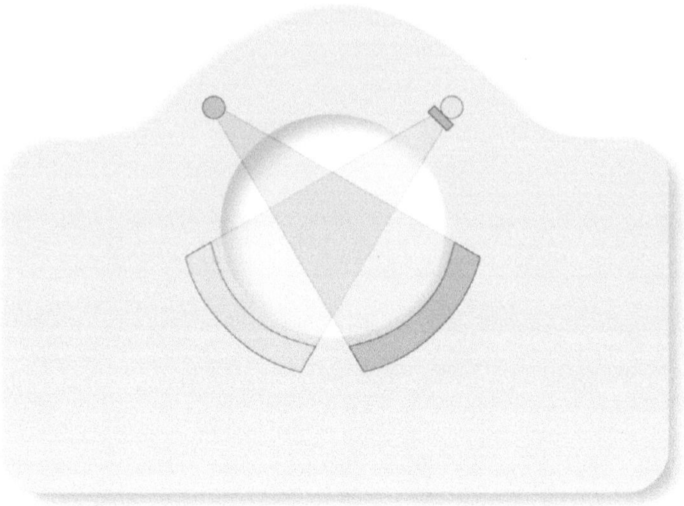

FIGURE 2.3 Schematic illustration of a Dual Source DECT scanner.

2.3.3 Dual Source CT

The first scanner with two independent imaging chains for simultaneous imaging was developed by Siemens AG (Forchheim, Germany). The original intent was to acquire projection data rapidly for cardiac imaging. The research community soon recognized that the two imaging chains could be operated at two different energies simultaneously to enable dual energy imaging. Figure 2.3 shows a schematic illustration of a dual source CT. The combination of two source/detector pairs, orthogonal to each other, allows each slice to be scanned simultaneously at the two energies. In the earlier models, the typical energy pairs used were 80/140 kVp and 100/140 kVp. In the newer models, other energy pairs (e.g., 70/150 kVp) are possible. It is also possible to increase the spectral separation between the two sources by filtering the high-energy x-ray beam with a tin filter, which acts as a high-pass filter.

2.3.4 Rapid Energy Switching DECT

Single source CT scanners can be turned into a DECT using rapid kVp switching at the x-ray source. General Electric's Gemstone Spectral Imaging CT (GE Healthcare, Waukesha, WI, USA), which is schematically illustrated in Figure 2.4, was the first scanner to implement this technology. As shown in this figure, the x-ray projections alternate between low- and high-energy scans and the temporal registration between them is nearly perfect. Typically, 80/140 kVp scan pairs are used for low- and high-energy components. Implementation of this technology requires innovation of both the x-ray source side as well as the detector side. It is easy to understand why such DECT projection data requires very fast switching between low- and high-energy spectra. However, the detector must also be modified to accommodate ultra-fast sampling because the data stream now is twice as rich. In the GE implementation, fast sampling is achieved using a proprietary, garnet-based scintillator detector. This detector system has very low afterglow for spectral separation of each successive projection.

2.3.5 Layered Detector DECT

In the DECT implementations discussed so far, the dual energy projections are acquired by changing the energy of the beam on the x-ray source side. The next two implementations deviate

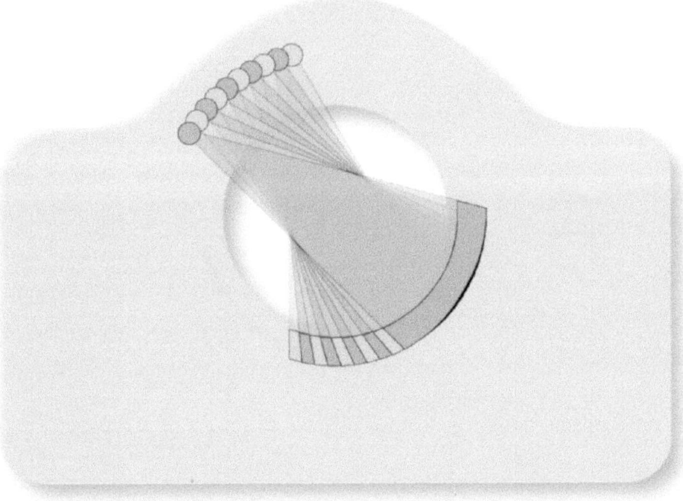

FIGURE 2.4 Schematic illustration of a fast kVp switching DECT scanner.

from this paradigm and implement detector-side multispectral scanning. Figure 2.5 schematically shows a layered or sandwich detector DECT called IQon™ (Philips Healthcare, Andover, MA, USA). It has an imaging chain with a single source-detector combination. The scanner takes advantage of the fact that the x-ray beam is polyspectral. In this design, the spectral separation is achieved at the level of the detector using a highly specialized detector array that consists of two layers that are sensitive to two different energies. The first layer preferentially absorbs the low-energy photons and second layer absorbs the remaining high-energy photons. The thickness of these layers is adjusted in such a manner that each layer absorbs approximately 50% of the incident photons.

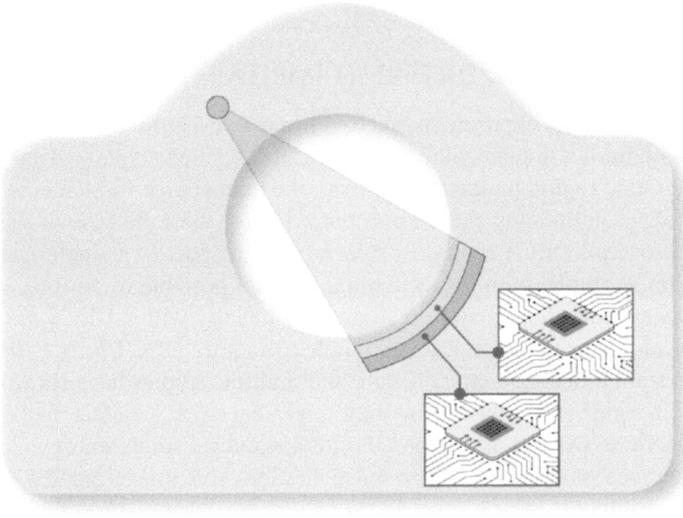

FIGURE 2.5 A sandwich detector DECT.

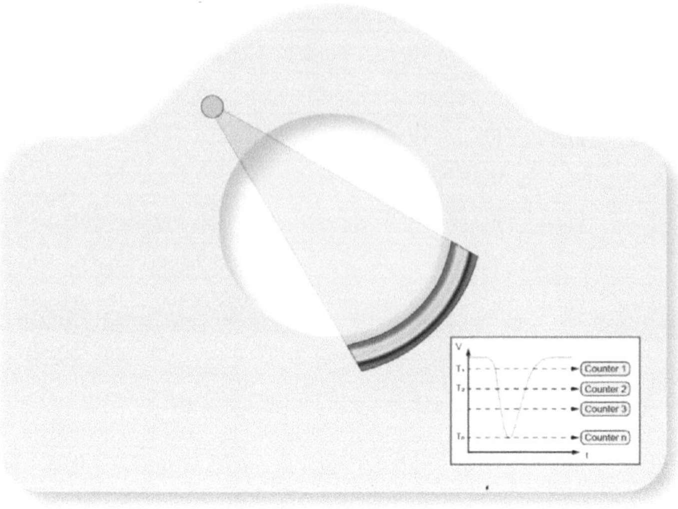

FIGURE 2.6 A photon-counting, multispectral CT scanner.

2.3.6 Photon Counting CT

One can take the concept of leveraging the polyspectral x-ray beam even further. There are advanced detectors that can detect each incoming x-ray photon, measure their energy, and sort them into energy bins. In this manner, these detectors, which are typically referred to as photon-counting detectors, can sort the incident x-ray beam into a set of energy bins enabling truly multispectral imaging. The energy bins are selectable, and this type of selectivity can then be used to detect and classify materials based on their spectral response (e.g., by leveraging the k-edge of contrast materials such as gadolinium). Figure 2.6 schematically illustrates a photon-counting scanner. Such scanners are not available for routine clinical use at this time as they are still under development. However, early results from research prototypes have shown that such scanners hold tremendous promise in tissue characterization and dose reduction.[1]

2.4 RADIATION DOSE FOR DIFFERENT IMPLEMENTATIONS

Minimizing patient radiation exposure is an important consideration in radiology.[2] The precise doses associated with the six implementations of DECT described above will vary depending on the equipment and anatomic region imaged. In general, the dual source implementation of DECT may be configured so that each imaging chain uses approximately half the dose of a single-energy scan. This will make the overall DECT scan dose neutral with respect to a single-energy scan. In other implementations, for example, with kV switching, it is not possible to do tube current modulation during the scan. As a result, there may be a slight dose penalty with a DECT scan.

In routine clinical practice, however, it is possible to acquire DECT images that have essentially the same dose exposure as a single-energy scan, and multiple studies have shown that DECT imaging does not result in significantly more dose than single-energy CT. In fact, one study demonstrated a 10% and 12% decrease in dose as compared with a standard single-energy CT acquisition, with no significant difference in objective image noise or subjective image quality.[3] Other studies have corroborated these results.[4,5]

Therefore, risk of significantly higher radiation dose should not be an overriding concern when ordering a dual energy CT scan.

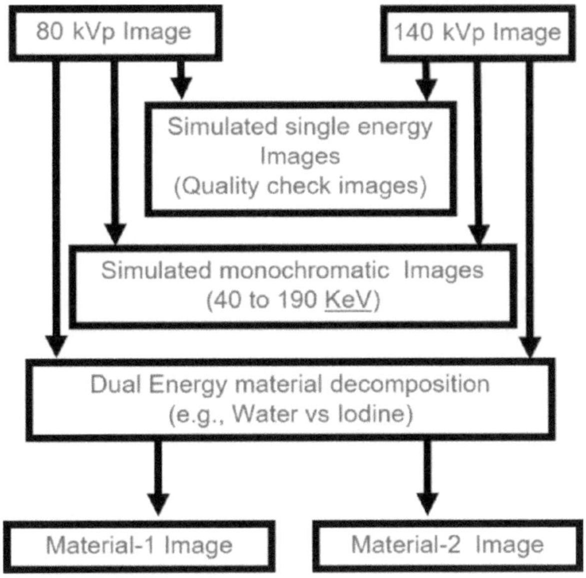

FIGURE 2.7 DECT post-processing algorithm.

2.5 IMAGE PROCESSING

Irrespective of the technical implementation, all DECT scanners enable acquisition of a low- and high-energy image for the same anatomy. These images are then combined using post-processing algorithms to elucidate different features of the anatomy being imaged. For example, one can use DECT to optimize image contrast, differentiate between various materials, determine the quantity of a given material in each voxel, or produce the so-called virtual monochromatic images.[6] Figure 2.7 shows a typical post-processing suite of applications that is available with most DECT scanners.

At the simplest level, linear image fusion may be used to produce weighted-average images that simulate standard single-energy acquisitions at the equivalent photon energies. Next, using linear models, one can derive the photoelectric and Compton scattering components of the attenuation from dual energy data. Since the measured attenuation is a combination of these two dominant physical processes, and the energy dependence is known a priori, one can derive virtual monoenergetic images by extrapolating the attenuation for each voxel to a defined energy. This is a way to improve image contrast and reduce beam-hardening artifacts.

We now describe the details of generating virtual non-contrast (VNC) images using material decomposition. The low- and high-energy data sets acquired during DECT encode the tissue attenuation at two energies. Post-processing algorithms for discriminating between two different materials exploit the differences in attenuation values at the two acquired energies. These algorithms assume each voxel consists of only two types of preselected materials such as water and iodine, calcium or another high atomic number material. Knowing the photoelectric and Compton scattering attenuation of these material pairs (e.g., water and iodine) from the tables published by the National Institute of Standards and Technology, these algorithms compute the proportion of these materials in each voxel that will generate the overall attenuation obtained at the two energies observed. In this manner, the two energy pairs representing low- and high-energy components are transformed into "virtual" images representing the two materials. For example, one can derive a VNC image and a virtual iodine image from a contrast-enhanced DECT. Both images, respectively, hold quantitative information on the presence of the selected materials used for decomposition. Using imaging blending techniques, one can display a combination of these two images such that, for example, the VNC image is displayed in shades of gray while the iodine content is overlaid in shades of red.

In summary, the following types of post-processed images are feasible with DECT.

- Material decomposition images created using two or three material decomposition algorithms. Any two materials may be used as pairs in this decomposition process. Typical material pairs that are used are listed below:
  - Water–Iodine pair, that may be used to generate a VNC image and an iodine overlay image
  - Water–Calcium pair
  - Calcium–Iodine pair
- Virtual monochromatic images. These typically range from 40 to 190 keV energy levels.
- Quantitative images based on effective atomic number (Z values). These images provide concentration of a chosen material, typically iodine, in each voxel.

In the next section, we illustrate some typical applications of DECT and these post-processing techniques in head and neck imaging.

2.6 APPLICATIONS OF DECT IN NEUROIMAGING

2.6.1 Material Decomposition

As mentioned earlier, a material decomposition algorithm converts the low- and high-energy images into a pair of images that represent two preselected materials. Such decomposition may be used to differentiate materials that have the same intensity on a single-energy image. For example, both hemorrhage and dilute contrast are hyperdense on a non-contrast head CT. Therefore, on a scan performed after a catheter intervention, it may be difficult to differentiate between contrast extravasation and hemorrhagic conversion of a stroke. DECT may be used to differentiate between these two materials. Other applications of this technique, to name a few, include automatic bone removal, differentiation of dilute contrast from diffuse mineralization, characterization of different components of a calcified atherosclerotic plaque, and characterization of kidney stones. We describe some typical use cases of material decomposition.

2.6.1.1 Automatic Bone Removal

While iodinated contrast and bone are both hyperdense on a single-energy scan, their spectral signature is very different on a dual energy CT. This fact may be used to remove bone from a contrast-enhanced CT angiogram. The underlying algorithm in bone subtraction is primarily a material decomposition between calcium and iodine material pairs. Figure 2.8 shows maximum intensity projections of a CT venogram where the bone has been removed using the spectral signature of calcium.

2.6.1.2 Differentiating Hemorrhage from Iodinated Contrast

Figures 2.9 and 2.10 show two cases of strokes in the left middle cerebral artery (MCA) territory after catheter-assisted thrombectomy and intra-arterial therapy. For the patient depicted in Figure 2.9, on post-procedure single-energy CT images (Figure 2.9A), there is a focal mixed hyper- and hypo-density within the left MCA territory (arrowhead) and linear hyperdensity in the subarachnoid space (arrow). The mixed density is concerning for hemorrhagic conversion of an ischemic stroke while the linear hyperdensity is concerning for subarachnoid hemorrhage. The VNC image Figure 2.9B shows an area of hypoattenuation in left lentiform nuclei consistent with developing infarction. The hyperdensity in this region maps to the iodine overlay image (Figure 2.9C), confirming contrast staining of the infarcted territory because the blood–brain barrier has been disrupted. The subarachnoid hyperdensity in the posterior left MCA territory has corresponding hyperdensity

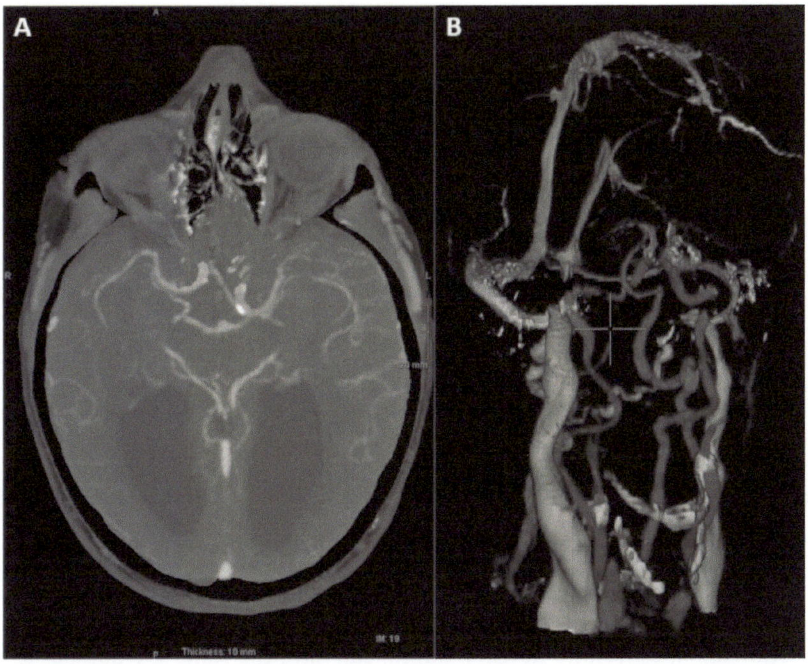

FIGURE 2.8 (A) Axial maximum intensity projection (MIP) image through the brain from a head and neck CT venogram after DECT bone removal, and (B) Right-lateral oblique view of the venogram after bone removal.

on both iodine overlay and VNC images suggesting that it represents a mixture of iodine and blood products, likely iatrogenic from the intervention.

Figure 2.10A shows another post-procedure single-energy CT image after an attempted thrombectomy on a different patient. In this image, the left MCA is hyperdense. In addition, there is another area of hyperdensity in the brain parenchyma that could be hemorrhage or contrast staining. In order to distinguish between these two possibilities, a VNC was generated (Figure 2.10B). The VNC images show faint hyperdensity in the left MCA that likely represent residual intraluminal thrombus within the entire M1 segment. The area of parenchymal hyperdensity on the single-energy

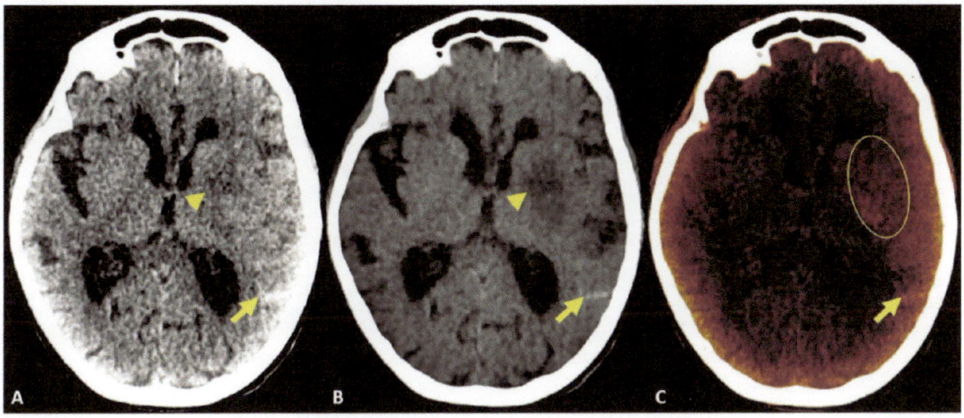

FIGURE 2.9 Non-contrast dual energy head CT after intra-arterial therapy for left MCA stroke. (A) Single-energy image. (B) Corresponding virtual non-contrast image. (C) Iodine overlay image.

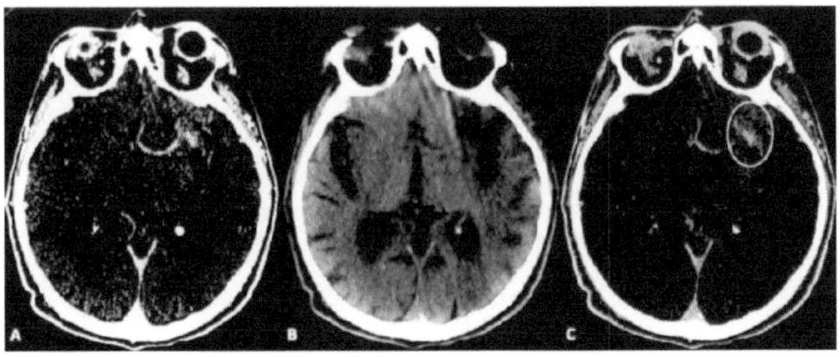

FIGURE 2.10 Arterial contrast staining and contrast extravasation after intra-arterial therapy for an acute left MCA stroke. (A) Post-procedure single-energy CT image. (B) Virtual non-contrast image. (C) Iodine overlay image.

image appears as hypodense on the VNC image, with the hyperdensity mapped on the iodine overlay image (Figure 2.10C). These findings represent an acute infarct with contrast staining marked by the ellipse in Figure 2.10C.

2.6.1.3 Differentiating Hemorrhage from Calcification

Diffuse mineralization, especially in early stages, can have the same CT number as acute hemorrhage. This typically does not pose a clinical dilemma because mineralization, and more specifically parenchymal calcification, occurs in characteristic regions within the brain parenchyma, e.g., in bilateral lentiform nuclei. Very often, prior CT scans are available, and they readily confirm the presence calcification as they remain stable of months and years while hemorrhage evolves over a time period of hours and days. In the setting of acute trauma, however, when prior head CT scans are not available, differentiating acute intracranial hemorrhage from incidental calcification may become important. Dual energy CT may be used for this purpose.

Figure 2.11 shows a 54-year-old woman who was imaged after acute trauma to the head. The single energy (Figure 2.11A) shows a focal hyperdensity in the right thalamus that is concerning for acute, post-traumatic intracranial hemorrhage. The position of this hyperdensity is somewhat atypical for intraparenchymal mineralization. At the same time, being deep within the brain, it is also atypical for a hemorrhagic contusion. A DECT image was performed and the images were post-processed to generate Virtual Non-calcium (VNCa) and Virtual Calcium (VCa) images shown in

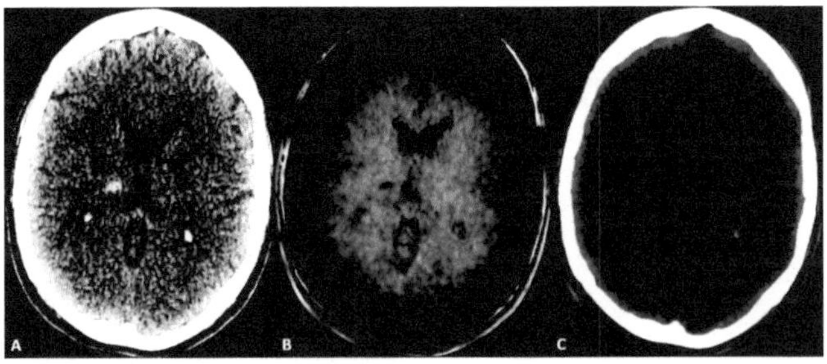

FIGURE 2.11 Calcium subtraction in a 54-year-old woman assessed for intracranial injury in the setting of acute trauma. (A) Single-energy equivalent of unenhanced DECT, showing a hyperdense region in the right thalamus which may be hemorrhage or calcification. (B) Virtual-non-calcium image does not contain any hyperdensity in the right thalamus, ruling out hemorrhage. (C) Calcium-overlay image shows that the hyperdensity in question represents calcium.

Figure 2.11B and 2.11C, respectively. As can be seen, the focus of hyperdensity on the single-energy image corresponds to an area of hypodensity on the VNCa image. The hyperdensity is completely mapped on the calcium image, confirming that this hyperdensity is an area of calcification. A repeat CT confirmed this finding of DECT.

2.6.1.4 Tumor Characterization

On a single-energy, contrast-enhanced CT it is not possible to assess the degree of enhancement in a lesion such as a tumor or a metastasis; while it is routine to say that a particular lesion is enhancing, one cannot partition the observed hyperdensity between the intrinsic hyperdensity of the mass and that from contrast enhancement. DECT offers the ability to make such distinction. Assessment of the degree of enhancement of a lesion allows us to characterize its vascularity and its intrinsic tissue blood volume. This property could be used to assess response of a tumor to therapy, differentiate between benign and malignant etiologies, or different types of tumors.

Figure 2.12 shows one such scenario. This patient, who had a known history of both lung cancer and multiple myeloma, was found to have a lytic lesion in the left aspect of a thoracic vertebral body that was invading the posterior elements as well as perivertebral soft tissues. From a single DECT acquisition, VNC and contrast-enhanced views were obtained. As can be seen, the degree of overall enhancement is low, making this entity more likely to be secondary to multiple myeloma rather than a lung cancer metastasis. While useful, a word of caution is apropos when comparing the degree of enhancement to assess response to therapy. The overall contrast uptake is dependent of the time of image acquisition with respect to the start of contrast injection. It is also dependent on physiologic factors such as heart rate and ejection fraction. Therefore, small change in the quantitative degree of iodine uptake should be interpreted cautiously.

2.6.2 Virtual Monochromatic Images

As mentioned previously, low- and high-energy data sets acquired by DECT may also be converted into virtual monochromatic images that simulate images as if they were acquired using an x-ray beam with a single photon energy. They are referred to as "virtual" because simulated images cannot account for all the non-linear effects of the polychromatic nature of the x-ray beam and are not equivalent to "true" monochromatic x-ray images. Nonetheless, they can be used to mitigate some of the artifacts that arise from beam polychromaticity.

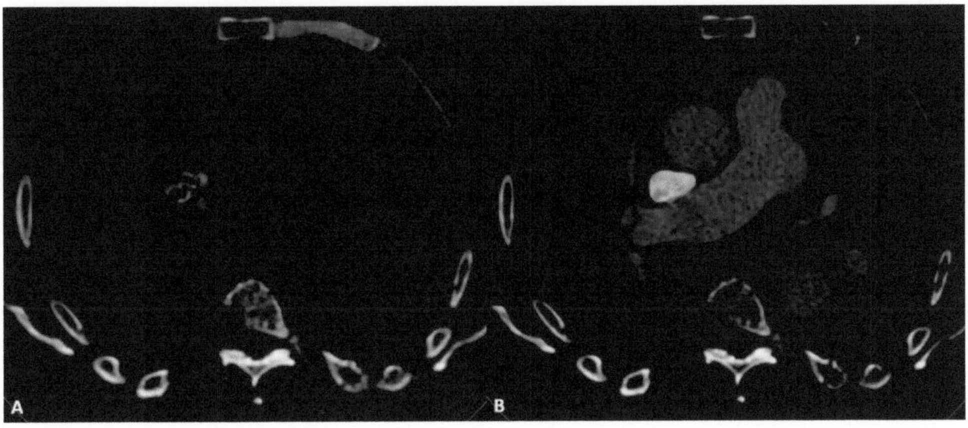

FIGURE 2.12 Tumor characterization by degree of enhancement. (A) Virtual non-contrast image shows tumor invading vertebral body. (B) Iodine-overlay image clearly visualizes the distribution of contrast uptake in the tumor.

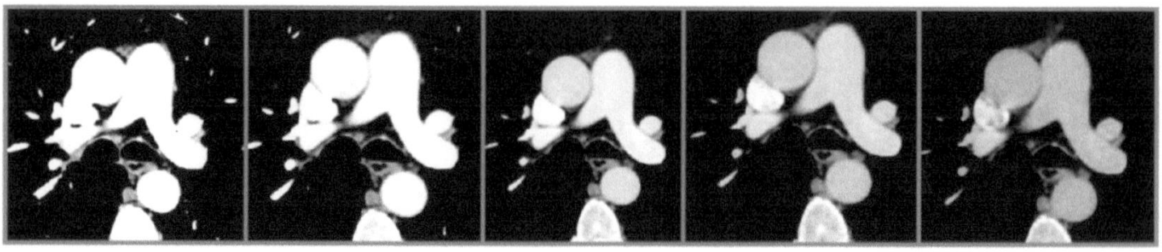

FIGURE 2.13 Apparent brightness of iodine as a function of the monochromatic beam energy.

Figure 2.13 shows images of the ascending and descending aorta at the left of the main pulmonary artery trunk. As can be seen, and as would be expected, the intensity of iodine increases as the virtual energy level approaches the k-edge of iodine (33.4 keV). We briefly describe how this feature can be used to mitigate metal and beam-hardening artifacts, and to improve the contrast resolution of an image.

2.6.2.1 Metal and Beam-Hardening Artifact Reduction

Virtual monoenergetic images, which simulate a monochromatic x-ray beam, rely on decomposition of the acquired low- and high-energy images into photoelectric and Compton scattering components. These components are then used to generate a simulated image at a desired energy level. As the name implies, these images should overcome some of the limitations of a polychromatic x-ray beam. For example, the beam-hardening artifact in CT results from the fact that the low-energy photons in an x-ray beam are preferentially filtered out as the beam penetrates deeper into the tissues. For example, DECT can produce simulated beam energies as high as 190 keV; at such a high-energy, x-ray photons penetrate deeper through materials, reducing beam-hardening artifacts.

Figure 2.14 shows a single slice through the posterior fossa with characteristic beam-hardening artifacts through the brain stem at 120 kVp. As compared to the single-energy image, the beam-hardening artifacts through the brain stem are reduced in the virtual monochromatic images at higher monoenergetic levels. At low energy levels (Figure 2.14B), there is increased image noise and bone streak artifact, while preserving gray-white matter contrast. High energy levels (Figure 2.14D) suffer

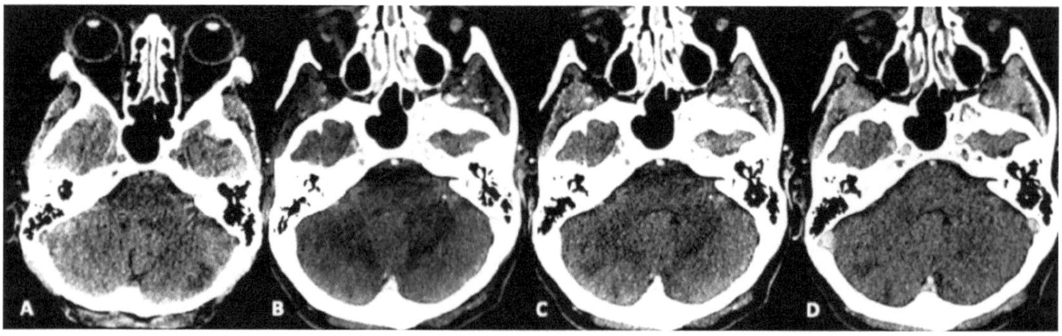

FIGURE 2.14 (A) Unenhanced, single-energy CT image at 120 kV through the skull base and posterior fossa; (B-D) corresponding DECT images at virtual monochromatic energy levels of 40, 75, and 140 kV, respectively.

less from artifacts but have reduced tissue contrast. Empirically, the optimal virtual monochromatic energy level is found to be approximately 70–75 keV (Figure 2.14C).

Metal artifacts are a result of inadequate beam penetration and may be reduced by increasing the beam energy. Simulated monochromatic images may be used to reduce the artifact emanating from dental hardware,[7] or in maxillofacial imaging to mitigate the effect hardware used for facial reconstruction.[8-10] Similarly, beam-hardening artifacts from dental implants or aneurysm clips may also be decreased by increasing the virtual monochromatic energy level of the DECT reconstruction.[11,12] Figure 2.15 shows an example of metal artifact reduction from bilateral mandibular reconstruction surgeries.

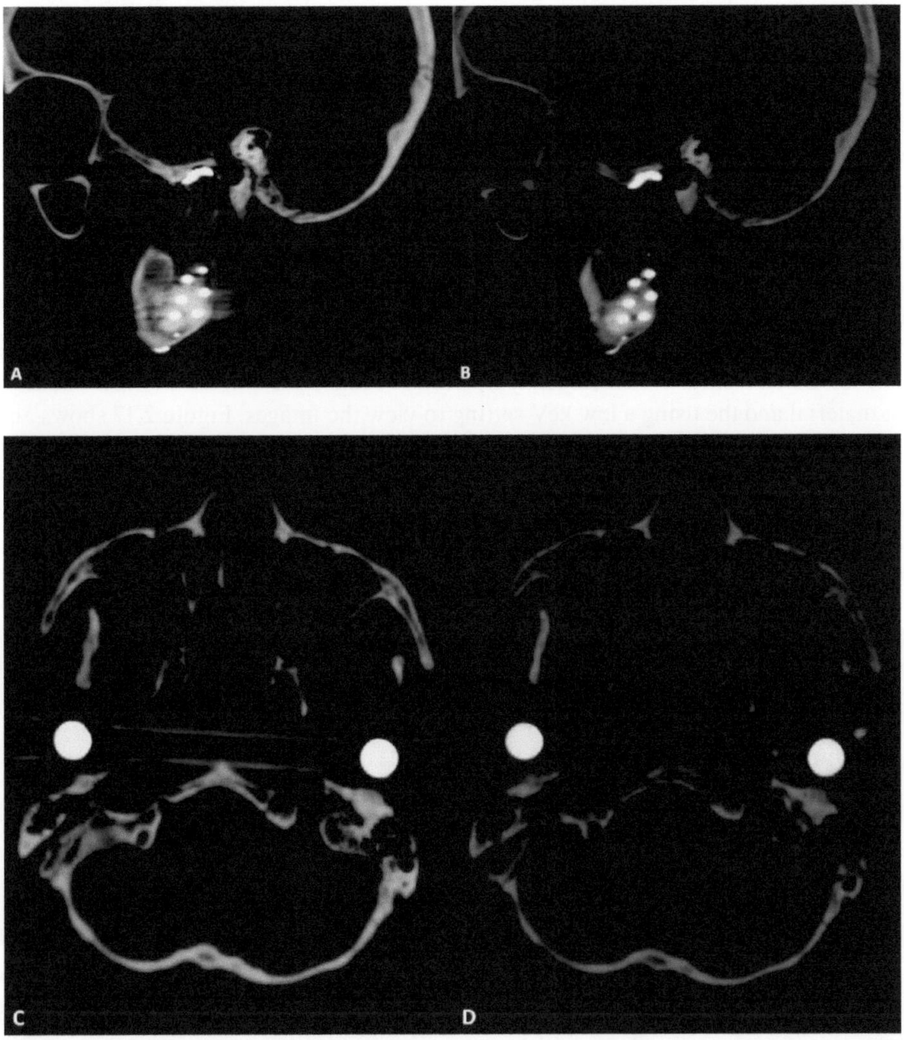

FIGURE 2.15 Metal artifact reduction from dental hardware. (A) Sagittal single-energy equivalent of DECT image shows metal artifacts around the mandibular reconstruction hardware despite aggressive window/level setting. (B) Reduction of metal-artifacts on sagittal 190 keV virtual-monochromatic image. (C) Severe metal artifacts in the axial plane of the single-energy acquisition. (D) Another example of a virtual-monochromatic image at 190 keV from the dual-energy acquisition that greatly reduces the metal artifacts.

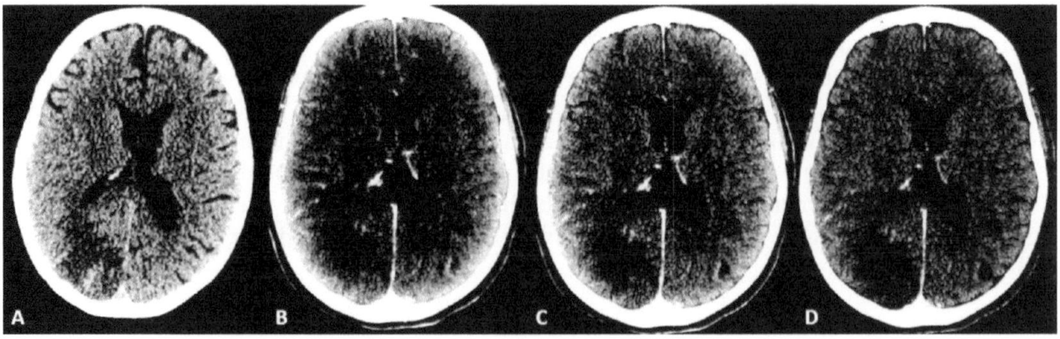

FIGURE 2.16 (A) Single-energy CT image at 120 kVp. (B-D) DECT images at virtual monochromatic energy levels of 40, 65, and 90 kV respectively at a supratentorial brain slice.

2.6.2.2 Accentuation of Contrast Enhancement

The virtual monochromatic energy level also affects the soft tissue contrast of an image. This feature may be used to accentuate gray-white differentiation in brain images, or in improving the visualization of tumors and other pathology in head and neck imaging. Figure 2.16 shows an example of one such application. As can be seen, at low energy levels, there is increased image noise while preserving gray-white matter contrast is improved. At high energy levels, the image noise and artifacts are reduced, but the tissue contrast is also decreased. Pomerantz et al.[13] have determined the optimal virtual monochromatic energy level to be approximately 65 keV.

Increased soft tissue contrast, especially at the low keV levels, may also be used to boost visualization of iodinated contrast. This fact may be used to reduce the amount of intravenously injected contrast material and the using a low keV setting to view the images. Figure 2.17 shows an example of a sagittal DECT image of the cervical spine after contrast administration. In Figure 2.17A, it is difficult to see the enhancing structures in the central canal. A color overlay of the iodinated contrast, which can be individual window-leveled, makes the visualization much clearer. For example, one can see the anterior spinal artery along the ventral surface of the spinal cord and be reassured that the degenerative changes are not indenting the cord.

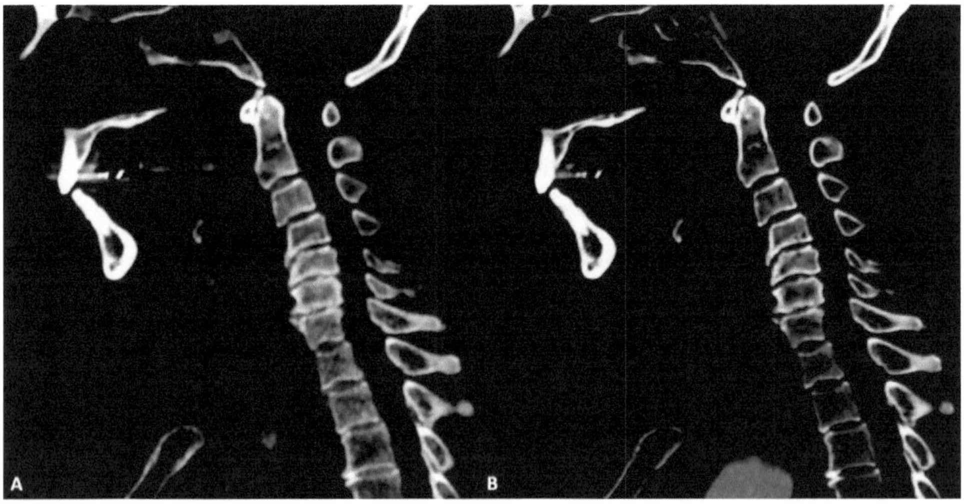

FIGURE 2.17 CT images of the cervical spine after low-volume contrast administration. (A) Unenhanced, single energy (B) Dual energy, with iodinated contrast overlay. Note the increased visibility of the anterior spinal artery along the ventral surface of the spinal cord in DECT compared to single energy CT.

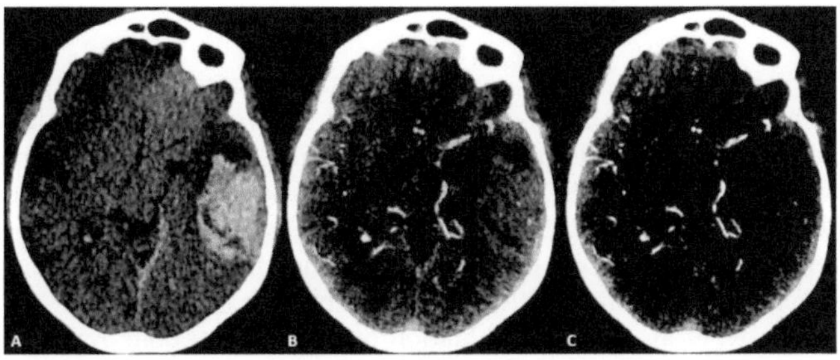

FIGURE 2.18 Spot and Diffuse signs at dual-energy CTA to assess expansion risk of an intracranial hemorrhage. (A) Virtual-non-contrast image is able to clearly show the location, shape, and size of the hematoma. (B) Iodine-overlay image shows three tiny "spot-signs"; the iodine content of these spot signs is measured. (C) Analysis of the iodine-only image in HU yields both the total amount of iodine present in the hematoma and the amount of iodine present in the focal spots. A combination of these metrics is used to compute the risk of hematoma expansion.

2.6.3 Quantitative Imaging

Traditional single-energy CT provides a single HU value for each voxel. With DECT, one can determine the proportion of materials in each voxel, assuming that the voxel is composed of only two types of materials. For example, one can quantitate the amount of iodine uptake by a tumor and this degree of enhancement may be used to assess response to therapy.

Another novel use of iodine quantitation is in predicting the risk of intracranial hematoma expansion. Multiple papers have described the so-called "spot sign" on single-energy CT. In addition, several other radiographic markers have also been proposed to assess increased risk of hematoma expansion, including initial hematoma volume,[14,15] patterns of attenuation within the hematoma on CT images,[16,17] and the spot sign on CT angiography.[18] Spot sign refers to the bright spots seen on (delayed) head CT images after contrast administration. These spots, which are thought to represent areas of contrast extravasation and active bleeding,[19] have been shown to be a marker of hematoma expansion. The conventional single-energy spot sign is highly specific for hematoma expansion; however, it has relatively low sensitivity.[20-22] Recent results that use quantitative imaging techniques show that DECT may be used to optimize spot sign detection and improve its sensitivity.[23]

On a single-energy scan, it may be difficult to observe the spot because of the relative difficulty of differentiating hyperdense hemorrhage from spotty or diffuse contrast extravasation from leaky blood vessels.[24,25] DECT can be used to quantitate the amount of iodine because of its ability to separate hemorrhage from iodinated contrast.[26-28] For example, iodine-only images obtained from DECT can differentiate hemorrhage from iodinated contrast staining and extravasation in the brain.[29]

Tan et al.[23] showed that quantification of iodine content in the hematoma may be used to identify a hematoma at high risk of expansion. Figure 2.18 shows an example of the methodology followed in this chapter. Using DECT, they measured iodine that is diffusely present in the hematoma (I_h). They also measured the amount of iodine in the brightest spot sign (I_{bs}) within the hematoma. Using a combination of I_h and I_{bs}, this chapter defines a new score called the I2-score that predicts the risk of hematoma expansion. We refer the reader to Tan et al.[23] for details.

2.7 CONCLUSION

DECT has several useful and promising applications in head and neck imaging, including artifact reduction, contrast accentuation, tumor characterization, and quantitative imaging. Thus, familiarity with the role of DECT in neuroradiology is crucial.

REFERENCES

1. Steidley JW. Exploring the spectrum – Advances and potential of spectral CT Phillips Netforum Community. 2008. Phillips Healthcare. Nov 5, 2013. http://clinical.netforum.healthcare.philips.com/us_en/Explore/White-Papers/CT/Exploring-the-spectrum-Advances-and-potential-of-spectral-CT
2. Henzler T, Fink C, Schoenberg SO, Schoepf UJ. Dual-energy CT: Radiation dose aspects. *Am J Roentgenol.* 2012;199:S16–25.
3. Tawfik AM, Kerl JM, Razek AA, et al. Image quality and radiation dose of dual-energy CT of the head and neck compared with a standard 120-kVp acquisition. *Am J Neuroradiol.* 2011;32:1994–1999.
4. Deng K, Liu C, Ma R, et al. Clinical evaluation of dual-energy bone removal in CT angiography of the head and neck: Comparison with conventional bone-subtraction CT angiography. *Clin Radiol.* 2009;64:534–541.
5. Johnson TR, Krauss B, Sedlmair M, et al. Material differentiation by dual energy CT: Initial experience. *Eur Radiol.* 2007;17:1510–1517.
6. Johnson TR. Dual-energy CT: General principles. *AJR Am J Roentgenol.* 2012;199:S3–8.
7. Tanaka R, Hayashi T, Ike M, Noto Y, Goto TK. Reduction of dark-band-like metal artifacts caused by dental implant bodies using hypothetical monoenergetic imaging after dual-energy computed tomography. *Oral Surg Oral Med Oral Pathol Oral Radiol.* 2013;115:833–838.
8. Bamberg F, Dierks A, Nikolaou K, Reiser MF, Becker CR, Johnson TR. Metal artifact reduction by dual energy computed tomography using monoenergetic extrapolation. *Eur Radiol.* 2011;21:1424–1429.
9. Guggenberger R, Winklhofer S, Osterhoff G, et al. Metallic artefact reduction with monoenergetic dual-energy CT: Systematic ex vivo evaluation of posterior spinal fusion implants from various vendors and different spine levels. *Eur Radiol.* 2012;22:2357–2364.
10. Lewis M, Reid K, Toms AP. Reducing the effects of metal artefact using high keV monoenergetic reconstruction of dual energy CT (DECT) in hip replacements. *Skeletal Radiol.* 2013;42:275–282.
11. Shinohara Y, Sakamoto M, Iwata N, et al. Usefulness of monochromatic imaging with metal artifact reduction software for computed tomography angiography after intracranial aneurysm coil embolization. *Acta Radiol.* 2014;55(8):1015–1023. Epub 2013 Nov 11.
12. Stolzmann P, Winklhofer S, Schwendener N, Alkadhi H, Thali MJ, Ruder TD. Monoenergetic computed tomography reconstructions reduce beam-hardening artifacts from dental restorations. *Forensic Sci Med Pathol.* 2013;9:327–332.
13. Pomerantz SR, Kamalian S, Zhang D, et al. Virtual monochromatic reconstruction of dual-energy unenhanced head CT at 65-75 keV maximizes image quality compared with conventional polychromatic CT. *Radiology.* 2013;266(1):318–325. doi: 10.1148/radiol.12111604. Epub 2012 Oct 16.
14. Takeda R, Ogura T, Ooigawa H, et al. A practical prediction model for early hematoma expansion in spontaneous deep ganglionic intracerebral hemorrhage. *Clin Neurol Neurosurg.* 2013;115:1028–1031.
15. Brouwers HB, Chang Y, Falcone GJ, et al. Predicting hematoma expansion after primary intracerebral hemorrhage. *JAMA Neurol.* 2014;71:158–164.
16. Barras CD, Tress BM, Christensen S, et al. Quantitative CT densitometry for predicting intracerebral hemorrhage growth. *AJNR Am J Neuroradiol.* 2013;34:1139–1144.
17. Boulouis G, Morotti A, Charidimou A, Dowlatshahi D, Goldstein JN. Noncontrast computed tomography markers of intracerebral hemorrhage expansion. *Stroke.* 2017;48:1120–1125.
18. Delgado Almandoz JE, Yoo AJ, Stone MJ, et al. Systematic characterization of the computed tomography angiography spot sign in primary intracerebral hemorrhage identifies patients at highest risk for hematoma expansion: The spot sign score. *Stroke.* 2009;40:2994–3000.
19. Phan CM, Yoo AJ, Hirsch JA, Nogueira RG, Gupta R. Differentiation of hemorrhage from iodinated contrast in different intracranial compartments using dual-energy head CT. *AJNR Am J Neuroradiol.* 2012;33:1088–1094.
20. Demchuk AM, Dowlatshahi D, Rodriguez-Luna D, et al. Prediction of haematoma growth and outcome in patients with intracerebral haemorrhage using the CT-angiography spot sign (predict): A prospective observational study. *Lancet Neurol.* 2012;11:307–314.
21. Del Giudice A, D'Amico D, Sobesky J, Wellwood I. Accuracy of the spot sign on computed tomography angiography as a predictor of haematoma enlargement after acute spontaneous intracerebral haemorrhage: A systematic review. *Cerebrovasc Dis.* 2014;37:268–276.
22. Du FZ, Jiang R, Gu M, He C, Guan J. The accuracy of spot sign in predicting hematoma expansion after intracerebral hemorrhage: A systematic review and meta-analysis. *PLoS One.* 2014;9:e115777.
23. Tan CO, Lam S, Kuppens D, et al. Spot and diffuse signs: Quantitative markers of intracranial hematoma expansion at dual-energy CT. *Radiology.* 2019;290(1):179–186. doi: 10.1148/radiol.2018180322.

24. Mericle RA, Lopes DK, Fronckowiak MD, Wakhloo AK, Guterman LR, Hopkins LN. A grading scale to predict outcomes after intra-arterial thrombolysis for stroke complicated by contrast extravasation. *Neurosurgery.* 2000;46:1307–1314; discussion 1314-1305.
25. Greer DM, Koroshetz WJ, Cullen S, Gonzalez RG, Lev MH. Magnetic resonance imaging improves detection of intracerebral hemorrhage over computed tomography after intra-arterial thrombolysis. *Stroke.* 2004;35:491–495.
26. Graser A, Johnson TR, Chandarana H, Macari M. Dual energy CT: Preliminary observations and potential clinical applications in the abdomen. *Eur Radiol.* 2009;19:13–23.
27. Ferda J, Novak M, Mirka H, et al. The assessment of intracranial bleeding with virtual unenhanced imaging by means of dual-energy CT angiography. *Eur Radiol.* 2009;19:2518–2522.
28. Gupta R, Phan CM, Leidecker C, et al. Evaluation of dual-energy CT for differentiating intracerebral hemorrhage from iodinated contrast material staining. *Radiology.* 2010;257:205–211.
29. Phan CM, Yoo AJ, Hirsch JA, Nogueira RG, Gupta R. Differentiation of hemorrhage from iodinated contrast in different intracranial compartments using dual-energy head CT. *AJNR Am J Neuroradiol.* 2012;33:1088–1094.

3 Clinical Perspective on Dual Energy Computed Tomography

Charis McNabney, Shamir Rai, and Darra T. Murphy
Department of Radiology, St. Paul's Hospital, Vancouver, British Columbia, Canada

CONTENTS

3.1 DUAL ENERGY COMPUTED TOMOGRAPHY

Computed tomography (CT) is a pivotal diagnostic resource in modern medical healthcare. Dual energy computed tomography (DECT) enhances the modalities potential and refers to the use of two photon spectra (typical maximum voltages 140 and 80 kVp) to obtain two CT data sets (Grajo et al. 2016; Johnson 2012).

Principals underpinning DECT are identical regardless of scanner type. Currently, there are three technical approaches recruited by major CT suppliers:

- Single Source CT is a unit with rapidly alternating voltage switching source with a single detector registering information from both energies (GE healthcare)
- Dual Source CT uses two x-ray tubes and two detectors to acquire dual energy data acquisition simultaneously (Siemens Medical Solutions)
- Dual-layer multi-detector scanner comprises top and bottom scintillator layers to capture low and high energy data, respectively (Philips Healthcare)

Conventional Single Energy CT (SECT) is performed at a fixed tube voltage and is useful for structural information of subjects only. Materials of a similar attenuation in SECT images are often indistinguishable with limited contrast, for example, calcium and iodine. Each DECT examination consists of two data sets of images from the same body part using two different energy levels (usually 80 and 140 kVp). DECT analyzes information via monochromatic evaluation or material decomposition. The addition of data from further energy spectra in DECT allows for materials to be differentiated based on the unique x-ray absorption characteristics of an element at different kilovoltage levels. Examples include soft tissue, fat, water, and iodine images with iodine and water images most utilized (Patel et al. 2013). Following differentiation, materials can be selected or removed. If selected, a material may be uniquely color-coded and maps superimposed on standard grayscale CT images for qualitative assessment (Mallinson et al. 2016). Histogram analysis based on DECT enables quantitative assessment of materials useful for comparison between studies (Uhrig et al. 2015). Energy-specific post-processing techniques applied to DECT data sets can produce routine diagnostic images known as virtual monochromatic images (VMIs), intended to replicate non-contrast images produced by SECT. A virtual monochromatic (VMC) energy spectrum can be produced, so anatomy may be viewed at different energy levels ranging from 40 to 190 keV. Data from both scanning energy levels contribute to the overall VMC image. The optimum energy (from the monochromatic energy spectrum) to view an image study varies based on indication; the lower energy spectrum offers superior soft tissue contrast whereas higher energy beams suffer less absorption and scatter of x-rays (attenuation) as they pass through metal and therefore less beam hardening. Post-processing software enables operators to select specific energy levels for viewing purposes (Patel et al. 2013; Yu & Christner 2011).

By virtue of DECT, material differentiation, identification, and quantification are now possible. Such capabilities are the basis of existing and future clinical applications.

3.2 ABDOMINAL IMAGING

3.2.1 Liver

DECT offers superior liver lesion detection and characterization compared to SECT.

Frequently, incidental low-attenuation liver lesions are identified on routine (single energy) CT contrast-enhanced abdominal studies. Owing to their size, lesions are often too small to be accurately characterized. Hypodense liver lesions usually represent benign cysts; however, hypodense metastases can mimic cysts. Further investigation is warranted in this situation for accurate lesion characterization, particularly amongst patients undergoing oncological assessment, due to lack of non-contrast study. DECT's capability to produce color overlay iodine maps and iodine tissue values, can help improve lesion conspicuity, so lesions are more distinct from background tissue. Following the administration of iodinated contrast, metastases demonstrate iodine uptake whereas cysts do not. Furthermore, iodine images give a more accurate assessment of enhancement compared to images from conventional contrast enhanced SECT (Patel et al. 2013; Silva 2011). Material differentiation and therefore the production of iodine images in DECT can further characterize hypodense lesions, avoiding the need for follow-up imaging such as magnetic resonance imaging (MRI), invasive proceedings (biopsy) and therefore prevent anxiety amongst patients involved in the diagnostic process (Grajo et al. 2016; Silva 2011).

A background of liver cirrhosis is both a predisposing factor for and a challenging background on which to detect hepatocellular carcinoma on conventional ultrasound, MRI, and CT (Mannelli & Rosenkrantz 2013). Post-processing of data in DECT offers superior lesion detection in cirrhotic patients compared to SECT and an alternative for patients with contraindications to MRI. DECT can produce a spectrum of monoenergetic images, which show increased contrast between lesions and background tissue at lower energies, meaning lesions are more distinct against background tissue. Furthermore, iodine images also play a critical role in lesion detection particularly when color-mapped and overlaid on grayscale CT images, to further increase lesion conspicuity (Grajo et al. 2016).

Hepatic steatosis, a condition where fat accumulates within liver cells, can impair liver iron content measurement on SECT. Advanced post-processing applications of DECT have improved quantification of hepatic iron deposition despite complication from a background of hepatic steatosis (Fischer et al. 2011).

Gallstones within the gallbladder that are composed purely of cholesterol may be hypodense to bile; other gallstones can calcify and be hyperdense and easily visible, but many gallstones are isodense to bile and therefore not visible on routine CT due to their composition. DECT can be helpful in determining the presence of isodense gallstones (Figure 3.1), which has clinical implications in terms of reducing the number of tests required for the patient and improving diagnostic accuracy.

3.2.2 Renal

DECT technique offers improved characterization of renal calculi and differentiation between renal cysts and enhancing cystic lesions.

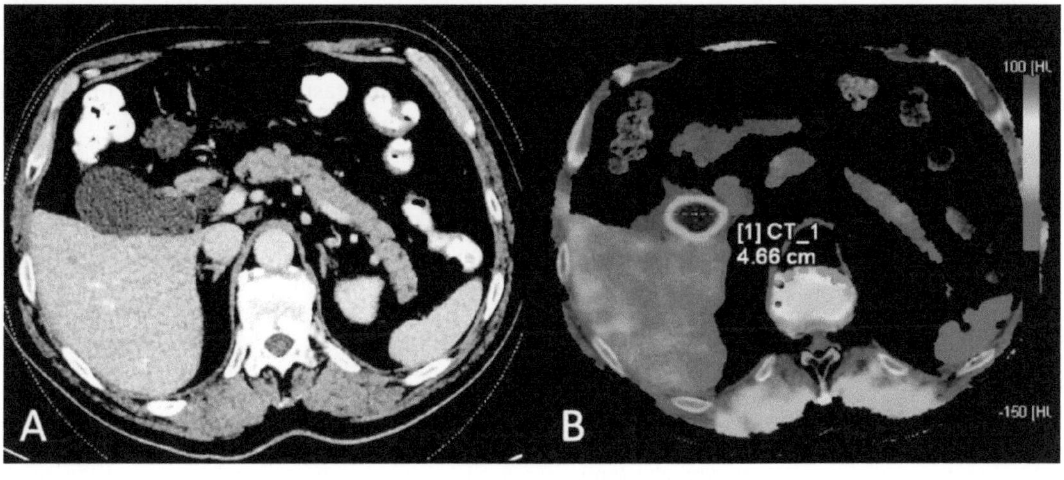

FIGURE 3.1 Gallstone in neck of gallbladder on conventional CT is difficult to see (A, left) as it is isodense to bile, whereas easy to detect using color mapping following DECT (B, right).

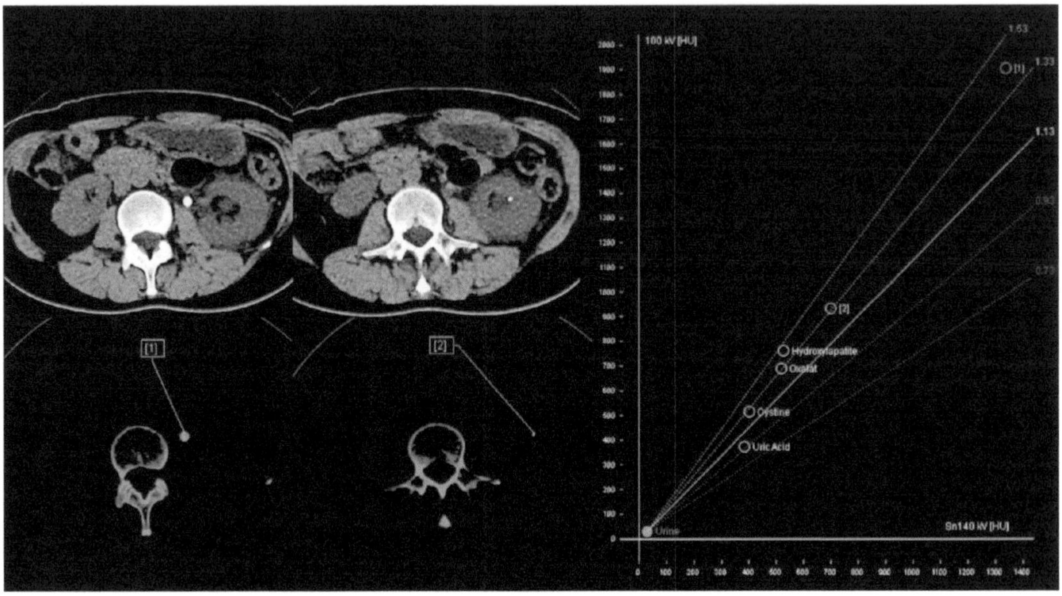

FIGURE 3.2 A patient with two renal calculi in the same kidney but of differing components, detectable by material decomposition at DECT.

In addition to determining renal stone size and location, DECT has recently been used to establish calculi composition of critical importance and influence for patient management. Uric acid calculi are treated medically whereas non-uric acid calculi (calcium, struvite, and cystine) tend to necessitate invasive approaches such as extracorporeal shockwave lithotripsy or percutaneous nephrolithotripsy (Kulkarni et al. 2013). The majority of renal stones contain two or more materials. DECT affords the ability for accurate quantification of uric acid and non-uric acid composition (Figure 3.2) to ensure proper management (Leng et al. 2016). DECT can also offer stone detection in nephrographic phase imaging and in contrast-filled collecting systems by the use of iodine subtraction techniques. This is not possible with SECT as contrast is likely to mask visualization of calculi; a further non-contrast study would be required to visualize calculi (Heye et al. 2012).

Classification of high-density renal lesions commonly found incidentally on a single-portal venous phase (contrast study) abdominal study is a diagnostic challenge. Differentials include hemorrhagic cyst or renal cell carcinoma; having vastly different prognosis and management, distinction is therefore critical. Dedicated dual-phase renal imaging (contrast and non-contrast images) are necessary for accurate classification of renal lesions to evaluate lesion enhancement as well as attenuation differences between enhanced and non-enhanced image acquisitions. DECT can facilitate by producing virtual unenhanced and iodine images from data sets acquired during initial contrast enhanced image acquisition, mitigating the need for an additional non-contrast study as would be required in conventional single CT. Renal cell carcinomas exhibit iodine uptake on iodine images (Heye et al. 2012). The contents of renal lesions, such as fat and calcification, can be identified on VMIs, which can be useful diagnosing benign renal lesions such as angiomyolipoma (Grajo et al. 2016; Jinzaki et al. 2014).

3.2.3 Pancreas

A subsect of pancreatic tumors are isoattenuating on SECT images, meaning they are indistinguishable from background pancreatic tissue and therefore likely to go undetected. Up to 11% of pancreatic ductal adenocarcinomas (PDAs) and 27% of pancreatic tumors under 2 cm are isoattenuating.

A recent study (Bhosale et al. 2015) suggested that DECT improves PDA lesion conspicuity at lower (50–70) kVps, compared to images acquired by routine (120 kVp) SECT, therefore improving PDA detection. Unfortunately, by the time many patients are diagnosed with pancreatic cancer, their disease is too advanced for surgery, the only curative option. Early diagnosis by improved visualization of PDA with DECT could therefore significantly impact patient prognosis (Bhosale et al. 2015). Insulinomas are small tumors of the pancreas, often difficult to localize on SECT. A recent study reported increased insulinoma detection from 68.8% with conventional SECT to 95.7% using both VMIs and an iodine map produced from DECT data sets (Lin et al. 2012).

3.3 CEREBROVASCULAR IMAGING

3.3.1 Distinguishing Enhancing Tumor from Acute Hemorrhage

Identifying the cause of intracranial hemorrhage is critical for patient management. CT angiography (CTA) is often used to establish whether vascular anomalies or enhancing tumor are culpable amongst other differentials. Acute hemorrhage and enhancing tumor are often indistinguishable when they exist concurrently, as both having high attenuation on SECT postcontrast images. Acute hemorrhage could therefore mask contrast enhanced tumor. By material differentiation and identification, DECT can produce an iodine map to identify and distinguish enhancing tumor from underlying hematoma. DECT can allow detection of tumor in the acute stage of bleeding, eliminating the need for a follow-up study at a later date, and potentially improving patient management (Kim et al. 2012).

3.3.2 Hemorrhage Transformation of Stroke from Background Contrast

Early recognition of hemorrhagic transformation of a stroke is critical. It is a major complication of reperfusion therapy such as thrombolysis and tends to occur 12–24 hours following treatment. An initial CT brain scan is performed to diagnose stroke and may have involved contrast to assess related vessels. In the follow-up scan, differentiating acute hemorrhage from residual contrast from the initial scan, can pose a diagnostic challenge in single energy non-contrast CT. DECT can help accurately distinguish intraparenchymal hemorrhage from iodinated contrast medium, by means of iodine mapping (Gupta et al. 2010) (Figure 3.3).

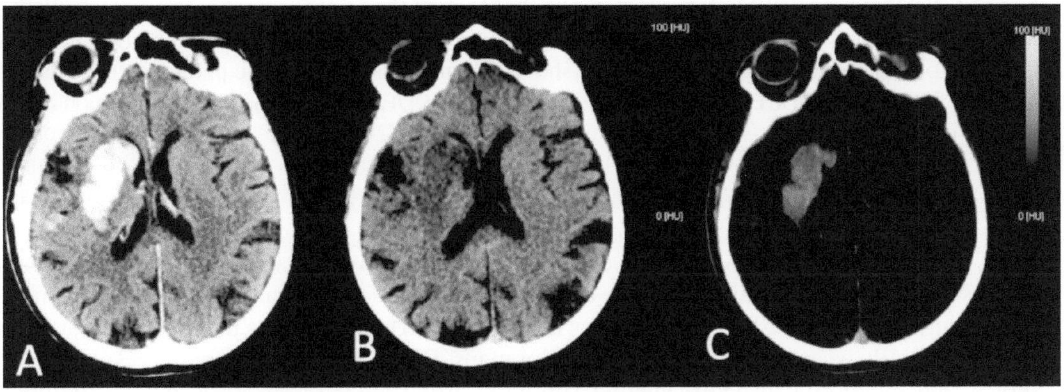

FIGURE 3.3 A contrast enhanced CT brain examination shows increased density on the monochromatic images (A), whereas the DECT with iodine subtraction (B) and an iodine map (C) shows that this is not hemorrhage but contrast staining in a patient with a right basal ganglia infarct presenting with a clinical stroke.

3.3.3 Calcium and Bone Subtraction

Visualization of head and neck vascular anatomy with CT angiogram is often obscured by calcified atheromatous plaque or beam hardening artefact from the skull and is therefore problematic when assessing affected vessels for disease. Using material analysis, calcium can be subtracted from osseous plaques and so vessel lumen is best depicted. This technique is clinically important for identifying carotid plaque components, assessing the degree of luminal narrowing and caliber (Hsu et al. 2016).

3.4 CARDIAC AND VASCULAR IMAGING

3.4.1 Calcium Score Calculation

Coronary artery calcium (CAC) scoring has become an established method of cardiovascular risk assessment for both symptomatic and asymptomatic patients. The addition of CAC scoring to coronary CTA facilitates more accurate mortality prediction than CT coronary angiography alone. CAC score is typically assessed on a non-contrast study prior to a contrast study in SECT, owing to the difficulty identifying and quantifying calcium in the presence of iodine in a contrast study. DECT has enabled non-contrast equivalent VMIs to be extracted from data obtained during a contrast study, removing the need for a separate non-contrast study. Specifically, iodine is removed from the coronary vessel and calcium remains. CAC scores derived from VMIs have been shown to correlate well with those obtained from true non-contrast studies and therefore DECT has the potential to serve as a lower dose equivalent (Yamada et al. 2014).

3.4.2 Characterization of Atherosclerotic Plaque

Clinical studies have shown that the composition of atherosclerotic plaque has more significant effect on a patients' condition than the degree of stenosis (Haghighi et al. 2015). Most cases of acute coronary syndrome occur as a result of rupture of vulnerable coronary plaques, which typically have a lipid-rich core and thin fibrous cap. It is therefore important to identify the contents of atherosclerotic plaques to establish high-risk lesions prior to rupture. This is currently difficult to achieve with conventional CT due to overlap in attenuation values between higher risk lipid rich and lower risk fibrotic plaques (Vliegenthart et al. 2012). Several studies have demonstrated that DECT offers superior characterization of non-calcific atherosclerotic plaque in cadaveric specimens than SECT (Obaid et al. 2014; Tanami et al. 2010). Much of the improvement in characterization of non-calcified plaque is however lost when imaging live patients, with temporal resolution has been named as one of the limiting factors. DECT shows potential for non-calcific plaque differentiation; however, further studies are required to validate the role of DECT in plaque characterization of live patients (Obaid et al. 2014).

3.4.3 Acute Chest Pain

DECT can identify obstructive cardiac disease as well as conventional CT; however, its roles in patients with acute chest pain relates to the fact that DECT can evaluate myocardial segments more accurately than SECT. DECT portrays myocardial perfusion defects more conspicuous than SECT, especially when presented as iodine color maps. DECT has superior spatial resolution that SPECT and therefore can detect smaller sub-endocardial areas of severe ischemia/infarction. Adenosine stress first-pass dual-energy myocardial perfusion CT could identify 100% of myocardial segments versus 88% of segments seen in stress dynamic real-time myocardial perfusion SECT (Weininger et al. 2012).

3.4.4 Assessment of Coronary Stenosis

CT coronary angiography has been deemed an effective gatekeeper to invasive coronary angiography. Despite technological advances in single energy CTCA, the technique is limited in high-risk patients with diffusely calcified vessels, with calcification having the greatest impact on diagnostic accuracy due to artifactual distortion (Brodoefel et al. 2008). When calcium scores exceed 400, artefacts can lead to overestimation of the degree of luminal encroachment (Ong et al. 2006). Specifically, blooming and beam hardening artefacts from densely calcific coronary lesions on SECT lead to imprecise quantification of coronary stenosis. DECT aims to offer a more accurate assessment of plaque and potentially improve overall diagnostic performance by means of monochromatic evaluation of coronary arteries, complemented by material decomposition; VMC evaluation of coronary vessels at higher energy levels aims to reduce blooming and beam hardening artefacts, whereas material decomposition, specifically subtraction of calcium, with only iodine remaining to offer a more precise quantification of coronary stenosis where calcific plaque is present. This may lead to a reclassification of the severity of lesions in coronary artery disease and prevent unnecessary referral for invasive angiography. This may also mean that intermediate to high-risk patients can be included in DECT coronary angiography studies (Cademartiri et al. 2007; Ruzsics et al. 2008).

3.5 MUSCULOSKELETAL IMAGING

3.5.1 Gout Imaging-Urate Detection and Analysis

Gout is a common form of inflammatory arthritis caused by deposition of monosodium urate (MSU) crystals in joints and surrounding soft tissues. Acute attacks present with acute excruciating joint pain. Gold-standard diagnosis of gout is by means of joint aspiration during an acute attack and fluid analysis to detect MSU crystals. The process can be painful, technically difficult, and carries a risk of introducing infection. Occasionally, the paucity of synovial fluid makes for a non-diagnostic procedure (Newberry et al. 2016). Difficulty arises when diagnosing gout because it can mimic other diseases and the conventional repertoire of investigations is neither sufficiently sensitive nor specific. Serum urate levels are not always raised in patients presenting with gout and may be raised in asymptomatic patients (Schlesinger et al. 2009). Similarly, imaging modalities such as ultrasound, MRI, and conventional CT do not deliver certainty of diagnosis during the acute phase and therefore are not incorporated into routine clinical practice (McQueen et al. 2011).

DECT has repeatedly been proven to be a useful noninvasive, accurate, and reliable diagnostic tool in the setting of acute gout. Moreover, DECT enables gout to be distinguished from infection or malignancy. DECT enables MSU deposits (tophi) to be identified, mapped, and rates followed throughout the course of gout (Figure 3.4). Color mapping allows obvious displays of urate deposits separate to surrounding bone and soft tissue (Mallinson et al. 2016). Volumetric assessment of gouty tophi can also be ascertained, allowing for comparison of data from serial scans, of particular importance for clinicians hoping to establish the efficacy of prophylactic urate-lowering therapies (Choi et al. 2012). Data from five major randomized control trials has a reported sensitivity of 78–100% and specificity of 89–100% for gout detection in DECT, significantly better than conventional investigations (Choi et al. 2009; Choi et al. 2012; Dalbeth & Choi 2012; Glazebrook et al. 2011; Manger et al. 2012).

Furthermore, a study by Choi et al. (2009) demonstrated that DECT was four times more effective at identifying rate deposits than clinical examination. Gout, as opposed to hyperuricemia is linked to a higher risk of death from all causes as well as cardiovascular disease, nephropathy, and joint destruction (Kuo et al. 2009). Rising rates of the sequelae from gout are prompting the need for an expeditious and accurate diagnosis of gout. DECT has emerged as leading technology, capable of meeting increased demand (Mallinson et al. 2016).

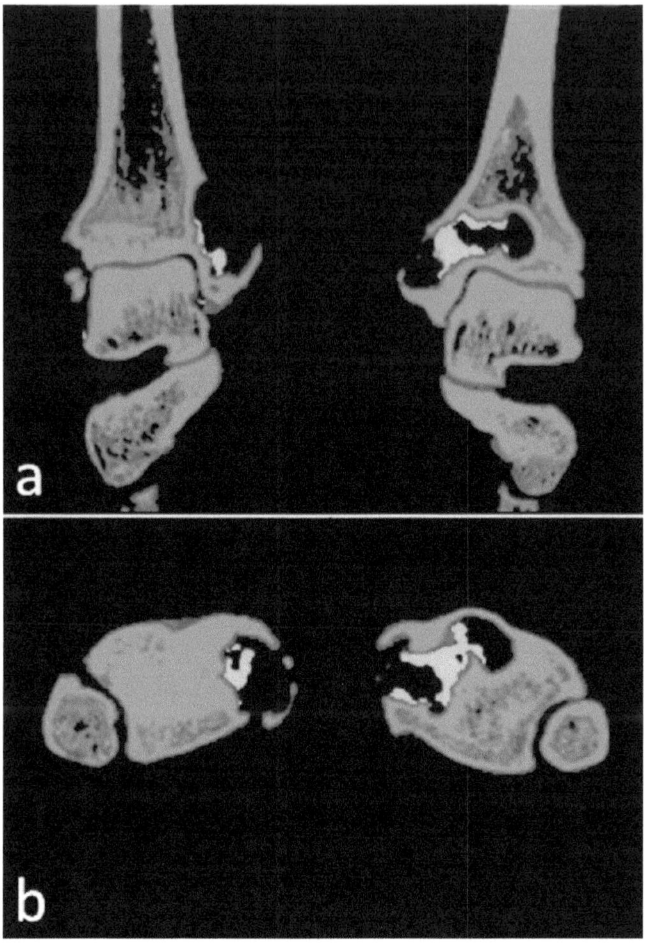

FIGURE 3.4 DECT evaluation in (a) coronal and (b) transverse axial planes in a patient with painful ankles showing chronic cystic lesions in the medial malleoli with uric acid deposition color-coded green in this example of acute-on-chronic gout.

3.5.2 Bone Marrow Edema Detection

Bone marrow edema secondary to trauma has traditionally been diagnosed on MRI with low signal on T1 and high signal on T2 fat-suppressed images. MRI is limited in the setting of trauma due to long acquisition scan times, prolonged and potentially painful patient positioning, patient contraindications, and variable "out-of-hours" availability. Conventional CT lacks the ability to detect bone marrow edema because attenuation changes caused by the edema are subtle (Alabsi et al. 2017). Non-calcium images (VNCa) produced by DECT have been validated by numerous studies for the detection of bone marrow edema (Bierry et al. 2014; Guggenberger et al. 2012; Pache et al. 2010; Wang et al. 2013). Color maps applied from DECT increase visibility and detection of subtle bone marrow edema (Mallinson et al. 2016) (Figure 3.5). Further research is required to validate the use of DECT in the setting of suspicion for minimally displaced hip fracture when no fracture is identified on pelvic radiograph. There are limitations for use of DECT for detection of small lesions with limited marrow edema, present adjacent to cortical bone; they are poorly visualized and can therefore be missed (Reddy et al. 2014).

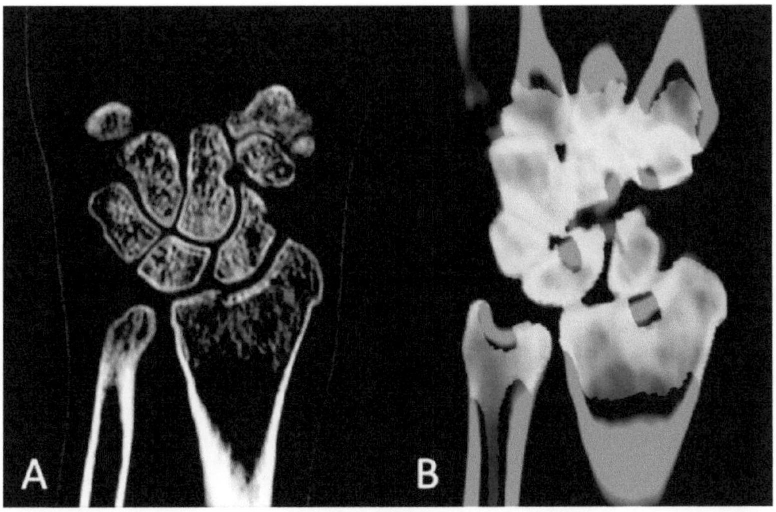

FIGURE 3.5 Monochromatic and DECT in a patient with a distal radius fracture. While the fracture is easily identified on the baseline CT, the extent of edema only becomes apparent with DECT.

3.5.3 Collagen Analysis: Ligaments, Tendons, and Intervertebral Discs

MRI is the gold-standard noninvasive assessment for tendons, menisci, and ligaments, whereas conventional CT evaluation of soft tissue is limited. CT arthrography following administration of intra-articular contrast injection can provide a reasonable assessment of some ligaments; however, the investigation is invasive and does not provide assessment of all ligaments. DECT does not require the use of intra-articular contrast injection. Instead tissue decomposition method employed by DECT can identify collagen, formulate a representative color-coded map, which can be fused to standard grayscale CT images within structures, to help with anatomic location and detection of pathological conditions (Mallinson et al. 2016).

Certain ligaments (such as anterior and posterior cruciate ligament, patellar ligament, and fibular collateral ligament) are clearly identified on DECT (Figure 3.6), while others are not so clearly depicted (Sun et al. 2008). DECT was found to accurately assess ligamentous injury secondary to penetrating injuries of the wrist and ankle in post-mortem subjects (Persson et al. 2008). DECT was compared to MRI for examination of anterior cruciate ligament (ACL) tears in porcine models. DECT had a similar sensitivity and specificity to MRI for determining partial ACL tears; however, neither demonstrated sufficient sensitivity for detection of partial ACL tears. MRI had superior sensitivity and specificity to detect full ACL tears when compared to DECT. Further research and technical advances are required to enhance DECT's ability at ligamentous assessment (Fickert et al. 2012).

Tendons have not been as thoroughly investigated as ligaments. Studies have confirmed that DECT is able to visualize Achilles, plantar, flexor policies longus, flexor digitorum superficialis, and profundus, as well as extensor digitorum longus tendons (Deng et al. 2009; Mallinson et al. 2013). A study by Deng et al. (2009) reported image quality of the hand is superior on DECT compared to conventional CT, particularly because beam hardening artefacts are reduced between the phalanges. Furthermore, all tendons within the hand were visualized by DECT.

3.5.4 Future Applications

Pilot studies have indicated potential for DECT arthrography (to evaluate joints); however, larger patient trials and refinement of post-processing techniques are required to prove clinical efficacy. Similarly, DECT's use in the detection and follow-up of metastases requires further validation,

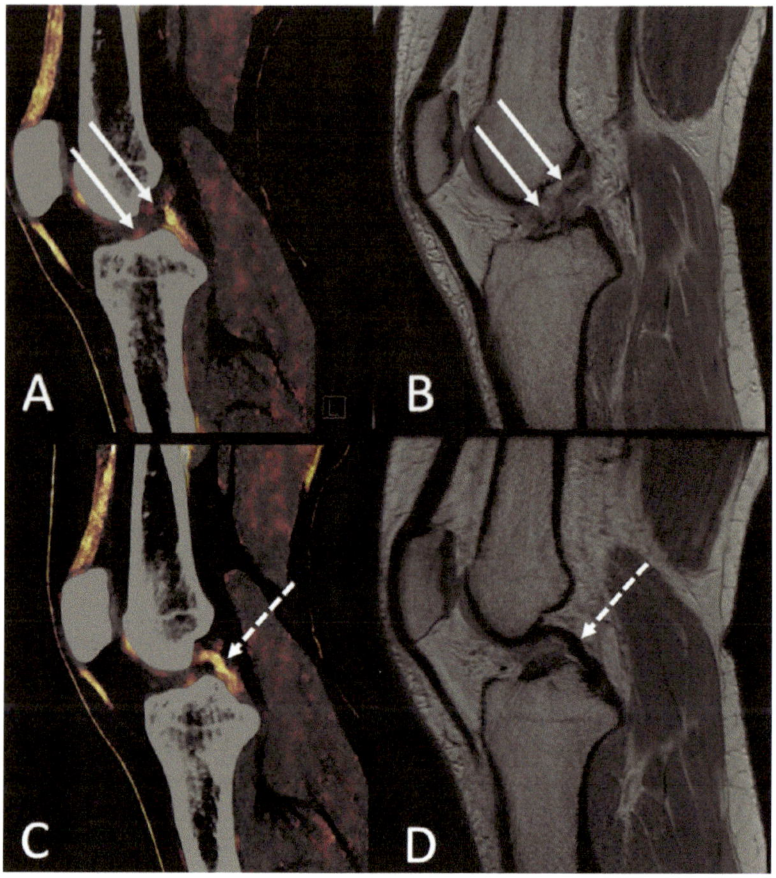

FIGURE 3.6 DECT images (A, C) of a patient post-knee pivot-shift twisting injury with subsequent imaging gold standard MRI correlation (B, D). The images A and B show correlation of a torn anterior cruciate ligament (white arrows) and the images C and D show correlation of an intact posterior cruciate ligament (dashed arrows).

particularly with respect to presentation of different tumor types and normal variants. DEXA scanning is considered the reference standard for assessment of osteoporosis; however, there are many reported limitations to this technique. A three-dimensional approach can help overcome some of these limitations. DECT with bone mineral density application represents a promising three-dimensional approach in the assessment of osteoporosis, with reduced radiation dose when compared to conventional CT (Mallinson et al. 2016).

3.6 ARTEFACT REDUCTION

3.6.1 Metallic Prosthesis

Metal within prosthesis causes streak artefacts in CT imaging due to photon starvation, photon scatter, and excessive beam hardening. Beam hardening is due to the absorption or scatter of x-rays from the scanning beam by the metallic prosthesis, so less x-rays are registered at the detector (Barrett & Keat 2004). Conventional CT acquisition and reconstruction techniques can be applied to minimize artefact from metallic prosthesis, often at the expense of an increased radiation dose. Despite best attempts, artefacts related to metallic prosthesis in conventional CT still remain problematic (Nicolaou et al. 2012). For example, in patients with hip prosthesis, visualization of tissue adjacent

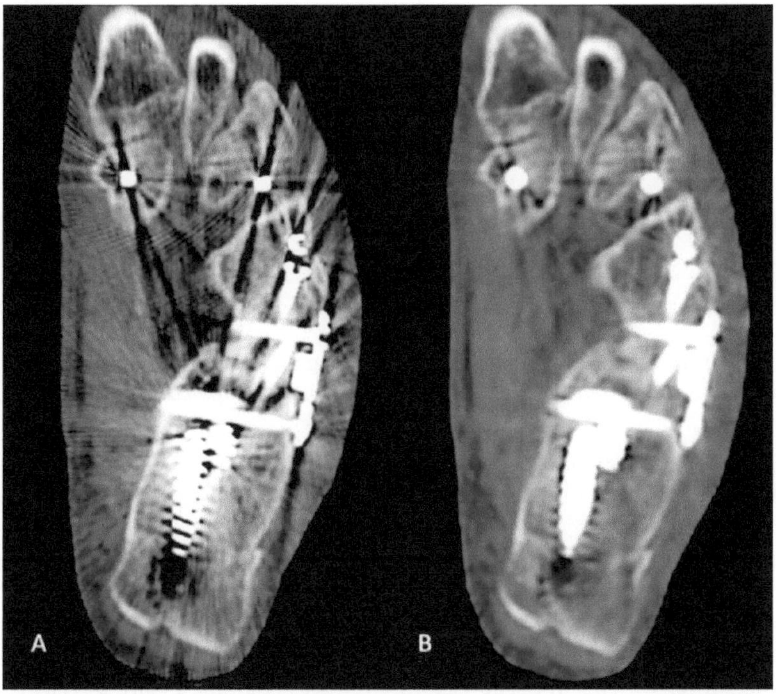

FIGURE 3.7 CT images of the axial hindfoot showing the difference in beam-hardening (or 'streak') artefact between conventional (A) and dual energy (B) CT images with metallic hardware.

to the prosthesis becomes impaired, including pelvic organs which potentially results in missed findings (Elmpt et al. 2016). Radiologists are frequently asked to assess metallic prosthesis for periprosthetic fractures, infection, aseptic loosening, metallic failure and fractures, pseudotumors, and recurrence of tumors (sarcomas) (Roth et al. 2012). MRI is also beneficial for assessment of metallic prosthesis due to superior soft tissue detail surrounding the prosthesis and sensitivity for bone edema; however, images are also prone to distortion related to metallic prosthesis (Suh et al. 1998).

Artefact reduction is achieved in DECT by energy specific post-processing techniques applied to DECT data sets, enabling the generation of a VMC energy spectrum. VMIs are less susceptible to beam hardening artefacts (Figures 3.7–3.9). Higher energy beams suffer less absorption and scatter

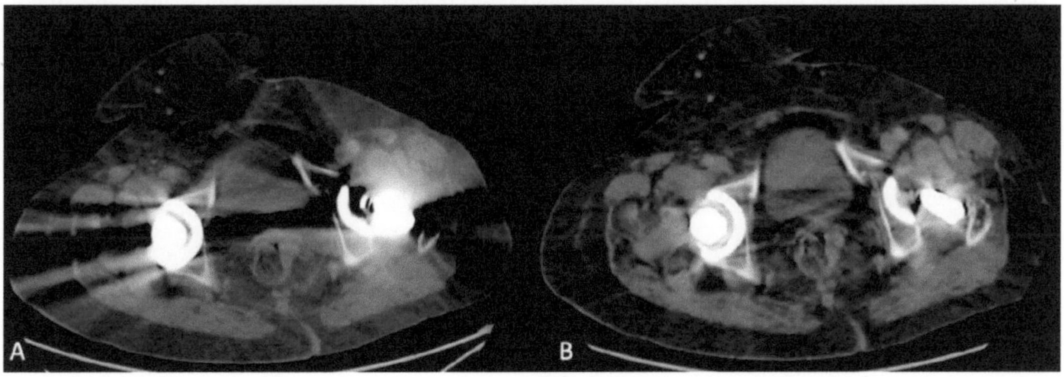

FIGURE 3.8 CT images of the axial pelvis showing the difference in beam-hardening (or 'streak') artefact between conventional (A) and dual energy (B) CT images with metallic hardware.

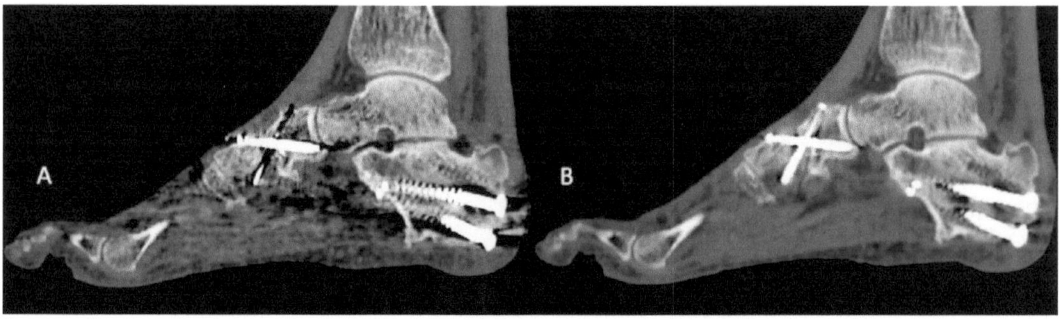

FIGURE 3.9 CT images of the sagittal whole foot showing the difference in beam-hardening (or 'streak') artefact between conventional (A) and dual energy (B) CT images with metallic hardware.

(attenuation) of x-rays as they pass through metal and therefore less beam hardening. The optimum energy (from the monochromatic energy spectrum) to view an image study varies based on factors such as patient and prosthetic size. Post-processing software enables operators to select specific energy levels with least ensuing beam hardening for viewing purposes (Yu & Christner 2011).

The preferred energy level to obtain optimal image for an implant is between 105 and 133 keV. When reconstructed monoenergetic images of different keV values are compared, the amount of streak artefact decreases and therefore surrounding soft tissue visibility increases with increasing keV, until a point after which soft tissue visibility reduces (Bamberg et al. 2011).

Various studies have confirmed the use of DECT in metal artefact reduction (Bamberg et al. 2011; Guggenberger et al. 2012; Zhou et al. 2011). A study by Bamberg et al. (2011) compared images from high energy DECT images with those of conventional CT images in 31 patients with prosthesis. Higher energy monoenergetic kiloelectron-volt DECT images were noted to bring about superior image quality in 29 out of the 31 patients and superior diagnostic quality in 27 out of 31 patients when compared to lower energy monoenergetic kiloelectron-volt images. Of paramount significance, decisive diagnostic features, such as periprosthetic fractures and loosening of a screw, were only visible on higher energy monoenergetic kiloelectron-volt DECT image reconstructions. The optimum viewing kiloelectron-volt energy varied based on the size and composition of the prosthesis. DECT enables metal artefact to be reduced, image quality improved, and increased diagnostic yield compared to conventional CT images (Bamberg et al. 2011).

3.6.2 Intracranial Prosthesis

Intracranial aneurysm may be treated with aneurysm clipping or coiling. Follow-up scans may be required to assess for aneurysm recurrence or residual aneurysm filling. Clips and coiling implanted devices cause beam hardening and streak (BHS) artefact, interfering with visualization of aneurysm and adjacent vessels often rendering assessment difficult, if not impossible. VMIs reduce BHS artefacts when viewed at higher energies increments, 110 keV for assessment of vascular lumen or aneurysm residual, adjacent to clip or coil, with the highest energy levels (140 keV) reserved for evaluation of metallic hardware itself (Shinohara et al. 2014).

3.6.3 Pixel Mis-Registration in Conventional CT

A multiphase CT protocol constitutes unenhanced image acquisition followed by IV contrast administration for acquisition of enhanced images. Due to unpreventable breathing or motion artefacts, the images may vary significantly on a pixel by pixel basis, predisposing to pseudoenhancement when in fact there is no enhancement. By contrast, following the emission of two different photon energies with DECT, both data sets are acquired almost simultaneously. Both reconstructed VMI (unenhanced) and iodine-specific images are generated from the simultaneously acquired data sets, meaning that motion artefact is limited and therefore a more accurate assessment of enhancement obtained (Heye et al. 2012).

3.6.4 Coronary Stenosis

Blooming and beam hardening artefacts caused by severe calcified plaque in conventional CT coronary angiography can obscure the underlying vessel lumen and lead to imprecise quantification of the calcific lesion. Coronary stenosis may be overestimated and patients may be inappropriately referred for invasive angiography (Cademartiri et al. 2007). By means of monochromatic analysis of data, blooming and beam hardening artefacts are reduced. DECT aims to offer a more accurate assessment of coronary artery disease and therefore increase the positive predictive value of diagnosis (Ruzsics et al. 2008). Likewise, the metallic material within coronary stents can cause beam hardening and blooming artefacts on CT coronary angiography images and subsequently an underestimation in stent lumen. DECT can mitigate artefacts associated with metallic stenting and therefore lead to more accurate assessment of stent lumen patency; however, larger studies are required to prove a significant benefit with DECT over conventional CT (Zou & Silver 2009).

3.7 ONCOLOGY IMAGING

3.7.1 Improved Lesion Characterization

DECT is advantageous for liver, renal, and pancreatic lesion detection in aforementioned abdominal imaging section (Heye et al. 2012).

3.7.2 Improved Lesion Conspicuity

Contrast to noise ratio is the most important factor for an image interpreter when distinguishing a lesion from a background of normal tissue. Lower energy VMI in DECT enhances contrast between lesions and background tissue, improving lesion conspicuity and potentially allowing for increased lesion detection (Patel et al. 2013). If lesions are better observed, tumor margin delineation is better defined and size measurements are more accurate. This is crucial for monitoring solid lesion response to therapy, particularly for patients enrolled in clinical trials, as per WHO and RECIST criterion. Moreover, the extent of disease within an organ and association with adjacent vasculature can be more accurately assessed, to better inform treatment strategy, particularly for staging and surgical implications (Grajo et al. 2016).

3.7.3 Evaluation of Tumor Response to Therapy

Assessment of early treatment response is vital prior to adjusting, continuing, or discontinuing treatment regimes, to maximize benefits and minimize oncological treatment associated risks (Canellas et al. 2016). Treatment by newer cancer target therapies restricts growth as opposed to tumor regression as in more conventional therapies. Target therapy treated lesions may not exhibit a significant size reduction and therefore conventional methods of serial size measurement are not reliable (Meerten et al. 2009). Lesions, such as hepatocellular and renal cell carcinoma, often contain both tumor and hemorrhage/thrombus, meaning arbitrary size and volumetric measurements are not representative of tumor burden. Furthermore, following treatment lesions can be a mixture of necrotic tissue and tumor, which appear heterogenous and indistinguishable on SECT. DECT offers the potential to examine viable tumor at a functional level. Qualitative iodine maps and quantitative iodine tissue values processed from DECT data sets offer the potential for detection of residual or recurrent disease (Grajo et al. 2016; Lee et al. 2012).

3.7.4 Oncology-Related Comorbidities

Not only is DECT useful for the diagnostic process but also detecting oncology-related complications and comorbidities. DECT by means of Blood Flow images has a higher sensitivity for diagnosing pulmonary embolism compared to conventional multidetector computed tomography (MDCT). DECT can be used to assess iodine distribution in pulmonary parenchyma and contrast medium in bowel wall to diagnose pulmonary embolism and bowel ischemia respectively (De Cecco et al. 2012).

DECT has numerous advantages for oncological imaging, including enhanced lesion detection and characterization, allows for treatment planning, evaluation of response to therapy as well as detection of oncological-related pathology. The potential of DECT in oncology has not yet been fully exploited.

3.8 SAFETY AND DECT

3.8.1 Minimizing Contrast Media Risk

Contrast induced nephropathy (CIN) is a serious adverse event that may result from the administration of iodinated contrast media in CTA. Treatment is not definitive but instead supportive in nature, with prevention being the cornerstone of management (Mohammed et al. 2013). The dose-effect relationship between administered contrast medium volume and incurring renal toxicity is well cited. By virtue of low energy monochromatic imaging in DECT, up to 50% less iodinated contrast volume is required compared to SECT to produce images without compromising image interpretability (Raju et al. 2014). Risk factors for CIN are including baseline renal function, diabetes, heart failure, male sex, hypertension, and anemia (Mohammed et al. 2013). Many of the risk factors for CIN overlap with and may be prevalent amongst patients with vascular disease, a significant indication for CTA. Therefore, reducing iodinated contrast volume will significantly reduce risk and subsequently incidence of CIN amongst an already at risk patient population (Mohammed et al. 2013).

As previously mentioned, incidental renal lesions are commonly found on single phase portal venous abdominal studies (contrast study) and therefore warrant further investigation for characterization. This is usually in the form of a further dedicated dual phase study, with the requirement for an additional contrast bolus to be administered and so placing the patient at further risk of kidney injury. DECT can avoid this because contrast and non-contrast images can be extracted from a contrast study data set, so the renal lesion can be characterized; therefore, mitigating the need for follow-up imaging (Heye et al. 2012).

3.8.2 Effective Dose Reduction

3.8.2.1 Eliminate Non-Contrast Examinations

If a non-contrast and contrast study are required in SECT, two separate irradiating studies are required. DECT has enabled iodine to be subtracted from contrast study data to reconstruct a non-contrast equivalent, VMI, removing the need to obtain a separate non-contrast study; therefore, no substantial increase in radiation dose and image acquisition time thereof. The image quality of VMIs and true unenhanced images are not significantly different (Heye et al. 2012). Contrary to belief, the radiation dose from DECT may be equivalent if not less than SECT, as the radiation voltage alters between low and high kVps during acquisition. DECT therefore has the potential to replace dual phase protocols and in doing so, significantly reduce radiation dose across patient populations of many medical disciplines, which employ dual phase CT studies (Mallinson et al. 2016).

3.8.2.2 Decreased Follow-up Studies

Sub-centimeter liver lesions often require patients to be re-called for further imaging for accurate characterization. Likewise, hyperdense renal cysts frequently appear on contrast enhanced abdominal studies cannot be accurately characterized and require follow-up imaging. DECT can remove the need for follow-up imaging by allowing for characterization of lesions by means of iodine material decomposition image, saving scan acquisition time, and reducing the overall radiation dose (Silva 2011).

Renal calculi may be suspected on abdominal single energy contrast CT studies if there are secondary signs of calculi are present. Differentiating contrast and calcified calculi can be difficult if not impossible on single energy studies. By means of material separation and differentiation applied to DECT data sets, contrast can be subtracted from the image and calcified calculi may be demonstrated. This is not possible in SECT and an additional irradiating non-contrast study would be required (Heye et al. 2012).

3.9 CONCLUSION

DECT is an innovative imaging modality with many established, evolving, and emerging indications. By virtue of DECT, material separation and tissue characterization is now possible and has facilitated increased lesion detection as well as characterization, imaging improvements at all stages of oncological care, all at comparable and on occasions reduced radiation doses. DECT can also overcome diagnostic challenges and can offer more material-specific information of significance within many medical disciplines. By means of DECT, management can be better informed from a single investigation. Further exciting applications and previously unavailable possibilities may now be ventured with DECT (Grajo et al. 2016).

REFERENCES

Alabsi, H. et al., 2017. Advancements in dual-energy CT applications for musculoskeletal imaging. *Current Radiology Reports*, 5(11), pp.649–614. Available at: http://link.springer.com/10.1007/s40134-017-0249-1.

Bamberg, F. et al., 2011. Metal artifact reduction by dual energy computed tomography using monoenergetic extrapolation. *European Radiology*, 21(7), pp.1424–1429. Available at: http://link.springer.com/10.1007/s00330-011-2062-1.

Barrett, J.F. & Keat, N., 2004. Artifacts in CT: Recognition and avoidance. *Radiographics*, 24(6), pp.1679–1691. Available at: http://pubs.rsna.org/doi/10.1148/rg.246045065.

Bhosale, P. et al., 2015. Quantitative and qualitative comparison of single-source dual-energy computed tomography and 120-kVp computed tomography for the assessment of pancreatic ductal adenocarcinoma. *Journal of Computer Assisted Tomography*, 39(6), pp.907–913. Available at: http://content.wkhealth.com/linkback/openurl?sid=WKPTLP:landingpage&an=00004728-201511000-00013.

Bierry, G. et al., 2014. Dual-energy CT in vertebral compression fractures: Performance of visual and quantitative analysis for bone marrow edema demonstration with comparison to MRI. *Skeletal Radiology*, 43(4), pp.485–492. Available at: http://link.springer.com/10.1007/s00256-013-1812-3.

Brodoefel, H. et al., 2008. Dual-source CT: Effect of heart rate, heart rate variability, and calcification on image quality and diagnostic accuracy. *Radiology*, 247(2), pp.346–355. Available at: http://pubs.rsna.org/doi/10.1148/radiol.2472070906.

Cademartiri, F., La Grutta, L. & Runza, G., 2007. Influence of convolution filtering on coronary plaque attenuation values: Observations in an ex vivo model of multislice computed tomography coronary angiography | springerLink. *European Radiology*, 17(7), pp.1842–1849.

Canellas, R. et al., 2016. Characterization of Portal Vein Thrombosis (Neoplastic Versus Bland) on CT Images Using Software-Based Texture Analysis and Thrombus Density (Hounsfield Units). *American Journal of Roentgenology*, 207(5), W81–W87. http://doi.org/10.2214/AJR.15.15928

Choi, H.K. et al., 2009. Dual energy computed tomography in tophaceous gout. *Annals of the Rheumatic Diseases*, 68(10), pp.1609–1612. Available at: http://ard.bmj.com/cgi/doi/10.1136/ard.2008.099713.

Choi, H.K. et al., 2012. Dual energy CT in gout: A prospective validation study. *Annals of the Rheumatic Diseases*, 71(9), pp.1466–1471. Available at: http://ard.bmj.com/lookup/doi/10.1136/annrheumdis-2011-200976.

Dalbeth, N. & Choi, H.K., 2012. Dual-energy computed tomography for gout diagnosis and management. *Current Rheumatology Reports*, 15(1), pp.189–210. Available at: http://link.springer.com/10.1007/s11926-012-0301-3.

De Cecco, C.N. et al., 2012. Dual-energy CT: Oncologic applications. *American Journal of Roentgenology*, 199(5_supplement), pp.S98–S105. Available at: http://www.ajronline.org/doi/10.2214/AJR.12.9207.

Deng, K. et al., 2009. Initial experience with visualizing hand and foot tendons by dual-energy computed tomography. *Clinical Imaging*, 33(5), pp.384–389. Available at: http://linkinghub.elsevier.com/retrieve/pii/S0899707109000047.

Fickert, S. et al., 2012. Assessment of the diagnostic value of dual-energy CT and MRI in the detection of iatrogenically induced injuries of anterior cruciate ligament in a porcine model. *Skeletal Radiology*, 42(3), pp.411–417. Available at: http://link.springer.com/10.1007/s00256-012-1500-8.

Fischer, M.A. et al., 2011. Quantification of liver iron content with CT—added value of dual-energy. *European Radiology*, 21(8), pp.1727–1732. Available at: http://link.springer.com/10.1007/s00330-011-2119-1.

Glazebrook, K.N. et al., 2011. Identification of intraarticular and periarticular uric acid crystals with dual-energy CT: Initial evaluation. *Radiology*, 261(2), pp.516–524. Available at: http://pubs.rsna.org/doi/10.1148/radiol.11102485.

Grajo, J.R. et al., 2016. Dual energy CT in practice: Basic principles and applications. *Applied Radiology Journal*, 45(7), pp.6–12. Available at: http://appliedradiology.com/articles/dual-energy-ct-in-practice-basic-principles-and-applications.

Guggenberger, R. et al., 2012. Diagnostic performance of dual-energy CT for the detection of traumatic bone marrow lesions in the ankle: Comparison with MR imaging. *Radiology*, 264(1), pp.164–173. Available at: http://pubs.rsna.org/doi/10.1148/radiol.12112217.

Gupta, R. et al., 2010. Evaluation of dual-energy CT for differentiating intracerebral hemorrhage from iodinated contrast material staining. *Radiology*, 257(1), pp.205–211. Available at: http://pubs.rsna.org/doi/10.1148/radiol.10091806.

Haghighi, R. et al., 2015. DECT evaluation of noncalcified coronary artery plaque. *Medical Physics*, 42(10), pp.5945–5954. Available at: http://doi.wiley.com/10.1118/1.4929935.

Heye, T. et al., 2012. Dual-energy CT applications in the abdomen. *American Journal of Roentgenology*, 199(5_supplement), pp.S64–S70. Available at: http://www.ajronline.org/doi/10.2214/AJR.12.9196.

Hsu, C.-T. et al., 2016. Principles and clinical application of dual-energy computed tomography in the evaluation of cerebrovascular disease. *Journal of Clinical Imaging Science*, 6(1), pp.27–28. Available at: http://www.clinicalimagingscience.org/text.asp?2016/6/1/27/185003.

Jinzaki, M. et al., 2014. Renal angiomyolipoma: A radiological classification and update on recent developments in diagnosis and management. *Abdominal Imaging*, 39(3), pp.588–604. Available at: http://link.springer.com/10.1007/s00261-014-0083-3.

Johnson, T.R.C., 2012. Dual-energy CT: General principles. *American Journal of Roentgenology*, 199(5_supplement), pp.S3–S8. Available at: http://www.ajronline.org/doi/10.2214/AJR.12.9116.

Kim, S.J. et al., 2012. Dual-energy CT in the evaluation of intracerebral hemorrhage of unknown origin: Differentiation between tumor bleeding and pure hemorrhage. *American Journal of Neuroradiology*, 33(5), pp.865–872. Available at: http://www.ajnr.org/cgi/doi/10.3174/ajnr.A2890.

Kulkarni, N.M. et al., 2013. Determination of renal stone composition in phantom and patients using single-source dual-energy computed tomography. *Journal of Computer Assisted Tomography*, 37(1), pp.37–45. Available at: http://content.wkhealth.com/linkback/openurl?sid=WKPTLP:landingpage&an=00004728-201301000-00006.

Kuo, C.-F. et al., 2009. Gout: An independent risk factor for all-cause and cardiovascular mortality. *Rheumatology*, 49(1), pp.141–146. Available at: https://academic.oup.com/rheumatology/article/1790618/Gout.

Lee, Y.H. et al., 2012. Metal artefact reduction in gemstone spectral imaging dual-energy CT with and without metal artefact reduction software. *European Radiology*, 22(6), pp.1331–1340. Available at: http://link.springer.com/10.1007/s00330-011-2370-5.

Leng, S. et al., 2016. Dual-energy CT for quantification of urinary stone composition in mixed stones: A phantom study. *American Journal of Roentgenology*, 207(2), pp.321–329. Available at: http://www.ajronline.org/doi/10.2214/AJR.15.15692.

Lin, X.Z. et al., 2012. Dual energy spectral CT imaging of insulinoma—value in preoperative diagnosis compared with conventional multi-detector CT. *European Journal of Radiology*, 81(10), pp.2487–2494. Available at: http://linkinghub.elsevier.com/retrieve/pii/S0720048X11007741.

Mallinson, P.I. et al., 2013. Achilles tendinopathy and partial tear diagnosis using dual-energy computed tomography collagen material decomposition application. *Journal of Computer Assisted Tomography*, 37(3), pp.475–477. Available at: http://content.wkhealth.com/linkback/openurl?sid=WKPTLP:landingpage&an=00004728-201305000-00027.

Mallinson, P.I. et al., 2016. Dual-energy CT for the musculoskeletal system. *Radiology*, 281(3), pp.690–707. Available at: http://pubs.rsna.org/doi/10.1148/radiol.2016151109.

Manger, B. et al., 2012. Detection of periarticular urate deposits with dual energy CT in patients with acute gouty arthritis. *Annals of the Rheumatic Diseases*, 71(3), pp.470–472. Available at: http://ard.bmj.com/lookup/doi/10.1136/ard.2011.154054.

Mannelli, L. & Rosenkrantz, A., 2013. Focal lesions in the cirrhotic liver. *Applied Radiology Journal*, pp.1–6.

McQueen, F.M., Doyle, A. & Dalbeth, N., 2011. Imaging in gout—what can we learn from MRI, CT, DECT and US? *Arthritis Research & Therapy*, 13(6), 246. Available at: http://arthritis-research.biomedcentral.com/articles/10.1186/ar3489.

Meerton, E. et al., 2009. Pathological analysis after neoadjuvant chemoradiotherapy for esophageal carcinoma: the Rotterdam experience. *Journal of Surgical Oncology*, 100(1), 32-37. http://doi.org/10.1002/jso.21295

Mohammed, N.A. et al., 2013. Contrast-induced nephropathy. *Heart Views*, 14(3), pp.106–20. Available at: http://www.heartviews.org/text.asp?2013/14/3/106/125926.

Newberry, S.J. et al., 2016. Diagnosis of gout: A systematic review in support of an American College of Physicians Clinical Practice Guideline. *Annals of Internal Medicine*, 166(1), pp.27–36. Available at: http://annals.org/article.aspx?doi=10.7326/M16-0462.

Nicolaou, S. et al., 2012. Dual-energy CT: A promising new technique for assessment of the musculoskeletal system. *American Journal of Roentgenology*, 199(5_supplement), pp.S78–S86. Available at: http://www.ajronline.org/doi/10.2214/AJR.12.9117.

Obaid, D.R. et al., 2014. Dual-energy computed tomography imaging to determine atherosclerotic plaque composition: A prospective study with tissue validation. *Journal of Cardiovascular Computed Tomography*, 8(3), pp.230–237. Available at: http://linkinghub.elsevier.com/retrieve/pii/S1934592514001014.

Ong, T.K. et al., 2006. Accuracy of 64-row multidetector computed tomography in detecting coronary artery disease in 134 symptomatic patients: Influence of calcification. *American Heart Journal*, 151(6), pp.1323.e1–1323.e6. Available at: http://linkinghub.elsevier.com/retrieve/pii/S0002870306000573.

Pache, G. et al., 2010. Dual-energy CT virtual noncalcium technique: Detecting posttraumatic bone marrow lesions—feasibility study. *Radiology*, 256(2), pp.617–624. Available at: http://pubs.rsna.org/doi/10.1148/radiol.10091230.

Patel, B.N. et al., 2013. Single-source dual-energy spectral multidetector CT of pancreatic adenocarcinoma: Optimization of energy level viewing significantly increases lesion contrast. *Clinical Radiology*, 68(2), pp.148–154. Available at: http://linkinghub.elsevier.com/retrieve/pii/S0009926012003571.

Persson, A. et al., 2008. Advances of dual source, dual-energy imaging in postmortem CT. *European Journal of Radiology*, 68(3), pp.446–455. Available at: http://linkinghub.elsevier.com/retrieve/pii/S0720048X08002507.

Raju, R. et al., 2014. Reduced iodine load with CT coronary angiography using dual-energy imaging: A prospective randomized trial compared with standard coronary CT angiography. *Journal of Cardiovascular Computed Tomography*, 8(4), pp.282–288. Available at: http://linkinghub.elsevier.com/retrieve/pii/S1934592514001531.

Reddy, T. et al., 2014. Detection of occult, undisplaced hip fractures with a dual-energy CT algorithm targeted to detection of bone marrow edema. *Emergency Radiology*, 22(1), pp.25–29. Available at: http://link.springer.com/10.1007/s10140-014-1249-6.

Roth, T.D. et al., 2012. CT of the hip prosthesis: Appearance of components, fixation, and complications. *Radiographics*, 32(4), pp.1089–1107. Available at: http://pubs.rsna.org/doi/10.1148/rg.324115183.

Ruzsics, B. et al., 2008. Dual-energy CT of the heart for diagnosing coronary artery stenosis and myocardial ischemia-initial experience. *European Radiology*, 18(11), pp.2414–2424. Available at: http://link.springer.com/10.1007/s00330-008-1022-x.

Schlesinger, N., Norquist, J.M. & Watson, D.J., 2009. Serum urate during acute gout. *The Journal of Rheumatology*, 36(6), pp.1287–1289. Available at: http://www.jrheum.org/cgi/doi/10.3899/jrheum.080938.

Shinohara, Y. et al., 2014. Usefulness of monochromatic imaging with metal artifact reduction software for computed tomography angiography after intracranial aneurysm coil embolization. *Acta Radiologica*, 55(8), pp.1015–1023. Available at: http://journals.sagepub.com/doi/10.1177/0284185113510492.

Silva, A.C., 2011. Dual-energy (spectral) CT: Applications in abdominal imaging. *Radiographics*, 31, pp.1031–1046.

Suh, J.-S. et al., 1998. Minimizing artifacts caused by metallic implants at MR imaging: Experimental and clinical studies. *American Journal of Roentgenology*, 171(5), pp.1207–1213.

Sun, C. et al., 2008. An initial qualitative study of dual-energy CT in the knee ligaments. *Surgical and Radiologic Anatomy*, 30(5), pp.443–447. Available at: http://link.springer.com/10.1007/s00276-008-0349-y.

Tanami, Y. et al., 2010. Computed tomographic attenuation value of coronary atherosclerotic plaques with different tube voltage. *Journal of Computer Assisted Tomography*, 34(1), pp.58–63. Available at: http://content.wkhealth.com/linkback/openurl?sid=WKPTLP:landingpage&an=00004728-201001000-00011.

Uhrig, M. et al., 2015. Histogram analysis of iodine maps from dual energy computed tomography for monitoring targeted therapy of melanoma patients. *Future Oncology*, 11(4), pp.591–606. Available at: http://www.futuremedicine.com/doi/10.2217/fon.14.265.

van Elmpt, W. et al., 2016. Dual energy CT in radiotherapy: Current applications and future outlook. *Radiotherapy and Oncology*, 119(1), pp.137–144. Available at: http://linkinghub.elsevier.com/retrieve/pii/S0167814016001146.

Vliegenthart, R. et al., 2012. Dual-energy CT of the heart. *American Journal of Roentgenology*, 199(5_supplement), pp.S54–S63. Available at: http://www.ajronline.org/doi/10.2214/AJR.12.9208.

Wang, C.-K. et al., 2013. Bone marrow edema in vertebral compression fractures: Detection with dual-energy CT. *Radiology*, 269(2), pp.525–533. Available at: http://pubs.rsna.org/doi/10.1148/radiol.13122577.

Weininger, M. et al., 2012. Adenosine-stress dynamic real-time myocardial perfusion CT and adenosine-stress first-pass dual-energy myocardial perfusion CT for the assessment of acute chest pain: Initial results. *European Journal of Radiology*, 81(12), pp.3703–3710. Available at: http://linkinghub.elsevier.com/retrieve/pii/S0720048X10005760.

Yamada, Y., Jinzaki, M. & Okamura, T., 2014. Feasibility of coronary artery calcium scoring on virtual unenhanced images derived from single-source fast kVp-switching dual-energy coronary CT angiography—clinicalKey. *Journal of Cardiovascular Computed Tomography*, 8(5), pp.391–400.

Yu, L. & Christner, J., 2011. Virtual monochromatic imaging in dual-source dual-energy CT: Radiation dose and image quality. *Medical physics*, 38(12), pp.6371–6379.

Zhou, C. et al., 2011. Monoenergetic imaging of dual-energy CT reduces artifacts from implanted metal orthopedic devices in patients with factures. *Academic Radiology*, 18(10), pp.1252–1257. Available at: http://linkinghub.elsevier.com/retrieve/pii/S1076633211002571.

Zou, Y. & Silver, M.D., 2009. Elimination of blooming artifacts off stents by dual energy CT. In *SPIE Medical Imaging*. SPIE, p. 72581X–9. Available at: http://proceedings.spiedigitallibrary.org/proceeding.aspx?doi=10.1117/12.811696.

Part II

Spectral, Photon-Counting CT: Clinical Perspective and Applications

4 Imaging of the Breast with Photon-Counting Detectors

Stephen J. Glick and Bahaa Ghammraoui
Office of Science and Engineering Laboratories, CDRH,
U.S. Food and Drug Administration, Silver Spring, Maryland, USA

CONTENTS

4.1 BRIEF OVERVIEW OF X-RAY BREAST IMAGING

Breast cancer is the second most diagnosed cancer in women after skin cancer, and it is the second most deadly cancer in women after lung cancer. It is estimated that one out of every eight women will get breast cancer during their lifetime. Screening of asymptomatic women with mammography is in part responsible for the 39% reduction in breast cancer mortality observed in the past 30 years.[1] Nonetheless, conventional mammography has less than ideal performance, especially for women with dense breast tissue. It has been estimated that approximately 20–50% of breast cancers are missed when imaging women with dense breast tissue[2]; and in addition, 60–80% of biopsies performed based on suspicious lesions found in mammography are not cancer.[3] One of the primary limitations with mammography is the tissue superposition problem. That is, mammography is a 2D-imaging modality, and thus the complex breast structure overlaps within the mammogram making it sometimes difficult to visualize diagnostic features. Because of this, researchers in academia and industry have been developing 3D-breast imaging modalities, namely digital breast tomosynthesis (DBT) and dedicated breast CT (bCT). DBT is a form of limited-angle tomography where multiple projections are acquired as the x-ray tube follows a predefined trajectory covering an angular range of usually 50° or less. The projections are then reconstructed to obtain image slices through the breast. To date, there have been many prospective and retrospective clinical studies showing that use of DBT in general can increase cancer detection rates with similar or a decrease in false-positive rates.[4] There are currently four vendors that market FDA approved DBT devices.

Most clinical breast imaging systems use either direct-conversion or indirect-conversion, energy integrating detectors. As discussed in this chapter, use of photon-counting detectors in breast imaging systems offer a number of advantages over systems using energy integrating detectors. One company has developed both mammography and DBT systems using edge-on silicon photon-counting detectors in a multi-slit acquisition geometry[5–7]; however, to date there are no commercialization plans for the DBT system.

DBT is sometimes referred to as pseudo-3D because the limited-angle acquisition prohibits true 3D visualization of the breast. A number of studies investigating the imaging of the breast with conventional whole-body CT scanners were published in the 1980s and 1990s.[8–10] These studies used intravenously administered iodinated contrast agents and imaged patients in the prone position with foam blocks positioned to allow the breasts the hang freely. Although results were somewhat positive; a relatively large radiation dose to the chest was required, and subsequently bCT with whole-body CT systems has only been used for certain very limited cases. In the early 2000s, a number of researchers started to investigate CT of the breast using dedicated imagers employing energy integrating, indirect-conversion detectors and cone-beam acquisition geometries.[11] Currently, one company has received FDA approval to market their bCT device (Koning Inc, Rochester, NY). There are also a few prototype bCT systems using photon-counting detectors.[12,13] One of these prototypes uses a Cadmium-Telluride (CdTe) photon-counting detector with detector pixel size of 100 μm^2. There have been a handful of retrospective clinical trials performed comparing bCT to conventional mammography and breast MRI.[14,15] Some of these studies have indicated that dedicated bCT has potential for improving diagnostic accuracy; however, it's too early to make strong conclusions on the performance of bCT and additional clinical studies are needed.

In many cases, breast imaging with DBT or bCT can improve lesion detection and diagnosis over conventional mammography; however, performance is still limited for the dense breast. One approach that has been investigated for some time is the use of vascular contrast agents that can portray the tumor angiogenesis process to improve visualization and characterization of breast lesions. Iodinated contrast-enhanced imaging with either DBT or bCT has showed great potential for improving diagnostic accuracy. For example, Aminololama-Shaker et al.[16] analyzed 42 women with BI-RADS 4 and 5 category microcalcifications imaged with contrast-enhanced bCT. It was observed that visualization of one form of breast cancer, ductal carcinoma in situ (DCIS), with contrast bCT was similar to that of mammography, but greatly improved compared to un-enhanced bCT. One common approach for iodinated contrast-enhanced imaging with DBT or bCT is the temporal subtraction method, where images acquired from a precontrast scan are subtracted from those acquired postcontrast in an effort to eliminate background structure. However, a major limitation with the temporal subtraction method is that pre- and postcontrast scans can be difficult to align owing to patient motion. Furthermore, acquisition time and patient dose are higher using the temporal subtraction method. In Section 4.2.3 (Material Decomposition), the advantages of using photon-counting detector systems with iodinated contrast-enhanced imaging of the breast are discussed.

4.2 BENEFITS OF PHOTON-COUNTING DETECTORS VS. ENERGY INTEGRATING DETECTORS IN BREAST IMAGING SYSTEMS

4.2.1 Reduction of Electronic Noise

Most clinical breast imaging systems use energy integrating detectors for image acquisition. These types of detectors exhibit noise from three sources; quantum, electronic, and fixed pattern noise. Electronic noise, often referred to additive noise, arises from various sources in the analog electronics of the detector including amplifiers and gate and bias lines, and is generally uncorrelated with neighboring pixels. Since electronic noise is not dependent on the signal, it typically does not present a problem at higher x-ray fluence where quantum noise dominates. However, at lower x-ray fluence that might be used for low-dose imaging, it is possible that electronic noise can play a part in degrading image quality. Photon-counting detectors treat electronic noise as x-ray signals with energies located at the lower end of the spectrum. Therefore, in theory, it is possible to eliminate electronic noise altogether, although the lower energy threshold of the detector might be selected to allow some electronic noise to be measured.

As discussed in Chapter 10, one of the benefits of photon-counting detectors is the reduction of electronic detector noise. The impact of electronic detector noise in current clinical breast imaging systems (i.e., using energy integrating detectors) is unclear. Monnin et al.[17] have used a second-order fit of pixel variance to investigate the contribution of electronic noise in six clinical mammography systems. Figure 4.4 of their paper shows the fraction of pixel noise that can be attributed to electronic noise, as a function of photon fluence incident on the detector. From this data, it appears as if the electronic noise makes up approximately 10% of the total noise at typical photon fluences that are set by the automatic exposure control (AEC) software. Since DBT involves measurement of many projection images (up to 25), the photon fluence incident on the detector is typically much lower than with mammography. However, detectors designed for DBT systems use different readout schemes (varying gain) to minimize the influence of electronic noise. Zhao et al.[18] have empirically studied noise power spectra of an amorphous selenium detector designed for DBT, and suggested that this DBT system is essentially quantum noise limited.

Dedicated bCT systems place more challenges on minimizing electronic detector noise at low x-ray fluence. Typical bCT systems acquire 300 projection images, and although radiation dose is typically higher than a single full-field digital mammography (FFDM) or DBT acquisition, x-ray fluence on the detector behind the breast can be in the realm where the relative component of electronic noise is high. Yang et al.[19] investigated the fractional electronic noise using a prototype bCT with an energy integrating Varian 4030CB flat-panel imager. This detector was designed with two gain modes; low gain and dynamic gain. For a typical bCT scan acquired with the low-gain mode, electronic noise contributed 21% of the total pixel noise for a 10-cm diameter breast model and 44% for a 17-cm diameter breast model. For the scan acquired in dynamic-gain mode, electronic noise contributed 2.6% of the total pixel noise for a 10-cm breast, and 7.3% for a 17-cm breast. Although the dynamic gain mode effectively reduces the impact of electronic noise, it is somewhat challenging to use because the user has to spatially define where in the image the detector gain should be changed.

In summary, more research is needed to better understand how electronic noise affects image quality in breast imaging. Based on published reports, it appears as if the impact of electronic noise could be greater with bCT than for FFDM or DBT systems. Thus, bCT systems that use photon-counting detector technology might have advantages over conventional bCT systems when imaging at lower dose levels.

4.2.2 Energy Weighting

Since the number of secondary quanta produced from each x-ray absorbed in the detector is proportional to the absorbed x-ray energy, detectors operating in an energy integrating mode will inherently weigh detected photons proportional to their energy. This detector operating mode is suboptimal in breast imaging because tumor contrast is higher at lower energies (see Figure 4.1) where less inherent weighting is applied. This is not the case with photon-counting detectors; however, where all x-rays are weighted equivalently, regardless of their energy. Tapiovaara and Wagner[20] pointed out that if individual x-rays could be distinguished, then there exists an optimal energy weighting scheme that would give more weight to lower energy x-rays, thereby maximizing signal-to-noise ratio (SNR). Two approaches for energy weighting with photon counting bCT imaging systems

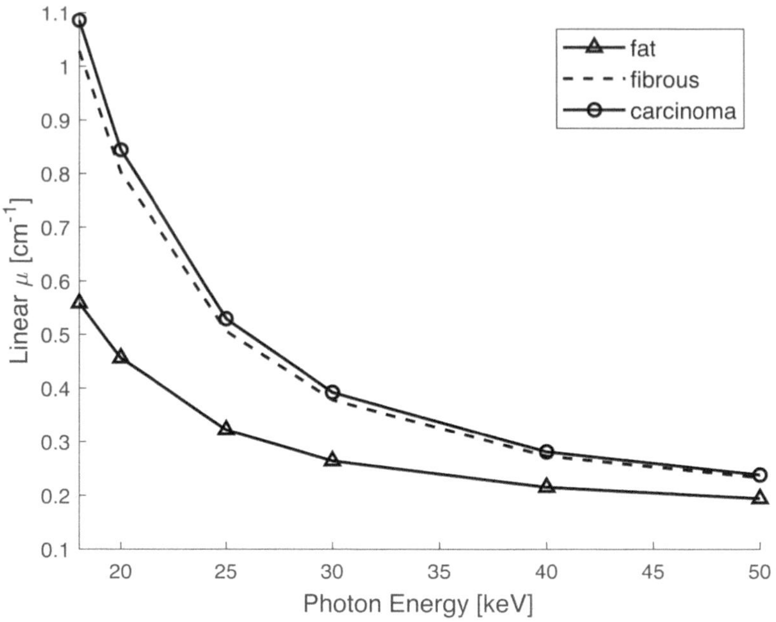

FIGURE 4.1 Linear attenuation coefficient as a function of photon energy for breast tissues: fat, fibrous, and breast carcinoma obtained from empirical measurements.[25]

have been explored; projection-based and image-based (see Figures 4.2 and 4.3). Shikhaliev[21] studied advantages of projection-based energy weighting using a laboratory benchtop spectral bCT system with a mulit-slit, multi-slice geometry and a CdTe photon-counting detector. Using phantoms, he reported that the contrast-to-noise ratio (CNR) for signals consisting of; carcinoma,

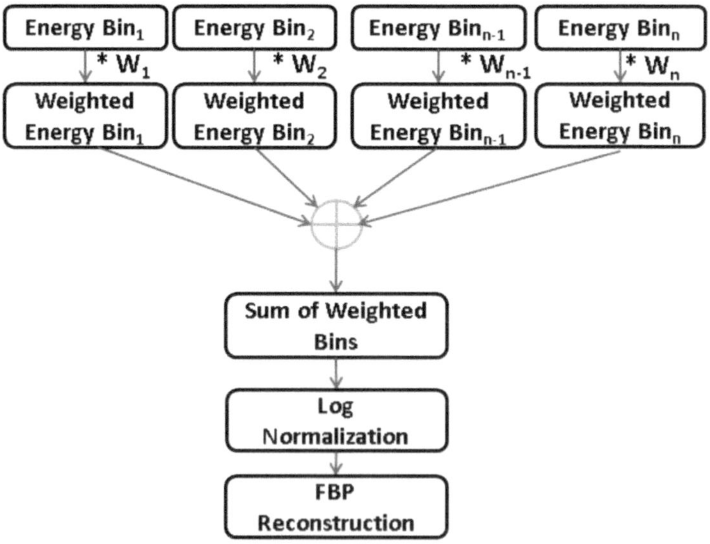

FIGURE 4.2 Flowchart describing the projection-based energy weighting technique. Reprinted from Kalluri K, Mahd M, Glick SJ. Investigation of energy weighting using an energy discriminating photon counting detector for breast CT. *Med Phys.* 2013;40:8, 081923, http://dx.doi.org/10.1118/1.4813901.

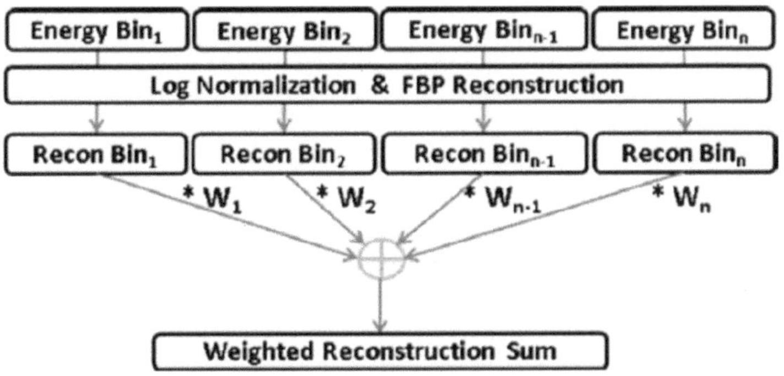

FIGURE 4.3 Flowchart describing the image-based energy weighting technique. Reprinted from Kalluri K, Mahd M, Glick SJ. Investigation of energy weighting using an energy discriminating photon counting detector for breast CT. *Med Phys*. 2013;40:8, 081923, http://dx.doi.org/10.1118/1.4813901.

blood, adipose tissue, iodine, and $CaCO_3$ increased by a factor of 1.16, 1.20, 1.21, 1.36, and 1.35 respectively over that measured with an energy integrating detector. One thing to note about this study is that 90 kV tube voltage was used, somewhat higher than what is typical for other bCT prototypes. Schmidt[22] studied an optimal image-based weighting method first proposed by Niederlohner et al.,[23] using computer simulations of bCT. They reported CNR improvement factors of 1.15, 1.50, and 1.31 for adipose tissue, $CaCO_3$, and an iodine lesion model respectively as compared to that obtained with energy integrating weighting. Although CNR improvements of image-based weighting were similar to that from projection-based weighting, image-based weighting was preferred because it minimized the cupping artifact due to beam-hardening that was observed with the projection-based weighting approach. Kalluri et al.[24] used a computer simulation study to investigate the performance improvement in energy weighting achieved with use of an energy discriminating photon-counting detector for bCT. They reported improvements in SNR of 1.31 and 1.17 for microcalcification and an iodine-enhanced mass respectively with projection weighting, and 1.41 and 1.15 for microcalcification and an iodine-enhanced mass respectively with image weighting. In addition, they performed a task-based assessment of microcalcification detection with bCT. This study showed a statistically significant difference between microcalcification detection using conventional bCT with an energy integrating detector (average area under (receiver operating characteristic, ROC) curve (AUC) of 0.732) and energy weighting with a photon-counting detector with three energy bins (AUC of 0.871). In summary, there appears to moderate improvements with use of energy weighting in bCT, although ultimately clinical studies are needed to investigate whether improvements observed with simulation and phantom studies would translate to that of clinical use.

4.2.3 Material Decomposition

One of the major benefits in imaging with energy discriminative detectors is the potential for quantitatively assessing the density of various materials in the object being imaged. Methods for material decomposition have been discussed extensively in other chapters of this book.

Chapters 5, 6, and 10 provide an in-depth discussion on material decomposition methods that become possible with use of photon-counting detectors. There are a number of potentially important clinical applications of material decomposition in breast imaging including estimation of the composition of adipose tissue, fibroglandular tissue, iodine contrast uptake, protein levels, water content, and chemical composition of microcalcifications.

Accurate estimation of adipose and fibroglandular tissue has become more important of late because of increasing awareness that women with dense breast tissue have increased risk for developing breast cancer.[26–28] Many states in the U.S. now require the reading radiologist to report the patient's estimated breast density. Currently, radiologists use the ACR BI-RADS® rating system to categorize patients into different density groups; however, agreement between radiologists using this approach has been shown to have high variability.[29,30] To reduce variability, several investigators have introduced software-based quantitative methods for estimating either area-based or volume-based breast density. Recently, it has been shown that spectral breast-imaging approaches using photon-counting detectors can provide unique advantages in estimating breast density.[31,32] At this point in time, there is one commercial system that uses edge-on geometry Si detectors that has demonstrated ability to estimate breast density using material decomposition methods.[31] Section 4.4.1 (Estimation of Breast Density) discusses a recent study to quantify volumetric breast density using material decomposition with a CdTe-based photon-counting detector.

For many years, breast imaging scientists have studied methods that use vascular contrast agents to image the tumor angiogenesis process, with the hope of improving characterization of lesions and their surrounding blood vessels. For instance, iodinated contrast-enhanced imaging of breast has been evaluated with various modalities including FFDM, DBT, and bCT.[33–35] One approach that has been discussed for iodinated contrast imaging is the temporal subtraction method, involving subtraction of two separate acquisitions, one before contrast administration, and one postcontrast. This method is challenging due to the problem of patient motion between the two scans, as well as increased acquisition times. Using both computer simulations and experimental phantom acquisitions, Ding et al.[36] have suggested that iodine mass thickness can be estimated using photon counting-based spectral mammography with only one scan, thereby eliminating many of the problems with the temporal subtraction method. Iodinated contrast-enhanced dedicated bCT has also been studied.[34] Current methods are particularly cumbersome because precontrast and postcontrast images of each breast typically need to be acquired.

Kalluri[37] demonstrated through computer simulations that photon counting based, iodinated contrast-enhanced bCT would have great potential for improving workflow compared to that with conventional systems using energy integrating detectors. In these studies, the linear attenuation coefficient within the breast was parameterized with three basis functions, $f_i(E)$, as a function of energy(E) representing adipose tissue, fibroglandular tissue, and a lesion with iodine uptake:

$$\mu(\vec{x},E)=\sum_{i}^{3} a_i\, f_i(E). \tag{4.1}$$

With these basis functions, the discrete-object, discrete data mean model can be represented as:

$$\lambda_k\,(A_i)=\int S_i(E)D(E)I_o(E)\exp\left(-\sum_{i=1}^{3} A_i\, f_i(E)\right)dE, \tag{4.2}$$

where:

$$A_i=\int a_i\, ds, \tag{4.3}$$

and $i = 1,2,3$ represents the three tissue types. The terms $S_i(E)$, $D(E)$, and $I_o(E)$ represent the energy bin sensitivity, the detector absorption efficiency, and the polychromatic x-ray photon fluence respectively.

Eq. (4.2) was then solved for the A_i's using a penalized maximum-likelihood (PML) algorithm with a gamma prior. Computer simulation was used to evaluate the material decomposition method. The simulation modeled an ideal cadmium zinc telluride (CZT) photon-counting detector based bCT system with three energy bins. An anthropomorphic breast phantom[38] based on CT reconstructions of fresh surgical mastectomy specimens was used with a single iodinated lesion inserted in random locations using the lesion model of de Sisternes et al.[39] After estimation of the A_i's for each material: adipose tissue, fibroglandular tissue, and iodine; cone-beam filtered backprojection was used to generate material images. Shown in Figure 4.4 are reconstructed images resulting from the simulation study. Reconstructed slices in the each row represent adipose tissue (1st row), fibroglandular tissue (2nd row), and iodine uptake (3rd row). Reconstructed slices in the 1st column represent the true phantom images of each material. Reconstructions in the 2nd column represent the material images using a maximum likelihood estimate of the A_i parameters, whereas reconstructions in the 3rd and 4th column represent material images with PML using different weightings on the gamma prior. This study clearly demonstrated the potential for estimating different tissue types using a photon counting based bCT system.

Another potential breast imaging application for material decomposition is determining the chemical composition of the lesion to differentiate between malignant from benign lesions. Previous reports using optical spectroscopy on excised lesions suggested that accuracy of lesion analysis

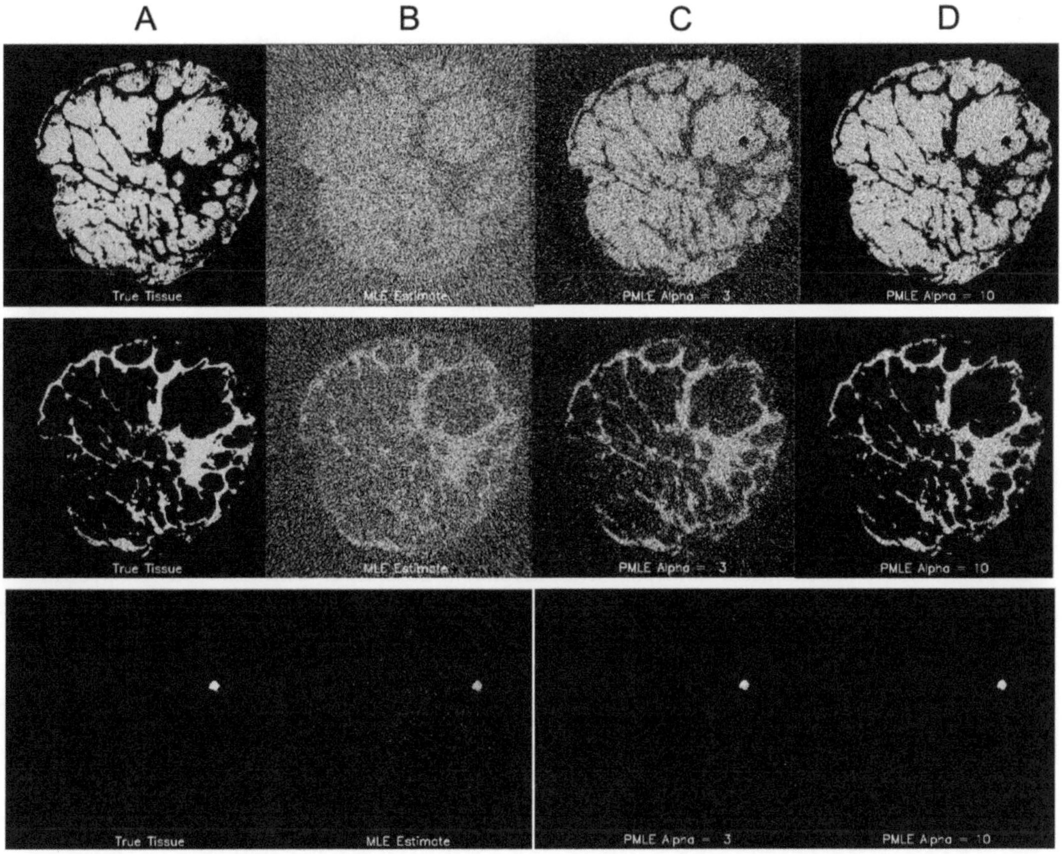

FIGURE 4.4 Example images from simulation study of material decomposition for iodinated contrast-enhanced breast CT with a CZT photon-counting detector. The true anthropomorphic breast phantom is shown in column (A) and consisted of three materials; (top) adipose tissue, (middle) fibroglandular tissue, and (bottom) iodine. Results from three reconstruction methods are shown; column (B) maximum-likelihood with no regularization, (C and D) penalized maximum-likelihood with different weighting on the gamma prior.

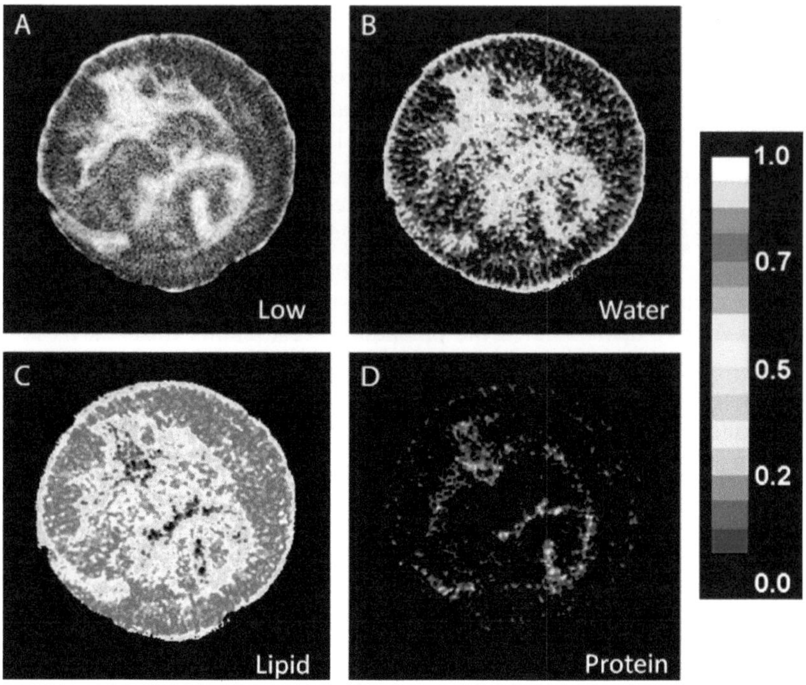

FIGURE 4.5 (A) CT reconstruction of a breast specimen, and reconstructed slices obtained with material decomposition representing, (B) the water image, (C) the lipid image, and (D) the protein image. Reprinted with permission from Ding H, Klopfer MJ, Ducote JL, Masaki F, Molloi S. Breast tissue characterization with photon-counting spectral CT imaging: A postmortem breast study. *Radiology*. 2014;272(3):731–738.

might be improved by quantitatively estimating the water, lipid, and protein contents of a lesion.[40] Ding et al.[41] imaged nineteen pairs of postmortem breasts with a CZT based photon counting bCT system, characterizing the feasibility of estimating water, lipid, and protein contents using a dual-energy material decomposition technique. Figure 4.5 shows the CT image (Figure 4.5A) of one postmortem breast specimen along with corresponding material decomposition images for water (Figure 4.5B), lipid (Figure 4.5C), and protein (Figure 4.5D). Results from this study indicated that composition of breast tissue in terms of water, lipid, and protein can be accurately characterized (in comparison with chemical analysis) at a reasonable dose level with CZT based spectral CT. Recently Drukker et al.[42] conducted a clinical study with 109 women analyzing water, lipid, and protein content BIRADS 4 and 5 lesions. This first of its kind clinical study concluded that three-material image analysis has the potential to reduce unnecessary biopsies.

Other efforts that use material decomposition to classify malignant and benign calcified lesions, as well as to discriminate solid masses and cysts are described in Section 4.4.2 (Classification of Microcalcifications).

4.3 DETECTOR DESIGN REQUIREMENTS FOR BREAST IMAGING SYSTEMS

4.3.1 Count-Rate Requirements

One challenge with the operation of semiconductor based photon-counting detectors used for x-ray imaging is their limited count-rate capabilities. Due to the varying arrival time intervals between incident x-rays and the limited detector pulse resolving time, detected x-rays can generate overlapping pulses that can be recorded as a single count with erroneous energy. This process is referred to as pulse pileup, and can result in degradation of image quality including loss of counts (dead time loss) and degradation of the recorded energy spectrum. In addition to pulse pileup, high count rates incident on semiconductor detectors can result in buildup of charge within the detector resulting in collapse or degradation of the applied electric field across the detector, a phenomena called polarization. It is possible to design photon-counting detectors such that the charges generated by an absorbed x-ray are removed at a sufficiently high rate to minimize count-rate limitations, although there are a number of design tradeoffs that must be considered. A recent review paper suggested that maximum count rates achievable with photon-counting detectors are in the range of $1–200 \times 10^6$ counts per s-mm^2.

For modern-day CT scanners, typical count rates for rays traversing through the center of the body are approximately on the order of $1. \times 10^8$ x-rays/s-mm^2, whereas the peak flux near the periphery of the body can reach $1. \times 10^9$ x-rays/s-mm^2. Thus, clinical CT detectors must be able to operate at high flux with little degradation in energy resolution or count-loss.

As discussed in detail in Chapters 16–18, one challenge with the operation of semiconductor-based photon-counting detectors used for x-ray imaging is their limited count-rate capabilities. Therefore, it is important to be able to estimate clinical count rates required for breast imaging modalities. A recent review paper suggested that maximum count rates achievable with state-of-the-art photon-counting detectors are approximately $2. \times 10^8$ photons per s-mm^2. One can estimate required count rates in mammography and bCT by using the following analysis.

From Nosratieh et al.[43] DgN dose coefficients (units of mGy/mGy) are available for contemporary mammography systems. Given a desired mean glandular dose (MGD), D provided to the breast of interest, and the DgN coefficient supplied from Ref. 43 the air kerma, K, incident on the breast can be computed as:

$$K = \frac{D}{DgN}. \tag{4.4}$$

To convert this air kerma to photon fluence, one can use Eq. 1.22b from Ref. 44 that provides an expression for the photon fluence per mGy air kerma:

$$\xi(E) = \beta\left[a + b\sqrt{E}\ln(E) + {c}/{E^2}\right]^{-1}, \tag{4.5}$$

where $\xi(E)$ is in units of photons/mm^2/mGy, $a = -5.0233 \times 10^{-6}$, $b = 1.8106 \times 10^{-7}$, $c = 0.0088$ ($r^2 = 0.9996$), and E is the unit of energy (keV). The constant β is equal to 114.3, and is a conversion factor from units of exposure to air kerma. Given the normalized x-ray spectra, $\hat{S}(E_i)$, defined at discrete energies $i = 0,1....N$ (with 0.5 or 1.0 keV intervals), the photon fluence incident on the breast, I_o, would be:

$$I_o = \sum_i^N \alpha\, \hat{S}(E_i), \tag{4.6}$$

where:

$$\alpha = \frac{K}{\sum_i \left({\hat{S}(E_i)}/{\xi(E_i)} \right)}. \tag{4.7}$$

Consider the imaging of a 5.0-cm thick, high-density breast with 25% fibroglandular composition. Suppose a W/Rh (filter/target) x-ray tube is used with 29 kV and HVL = 0.541 cm. From Ref. 43, the DgN (mGy/mGy) for these settings is 0.307. Thus from Eq. (4.4), the desired air kerma incident on the breast, K, would be 3.91 mGy to provide an MGD of 1.2 mGy. Using Eqs. (4.5–4.7) and the inverse-square law, the photon fluence incident on the detector, I_o can be computed as

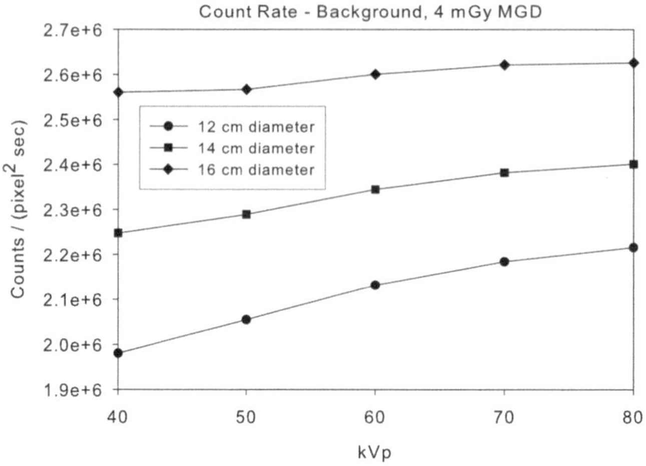

FIGURE 4.6 Estimated photon count-rate incident on the detector as a function of kVp setting for a breast CT scanner imaging three size cylindrical shaped breast models with 4 mGy MGD. The count rate here is in the background region of the projection image (where x-rays do not traverse through the breast). See text for more details.

approximately 17×10^6 photons/mm^2. Given that a typical digital mammography scan is 500 msec, the flux (per sec) would be approximately 3.4×10^7 photons/mm^2/sec. This flux should be feasible to measure with a high-performance photon-counting detector without significant degradation from pulse pileup or polarization effects.

Using a similar approach, typical count rates for dedicated bCT systems can also be determined. Figures 4.6 and 4.7 show calculated x-ray flux (counts per pixel per second) on the detector behind the middle of the breast (Figure 4.6), and in a background region where x-rays do not intersect the breast (Figure 4.7). X-ray flux is shown as a function of kVp for settings ranging from 40 to 80 kVp. These data were generated by modeling a bCT system with a tungsten anode spectra, Al x-ray filter of thickness 3 mm, 4 mGy MGD, a 200-μm detector pixel size and a source-to-detector distance of 86.1 cm. The breast was modeled as a cylinder with diameters of 12, 14, and 16 cm, and a 50/50

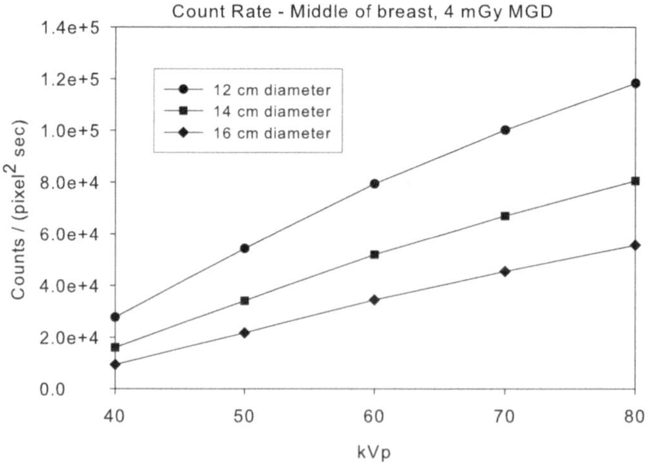

FIGURE 4.7 Estimated photon count-rate incident on the detector as a function of kVp setting for a breast CT scanner imaging three size cylindrical shaped breast models with 4 mGy MGD. The count rate here is in a region behind the middle of the breast (where x-rays traverse through the middle of the breast). See text for more details.

it typically requires two scans at two different time points, and the delay between scans can result in motion artifacts.

New advances in spectral mammography using energy discriminating photon counting-based detectors have opened up the possibility of accurately estimating volumetric breast density with only one mammography scan. Recent publications have suggested that one commercial system (Philips MicroDose SI) that uses Si-based photon-counting detectors can provide accurate estimates of breast density.[31]

Due to the low-quantum efficiency of Si, this system orients the Si detectors in an edge-on geometry, and requires the image acquisition by scanning a linear detector across the field-of-view. Although this approach is promising, challenges include a rather large x-ray tube loading and longer acquisition times that increase the possibility of artifacts due to breast motion.

Another, possibly more appealing idea would be the development of a flat-panel energy discriminating photon-counting detector that does not require a scanning acquisition geometry. Unlike Si, CdTe and CZT are two potentially useful materials with high-quantum efficiency that can be operated at room temperature. There are currently several nuclear medicine gamma cameras based on arrays of CdTe/CdZnTe detectors that have been developed, and there are also now several prototype CT scanners that are undergoing clinical testing. Unfortunately, at this time, there are no commercial spectral mammography systems that use these detector materials. To provide motivation in developing such a spectral mammography system, Ghammraoui et al.[32] have used a one-pixel CdTe spectral detector (Amptek XR-100T) to investigate CdTe based spectral mammography, and its ability to provide accurate estimates of volumetric breast density. In this laboratory study, a benchtop system was used to record a pencil-beam x-ray source through a 4-cm thick phantom consisting of breast-like tissue consisting of 50% adipose and 50% fibroglandular tissue (i.e., 2 cm of adipose tissue and 2 cm of fibroglandular tissue). X-rays were recorded into 2, 4, and 8 energy bins, and material decomposition was performed to estimate breast density. In Figure 4.10, there are scatter plots showing estimates of adipose and glandular thickness from 100 sample measurements at varying dose. X-rays were recorded into two energy bins after traversing through a 4-cm thick phantom with 50/50 glandular/adipose mass fraction (the true thickness of adipose and glandular phantom material was 2 cm each). It was observed that the thickness of each material could be accurately estimated with low bias and decreasing standard deviation with increasing dose. This study concluded that photon-counting spectral mammography systems using CdTe have great potential for accurately estimating volumetric breast density.

4.4.2 Classification of Microcalcifications

Although screening mammography has been very successful in reducing breast cancer mortality, there are still many false positives, resulting in unnecessary breast biopsies.[54] One type of malignant breast lesion, DCIS is usually diagnosed with the presence of microcalcifications. Studies have shown that there are two major types of microcalcifications; Type I consists of calcium oxalate dihydrate ($CaC_2O_4 - 2H_2O$, crystal name: weddellite), which are primarily found in benign ductal cysts, and Type II microcalcifications are composed of predominantly calcium phosphates ($Ca_5 (PO_4)_3(OH)$) mainly hydroxyapatite, mostly observed in proliferative cancerous lesions. Truong et al.[55] studied a series of breast biopsies and observed that if a calcified lesion contained only Type I calcifications, then it was highly likely to be benign. These Type I calcified lesions represented approximately 12% of benign breast biopsies studied. Therefore, any methods that can predict in vivo the chemical composition of a microcalcification might be able to be used to reduce unnecessary biopsies. Although Type I and Type II microcalcifications have different linear attenuation coefficients with respect to energy, it is difficult to differentiate the types based on x-ray attenuation

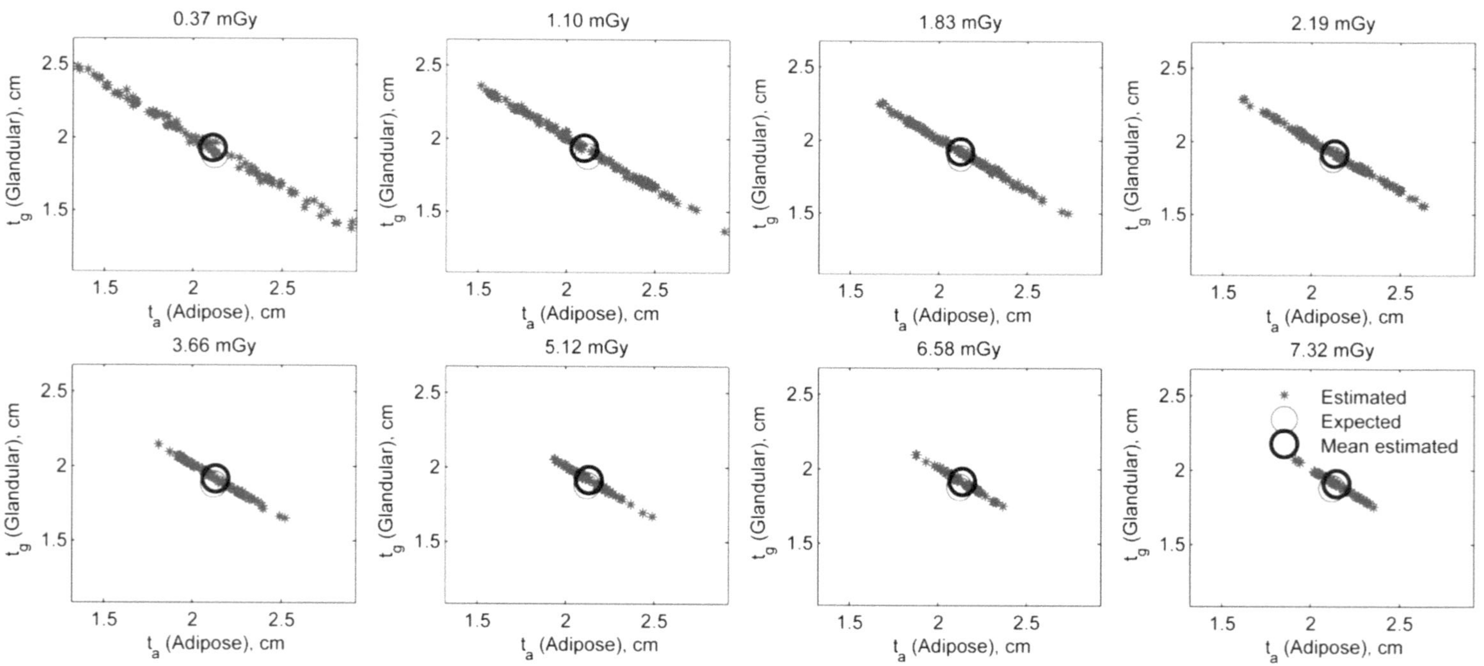

FIGURE 4.10 Scatter plots showing estimated thickness (estimates indicated by asterisk symbols) from 100 sample measurements using a one-pixel CdTe photon-counting detector with two energy bins. X-rays traveled through a 4-cm thick phantom with 50/50 fibroglandular/adipose mass fraction. Thin and thick circles represent the mean value of the estimates and the true mean value respectively. Reprinted from Ghammraoui B, Badal A, Glick SJ. Feasibility of estimating volumetric breast density from mammographic x-ray spectra using a cadmium telluride photon-counting detector. *Med Phys*. 2018;45:3604–3613. doi:10.1002/mp.13031. Copyright 2018 by the Copyright Clearance Center. Reprinted with permission.

alone. One possible approach for classifying calcification type is photon-counting spectral mammography using material-decomposition methods.

Ghammraoui et al.[56] have recently conducted computer simulation studies to investigate the feasibility of classifying microcalcifications with energy discriminating photon-counting detectors. More specifically, they investigated a dual-energy approach to differentiate between Type I calcifications consisting of calcium oxalate dihydrate that are more often associated with benign lesions, and Type II calcifications consisting of hydroxyapatite that are predominantly associated with malignant tumors. A realistic mammography x-ray spectrum was used to model attenuation through a compressed breast phantom consisting of 50% fibroglandular and 50% adipose tissue. Varying phantom thicknesses were studied, and calcifications of varying chemical composition and size were embedded into the phantom. Calcification sizes were randomly selected from a range of 200–600 μm with weight density of 2.1 g/cm^3 to model realistic breast calcifications. The simulation modeled an ideal detector, where each pixel measurement is independent (i.e., charge sharing and characteristic x-ray emission were not simulated). X-ray spectra were scaled to model different dose levels ranging from clinical dose levels to 25 mGy MGD. In addition, multiple noise realizations for each situation were studied to evaluate the precision of each measurement. The performance in differentiating Type I and Type II microcalcifications was assessed using ROC analysis. Results were reported for single microcalcifications, as well as for the average of ten microcalcifications. The latter being justified because most DCIS lesions exhibit clusters of microcalcifications, typically between 10 and 20. Shown in Figure 4.11 is the area under the ROC curve (AROC) indicating the performance in differentiating single calcification types, as well as for differentiating clusters of ten calcifications of each type. Also shown in Figure 4.11 are results when using different splitting energy values (i.e., dividing the low- and high-energy windows). It can be observed that differentiating between Type I and Type II single calcifications can be achieved with moderate accuracy. However, simultaneously analyzing ten calcifications within a cluster provided very high performance. In this case, the AROC was greater than 99% for radiation dose levels of greater than 4.8 mGy. These results are encouraging and suggest that a photon-counting detector based mammography system could provide a feasible solution to differentiating some malignant and benign calcified lesions in the breast.

4.4.3 Discrimination Between Solid Masses and Cysts

Another exciting clinical application for energy discriminating, photon counting-based breast imaging systems is the discrimination between solid masses and cysts, with the aim of reducing the recall rate. Currently in the U.S., the recall rate (i.e., proportion of women undergoing screening mammography that are asked to have additional imaging studies based on suspicious regions in the mammogram) is approximately 10% (the recall rate in Europe is considerably lower). Approximately 37% of recalls are based on visualization of benign mass lesions in the screening mammogram. A large proportion of these mass lesions (approximately 35%) are determined to be benign cysts based on follow-up ultrasound studies. Diagnosis of these benign cysts on screening mammography would reduce patient anxiety, lower healthcare costs, and ultimately result in more women adhering to recommended mammography screening protocols. Fredenberg et al.[57] published the first studies analyzing linear attenuation coefficients for breast cyst fluid and solid masses, which was integral for the development of methods to differentiate cyst from solid mass lesions. Following this study, the same group developed a multi-energy calibration method and an algorithm based on maximum likelihood for differentiating the two tissue types[58] using a Si-photon counting based spectral mammography system (Philips MicroDose SI). This algorithm was tested in a clinical pilot study on women undergoing two-view mammography as part of their standard diagnostic workup. Analysis was performed on 119 lesions, 62 of which were solid lesions, and 57 of which were cystic lesions.

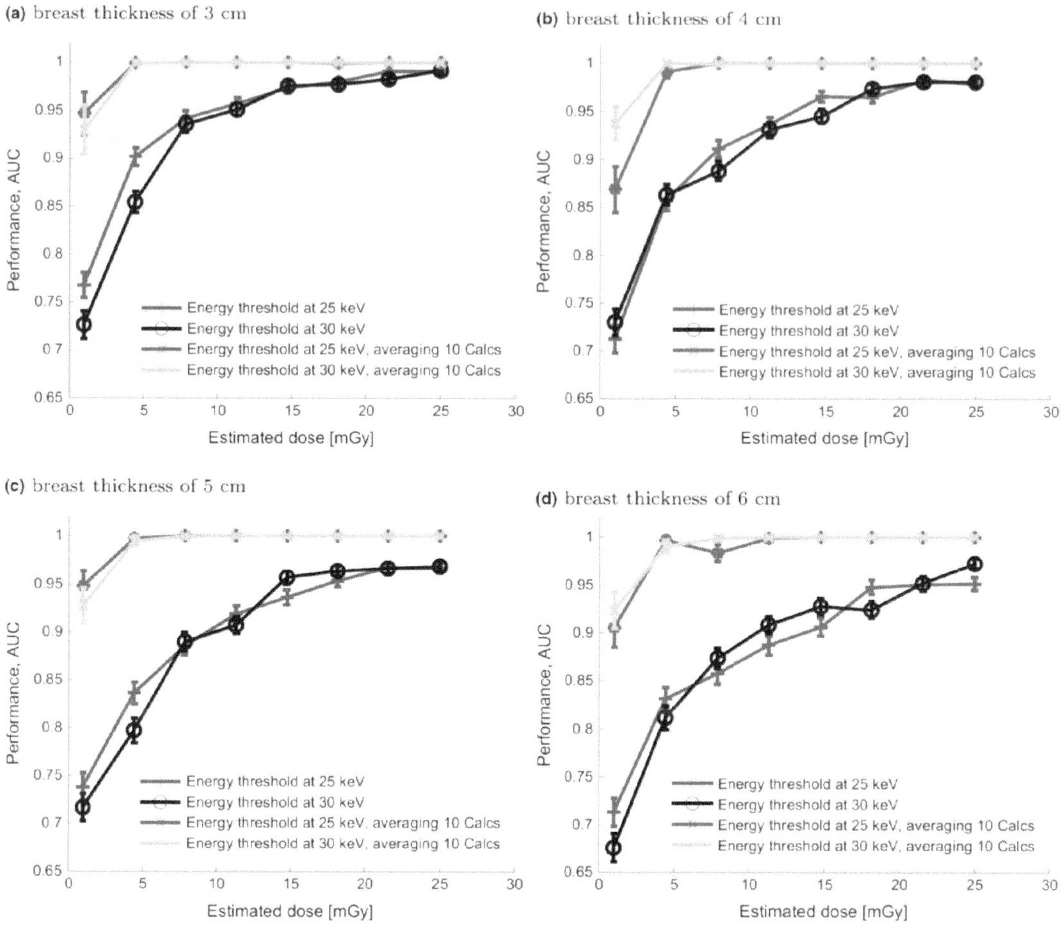

FIGURE 4.11 Area under the receiver operating curve (AROC) as a function of dose that portrays accuracy in classifying the two types of microcalcifications (weddellite vs. hydroxyapatite). Performance improves when averaging the estimated parameters over ten calcifications in a cluster. Shown are results with two different splitting energies. Reprinted from Ghammraoui B, Glick SJ. Investigating the feasibility of classifying breast microcalcifications using photon-counting spectral mammography: A simulation study. *Med Phys*. 2017;44:2304–2311. doi:10.1002/mp.12230. Copyright 2018 by the Copyright Clearance Center. Reprinted with permission.

Results suggested that spectral lesion characterization for reducing recalls of cystic lesions is feasible in a clinical setting for lesions with diameter of greater than 10 mm. The discrimination algorithm correctly classified 56% of cystic lesions greater than 10 mm at the 99% sensitivity level. Their analysis suggested that implementation of this approach in three UK breast imaging clinics would result in a 6% overall reduction in screening recalls. The authors suggested more studies are needed, including a multi-institutional trial to determine thresholds that would allow a safe classification of cystic lesions with spectral mammography.

DISCLOSURE AND ACKNOWLEDGMENTS

The authors have no relevant conflicts of interest to disclose. The mention of commercial products herein is not to be construed as either an actual or implied endorsement of such products by the Department of Health and Human Services.

The authors would like to acknowledge the contributions of Michael O'Connor Ph.D. and Kesava Kalluri Ph.D. to this chapter.

REFERENCES

1. Website. *American Cancer Society (2020): How Common is Breast Cancer?* https://www.cancer.org/cancer/breast-cancer/about/how-common-is-breast-cancer.html
2. Carney PA, Yankaskas C, Kerlikowske K, et al. Individual and combined effects of age, breast density, and hormone replacement therapy use on the accuracy of screening mammography. *Ann Intern Med.* 2003;138:168–175.
3. Carney PA, Parikh J, Sickles EA, et al. Diagnostic mammography: Identifying minimally acceptable interpretive performance criteria. *Radiology.* 2013;267(2):359–367.
4. Vedantham S, Karellas A, Vijayaraghavan GR, Kopans DB. Digital breast tomosynthesis: State of the art. *Radiology.* 2015;277(3):663–684.
5. Fredenberg E, Cederstrom B, Danielsson M. Energy filtering with x-ray lenses: Optimization for photon-counting mammography. *Radiat Prot Dosimetry.* 2010;139(1–3):339–342.
6. Fredenberg E, Lundqvist M, Aslund M, Hemmendorff M, Cederstrom B, Danielsson M. A photon-counting detector for dual-energy breast tomosynthesis. *Proc SPIE.* 2009;7258.
7. Berggren K, Cederstrom B, Lundqvist M, Fredenberg E. Characterization of photon-counting multislit breast tomosynthesis. *Med Phys.* 2018;45(2):549–560.
8. Nishino M, Hayakawa K, Yamamoto A, et al. Multiple enhancing lesions detected on dynamic helical computed tomography-mammography. *J Comput Assist Tomogr.* 2003;27(5):771–778.
9. Miyake K, Hayakawa K, Nishino M, et al. Benign or malignant?: Differentiating breast lesions with computed tomography attenuation values on dynamic computed tomography mammography. *J Comput Assist Tomogr.* 2005;29(6):772–779.
10. Yamamoto A, Fukushima H, Okamura R, Nakamura Y, Morimoto T. Dynamic helical CT mammography of breast cancer. *Radiat Med.* 2006;24:35–40.
11. Glick SJ. Breast CT. *Ann Rev Biomed Eng.* 2007;9:501–526.
12. Kalender WA, Kolditz D, Steiding C, et al. Technical feasibility proof for high-resolution low-dose photon-counting CT of the breast. *Eur Radiol.* 2017;27(3):1081–1086.
13. Cho H, Barber W, Ding H, Iwanczyk JS, Molloi S. Characteristic performance evaluation of a photon counting Si strip detector for low dose spectral breast CT imaging. *Med Phys.* 2014;41(9):091903.
14. Wienbeck S, Lotz J, Fischer U. Review of clinical studies and first clinical experiences with a commercially available cone-beam breast CT in Europe. *Clin Imag.* 2017;42:50–59.
15. O'Connell AM, Karellas A, Vedantham S. The potential role of dedicated 3D breast CT as a diagnostic tool: Review and early clinical examples. *The Breast J.* 2014;20(6):592–605.
16. Aminololama-Shakeri S, Abbey CK, Gazi P, et al. Differentiation of ductal carcinoma in-situ from benign micro-calcifications by dedicated breast computed tomography. *Eur J Radiol.* 2016;85(1):297–303.
17. Monnin P, Bosmans H, Verdun FR, Marshall NW. Comparison of the polynomial model against explicit measurements of noise components for different mammography systems. *Phys Med Biol.* 2014;59:5741–5761.
18. Zhao B, Zhao W. Imaging performance of an amorphous selenium digital mammography detector in a breast tomosynthesis system. *Med Phys.* 2008;35(5):1978–1987.
19. Yang K, Huang SY, Packard NJ, Boone JM. Noise variance analysis using a flat panel x-ray detector: A method for additive noise assessment with application to breast CT applications. *Med Phys.* 2010;37(7):3527–3537.
20. Tapiovaara M, Wagner, R. SNR and DQE analysis of broad spectrum x-ray imaging. *Phys Med Biol.* 1985;30(519).
21. Shikhaliev PM. Projection x-ray imaging with photon energy weighting: Experimental evaluation with a prototype detector. *Phys Med Biol.* 2009;54(16):4971–4992.
22. Schmidt TG. Optimal "image-based" weighting for energy-resolved CT [published online ahead of print 2009/08/14]. *Med Phys.* 2009;36(7):3018–3027.
23. Niederlohner D, Karg J, Giersch J, Anton G. The energy weighting technique: Measurements and simulations. *Nuc Instr Meth Phys Res A.* 2005;546:37–41.
24. Kalluri KS, Mahd M, Glick SJ. Investigation of energy weighting using an energy discriminating photon counting detector for breast CT. *Med Phys.* 2013;40(8):081923.
25. Johns PC, Yaffe MJ. X-ray characterisation of normal and neoplastic breast tissues. *Phys Med Biol.* 1987;32:675–695.
26. Boyd NF, Melnichouk O, Martin LJ, et al. Mammographic density, response to hormones, and breast cancer risk. *J Clin Oncol.* 2011;29(22):2985–2992.

27. Boyd NF, Martin LJ, Yaffe MJ, Minkin S. Mammographic density and breast cancer risk: Current understanding and future prospects. *Breast Cancer Res.* 2011;13(6):223.
28. Boyd NF, Martin LJ, Yaffe M, Minkin S. Mammographic density. *Breast Cancer Res.* 2009;11(Suppl 3):S4.
29. Redondo A, Comas M, Macia F, et al. Inter- and intraradiologist variability in the BI-RADS assessment and breast density categories for screening mammograms. *Br J Radiol.* 2012;85 (1019):1465–1470.
30. Ciatto S, Houssami N, Apruzzese A, et al. Categorizing breast mammographic density: Intra- and interobserver reproducibility of BI-RADS density categories. *Breast.* 2005;14(4):269–275.
31. Ding H, Molloi S. Quantification of breast density with spectral mammography based on a scanned multi-slit photon-counting detector: A feasibility study. *Phys Med Biol.* 2012;57(15):4719–4738.
32. Ghammraoui B, Badal A, Glick SJ. Feasibility of estimating volumetric breast density from mammographic x-ray spectra using a cadmium telluride photon-counting detector. *Med Phys.* 2018. doi: 10.1002/mp.13031.
33. Jong RA, Yaffe MJ, Skarpathiotakis M, et al. Contrast-enhanced digital mammography: Initial clinical experience. *Radiology.* 2003;228(3):842–850.
34. Prionas ND, Lindfors KK, Ray S, et al. Contrast-enhanced dedicated breast CT: Initial clinical experience. *Radiology.* 2010;256(3):714–723.
35. Chen SC, Carton AK, Albert M, Conant EF, Schnall MD, Maidment AD. Initial clinical experience with contrast-enhanced digital breast tomosynthesis. *Acad Radiol.* 2007;14(2):229–238.
36. Ding H, Molloi S. Quantitative contrast-enhanced spectral mammography based on photon-counting detectors: A feasibility study. *Med Phys.* 2017;44(8):3939–3951.
37. Kalluri KS. *Investigating improvements in breast CT using photon counting detectors* [PhD Thesis]. Lowell, MA: Department of Biomedical Engineering and Biotechnology, PhD Thesis, University of Massachusetts Lowell; 2013.
38. O'Connor JM, Das M, Didier C, Mahd M, Glick SJ. Generation of voxelized breast phantoms from surgical mastectomy specimens. *Med Phys.* 2013;40(4):041915.
39. de Sisternes L, Brankov JG, Zysk AM, Schmidt RA, Nishikawa RM, Wernick MN. A computational model to generate simulated three-dimensional breast masses. *Med Phys.* 2015;42(2):1098–1118.
40. Ding H, Ducote JL, Molloi S. Breast composition measurement with a cadmium-zinc-telluride based spectral computed tomography system. *Med Phys.* 2012;39(3):1289–1297.
41. Ding H, Klopfer MJ, Ducote JL, Masaki F, Molloi S. Breast tissue characterization with photon-counting spectral CT imaging: A postmortem breast study. *Radiology.* 2014;272(3):731–738.
42. Drukker K, Giger ML, Joe BN, et al. Combined benefit of quantitative three-compartment breast image analysis and mammography radiomics in the classification of breast masses in a clinical data set. *Radiology.* 2019;290(3):621–628. doi: 10.1148/radiol.2018180608:180608.
43. Nosratieh A, Hernandez A, Shen SZ, Yaffe MJ, Seibert JA, Boone JM. Mean glandular dose coefficients (D(g)N) for x-ray spectra used in contemporary breast imaging systems. *Phys Med Biol.* 2015;60(18):7179–7190.
44. Boone JM. X-ray production, interaction, and detection in diagnostic imaging. In: Beutel J, Kundel H, VAn Metter R, eds. *Handbook of Medical Imaging.* Bellingham, WA: SPIE; 2000.
45. Sempau J, Badal A, Brualla L. A PENELOPE-based system for the automated Monte Carlo simulation of clinacs and voxelized geometries-application to far-from-axis fields. *Med Phys.* 2011;38(11):5887–5895.
46. Glick SJ, Didier C. Investigating the effect of characteristic x-rays in cadmium zinc telluride detectors under breast computerized tomography operating conditions. *J Appl Phys.* 2013;114(14):144506.
47. Byng JW, Yaffe MJ, Jong RA, et al. Analysis of mammographic density and breast cancer risk from digitized mammograms. *Radiographics.* 1998;18(6):1587–1598.
48. Destounis S, Johnston L, Highnam R, Arieno A, Morgan R, Chan A. Using volumetric breast density to quantify the potential masking risk of mammographic density. *AJR Am J Roentgenol.* 2017;208(1):222–227.
49. Jeffreys M, Warren R, Highnam R, Smith GD. Initial experiences of using an automated volumetric measure of breast density: The standard mammogram form. *Br J Radiol.* 2006;79(941):378–382.
50. Marias K, Behrenbruch C, Highnam R, Parbhoo S, Seifalian A, Brady M. A mammographic image analysis method to detect and measure changes in breast density. *Eur J Radiol.* 2004;52(3):276–282.
51. Heine JJ, Carston MJ, Scott CG, et al. An automated approach for estimation of breast density. *Cancer Epidemiol Biomarkers Prev.* 2008;17(11):3090–3097.

52. Ducote JL, Molloi S. Quantification of breast density with dual energy mammography: A simulation study. *Med Phys.* 2008;35(12):5411–5418.
53. Ducote JL, Molloi S. Quantification of breast density with dual energy mammography: An experimental feasibility study. *Med Phys.* 2010;37(2):793–801.
54. Byers T, Wender R, Jemal A, Baskies A, Ward E, Brawley O. The American Cancer Society challenge goal to reduce US cancer mortality by 50% between 1990 and 2015: Results and reflections. *CA: A Cancer Journal for Clinicians.* 2016. *doi:103322/caac21348.*
55. Truong LD, Cartwright J, Jr., Alpert L. Calcium oxalate in breast lesions biopsied for calcification detected in screening mammography: Incidence and clinical significance. *Mod Pathol.* 1992;5(2):146–152.
56. Ghammraoui B, Glick SJ. Investigating the feasibility of classifying breast microcalcifications using photon-counting spectral mammography: A simulation study. *Med Phys.* 2017;44(6):2304–2311.
57. Fredenberg E, Dance DR, Willsher P, et al. Measurement of breast-tissue x-ray attenuation by spectral mammography: First results on cyst fluid. *Phys Med Biol.* 2013;58(24):8609–8620.
58. Erhard K, Kilburn-Toppin F, Willsher P, et al. Characterization of cystic lesions by spectral mammography: Results of a clinical pilot study. *Invest Radiol.* 2016;51(5):340–347.

5 Clinical Applications of Photon-Counting Detector Computed Tomography

Shuai Leng, Shengzhen Tao, Kishore Rajendran, and Cynthia H. McCollough
Department of Radiology, Mayo Clinic, Rochester, Minnesota, USA

CONTENTS

5.1 INTRODUCTION

X-ray detector is a major component of a clinical computed tomography (CT) system and has substantial impact on image quality as well as patient radiation dose, which consequently affects a wide range of clinical applications. Compared to the conventional scintillator-based CT detectors using an indirect conversion technology and integrating energy deposited by all received x-ray photons, photon-counting detectors (PCDs) possess many inherent advantages, which can be largely attributed to its direct conversion technology and energy discrimination capability. Although PCD technology has been widely utilized in nuclear medicine, its adoption in x-ray CT system has long been hampered due to the high-photon flux encountered in clinical CT imaging (1–6). However, various potential clinical benefits provided by the PCD technology have continued to motivate extensive research efforts in the past decade to bring PCDs into clinical CT practice, especially with the development of higher atomic number semiconductor materials and ultrafast application-specific integrated circuits (ASICs). In addition to several bench-top PCD-CT systems built for small animal imaging (7–17), systems that are capable of handling the high-photon flux encountered in clinical CT examinations have also been developed (18–22). Such systems provide researchers valuable opportunities to explore the potential of translating this technology into clinical practice. Using these systems, various studies involving phantoms, animals, and human subjects have demonstrated benefits of PCD-CT and its substantial impact on clinical practice (23).

In this chapter, we will discuss the potential clinical benefits of PCD-CT that have been demonstrated in a series of recent studies. These include increased iodine contrast-to-noise ratio (CNR) and dose efficiency, reduced electronic noise, reduced beam-hardening and metal artifacts, dose-efficient high-spatial resolution imaging, and simultaneous multi-energy data acquisition that enables differentiation and quantification of contrast agents and tissue types from a single scan. We will then discuss how these benefits can impact CT applications in each clinical area, such as neuro, chest, vascular, and musculoskeletal (MSK) imaging.

5.2 PCD-CT DATA SETS

We first introduce some concepts that are frequently used throughout this chapter. Typically, there are two types of data sets available for a PCD acquisition, that is, the energy threshold data and energy bin data, as shown in Figure 5.1. The energy threshold data represent the number of photons with energy higher than a user-defined energy threshold, up to the maximum photon energy determined by the x-ray tube potential. The energy bin data represent the number of photons between two nearby energy thresholds, which are obtained by subtracting the photon counts of two energy thresholds. For example, a PCD-CT scan performed at 140 kV with energy thresholds of 25 and 65 keV can generate two energy-threshold data sets, with photon energy ranges of [25, 140] keV and [65, 140] keV, respectively. Two energy bin data sets are then generated from the subtraction of the two threshold data, [25, 65] keV and [65, 140] keV. In this chapter, we refer to the lower-energy threshold data set (i.e., the [25 140] keV data set in this example) as the threshold-low (TL) data, and refer to the higher energy threshold data set (i.e., [65 140] keV data set) as the threshold-high

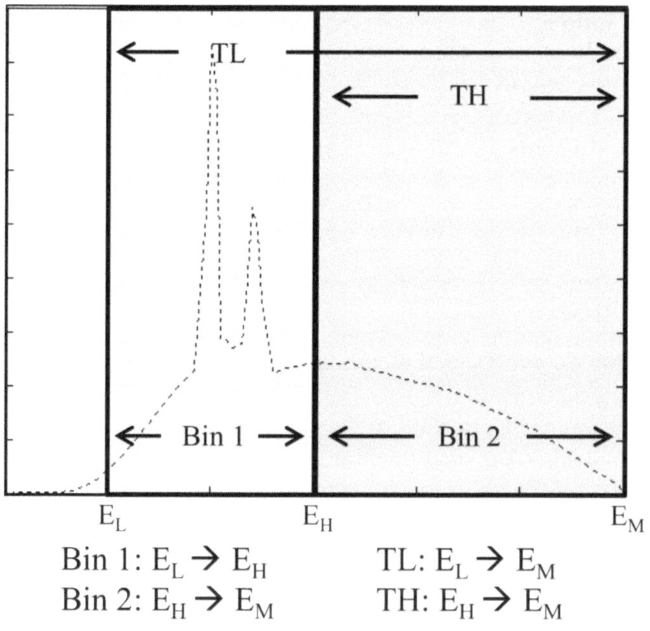

FIGURE 5.1 Photon-counting detector (PCD) data sets acquired with x-ray tube potential E_M and two energy thresholds (E_L and E_H). A total of four data sets can be generated: the two threshold data sets (TL and TH) correspond to photons with energies higher than the respective thresholds (E_L, E_H) but lower than the tube potential (E_M); the two bin data sets (Bin 1 and Bin 2) correspond to photons with energies between the two energy thresholds (Bin 1, E_L to E_H) or between the high energy threshold and the tube potential (Bin 2, E_H to E_M). Note that TH and Bin 2 data are identical. E_M = energy maximum; E_L = energy low; E_H = energy high; TL = threshold low; TH= threshold high. (Image reproduced from Yu et al. (26)).

(TH) data. The images reconstructed from these data sets are therefore referred as TL and TH images, respectively. The two energy bin data sets are referred as Bin 1 (i.e., [25, 65] keV) and Bin 2 (i.e., [65, 140] keV). Note that TH and Bin 2 are identical data sets.

5.3 PART I: BENEFITS OF PCD-CT

5.3.1 Reduced Electronic Noise

Image noise in CT mainly originates from two sources: quantum noise and electronic noise. The quantum noise, which is determined by the number of detected photons, can be traced back to the stochastic nature of x-ray photon interactions. On the other hand, the electronic noise mainly comes from the analog electronic circuits within the x-ray detection system and is therefore independent of the number of photons reaching detector. Generally speaking, the relative significance of quantum noise and electronic noise is determined by the incident photon flux or count rate. Mathematically, the number of detected photons can be treated as a random number with a Poisson distribution. Statistically, signal magnitude is proportional to photon count, N, while the standard deviation is proportional to $\sqrt{N}$, resulting a proportionally increased signal-to-noise ratio by a factor of $\sqrt{N}$. In the realm of high-photon flux, the number of photon reaching x-ray detector is relatively high. Therefore, the quantum noise dominates the total noise magnitude, and the effect of electronic noise is negligible. On the other hand, when there are fewer photons reaching detector, the magnitude of the electronic noise can be of similar order as, or, and in some cases, higher than the quantum noise. In modern energy integrating detector (EID)-based clinical CT systems, the electronic noise is usually negligible for majority of the imaging tasks. However, the effect of electronic noise can be observable for low-dose scans or morbidly obese patients where the number of detected photons is low (24, 25). In this case, the electronic noise can degrade image quality by causing streaking artifacts, particularly along highly-attenuating paths. Figure 5.2a shows the shoulder portion of an anthropomorphic thorax phantom scanned on the clinical EID-based CT system using a low-dose lung cancer screening protocol (26). Although the image is acquired using a very low-electronic noise EID detector, considerable streaking artifacts can still be observed between the shoulders of the phantom due to the electronic noise. These artifacts are further aggravated with gradually lowered radiation dose.

Different from the quantum noise that is determined by photon statistics, electronic noise is usually detected as a low-amplitude fluctuating signal. With PCD, the electronic noise can be interpreted as a photon with energy located at the lower-end of a typical x-ray spectrum. Consequently, by setting the low-energy threshold to be just above the energy associated with the amplitude of electronic noise signal (e.g., 25 keV), electronic noise can be readily excluded from the measured

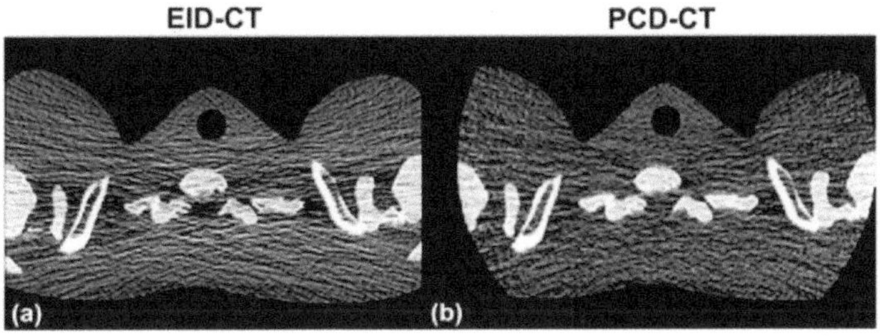

FIGURE 5.2 Images of the shoulder section of an anthropomorphic thorax phantom scanned on a clinical energy-integrating-detector (EID)-CT (a) and on a photon-counting-detector (PCD)-CT (b) using the same x-ray tube potential and radiation dose. Compared to the image acquired on an EID-CT, the PCD-CT image has noticeably less horizontal streaking artifacts and an overall more uniform appearance, which indicates that electronic noise has a more noticeable impact on the EID image than on the PCD image. (Image reproduced from Yu et al. (26)).

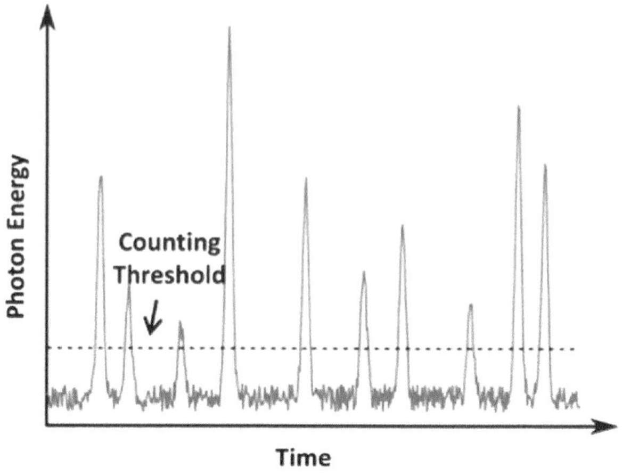

FIGURE 5.3 Illustration showing signals of individual x-ray photons detected using PCD with additive electronic noise. The PCD is able to discriminate the energy of each incident x-ray photon. Since the electronic noise is usually detected as a low-amplitude signal, it can be readily excluded from the measured counting data by setting a proper counting energy threshold to be just above the energy associated with the electronic noise amplitude. (Image reproduced from Leng et al. (23)).

count data. This principle is illustrated in Figure 5.3, which shows the low-amplitude electronic noise added on top of the detected x-ray photon signals represented as spikes of various amplitudes. Since a photon with an energy level lower than this threshold is very unlikely to be caused by a primary photon transmitted through the imaging object of interest, an energy threshold setting above this threshold will exclude electronic noise. Electronic noise, however, can have some impact on the detected energy spectrum as its signal amplitude is added to that of a detected photon, which artificially increases the energy of the detected photon.

Figure 5.2a and 2b compares the images of the same anthropomorphic phantom scanned on the clinical EID-CT and a research whole-body PCD-CT system using a low-dose lung cancer screening protocol with matched radiation dose (26). As shown, the images acquired on the PCD-CT features improved image uniformity and reduced streaking artifacts compared to the EID-CT. The advantage of PCD-CT in reduced electronic noise can be used to reduce overall image noise and improve image diagnostic quality in low-dose scanning. The results of a recent phantom study has shown that, for low-dose lung cancer screening, PCD-CT was able to provide better CT number stability and scan reproducibility, as well as reduced image noise, compared to an EID-CT (21). Alternatively, the reduced electronic noise can be used to improve radiation dose efficiency, as a lower-radiation dose can be used on a PCD to reach the same noise level as achieved with an EID-CT system using a higher-radiation dose level.

5.3.2 Improved Iodine CNR and Dose Efficiency

In the diagnostic x-ray energy range, the x-ray photons primarily interact with scanned objects through two physical mechanisms: the photoelectric effect and Compton scattering. Theoretically, the attenuation due to photoelectric effect increases with the effective atomic number (i.e., Z) of a material and decreases with the energy of incident x-ray photon E (i.e., $\mu_{PE} \propto Z^3/E^3$). On the other hand, the energy dependence of Compton effect is relatively flat within diagnostic energy range. Consequently, photoelectric effect contributes more to the attenuation of low-energy photons, while Compton scattering is the dominant effect accounting for high-energy photons. As a result, high-Z materials, such as iodine, have higher photon attenuation in the low-energy range due to the photoelectric effect, and therefore demonstrate higher signal or contrast in CT images.

Recall that for a conventional EID-CT system, the detector signal is proportional to the total energy of all detected x-ray photons. Due to the energy integrating nature of EID, lower-energy photons contribute less to the detector signal than the higher-energy photons. However, higher-energy photons have less information content from high-Z materials such as iodine, as the improved contrast of iodine is mainly explained by photoelectric interaction that manifests its effect in the low-energy range. Consequently, the underweighting of signal produced by lower-energy photons reduces the CNR of iodine signal in a CT system using EID. On the other hand, PCD counts each individual photon equally regardless of the photon energy, without the energy weighting in EID. Hence, the low-energy photons have a greater contribution to the image contrast for PCD-CT compared to EID-CT, which improves the iodine contrast and CNR (1–5, 27–35).

A recent study (18) has investigated the iodine contrast using anthropomorphic phantoms of different sizes to emulate newborn to large adult patients. The same phantoms were scanned on a clinical EID-CT system and a research whole-body PCD-CT system using different tube potentials of 80, 100, 120, and 140 kV with matching tube current-time product ranging from 50 to 550 mAs. Figure 5.4 shows the iodine CNR measured from images acquired with different

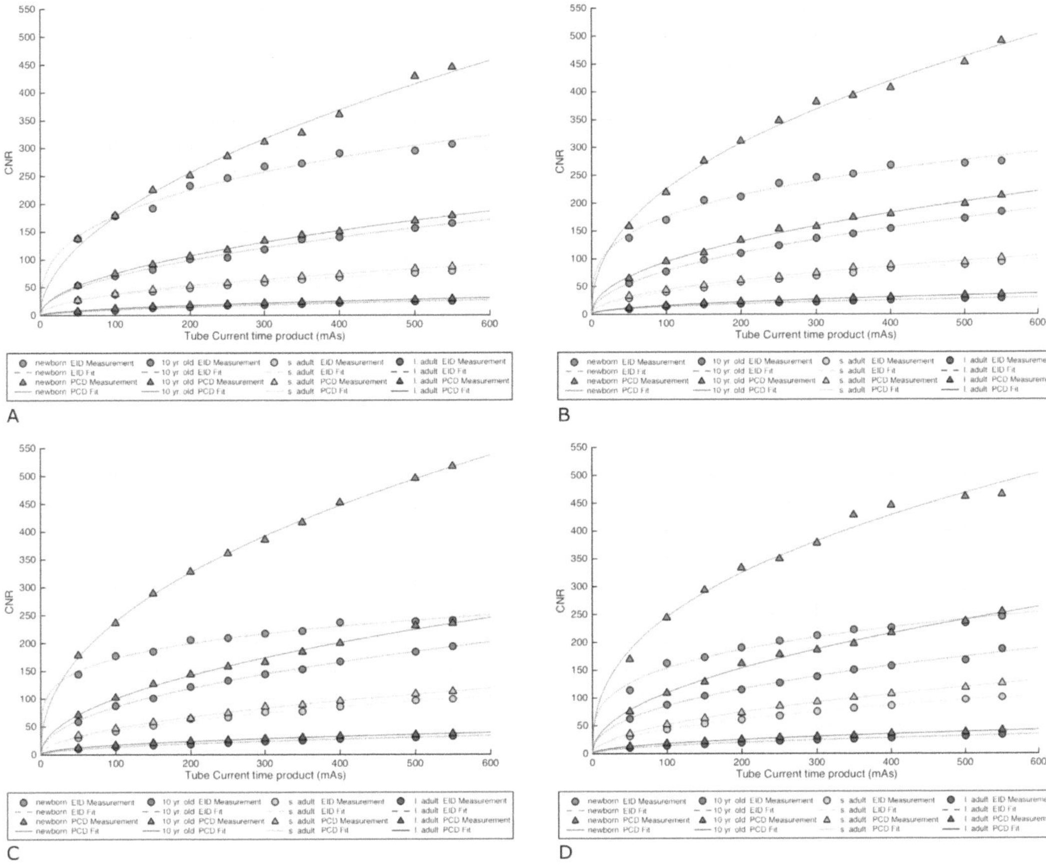

FIGURE 5.4 Comparison of CNR versus tube current-time product (mAs) for four anthropomorphic abdominal phantom sizes (new born, 10 year old, small adult, and large adult) between the EID images and the low-energy threshold (TL) images from the PCD acquired using a tube potential of 80 kV (A), 100 kV (B), 120 kV (C), and 140 kV (D). The iodine CNR in the PCD (TL) images was consistently greater than the iodine CNR in the EID images; s. adult indicates small adult; l. adult indicates large adult. (Images reproduced from Gutjahr et al. (18)).

tube potentials comparing EID versus PCD-CT. As shown, the PCD-CT demonstrated improved CNR than EID-CT for different patient sizes ranging from small to large subject habitus. This improvement was independent of radiation dose or tube current-time product. The improved iodine CNR is more pronounced for higher tube potentials, such as 120 or 140 kV. Note that the higher tube potentials are especially relevant when imaging moderately-sized to large patients.

In addition to the native uniform count weighting, other weighting schemes can also be used for the PCD data due to its energy discrimination capability. The CNR for a given material can be further increased by designing an optimal weighting scheme for the different narrow energy-bin data sets available from a single PCD scan (36, 37). Such schemes typically weight each energy-bin data set according to their contrast level and noise variance. The weighted energy-bin images are then combined to yield a final image with improved CNR. In general, the amount of CNR improvement depends on the object size and material, the x-ray tube potential, the PCD energy-threshold settings, and the energy response of the PCD (37).

For a given radiation dose level, the higher iodine contrast on a PCD-CT system will result in improved iodine CNR and therefore better image quality. Alternatively, if the same iodine CNR is desired, the PCD-CT system acquisition can be altered to either reduce radiation dose or reduce the volume of injected iodine contrast agent, hence reducing the risk of hypersensitivity reaction for sensitive patient population.

5.3.3 Beam Hardening/Metal Artifact Reduction

As photons pass through the scanned object, low-energy photons are preferentially attenuated compared to high-energy photons. Since poly-energetic beams are used in CT, this causes the effective photon energy to be shifted toward the higher end of the spectrum, a phenomenon known as beam hardening. This introduces artifacts, which are typically dark areas adjacent to highly attenuating objects such as cortical bone, affecting the image appearance and CT number accuracy for nearby soft tissues. In the presence of foreign object such as metal implants, severe image streaking artifacts together with dark/bright regions can be observed across the image (38, 39). These metal artifacts have a characteristic appearance, and are caused by multiple physical mechanisms, including x-ray scattering, photon starvation, as well as beam hardening effect. The severity of metal artifacts can vary according to the atomic number, density, and shape of the metal, as well as the surrounding anatomy and scan acquisition/reconstruction parameters. In many cases, the resulting metal artifacts can dramatically obscure critical structures, and result in a significant reduction in diagnostic confidence in various clinical tasks, such as distinguishing pathologic findings from normal structures.

Since each individual photon is sorted according to its energy in a PCD-CT acquisition, an energy-bin image can be reconstructed using only higher-energy photons. Compared to the conventional EID-CT image or the low-energy threshold image in a PCD acquisition, the high-energy bin image is more immune to beam hardening effect in areas around dense bones. Figure 5.5 shows the images of a cadaver head acquired on a clinical EID-CT system (a, d), together with the low-energy bin and high-energy bin images acquired on a research whole-body PCD-CT system (18). The high-energy image acquired on the PCD-CT (Figure 5.5c) shows clearer and sharper interface between skull and brain compared with the EID images (Figure 5.5a) and the low-energy bin PCD image (Figure 5.5b) due to less beam hardening effect and reduced calcium blooming from skull. The high-energy bin image around posterior fossa acquired on PCD-CT (Figure 5.5f) also showed considerably less beam hardening induced streaking between left and right petrous portion of temporal bones compared to the EID image (Figure 5.5d) and low-energy bin PCD images (Figure 5.5e). In this example, only water beam-hardening corrections were applied to the images as part of the normal image reconstruction, while the second-order bone beam-hardening corrections were not applied, in order to demonstrate that beam-hardening artifacts that normally require algorithmic correction were not present in the uncorrected high-energy bin PCD image.

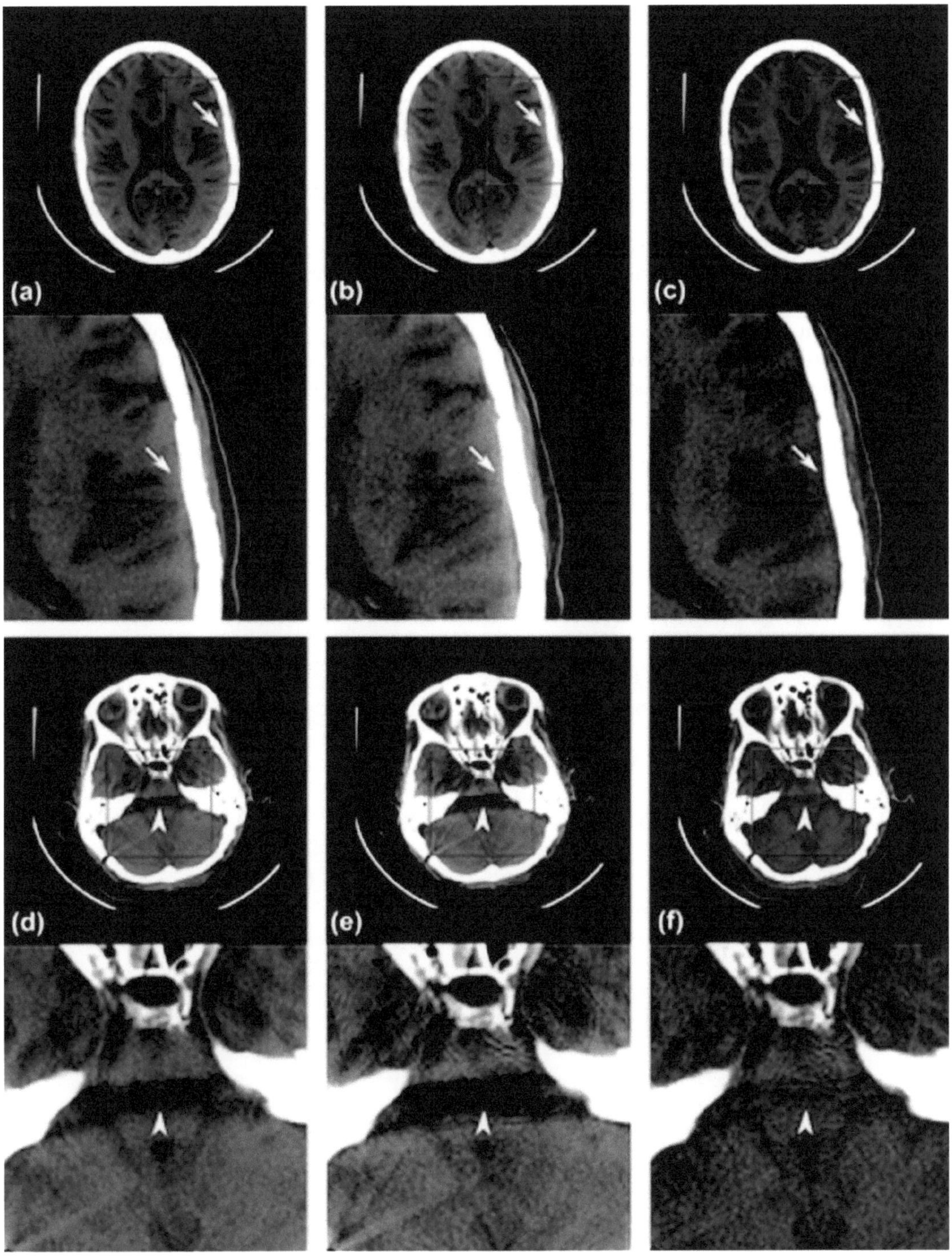

FIGURE 5.5 Images of a cadaver head scanned with a clinical energy-integrating-detector (EID)-CT (a, d) and a research whole-body photon-counting-detector (PCD)-CT (b, c, e, f) system. The high-energy threshold images from the PCD-CT (c, f) have less blooming artifacts (arrows) and beam-hardening artifacts (arrow heads) than the EID-CT images and low-energy threshold PCD-CT images (b, e). (Images reproduced from Gutjahr et al. (18)).

However, the use of high-energy bin signal to reduce beam hardening effect is at the cost of increased image noise and reduced dose efficiency, since the lower-energy photons are not used in the generation of high-energy bin image. This can be especially problematic for imaging with the presence of metal implant, as the dense metal can typically cause photon starvation and introduce severe streaking artifacts. To improve dose efficiency, the incident x-ray beam can be further hardened using additional filtration such as a tin filter, which increases the relative percentage of photons in the high-energy bin. The combination of using the high-energy bin image and tin filtration can further reduce metal artifacts, as well as image noise, thus providing improved delineation for tissue regions that would otherwise be affected by prominent metal artifact (40). Figure 5.6 shows the images of a 3D-printed vertebrae containing metallic pedicle screws acquired on a research whole-body PCD-CT system without (Figure 5.6A, B) and with (Figure 5.6C, D) the additional 0.4 mm tin beam filtration. Compared to the TL images that use the full energy spectrum (Figure 5.6A), the TH image (Figure 5.6B) shows reduced metal artifacts. The combination of additional beam filtration and TH image can further reduce image artifact, while keeping the image noise level close to that of the TL images before adding the beam filtration.

Figure 5.7 shows an example of patient images acquired on a clinical EID-CT system with 120 kV tube potential, compared with the TH image acquired on the PCD-CT system with 140 kV tube potential and added tin filtration (Sn140) (40). The patient had posterior rod and screw fixation of L2-L5 and a posterolateral bone graft. As shown in Figure 5.7C, D, the TH Sn140 kV PCD-CT images have

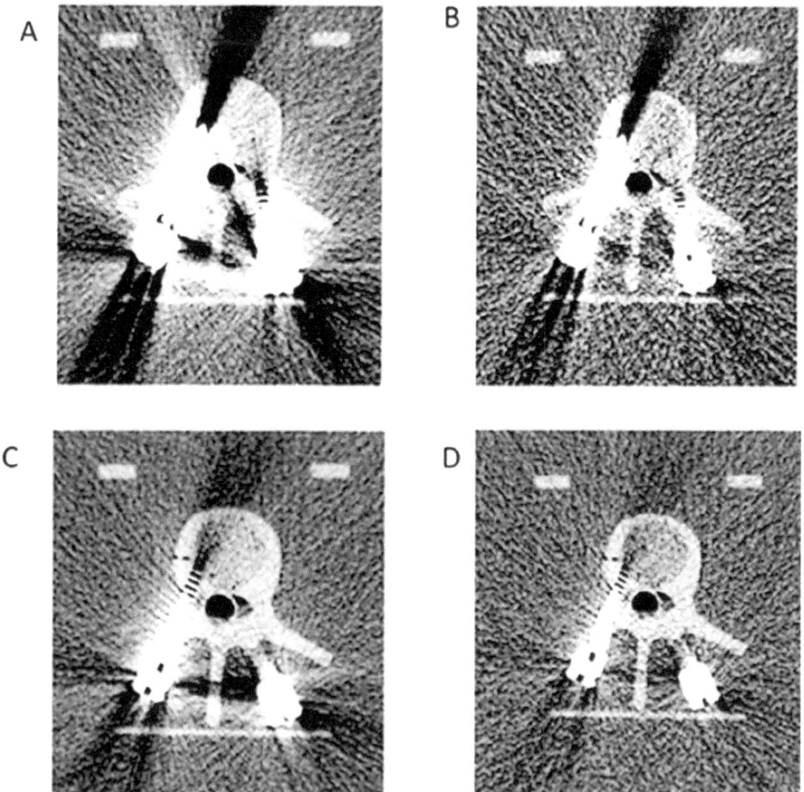

FIGURE 5.6 Images of a 3D-printed vertebrae containing metallic pedicle screws acquired without (A, B) and with (C, D) a 0.4 mm tin filter. (A, C): TL images acquired using the full energy spectrum. (B, D): TH images acquired using only higher-energy photons. W/L = 400/40 HU. (Images reproduced from Zhou et al. (40)).

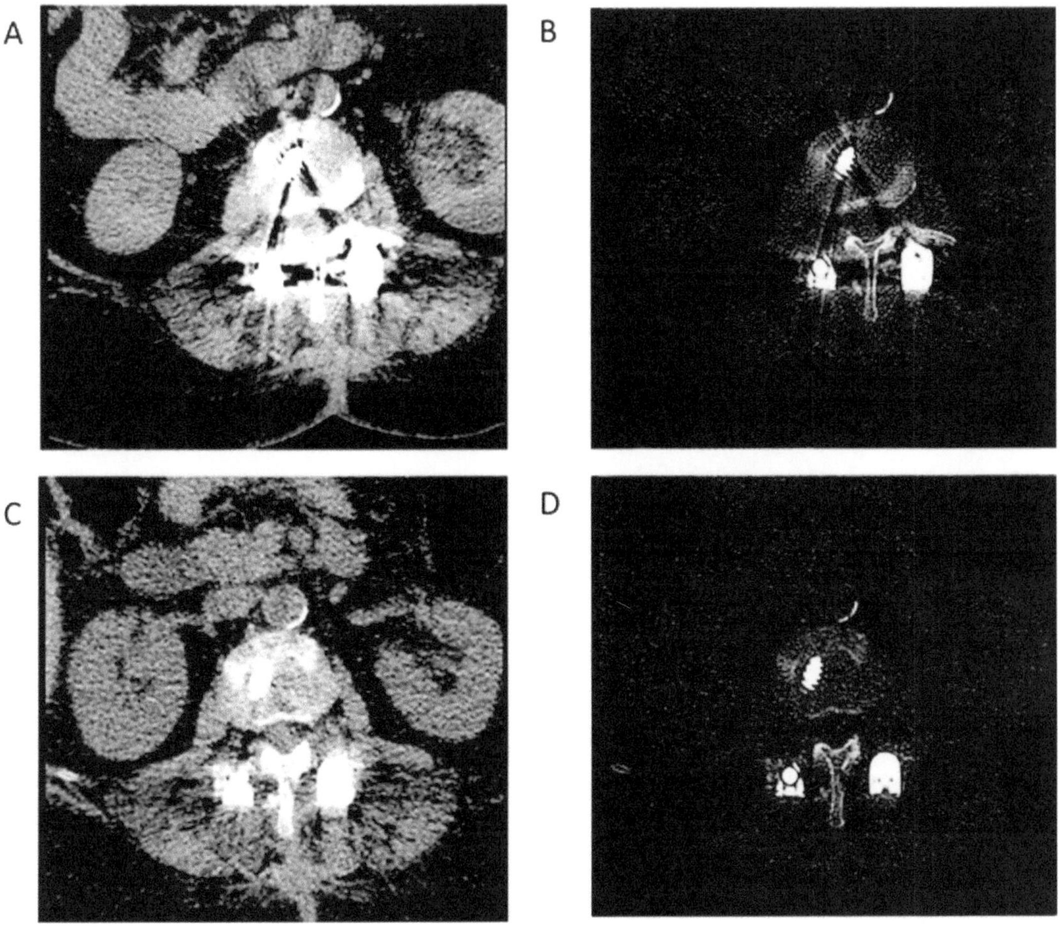

FIGURE 5.7 59-year-old female with posterior rod and screw fixation of L2-L5 and a posterolateral bone graft demonstrating improved visualization of critical anatomic structures of the spine with energy threshold high (TH) Sn140 kV PCD-CT (B, D), compared to the commercial energy-integrating-detector (EID)-CT (A, C) scanner. (A, C): Images reconstructed using soft tissue kernel, and (B, D): Images reconstructed using bone kernel. The metal artifact reduction on PCD enables visualization of anatomical structures that were obscured by the metal artifact on EID, such as central canal, neural foramina, and nerve roots. The metal artifact reduction is predominantly evident with the soft tissue algorithm (A vs. C) than with the bone algorithm (B vs. D). (Images reproduced from Zhou et al. (40)).

reduced metal artifact compared to the clinical EID-CT images (Figure 5.7A, B), and therefore demonstrate improved visualization of the central canal, neural foramina, and nerve roots. The metal artifact reduction is predominantly evident with the soft tissue reconstruction kernel (A vs. C) than with the bone reconstruction kernel (B vs. D). Note that, different from the true monochromatic x-ray imaging (such as that based on synchrotron source), the use of PCD high-energy bin and additional filtration can only reduce beam hardening and metal artifact but not completely eliminate them, since the narrow energy bin images are still reconstructed from a polychromatic x-ray spectrum with finite width.

5.3.4 Ultra-High Resolution Imaging Using Photon-Counting Detectors

In conventional EID-CT detectors, a reflective layer (septa) with a finite thickness is incorporated between each scintillating detector pixel, along the detector row and channel directions. Since scintillating detectors create visible light in the process of x-ray detection, the septa is designed

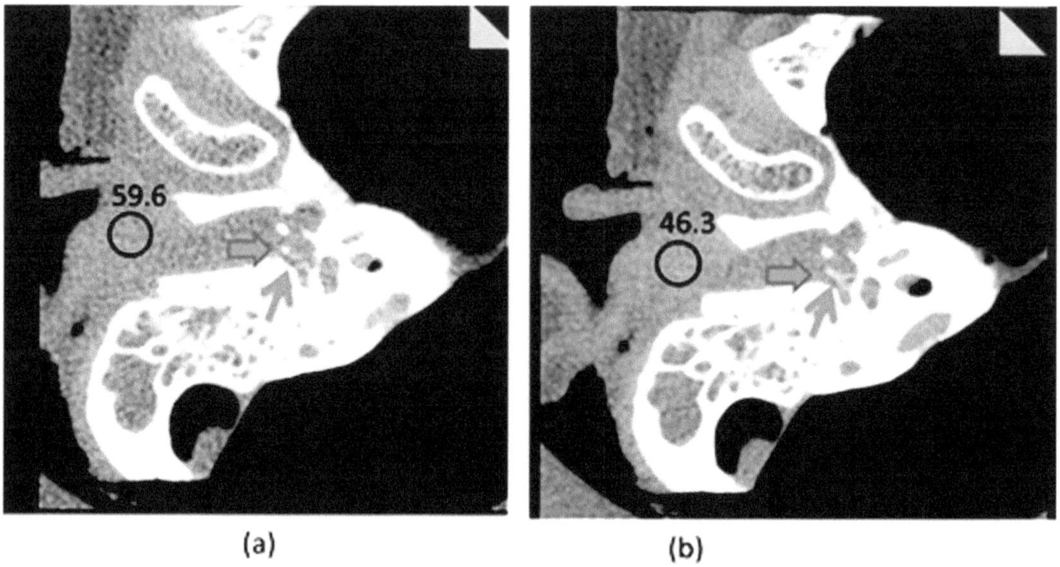

FIGURE 5.8 Cadaveric temporal bone specimen scanned using (a) EID-UHR and (b) PCD-UHR. The PCD-UHR exhibited lower-image noise, and better delineation of the stapes superstructure. (Image reproduced from Leng et al. (41)).

to prevent leakage of visible light between adjacent detector pixels. While it is possible to create smaller EID pixels, there is a physical limit to the thickness of the septa. Smaller detector pixels with a finite-width septa lead to reduced geometric dose efficiency, a consequence of the reduced detector fill factor (41). Clinically, comb or grid filters are placed near the detector to reduce the pixel aperture, resulting in smaller pixel size for ultra-high resolution (UHR) imaging. Though this approach is routinely used for specific imaging tasks such as the CT of inner ear, it is a dose-inefficient approach. Since the UHR filter is placed in front of the detector array, x-rays blocked by the filter have already passed through the patient, contributing to patient dose. This limitation could be overcome in the direct conversion PCD technology, where no septum between detector pixels is necessary, thereby allowing the design of smaller pixel sizes without losing fill factor and dose efficiency. Typical detector pixel sizes ranging from 55 to 1000 μm (pixel pitch) have been reported in the literature (42–44).

Cadaveric specimen scans (Figure 5.8) performed using a whole-body PCD-CT system demonstrated about 30% noise reduction using PCD-based UHR acquisition (32 × 0.25 mm collimation) compared to traditional comb filter-based EID-UHR imaging. At matched noise levels between PCD-UHR and EID-UHR, this translates to a 50% reduction in radiation dose (41).

5.3.5 Simultaneous High-Resolution and Multi-Energy CT

In clinical CT, high resolution (UHR) and dual-energy CT (DECT) data acquisition typically involves two separate scans. UHR-CT is limited to specific applications with high contrast, such as inner ear imaging. Dual-energy CT used for material differentiation and quantification is seldom performed using UHR mode with concerns on image noise and dose efficiency. PCD-CT offers the combined benefits of both UHR and DECT in a single acquisition. Smaller detector pixels allow high resolution imaging, while the energy discrimination capability (two or more energy bins) at the pixel level allows for multi-energy imaging. Some clinical examinations may require both high-resolution and multi-energy capabilities (19). For example, MSK imaging that

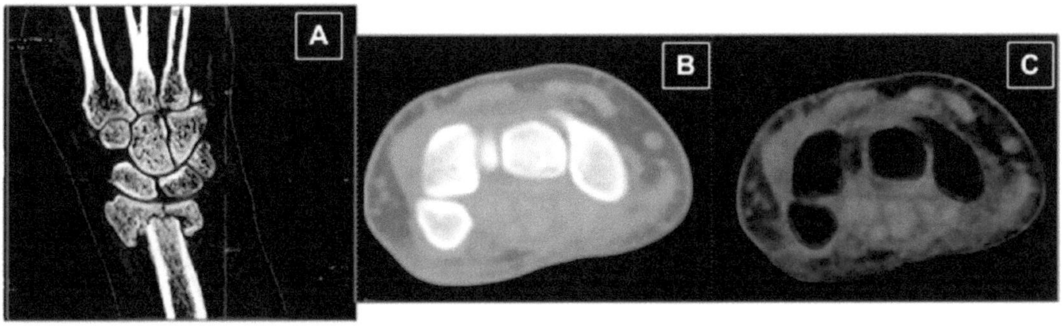

FIGURE 5.9 High-resolution and multi-energy imaging of the wrist. (A): PCD-UHR image reconstructed using V80 kernel at 0.25 mm slice thickness. (B): PCD-CT UHR image reconstructed using a quantitative smooth kernel (Q40). (C): Virtual non-calcium image for edema detection and quantification.

needs high spatial resolution for visualizing bone trabeculae and microfractures could also benefit from virtual non-calcium images to diagnose bone edema. The simultaneous high-resolution and multi-energy capability of PCD-CT is demonstrated using a wrist case in Figure 5.9. A patient was consented and scanned on the whole body PCD-CT at our institute. Two sets of images were reconstructed from the same scan: (1) a high-resolution images using a sharp kernel (V80) and the thinnest slice thickness (0.25 mm); (2) a dual-energy image set reconstructed with a quantitative smooth kernel (Q40), from which virtual non-calcium images were generated for bone edema detection and quantification.

5.3.6 PCD-CT of Novel CT Contrast Agents

The ability of PCD-CT to simultaneously discriminate multiple tissue types or contrast materials using their spectral signatures provides an opportunity for the development of new contrast agents and imaging techniques. Nanoparticle-based contrast agents have demonstrated longer blood pool retention (45), and have been successfully used as blood pool contrast agents to image leaky blood vessels in an animal tumor model (46). Several reports using heavy-metal based nanoparticles (gold (10), ytterbium (47), and gadolinium (48)) as potential CT contrast agents have also been published. Individualized nanoparticles that are functionalized and antibody-conjugated to target a specific tissue type or region of interest (e.g., cancerous cells, fibrotic collagenous tissue, macrophages) have been used in combination with PCD-CT to facilitate molecular imaging. This relies on the ability of PCD-CT to measure the K-edges of those high-Z materials that fall within the diagnostic CT energy range. The user-defined energy thresholds in PCD-CT can be placed close to the K-edge energy of high-Z contrast materials in order to capture the discontinuity in attenuation profile, as shown in Figure 5.10. This helps distinguish the K-edge of one material from other materials (e.g., bone, soft tissue, second contrast agent) and more importantly, quantify the concentration of the contrast materials in a given target site using material decomposition techniques. This approach has been mainly tested on rodents imaged using small-animal PCD-CT scanners.

Despite the promising outcomes of this approach, translation to large animals and subsequently to human trials remains challenging due to the pending evaluation of *in vivo* biocompatibility of these nanoparticles, high cost of raw material (e.g., gold) and manufacturing, and manufacturing variability for producing large volumes of nanoparticles for large animal or human imaging.

Due to the ability of PCD-CT to capture the spectral signature of multiple K-edge materials in the same acquisition, new reports (49, 50) have emerged demonstrating the potential for multiphase

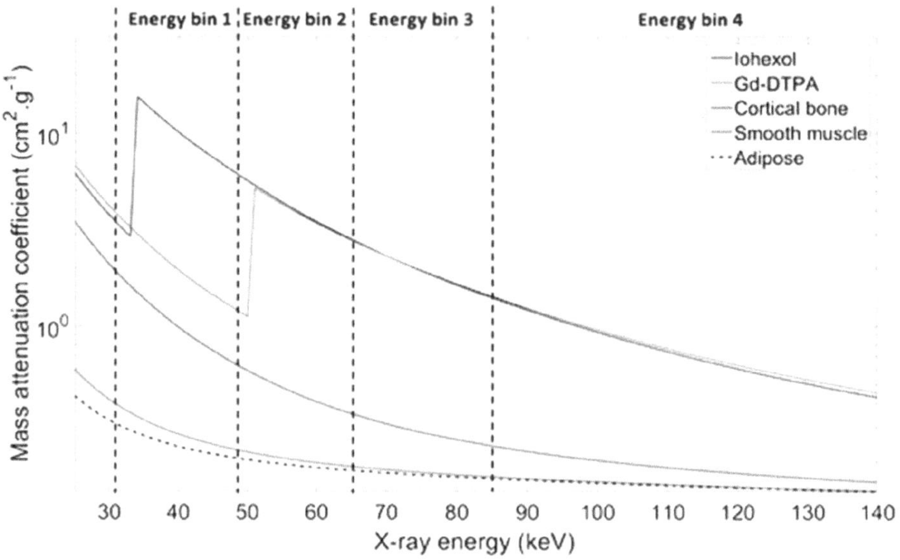

FIGURE 5.10 Energy threshold selection and energy bin placement based on K-edge of contrast materials. Bin 1 encompasses the iodine K-edge at 33 keV while Bin 2 accommodates the Gd K-edge at 50 keV.

imaging using single scan and multi-contrast materials. The traditional approach to biphasic imaging involves one contrast injection and two CT scans, occurring at different delays after injection for arterial and venous phase imaging. PCD-CT aims to accomplish multiphase imaging using a single scan and two contrast agents, each administered using a separate injection at a different time prior to the scan. A single PCD-CT scan occurring tens of seconds after the injection of the initial contrast agent (e.g., iodine) and shortly after the injection of the 2nd contrast agent (e.g., gadolinium) would capture both contrast agents but in different phases (e.g., iodine would have reached the venous phase, while gadolinium would still be in the arterial phase). Individual material maps obtained using material decomposition could then be used to highlight the different enhancement phases (e.g., arterial and venous phases).

Studies were reported using a sample patient data set and simulated iodine and gadolinium injections to evaluate the feasibility of this approach for biphasic (arterial and portal venous) liver scanning (49). In particular, this study evaluated contrast enhancement in the arterial and portal venous phases for different types of liver lesions assuming a scan at a single time point. This approach was possible due to the ability of PCD-CT to detect the K-edge of gadolinium, one of the contrast agents used in the study. Multi-contrast CT imaging and the development of novel nanoparticle-based PCD-CT contrast agents are relatively new areas of multidisciplinary research, and reports involving different PCD-CT systems and contrast agents continue to evaluate potential diagnostic values (50, 51). The clinical need for multi-contrast imaging, such as radiation dose reduction or improved diagnosis remains to be further evaluated.

5.4 PART II: POTENTIAL IMPACTS ON CLINICAL CT PRACTICE

With the benefits described in the previous section, PCD-CT can potentially generate substantial impacts in clinical practice. These can be achieved by either improving routine clinical examinations that are currently performed or creating new examinations using the unique features of PCD-CT. Most benefits of PCD can be directly translated into a broad range of clinical applications. For example, the reduced electronic noise can benefit all clinical examinations, although the benefits are more obvious in low-dose scans or obese patients. The increased iodine CNR can benefit all contrast enhanced CT scans, which account for a large portion of all CT examinations performed. In this section, we will review the impact PCD-CT has for each clinical area.

5.4.1 Musculoskeletal (MSK) Imaging

Many MSK CT applications, such as lower- and upper-extremity imaging, require high-imaging resolution to depict small anatomical structures and fine fractures. Such high resolution imposes a stringent requirement on CT systems. Due to the existence of septa, the detector size on conventional EID cannot be too small without significant loss of dose efficiency. The use of an attenuating comb filter on top of the detector array to reduce the detector aperture size sacrifices the geometrical dose efficiency. Therefore, the dose-efficient, high-resolution PCD-CT imaging mode can play a critical role in MSK applications (19). PCDs are able to eliminate the septa required by EIDs due to direct conversion from x-ray photon to electronic signal. Consequently, the detector pixel size can be further decreased without compromising geometrical dose efficiency. On a research whole-body PCD-CT system, a detector pixel size of 0.25 mm at isocenter can be achieved (19, 41, 52). Several phantom, cadaveric, and in vivo studies have been performed to evaluate the imaging performance using this system. These studies have demonstrated a 150-micron limiting spatial resolution using the UHR mode of this system. In addition, a 29% noise reduction can be achieved using PCD-UHR mode compared to EID-UHR with the same radiation dose. This translates to 50% dose reduction using PCD-CT to achieve the same noise levels between PCD-UHR and EID-UHR (19). The capability of PCD at dose efficient high-resolution imaging is especially relevant for high-resolution MSK CT applications such as when imaging hand, wrist, elbow, shoulder, foot, ankle, and knee. Figure 5.11 shows an example of wrist CT images acquired on the PCD-CT system using the UHR mode. Note that the fine trabecular bone structures can be well visualized. In addition, conventional EID-UHR is limited to extremities where the thin body parts have limited attenuation. For large body regions like shoulders and hips, high attenuation prohibits the application of EID-UHR due to its reduced dose efficiency. Consequently, these scans have to be limited to standard imaging methods, leaving an unmet need for high-resolution techniques. This, however, is not a limitation

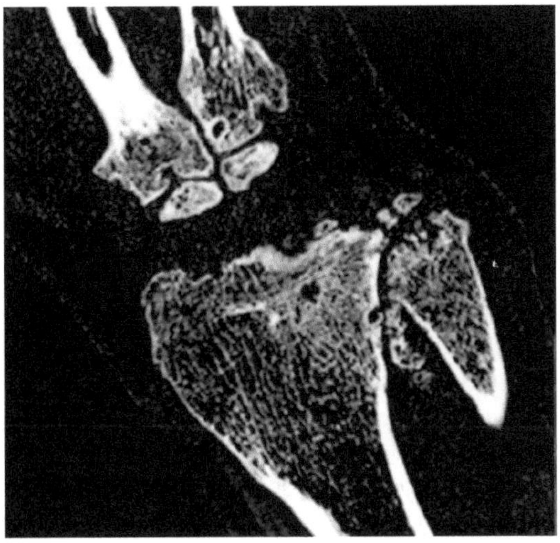

FIGURE 5.11 Example of patient's wrist images acquired using the UHR mode available on a research whole-body PCD-CT system. The high-spatial resolution performance enables accurate delineation of trabecular bone structures. (Image reproduced from Leng et al. (23)).

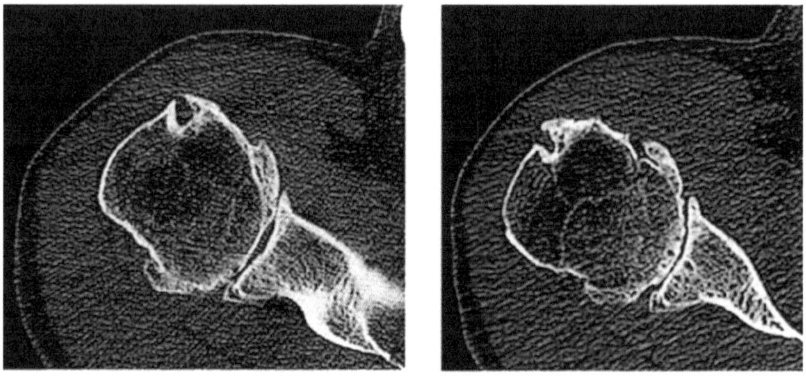

FIGURE 5.12 Shoulder images from the same patient acquired on a clinical EID-CT (a) and a research whole-body PCD-CT (b) with matched radiation dose. Image locations were selected to be as similar as possible. The PCD image shows sharper cortex and trabecular bone, and subchondral cysts and sclerosis compared with the EID image. (Image reproduced from Leng et al. (19)).

of the dose-efficient high-resolution mode in PCD-CT. Figure 5.12 shows an example of shoulder images acquired from the same patient on a conventional EID-CT (0.6 mm detector size at isocenter) and a research whole-body PCD-CT system with the Sharp mode (0.25 mm detector pixel size at isocenter) using matched radiation dose (19). The PCD-CT image demonstrates sharper cortex and trabeculae bones, and subchondral cysts and sclerosis compared to the EID-CT.

The simultaneous high-resolution and multi-energy imaging is also of great interest in MSK imaging, with the high-resolution images used for standard diagnosis of bone fractures while the multi-energy images used for bone edema detection and quantification, as shown in Figure 5.9. In addition, the capability of PCD in metal artifact reduction can also be particularly relevant for MSK imaging. Metal implants are common in MSK CT examinations, which can present a challenge by causing significant streaking and image non-uniformity. A previous clinical study has demonstrated significantly reduced metal artifacts severity and improved diagnostic confidence by using TH images acquired on a research whole-body PCD-CT with additional beam filtration, compared with clinical EID based CT systems (40). Figure 5.13 shows examples of ankle images acquired on a 69-year-old male with left tibiotalar arthrodesis with lateral plate and screw fixation. The TH image acquired on a PCD-CT images with Sn filtration (C, D) have reduced metal artifact compared to the EID-CT images (A, B). Note the improved visualization of the implant trabecular interface, cortex, trabecula, and soft tissue in the distal tibia near the tibiofibular joint on PCD-CT.

5.4.2 Vascular Imaging

CT angiography is a well-established technique that has been frequently utilized for the noninvasive evaluation of vasculature, detection of cerebral aneurysms, arterial stenosis, and other vascular anomalies. It is also widely used for preoperative evaluation.

Due to its energy discriminating capability, PCD-CT can remove the energy weighting on detected photons used in conventional EIDs and therefore improve iodine contrast as well as soft tissue contrast (18, 44). The better iodine contrast provided by PCD-CT can enable the use of higher tube potential, for example, 140 kV, for a brain CTA examination while providing comparable iodine contrast as the conventional EID system with 120 kV tube potential (53). The higher tube potential can help reducing the beam-hardening artifacts typically observed near the base of skull, cervical vertebrae, and dense calcified plaques, while maintaining the required iodine to soft tissue contrast. These beam-hardening artifacts can compromise the arterial enhancement and degrade

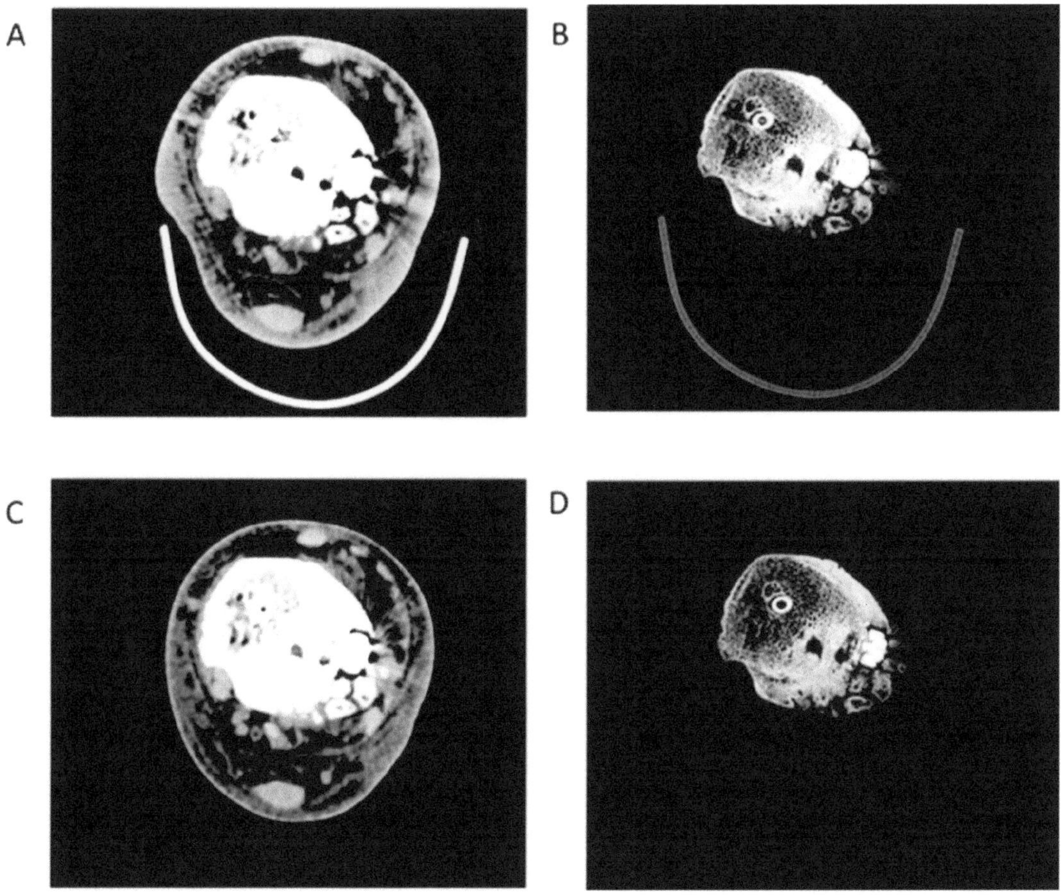

FIGURE 5.13 69-year-old male with left tibiotalar arthrodesis with lateral plate and screw fixation showing improved metal artifact reduction of the ankle with threshold high (TH) Sn140 kV PCD-CT. EID-CT 120 kV (A, B) and TH Sn 140 kV PCD-CT (C, D) are shown. The TH Sn 140 kV PCD-CT images (C, D) have reduced metal artifact compared to the EID-CT images (A, B) demonstrating improved visualization of the implant trabecular interface, cortex, trabecula, and soft tissue in the distal tibia near the tibiofibular joint. (A, C): Soft tissue algorithm kernel (WW/WL = 400/40 HU). (B, D): Bone algorithm kernel (WW/WL = 1500/450 HU). (Images reproduced from Zhou et al. (40)).

diagnostic image quality. CT angiography also benefits from PCD's simultaneous high-resolution and multi-energy capability with a single scan, where a sharp reconstruction kernel could be used to generate high-resolution CT images for visualizing small vessels, while a quantitative kernel followed by post-processing could be used for dual-energy analysis. The spectral information available via PCD-CT can enable multi-energy applications such as iodine quantification and virtual-monoenergetic imaging (VMI), which can be used to differentiate between high attenuating tissues such as iodine and calcified plaques, and therefore provide valuable additional information complementary to the conventional CT images.

Figure 5.14 shows examples of multiplanar reconstructions of the internal carotid artery of a patient who underwent head and neck CTA examinations on a conventional EID-CT with 120 kV tube potential and a research PCD-CT with 140 tube potential (53). The iodine contrast in PCD images is comparable to that of EID, even with higher tube potential for PCD scan, due to the

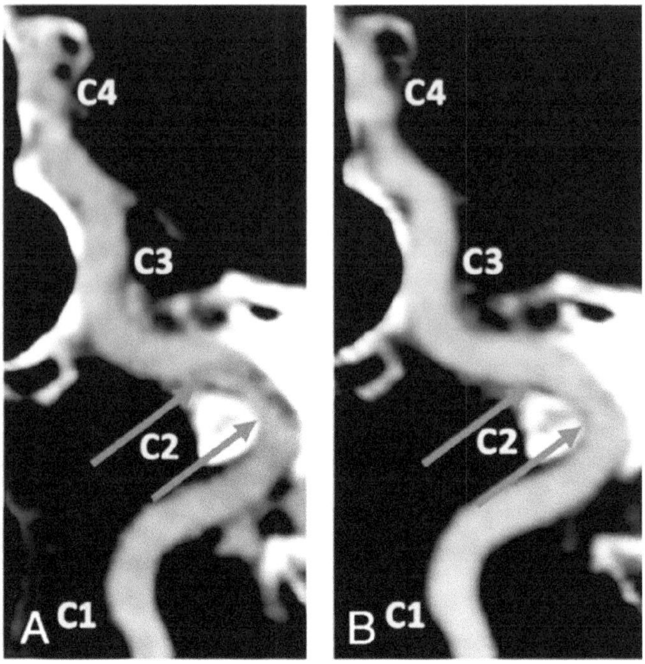

FIGURE 5.14 Multiplanar reconstructions of the internal carotid artery (ICA) of a 55-year-old woman who underwent CTA examinations on a conventional EID-CT (A) and a research PCD-CT system (B). Note the reduced lumen enhancement within the ICA petrous segment (C2) in (A) as pointed out by arrows, which may be mistaken for pathology. These artifacts are absent in the PCD-CT image (B). (Image reproduced from Symons et al. (53)).

removal of energy weighting. In addition, the use of higher tube potential reduces beam-hardening artifact. Note the reduced lumen enhancement around C2 spine in (A) as pointed out by arrows, which may be mistaken for pathology. These artifacts are absent in the PCD-CT image (B) due to better resistance to beam-hardening artifact.

Figure 5.15 shows images from a single head CTA examination using PCD-CT (19). PCD-CT can not only provide high-spatial resolution single-energy image typically used for anatomical imaging (Fig. 5.15A), but also provide dual-energy processed images such as bone removal, as shown in Fig. 5.15B, C.

5.4.3 Thoracic Imaging

Evaluating interstitial lung disease (ILD) using CT warrants high-resolution imaging. Current CT techniques for lung imaging have improved the understanding of ILD and the diagnostic performance for evaluating chronic obstructive pulmonary diseases and airway diseases (54). With the UHR capability offered by PCD-CT at routine dose levels, additional benefits could be expected in terms of clinical diagnosis. A prospective study (54) performed at our institute compared routine EID-based chest CT with the high-resolution PCD-CT. To maximize the benefits from the high-resolution acquisition mode, a dedicated sharp kernel and a large matrix reconstruction are required. In the patient study, a Q65-sharp kernel and a 1024 × 1024 matrix for image reconstruction was employed for PCD-CT data. Three chest radiologists assessed morphological features such as bronchi, lung nodules, ground glass opacities, and airways using the high-resolution PCD-CT images and conventional EID-CT images. The high-resolution (Q65/1024) PCD-CT images demonstrated improved visualization of fourth order bronchi and improved accuracy in nodule measurements compared to the conventional EID images. Figure 5.16 shows chest CT images obtained using a

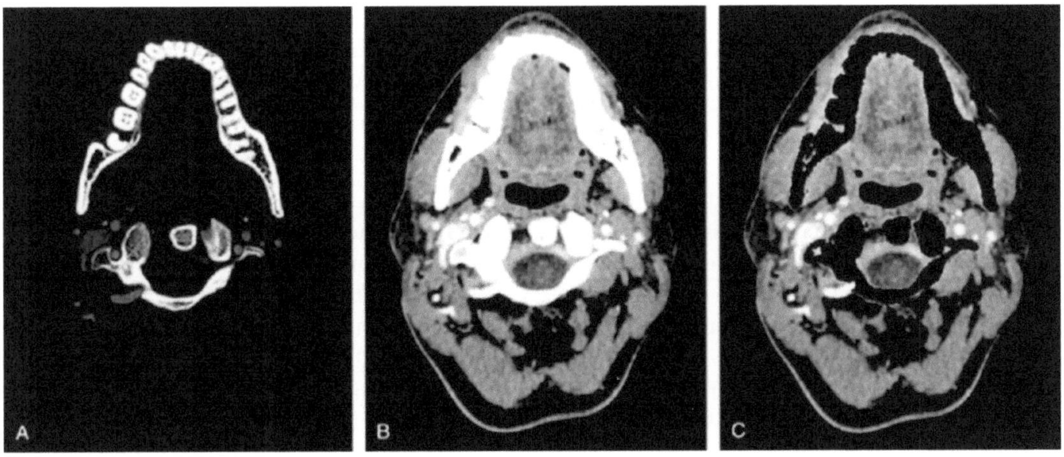

FIGURE 5.15 Images from a single head CTA examination using PCD-CT can provide both a high–spatial-resolution single-energy image (A), and a dual-energy processed image before (B) and after bone removal (C). Display settings: W/L = 1800/400 HU bone window for (A), W/L = 40/300 HU soft tissue window for (B) and (C). (Image reproduced from Leng et al. (19)).

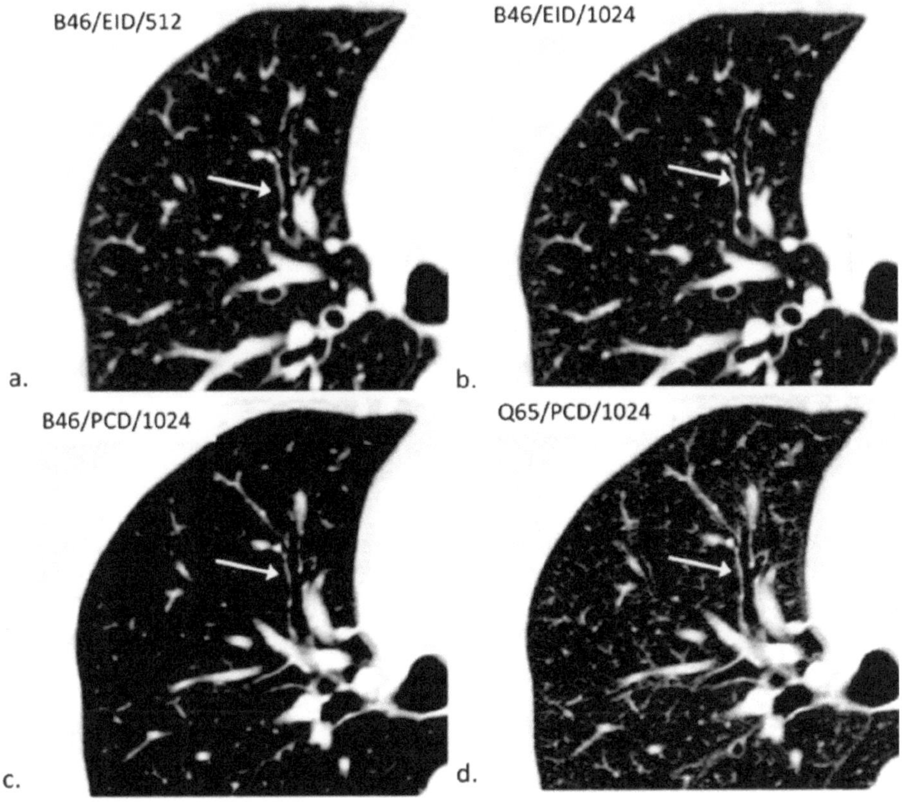

FIGURE 5.16 An 80-year-old patient evaluated for hemoptysis. B46/EID/512 (a), B46/EID/1024 (b), B46/PCD/1024 (c), and Q65/PCD/1024 (d) images demonstrating improved visualization of the fourth-order bronchial wall in the Q65/PCD/1024 (d) image compared with clinical reference (a). (Image reproduced from Bartlett et al. (54)).

conventional EID system and a PCD-CT system. The EID data were also reconstructed at 1024 × 1024 matrix for comparison. The Q65 PCD-CT images reconstructed using 1024 × 1024 matrix demonstrated improved bronchial wall delineation in a patient evaluated for hemoptysis.

5.4.4 Neuroimaging

CT has been playing an important role in neuroimaging. To date, brain CT imaging remains the diagnostic modality of choice in cases of trauma and other acute neurological disorders due to its accuracy, reliability, safety, and wide availability. However, conventional CT faces several challenges in neuroimaging. In non-contrast brain CT, for example, the contrast between gray-to-white matters is relatively limited, compromising the ability to assess the hypoattenuation as well as loss of GM-WM differentiation observed in early ischemic brain. In addition, the presence of high-attenuating skull can cause beam-hardening artifacts, which degrade the image quality of brain CT examinations, reduce the GM-WM differentiation, and potentially mimic intracranial hemorrhage.

Due to its capability of removing the energy weighting on the detected signal, PCD-CT may have improved soft tissue contrast. This advantage, together with better noise performance, allows improved differentiation between gray and white matters in a non-contrast head CT examination (55). Figure 5.17 compares examples of non-contrast brain CT images of a 59-year-old woman

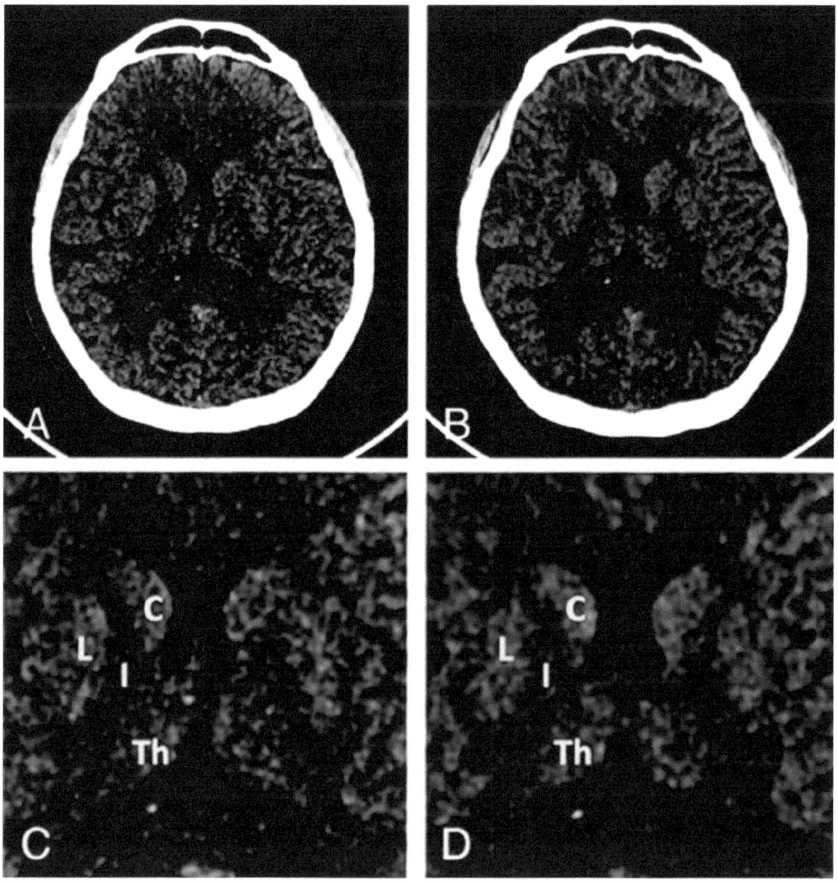

FIGURE 5.17 Non-contrast brain CT images of a 59-year-old woman acquired on a clinical EID-CT (A, C) and a research PCD-CT (B, D). (A, B): Axial EID/PCD reconstruction at the level of the basal ganglia. (C, D): Zoomed in images at the same level as (A, B). I, internal capsule; L, lentiform nucleus; Th, thalamus. (Image reproduced from Pourmorteza et al. (55)).

acquired on a conventional EID-CT and a research PCD-CT, which shows that the PCD images have reduced image noise and improved gray-matter and white-matter differentiation. In addition, studies have also demonstrated that the TH image from the PCD scan can be used to reduce skull-induced beam hardening effect.

The ability of reducing metal artifacts by combining TH in PCD and additional tin filtration can be particularly helpful for spine imaging. The presence of metal implant would otherwise cause severe image artifact and obscure anatomy of interest, such as central canal, neural foramina, and nerve roots, as shown in Figure 5.7 (40). Image quality may be further improved by combining the PCD-CT with post-processing based metal artifact reduction technique.

5.5 CONCLUSION AND OUTLOOK

In this chapter, we have reviewed the potential benefits of PCD and its impact in clinical CT imaging. Given the unique capability of counting individual photon and discriminating its energy, PCD has unique benefits over conventional energy integrating detector, such as reduced electronic noise, increased contrast and contrast-to-noise ratio, reduced beam-hardening and metal artifacts, and simultaneous high-resolution and multi-energy imaging. These benefits have a broad impact on clinical CT examinations in terms of image quality and radiation dose. Certain benefits, such as the high resolution, will benefit specific examinations and clinical areas more than the others. In addition to the improvement to current examinations, there are also substantial opportunities for PCD-CT to enable new clinical applications, such as nanoparticles and multi-contrast imaging.

Currently, widespread use of PCD-CT in clinical imaging is restricted since there is only a limited number of research PCD-CT systems capable of scanning patients, with no commercial scanners available. Applications of this technology will likely be expanded once commercial scanners are available with large scale manufacturing techniques. In addition, extensive ongoing research activities and technical developments to improve PCD performance will also broaden the horizon of clinical applications.

REFERENCES

1. Bennett JR, Opie AM, Xu Q, et al. Hybrid spectral micro-CT: System design, implementation, and preliminary results. *IEEE Trans Biomed Eng.* 2014;61(2):246–253.
2. Iwanczyk JS, Nygard E, Meirav O, et al. Photon counting energy dispersive detector arrays for x-ray imaging. *IEEE Trans Biomed Eng.* 2009;56(3):535–542.
3. Schlomka JP, Roessl E, Dorscheid R, et al. Experimental feasibility of multi-energy photon-counting K-edge imaging in pre-clinical computed tomography. *Phys Med Biol.* 2008;53(15):4031–4047.
4. Shikhaliev PM. Energy-resolved computed tomography: First experimental results. *Phys Med Biol.* 2008;53(20):5595–5613.
5. Taguchi K, Iwanczyk JS. Vision 20/20: Single photon counting x-ray detectors in medical imaging. *Med Phys.* 2013;40(10):100901.
6. Xu C, Danielsson M, Karlsson S, Svensson C, Bornefalk H. Preliminary evaluation of a silicon strip detector for photon-counting spectral CT. *Nucl Instrum Methods Phys Res Section A: Accelerators, Spectrometers, Detectors and Associated Equipment.* 2012;677:45–51.
7. Aamir R, Chernoglazov A, Bateman CJ, et al. MARS spectral molecular imaging of lamb tissue: Data collection and image analysis. *J Instrum.* 2014;9(02):P02005.
8. Anderson NG, Butler AP, Scott NJ, et al. Spectroscopic (multi-energy) CT distinguishes iodine and barium contrast material in MICE. *Eur Radiol.* 2010;20(9):2126–34.
9. Bornefalk H, Danielsson M. Photon-counting spectral computed tomography using silicon strip detectors: A feasibility study. *Phys Med Biol.* 2010;55(7):1999–2022.
10. Cormode DP, Roessl E, Thran A, et al. Atherosclerotic plaque composition: Analysis with multicolor CT and targeted gold nanoparticles. *Radiology.* 2010;256(3):774–782.
11. Koenig T, Zuber M, Hamann E, et al. How spectroscopic x-ray imaging benefits from inter-pixel communication. *Phys Med Biol.* 2014;59(20):6195.

12. Liu X, Gronberg F, Sjolin M, Karlsson S, Danielsson M. Count rate performance of a silicon-strip detector for photon-counting spectral CT. *Nucl Instrum Meth A*. 2016;827:102–106.
13. Rajendran K, Lobker C, Schon BS, et al. Quantitative imaging of excised osteoarthritic cartilage using spectral CT. *Eur Radiol*. 2017;27(1):384–392.
14. Ronaldson JP, Zainon R, Scott NJ, et al. Toward quantifying the composition of soft tissues by spectral CT with Medipix3. *Med Phys*. 2012;39(11):6847–6857.
15. Touch M, Clark DP, Barber W, Badea CT. A neural network-based method for spectral distortion correction in photon counting x-ray CT. *Phys Med Biol*. 2016;61(16):6132–6153.
16. Xu Q, Yu H, Bennett J, et al. Image reconstruction for hybrid true-color micro-CT. *IEEE Trans Biomed Eng*. 2012;59(6):1711–1719.
17. Zainon R, Ronaldson JP, Janmale T, et al. Spectral CT of carotid atherosclerotic plaque: Comparison with histology. *Eur Radiol*. 2012;22(12):2581–2588.
18. Gutjahr R, Halaweish AF, Yu Z, et al. Human imaging with photon counting-based computed tomography at clinical dose levels: Contrast-to-noise ratio and cadaver studies. *Invest Radiol*. 2016;51(7):421–429.
19. Leng S, Rajendran K, Gong H, et al. 150-μm spatial resolution using photon-counting detector computed tomography technology: Technical performance and first patient images. *Invest Radiol*. 2018;53(11):655–662.
20. Pourmorteza A, Symons R, Sandfort V, et al. Abdominal imaging with contrast-enhanced photon-counting CT: First human experience. *Radiology*. 2016;279(1):239–245.
21. Symons R, Cork TE, Sahbaee P, et al. Low-dose lung cancer screening with photon-counting CT: A feasibility study. *Phys Med Biol*. 2016;62(1):202–213.
22. Yu Z, Leng S, Jorgensen S, et al. Initial results from a prototype whole-body photon-counting computed tomography system. *Proc SPIE Int Soc Opt Eng*. 2015;9412. pii: 94120W.
23. Leng et al. Photon counting detector CT: System design and clinical applications of an emerging technology. *Radiographics*. May 6, 2019,39(3):729–743. https://doi.org/10.1148/rg.2019180115.
24. Duan X, Wang J, Leng S, et al. Electronic noise in CT detectors: Impact on image noise and artifacts. *AJR Am J Roentgenol*. 2013;201(4):W626–632.
25. Liu Y, Leng S, Michalak GJ, et al. Reducing image noise in computed tomography (CT) colonography: Effect of an integrated circuit CT detector. *J Comput Assist Tomogr*. 2014;38(3):398–403.
26. Yu Z, Leng S, Kappler S, et al. Noise performance of low-dose CT: Comparison between an energy integrating detector and a photon counting detector using a whole-body research photon counting CT scanner. *J Med Imaging*. 2016;3(4):043503.
27. Kappler S, Glasser F, Janssen S, Kraft E, Reinwand M. A research prototype system for quantum-counting clinical CT. *Proc SPIE Int Soc Opt Eng*. 2010;7622:76221Z.
28. Persson M, Huber B, Karlsson S, et al. Energy-resolved CT imaging with a photon-counting silicon-strip detector. *Phys Med Biol*. 2014;59(22):6709–6727.
29. Shikhaliev PM. Computed tomography with energy-resolved detection: A feasibility study. *Phys Med Biol*. 2008;53(5):1475–1495.
30. Shikhaliev PM. Photon counting spectral CT: Improved material decomposition with K-edge-filtered x-rays. *Phys Med Biol*. 2012;57(6):1595–1615.
31. Shikhaliev PM. Soft tissue imaging with photon counting spectroscopic CT. *Phys Med Biol*. 2015;60(6):2453–2474.
32. Shikhaliev PM, Fritz SG. Photon counting spectral CT versus conventional CT: Comparative evaluation for breast imaging application. *Phys Med Biol*. 2011;56(7):1905–1930.
33. Shikhaliev PM, Fritz SG, Chapman JW. Photon counting multienergy x-ray imaging: Effect of the characteristic x rays on detector performance. *Med Phys*. 2009;36(11):5107–5119.
34. Silkwood JD, Matthews KL, Shikhaliev PM. Photon counting spectral breast CT: Effect of adaptive filtration on CT numbers, noise, and contrast to noise ratio. *Med Phys*. 2013;40(5):051905.
35. Tümer T, Clajus M, Visser G, et al. Preliminary results obtained from a novel CdZnTe pad detector and readout ASIC developed for an automatic baggage inspection system. Nuclear Science Symposium Conference Record, Vol 1. 2000:pp. 4/36–4/41.
36. Giersch J, Niederlohner D, Anton G. The influence of energy weighting on x-ray imaging quality. *Nucl Instrum Meth A*. 2004;531(1–2):68–74.
37. Schmidt TG. Optimal "image-based" weighting for energy-resolved CT. *Med Phys*. 2009;36(7):3018–3027.
38. Glover GH, Pelc NJ. An algorithm for the reduction of metal clip artifacts in CT reconstructions. *Med Phys*. 1981;8(6):799–807.

39. Grosse Hokamp N, Hellerbach A, Gierich A, et al. Reduction of artifacts caused by deep brain stimulating electrodes in cranial computed tomography imaging by means of virtual monoenergetic images, metal artifact reduction algorithms, and their combination. *Invest Radiol.* 2018;53(7):424–431.
40. Zhou W, Bartlett DJ, Diehn FE, et al. Reduction of metal artifacts and improvement in dose efficiency using photon-counting detector computed tomography and tin filtration. *Invest Radiol.* 2018.
41. Leng S, Yu Z, Halaweish A, et al. Dose-efficient ultrahigh-resolution scan mode using a photon counting detector computed tomography system. *J Med Imaging (Bellingham).* 2016;3(4):043504.
42. Roessl E, Proksa R. K-edge imaging in x-ray computed tomography using multi-bin photon counting detectors. *Phys Med Biol.* 2007;52(15):4679–4696.
43. Walsh MF, Nik SJ, Procz S, et al. Spectral CT data acquisition with Medipix3.1. *J Instrum.* 2013;8(10):P10012.
44. Yu Z, Leng S, Jorgensen SM, et al. Evaluation of conventional imaging performance in a research whole-body CT system with a photon-counting detector array. *Phys Med Biol.* 2016;61(4):1572–1595.
45. Annapragada AV, Hoffman E, Divekar A, Karathanasis E, Ghaghada KB. High-resolution CT vascular imaging using blood pool contrast agents. *Methodist Debakey Cardiovasc J.* 2012;8(1):18–22.
46. Ghaghada KB, Sato AF, Starosolski ZA, Berg J, Vail DM. Computed tomography imaging of solid tumors using a liposomal-iodine contrast agent in companion dogs with naturally occurring cancer. *PLoS One.* 2016;11(3):e0152718.
47. Pan D, Schirra CO, Senpan A, et al. An early investigation of ytterbium nanocolloids for selective and quantitative "multicolor" spectral CT imaging. *ACS Nano.* 2012;6(4):3364–3370.
48. Badea CT, Holbrook M, Clark DP, Ghaghada K. Spectral imaging of iodine and gadolinium nanoparticles using dual-energy CT. *SPIE Medical Imaging: SPIE*, 2018; p. 7.
49. Muenzel D, Daerr H, Proksa R, et al. Simultaneous dual-contrast multi-phase liver imaging using spectral photon-counting computed tomography: A proof-of-concept study. *Eur Radiol Exp.* 2017;1(1):25.
50. Symons R, Cork TE, Lakshmanan MN, et al. Dual-contrast agent photon-counting computed tomography of the heart: Initial experience. *Int J Cardiovasc Imaging.* 2017;33(8):1253–1261.
51. Cormode DP, Si-Mohamed S, Bar-Ness D, et al. Multicolor spectral photon-counting computed tomography: In vivo dual contrast imaging with a high count rate scanner. *Sci Rep.* 2017;7(1):4784.
52. Pourmorteza A, Symons R, Henning A, Ulzheimer S, Bluemke DA. Dose efficiency of quarter-millimeter photon-counting computed tomography: First-in-human results. *Invest Radiol.* 2018;53(6):365–372.
53. Symons R, Reich DS, Bagheri M, et al. Photon-counting computed tomography for vascular imaging of the head and neck: First in vivo human results. *Invest Radiol.* 2018;53(3):135–142.
54. Bartlett DJ, Koo CW, Bartholmai BJ, et al. High-resolution chest computed tomography imaging of the lungs: Impact of 1024 matrix reconstruction and photon-counting detector computed tomography. *Invest Radiol.* 2019;54(3):129–137.
55. Pourmorteza A, Symons R, Reich DS, et al. Photon-counting CT of the brain: In vivo human results and image-quality assessment. *AJNR Am J Neuroradiol.* 2017;38(12):2257–2263.

6 Clinical Perspectives of Spectral Photon-Counting CT

Salim Si-Mohamed, Loic Boussel, and Philippe Douek
Radiology Department of Cardiothoracic and Vascular Imaging, Louis Pradel Hospital, Hospices Civils de Lyon, Lyon, France
CREATIS Laboratory, Claude Bernard Lyon 1 University, Lyon, France

CONTENTS

6.1 INTRODUCTION

Computed tomography (CT) is the most widely used imaging method in the world and has transformed patient care. A recent notable development in the field of CT is the analysis of spectral information of the X-rays that have passed through the subject. Although this concept has been discussed since CT was invented (1–3), the technology to accurately record this information has only become available over the past decade. Conventional CT scanners integrate all the signals from the detected transmitted X-ray photons into a single attenuation signal without recording any information on their individual energies. A variety of systems that are given the term dual-energy CT (DECT) and use energy-integrating detectors (EIDs) have been introduced clinically that begin to exploit the benefits of spectral detection by acquiring two energetically distinct datasets. Nevertheless, DECT systems do not typically have improved spatial resolution compared to single energy CT scanners, which is still limited by the scintillators used to convert photons into light that spread the signal spatially, and by the noise resulting from the signal integration process and the associated detection electronics. Furthermore, DECT systems only perform a two-point analysis of the X-ray attenuation, which improves tissue characterization and allows quite precise iodine quantification, but is insufficient to accurately discriminate between iodine and calcium, especially at low-radiation dose. In addition, many DECT systems expose the patient to two-energy beams that can result in potentially high-radiation exposure, and motion can create issues for aligning the two datasets. Finally, no specific contrast agent has been developed for DECT due to the lack of sensitivity of such systems for specific material imaging (4).

Recently, systems based on photon-counting detectors (PCDs), termed spectral photon-counting detectors CT (SPCCT) or multicolor SPCCT (5), have been introduced in the field of CT imaging. These PCDs are the subject of ongoing research and development in CT systems (4, 6–9). They have the capability of energy discrimination based on analysis of the pulse height of each detected photon of the transmitted X-ray spectrum and the count of their number above different energy thresholds or in multiple energy windows (6). The number of energy bins (windows) depends on the design of the detection chain of the PCDs, and the energy thresholds can be selected depending on the chosen application. Hence, the transmitted spectrum is divided into several energy bins leading to better sampling of the X-ray spectrum than DECT. This characteristic allows detection of K-edges within certain energy windows and to distinguish simultaneously between different attenuation profiles, for instance those specific to different contrast agents, allowing multi-contrast agent imaging (5). In addition, due to their architecture and detection mechanism, PCDs can provide improved spatial resolution and reduced radiation dose compared to conventional CT (10).

SPCCT systems are being investigated for preclinical and clinical CT applications as the next step to derive more information from transmitted X-ray photons. In this chapter, we describe our experience using experimental spectral photon-counting CT (SPCCT; Philips, Haïfa, Israel) in vitro and in vivo. In addition, potential SPCCT clinical applications are introduced.

6.2 POTENTIAL CLINICAL APPLICATIONS

6.2.1 High-Resolution Lung Imaging

High-resolution CT is mandatory for exploration of the lung, in particular for early diagnosis of interstitial lung diseases or lung cancer (12). Improving the overall quality of image while decreasing the radiation dose is considered as the evolution of CT imaging. Hence, SPCCT can play an important role in this evolution due to the greater spatial resolution and noise efficiency expected of its detectors, as illustrated recently by us and others (13)(Figure 6.1).

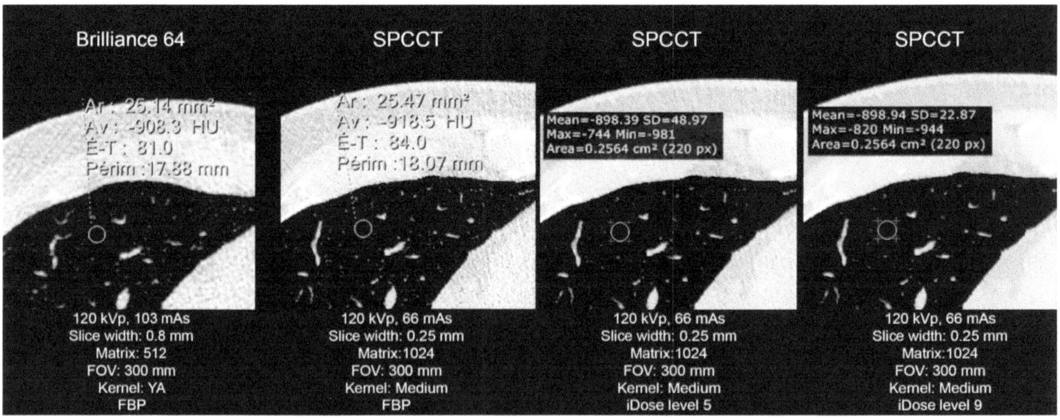

FIGURE 6.1 High-resolution SPCCT imaging of a human lung scanned on a full field-of-view SPCCT system (Haifa, Israel, Philips), in comparison to a standard CT imaging (Brilliance 64, Philips). The images demonstrated an excellent overall image quality with greater depiction of the distal airways in comparison to a standard CT imaging, even in lower radiation dose conditions. Iterative reconstruction adapted to SPCCT data allowed a reduction in image noise while maintaining an overall good image quality (Aknowledgment to Dr. Sara Boccalini for the figure).

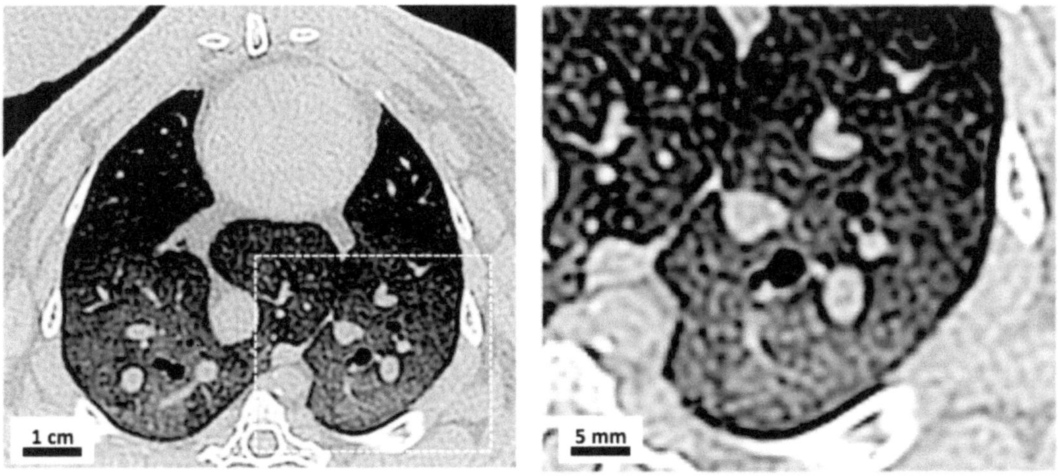

FIGURE 6.2 High-resolution SPCCT imaging of a rabbit lung (field-of-view: 160 mm, matrix size: 640 × 640 mm, voxel size: 0.25 × 0.25 × 0.25 mm). The images demonstrated an excellent overall image quality with a high depiction of the distal airways, as demonstrated by Kopp et al. (14).

A recent study by Kopp et al. (14) has demonstrated that SPCCT is a promising tool for evaluating size and shape of lung nodules in a phantom model. In this study, the authors demonstrated that SPCCT provides a higher spatial resolution allowing for a greater assessment of lung nodules in comparison to a last-generation clinical CT. In addition, they demonstrated the feasibility of SPCCT imaging in an animal (Figure 6.2), giving then a promising outlook to the capabilities of high-resolution SPCCT for pulmonary imaging.

6.2.2 Perfusion Organ Imaging

SPCCT has the potential to overcome the limitations of other imaging techniques in real quantitative perfusion analysis and specific imaging of inflammation with non-radioactive targeted probes. Indeed, conventional CT and magnetic resonance imaging (MRI) cannot perform absolute quantitative assessment of perfusion impairment, for example in stroke and myocardial infarction. While positron emission tomography (PET) can handle these tasks, it necessitates a complex and costly infrastructure to generate the specific probes. Finally, CT is widely available even in emergency settings unlike PET and MRI. This last element is of key importance when considering acute neuro- and cardiovascular diseases.

6.2.2.1 Lung Perfusion

Lung perfusion is an important functional parameter to evaluate the lung arteriolar compartment. To do so, the gold standard modality is represented by the scintigraphy via the detection of diffusible radiotracer, that because of their large size, will be retained in the pulmonary parenchyma capillaries, making it a good marker of the perfusion, that is, the flow per unit of lung tissue. With CT or MRI, the contrast agents behave differently because of their much smaller size making them non diffusible and distributed in the vascular and interstitial tissue. Their concentration within a volume reflects the perfused blood, which is not, *stricto sensu*, perfusion imaging (15). Hence, their analysis could be described as microangiography imaging, or lung parenchymogram. Despite this difference, the perfusion blood volume represented by the iodine distribution volume have been proven to be a surrogate marker for lung perfusion imaging, making the CT or MRI suitable modalities for this indication (16–20). Over the past 10 years, DECT technology has emerged as a new imaging modality for lung perfusion imaging via the possibility to generate the so-called iodine images, with the additional values to be quantitative and specific (21, 22). With the introduction of SPCCT and its capabilities, a new lung evaluation pathophysiological paradigm with targeted contrast materials carrying a payload with a compatible K-edge including among others, gold, bismuth, gadolinium, or ytterbium can thus be developed and can deliver additional, new contrast with clinically "perfusions and ventilation" relevant new information. The use of such contrast agent may have the potential to allow multi-contrast agents protocol taking benefit from the site of injection or the biodistribution of such contrast agents.

The feasibility of lung perfusion imaging using SPCCT was shown either with a blood pool contrast agent based on a K-edge element, using gold nanoparticles that mimic scintigraphy (Figure 6.3) (23) or with a high-concentrated gadoteridol-based contrast agent (24) to allow lung "perfusion" imaging with smaller volume than what it would request with a standard contrast agent at 0.5 M or 1 M (Figure 6.4).

In addition, SPCCT may have the unique advantage of a high-spatial resolution of the lung tissue, with visualization of small structure such as the bronchus, vessels in combination with the perfusion blood volume imaging. As a result, perfusion abnormalities can be confronted to the morphological analysis of the underlying lung tissue, with a potential improved characterization of vascular damages. In addition, the contrast materials images can allow the quantification of the perfused blood volume in a volume of interest, such as the pulmonary lobes. Hence, these images would beneficiate from a perfect co-registration, a specificity, a quantification ability, and a high-spatial resolution with the potential for a better evaluation of lung perfusion.

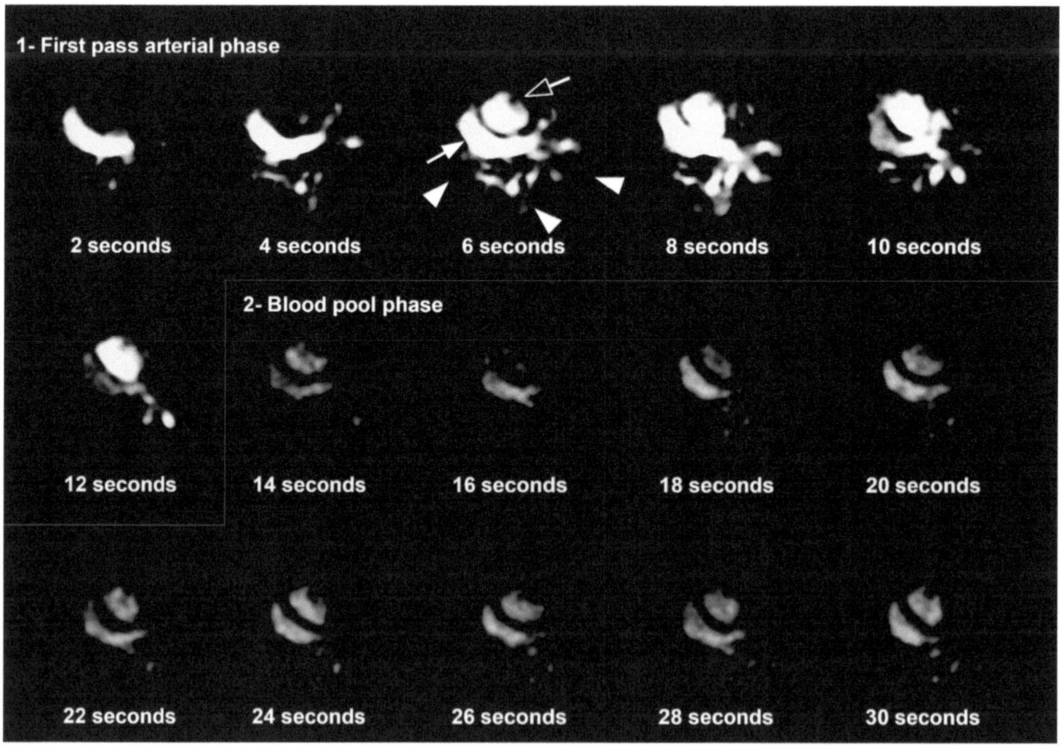

FIGURE 6.3 In-vivo SPCCT thoracic dynamic acquisitions after injection of gold nanoparticles (23). K-edge specific imaging of gold allowed the visualization of just the blood compartment (thoracic vessels, cardiac cavities, myocardial, and pulmonary perfusion) with the benefit of the removal of all other anatomical structures. Peak gold concentration decreased from 25.6 ± 0.8 mg/mL (right ventricle: arrow) to 17.1 ± 1.0 mg/mL and 16.7 ± 0.3 mg/mL (pulmonary artery, left ventricle: empty arrow) to 13.0 ± 0.9 mg/mL (aorta), 6.0 ± 0.7 mg/mL (myocardium), and 4.95 ± 0.94 mg/mL (lung: head arrow). After 30 seconds, mean concentration (6.7 ± 0.4 mg/mL) was similar between all systemic vessels as expected due to the blood pool effect of the gold nanoparticles.

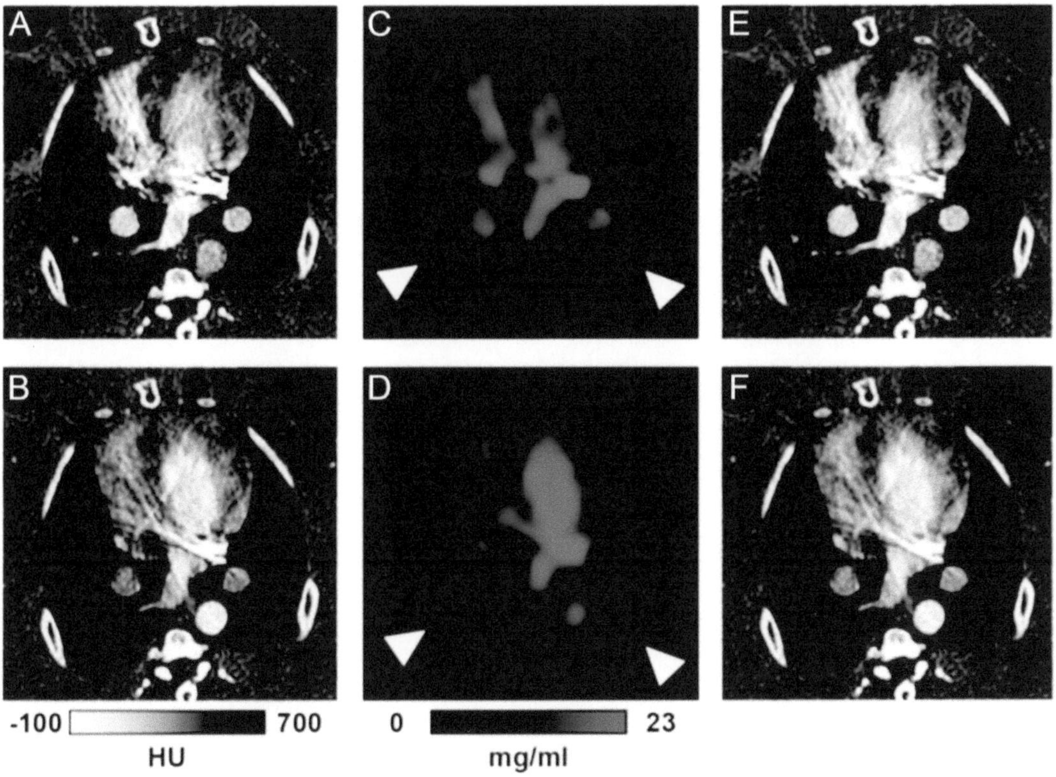

FIGURE 6.4 In-vivo SPCCT thoracic dynamic acquisition after injection of a 1.25 M solution based on gadoteridol, which is a macrocyclic complex of gadolinium, with a low viscosity and osmolality explaining the potential for high concentration (Bracco; Milan, Italy) (24). In vivo, conventional images allowed to see the enhancement in the cardiac cavities from the right ventricle (A) to the left (B) and also the blood vessels from the pulmonary artery (A) to the aorta (B). Conversely, the gadolinium K-edge images (C-D) allowed specific visualization of the blood compartment (head arrow) with the benefit of the removal of all other anatomical structures seen on the overlay images (E-F), that is, bone, soft tissue.

6.2.2.2 Renal Perfusion Imaging

Renal perfusion imaging has been validated to dynamically assess the renal perfusion with a standard CT technology (25) using gamma variate model. In that case, the iodine is used for its well-known linear correlation between tissue attenuation and concentration. Renal perfusion assessment is of great interest to diagnose and prevent the evolution of numerous conditions responsible for a low-renal perfusion toward vascular nephropathies. However, some patients are hypersensitive to iodinated agents. Moreover, these agents are contraindicated for use in patients with renal insufficiency, as their use in chronic kidney disease can lead to further reduction in kidney function, an event known as contrast-induced nephropathy. Nevertheless, iodine is the only contrast agent that has yet the potential for renal perfusion.

With SPCCT via K-edge imaging, the renal perfusion could be performed with other less nephrotoxic contrast agents. These contrast agents would have to be heavy atoms based such as it has been demonstrated in a proof-of-concept with a gadolinated contrast agent. In this study, the authors showed the feasibility of the SPCCT to measure renal perfusion with a gadolinated contrast agent compared to a simultaneous iodine injection as reference in a rabbit model (26). They demonstrated that SPCCT allows high-resolution in vivo dynamic dual contrast kidney perfusion imaging and quantification with gamma variate modeling using either conventional HU or gadolinium K-edge specific imaging (Figure 6.5).

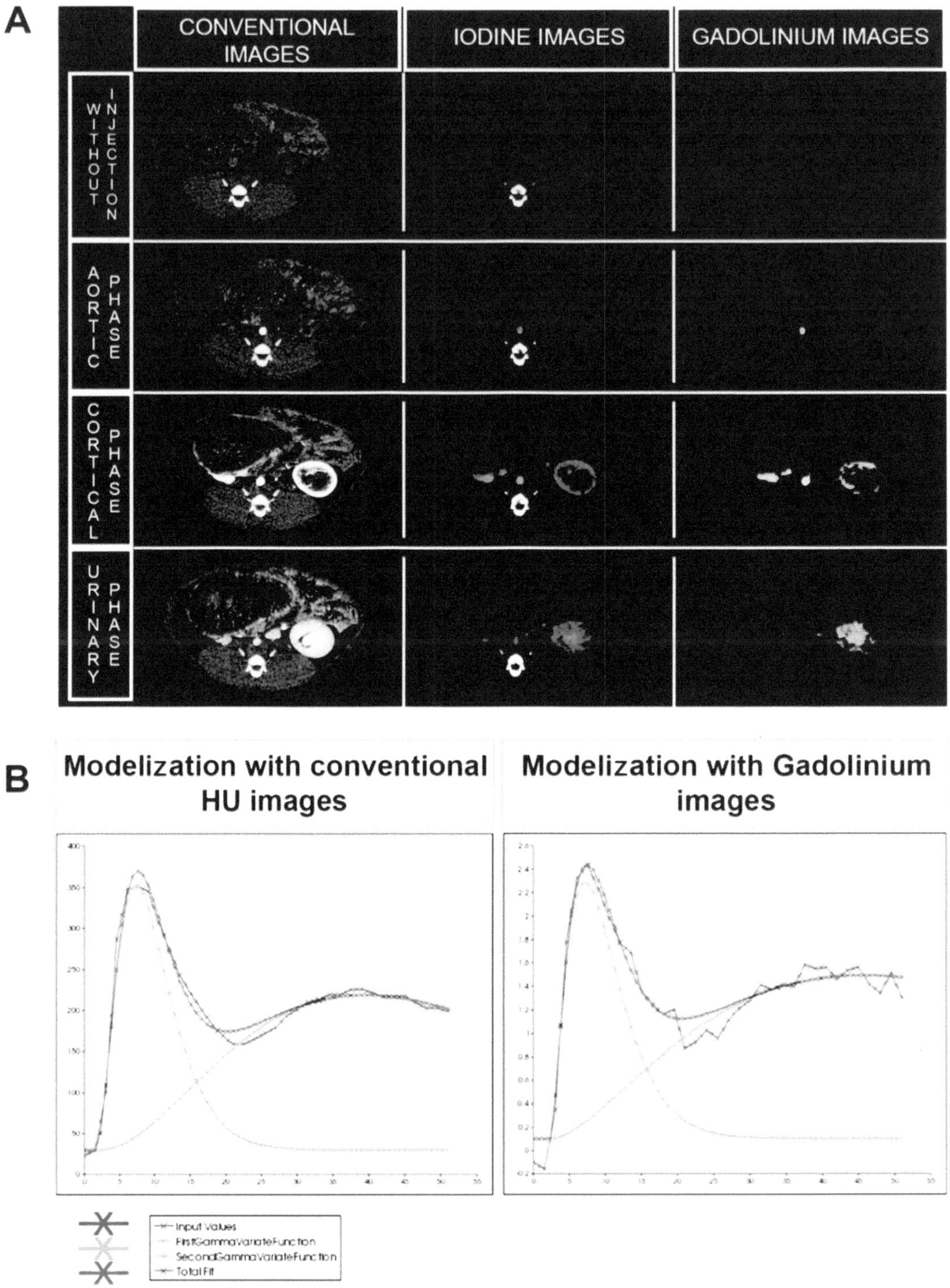

FIGURE 6.5 SPCCT provided high-resolution conventional HU, specific gadolinium K-edge and iodine material decomposition images of the cortex and the medulla (A). Gamma variate modelization graphs of the corresponding renal perfusion imaging using conventional images (B) and K-edge gadolinium images (C), where the mean transit time (MTT) were measured at 7.97 and 7.94 seconds respectively (26).

6.2.2.3 Brain Perfusion Imaging

Ischemic stroke (IS) is the third leading cause of death and the second most common cause of death worldwide, with considerable disability among survivors. Rapid evaluation of acute stroke patients will increase as the population ages and acute therapies expand. Thrombolytic therapy has led to a higher proportion of patients presenting to hospital early, and this, with parallel developments in imaging technology, has greatly improved the understanding of acute stroke pathophysiology. The main challenge of stroke imaging is the distinction of hypoperfused tissue into three operational compartments; tissue that will inevitably die (core), tissue that will in principle survive (oligemia), and tissue that may either die or survive (the ischemic penumbra).

PET shaped the concepts underlying modern acute stroke imaging and remains the gold standard. Based on validated thresholds, affected tissue can be classified as **core, penumbra, oligemia**. However, this method is not available in emergency practice for acute stroke management. Multiparametric MRI combining diffusion weighted imaging (DWI) with perfusion weighted imaging (PWI) has changed the management of acute stroke. DWI and PWI have revolutionized the diagnostic sensitivity of imaging ischemia. Expansion of the initial lesion within the area at risk occurs almost exclusively in those patients, who initially have a perfusion defect larger than the DWI lesion. However, one of the main limitations of MRI is the lack of absolute quantification of perfusion parameters and therefore the accurate distinction between penumbra and oligemia. In contrast, investigations of dynamic CT perfusion scanning have shown the feasibility and promise of this method for the rapid assessment of patients with acute stroke. Compared with other methods of cerebral perfusion imaging, CT perfusion imaging with intravenous infusion of iodinated contrast material offers a number of practical advantages. Dynamic CT perfusion scanning can provide better quantitative information about multiple hemodynamic parameters (e.g., cerebral blood flow (CBF), cerebral blood volume (CBV), time to peak enhancement, or mean transit time (MTT)) from one examination. Matched perfusion abnormalities on CBV and MTT maps correspond to areas of non-salvageable brain tissue and neuronal death, also known as core infarct. Mismatched areas of abnormal perfusion namely, areas of prolonged MTT and diminished CBF where CBV is relatively preserved correspond to areas of salvageable tissue. However, CT quantification needs to be improved for a better assessment of ischemic tissue viability. Furthermore, hyperdense lesions can frequently be observed on the CT obtained immediately after endovascular intervention, and it is sometimes difficult to differentiate intraparenchymal hemorrhage from contrast agent extravasation. DECT should already provide more accurate perfusion assessment of heterogeneous tissues than conventional CT perfusion but K-edge imaging should be more specific and accurate as previously explained. Spectral CT may further provide more accurate pattern of hemodynamic status, by direct and precise quantification of contrast agent concentrations in the different brain areas instead of current attenuation measurements with superposition of the contrast agent attenuation with inhomogeneous tissues densities.

Preliminary data showed that brain perfusion K-edge imaging of a gadolinated contrast agent in vivo in the rabbit brain was possible with SPCCT (Figure 6.6). The clear advantage of the photon-counting scanner approach is its specificity (K-edge imaging of gadolinium) and the possibility of quantitative follow-up. The limitation of course will be sensitivity, which limit will need be explored on the SPCCT in-vivo models.

6.2.3 Atherosclerosis Imaging

Atherosclerosis and its final complication, plaque ruptures and subsequent infarct in heart or brain is the main underlying pathology of cardiovascular diseases (CVD) and atherosclerosis is responsible for 70% of all cases of CVD. In order to reduce the risk of an acute event, unstable atherosclerosis has to be detected at an early stage of its development. A variety of factors contribute to the development and progression of atherosclerosis. The earliest steps in the development of coronary artery disease are thought to be the dysfunction of the

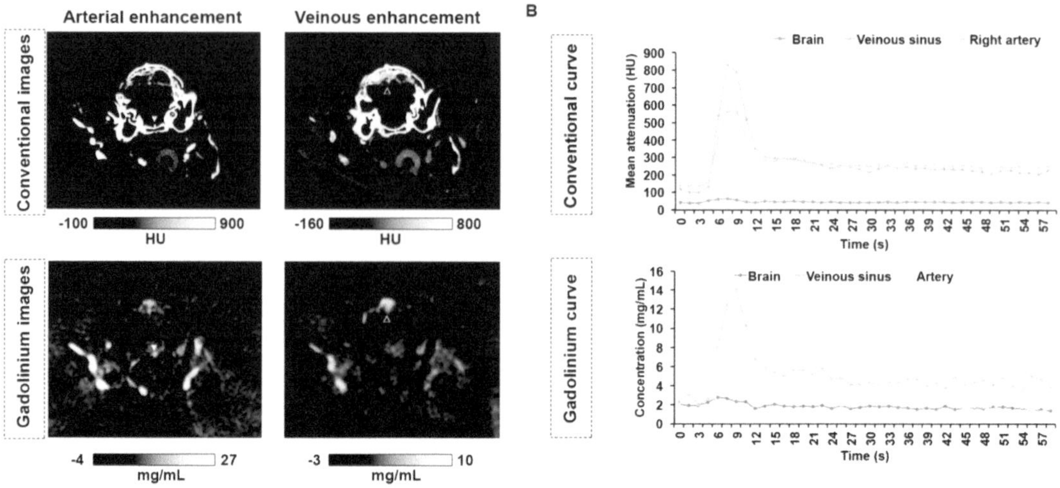

FIGURE 6.6 Spectral photon-counting CT imaging of the rabbit's brain during the arterial and venous phases and perfusion quantitative curves (top row: conventional images, bottom row: gadolinium K-edge images, white arrow: basilar artery, clear arrow: sinus venosus). To be noted that the absolute quantification of gadolinium is possible only with the material images measurement in mg/mL but not with the conventional ones in HU.

endothelium. This initial process is followed by molecular mechanisms that contribute to plaque development and progression: inflammation, macrophage infiltration, lipid deposition, calcification, extracellular matrix degradation, oxidative stress, cell apoptosis, and thrombosis (27, 28). However, atherosclerosis ultimately progresses to clinically over cardio- or neurovascular disease. These clinical manifestations are most often the result of an atherosclerotic plaque rupture. Therefore, identification of plaques at high risk of rupture is thus a major clinical concern.

Current treatment strategies (including medication, stenting, and surgical approach such as end-arterectomy) rely on the measurement of the plaque-related stenosis of the considered artery (29, 30). Standard and DECT are widely used to assess this degree of stenosis but their results are often impaired by their current spatial resolution (0.5 mm insufficient to image vessels smaller than 1 mm) and the presence of calcification within the plaque, particularly during coronary arteries examination. This excludes a large proportion of patients who are still referred to invasive techniques such as coronary angiography as MRI, which is less sensitive to calcification, cannot currently correctly assess the coronary arteries. In this field, the spectral analysis provided by SPCCT to separate between calcifications and contrast-enhanced vessel lumen could improve the quantification of the stenosis and strongly reduce the examination failure rate in patients with heavily calcified arterial wall (31). Similarly, SPCCT, by increasing the spatial resolution of the detectors by a factor of two, will strongly improve the accuracy of stenosis measurement in these small vessels.

Beside stenosis assessment, several clinical observations have emphasized the need for a more detailed analysis of the structure and biology of atherosclerotic plaques. The goal is to identify vascular remodeling and describe plaques with regard to specific criteria of vulnerability, such as a thin fibrous cap and a large lipid core. MR imaging approaches have been developed, and these approaches allow noninvasive characterization of the vessel wall but still with a lack of spatial resolution and a short anatomic coverage that limits the techniques to an analysis of a few plaques during the same examination. A preliminary ex-vivo study of coronary arteries on a preclinical limited field-of-view SPCCT prototype demonstrated a great potential for plaque component analysis (i.e., lipid, calcium, and fibrosis) by individually analyzing photoelectric, Compton scattering and iodine concentration (after contrast injection with K-edge technique) of each plaque components (32). In parallel, the explosive growth of biocompatible nanotechnologies now offers the possibility to build specific contrast agents embedding these atoms as a payload. For example, Cormode et al. have shown, using a similar prototype, that gold embedded in specific nanoparticles can be detected in unstable plaque (5). However, this prototype was not adequate for in-vivo applications because of its low count-rate capability, resulting in long scan times. But the technology has being scaled up recently to human sizes to prepare acquisition protocols for human scanning.

This technology would then allow for better assessing atherosclerotic plaque components and the level of intraplaque inflammation in order to adapt the preventive treatment for each patient. Furthermore, thrombus imaging and quantitative perfusion imaging allowed by SPCCT, will assist in the treatment decision in stroke or myocardial infarction, namely thrombolysis and reperfusion lesion prevention (i.e., by using cyclosporine) in emergency settings. Furthermore, monitoring tissue inflammation and perfusion recovery will allow us to assess the therapeutic response in these patients. Thus, a significant impact on clinical decisions in neurovascular and cardiovascular diseases is expected thanks to a relatively affordable and widely available imaging technique.

In conclusion, SPCCT has the potential for an innovative in vivo high-resolution spectral quantitative imaging of atherosclerotic carotid and coronary arteries, brain and myocardial tissue, with new photon-counting detectors technology using standard and new specific contrast media at a lower X-ray dose in order to overcome the current limitations in CT imaging, mainly spatial and spectral resolution and radiation dose.

6.2.3.1 Stent and Coronary Artery Imaging

Blooming artifacts in standard CT angiography images related to vascular calcifications and metallic stents impair correct visualization of the vascular lumen, reducing the possibility of diagnosis of coronary stenosis or in-stent restenosis. Indeed, blooming artifacts can cause under- or overestimation of the vessel lumen because of the thicker appearance of highly attenuating materials (33). Hence, there is a need for decreasing blooming artifacts, which are due mainly to highly attenuating material artifacts and the partial volume averaging effect. The higher spatial resolution inherent to SPCCT systems has the potential to reduce the partial volume effect and therefore might be expected to reduce blooming, as related recently by multiple studies in vitro (34–36). But a study investigated this capability also in vivo and confirmed the improvement of the visualization of stent architecture compared to a standard CT system (35). The authors have demonstrated that the apparent width of the metallic struts was smaller on SPCCT than on the standard CT for the stent (Figures 6.7 and 6.8). Thus, SPCCT enables improved visualization of stent metallic mesh owing to a significant reduction of blooming artifacts due to increased spatial resolution compared to conventional CT.

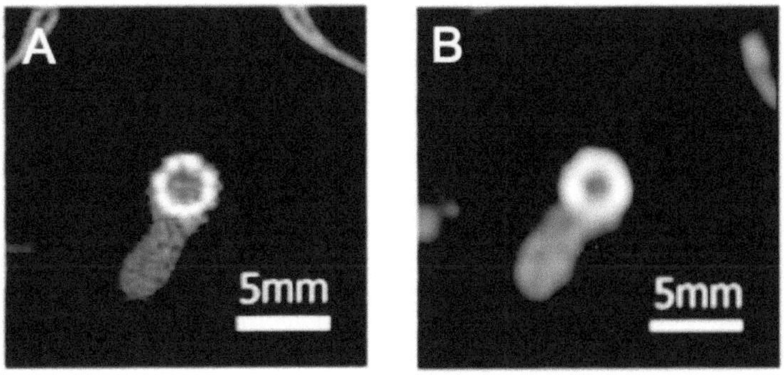

FIGURE 6.7 SPCCT (Philips, Haïfa, Israel) (A) and standard CT (Brilliance 64; Philips, Haïfa, Israel) (B) acquisitions of a stent placed in the aorta of a rabbit, under similar acquisition and reconstruction parameters (35).

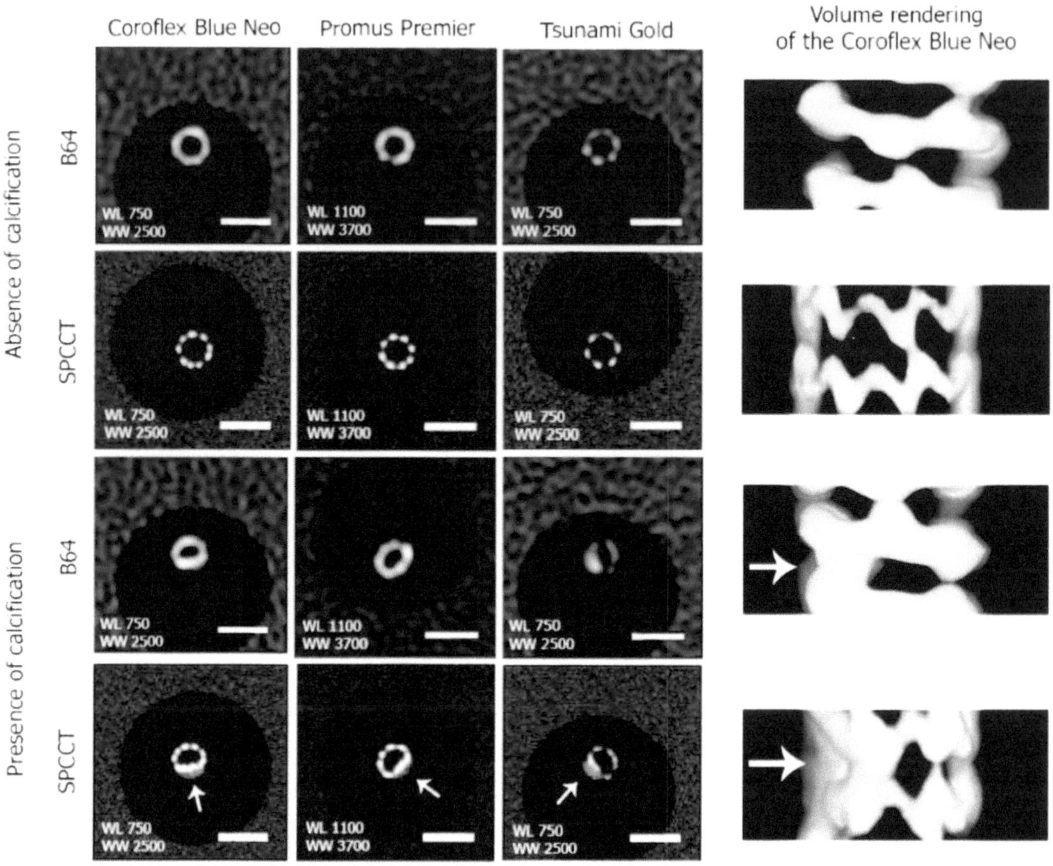

FIGURE 6.8 Representative conventional HU images acquired on the B64 and on the SPCCT at similar locations in the stents in the absence (top) and presence of calcification (bottom) (35). The smaller size of the photon-counting detectors results in an improved visualization of the stent metallic struts. On the SPCCT images the stents can be visually separated from the calcification (white arrows), while this separation is not possible on the B64 images due to larger detector size. The improved quality of SPCCT images allows clear visualization by volume rendering (right for the Coroflex Blue Neo stent) of the metallic mesh of the stent and its deformation due to the presence of the calcification insert, while this is not possible for B64. A 5-mm scale bar is shown on each conventional HU image.

In addition, given the great spatial resolution of the photon-counting detectors and their noise efficiency, the SPCCT technology presents the ability to improve the depiction of the lumen coronary arteries, even more in presence of vascular calcifications as discussed hereinbefore (Figure 6.9).

It is also possible to anticipate the possibility to perform a SPCCT coronary K-edge imaging using a gadolinated contrast agent (31) (Figure 6.10). In this study, the authors demonstrated that SPCCT allowed a full 3D-coronary SPCCT imaging with clear differentiation between calcification and gadolinium using spectral K-edge images. K-edge gadolinium images demonstrated exclusively the lumen with benefice of the removal of all the other structures, for example, calcified plaque, soft tissue, and with absence of blooming artefact. Mean lumen diameter measured on K-edge images were higher than measured on conventional CT images (2.0 ± 0.13 cm vs. 1.8 ± 0.1 cm, $p < 0.05$) in favor of blooming artefact suppression. Hence, SPCCT with a K-edge contrast agent may be a promising tool for better depiction of the lumen diameter quantification.

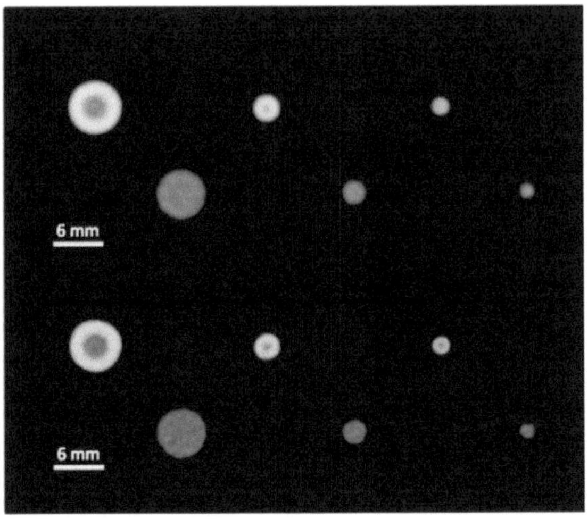

FIGURE 6.9 Representation of conventional images of a coronary phantom presenting a peripheral calcium-like ring and a lumen filling with an iodinated contrast agent (concentration at 21.4 mg/mL) (dual-layer DECT with high resolution on top row; SPCCT on the bottom row) (37). The sharpness and depiction between the calcifications and the lumen are better on the SPCCT images compared to high-resolution DECT in all the tubes even in the smaller one (0.5 mm diameter of the lumen), despite the higher noise on SPCCT images, related to the fact that they were reconstructed with standard FBP in comparison with the images of DECT that were reconstructed with iterative reconstruction method).

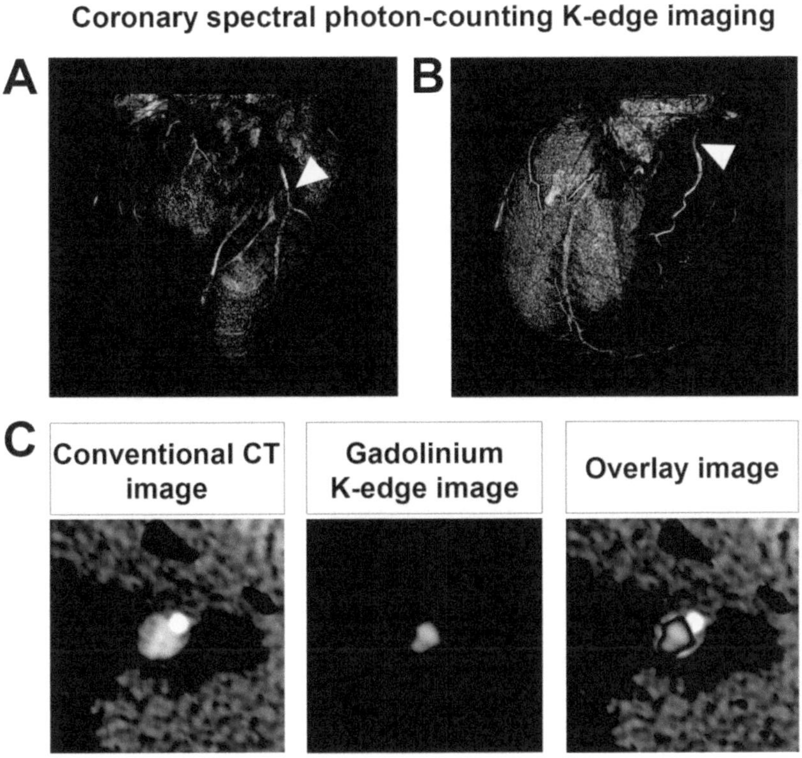

FIGURE 6.10 Representation of a full SPCCT acquisition of an ex-vivo heart with calcified coronary arteries. The injection of a gadolinated contrast agent demonstrated on the gadolinium images via the K-edge technique a better depiction for the lumen in presence of calcifications.

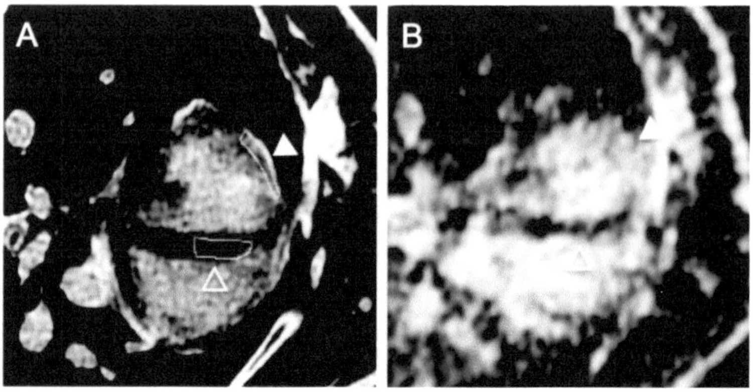

FIGURE 6.11 Late gadolinium enhancement SPCCT images of a rabbit myocardial infarction (A: conventional image, B: K-edge maps of gadolinium, empty head arrow: remote myocardium, full head arrow: infarcted myocardium). The K-edge images allow the quantification of the gadolinium in the infarcted zone for evaluation of the extracellular volume (Infarcted myocardium: 8.53 ± 1.66 mg/mL versus remote myocardium: 4.9 ± 1.56 mg/mL).

6.2.3.2 Myocardial Infarction

Conventional and Dual-energy CT with dual-source and detector assembly with their superior quality for imaging coronary arteries and functional cardiac imaging capability is increasingly used as a noninvasive imaging investigation. They have been proposed to detect myocardial perfusion defects, including following acute or chronic infarction (38). However, studies using CT data are susceptible to beam-hardening artefacts that may mimic perfusion defect. Furthermore, CT, as MRI, allows a visualization of the perfusion defect but not a real quantification of the perfusion. This quantification can be performed with PET but again with a poor accessibility and a high cost. Finally, the radiation dose in perfusion CT is currently too high for a clinical application of CT perfusion. Similarly, studies in animals and humans indicate that myocardial perfusion studies performed with CT accurately detect myocardial ischemia and infarcts compared with single photon emission computed tomography (SPECT), but includes a rather high-radiation exposure. Furthermore, the detection of myocardial late enhancement has been demonstrated with conventional CT (39). However, because of the poor contrast between normal and abnormal myocardium in late enhancement studies with conventional CT limits its clinical use and its potential in determining precisely the different components of reperfusion myocardial lesions.

Hence, the SPCCT has the potential to overcome these limitations in perfusion and delayed enhancement imaging by obtaining artifact-free accurate material-decomposition images for quantitative iodine and gadolinium contrast based perfusion measurement with K-edge imaging technique. Furthermore, SPCCT makes it possible to lower the dose and simulations have shown the amplitude of the putative benefit. Preliminary measurements have confirmed this potential (Figure 6.11), but a full prototype measurement is needed to fully validate these advantages. Reduced dose scanning procedures will thus open the use of SPCCT for myocardial perfusion imaging in clinical practice.

6.2.4 Simultaneous Multiphase CT Imaging

One of the main advantages of SPCCT is to image multiple contrast agents simultaneously due to specific discrimination, using their K-edge signatures and/or material decomposition. Indeed, by dividing the spectrum into well-chosen energy-based datasets, it would be possible to detect multiple elements such as gadolinium, gold, bismuth, ytterbium, and tantalum, whose K-edges are in the relevant energy range of the X-ray spectrum used, this latter being ~40–100 keV. Note that while the X-rays used in SPCCT range between ~25–120 keV, K-edge imaging requires sufficient number of photons above and below the K-edge; therefore, excluding elements whose K-edges are much below 40 or over 100 keV. This will potentially permit a new form of functional imaging, where multiple contrast agents with different pharmacokinetics are used simultaneously in the same biological system. For example, with the use of different contrast agents in the vascular system injected sequentially, within a single scan we would be able to image multiple uptake phases of a given tissue/organ; or the use of a combination of one non-specific and one specific contrast agent for the simultaneous imaging of the vascular lumen and vascular wall in pathologies such as atherosclerosis (5); or for the simultaneous imaging of the different biodistributions of two contrast agents, such as gold nanoparticles and iodine contrast agents, to probe different biological processes and diseases in a single scan (40); or for the visualization of iodinated contrast agent despite the presence of tantalum based liquid embolic agent such as onyx (Micro Therapeutics, Irvine, USA) (41) or blood in the brain (42); or for the simultaneous imaging of two different compartments (43, 44), such as the peritoneal cavity and the blood with the use of iodine and gadolinium contrast agents, to permit the differentiation of the peritoneal and blood enhancement of peritoneal metastasis (Figure 6.12) (44). Note that gold nanoparticles are a good candidate for K-edge imaging, as has been shown previously (5, 45–48). But they have the potential to circulate longer than iodinated contrast agents for improved blood pool imaging and possessing high biocompatibility (49, 50).

In addition, this will potentially permit a new form of protocol imaging, where two contrast agents with similar pharmacokinetic could be used simultaneously but with a different time of injection to

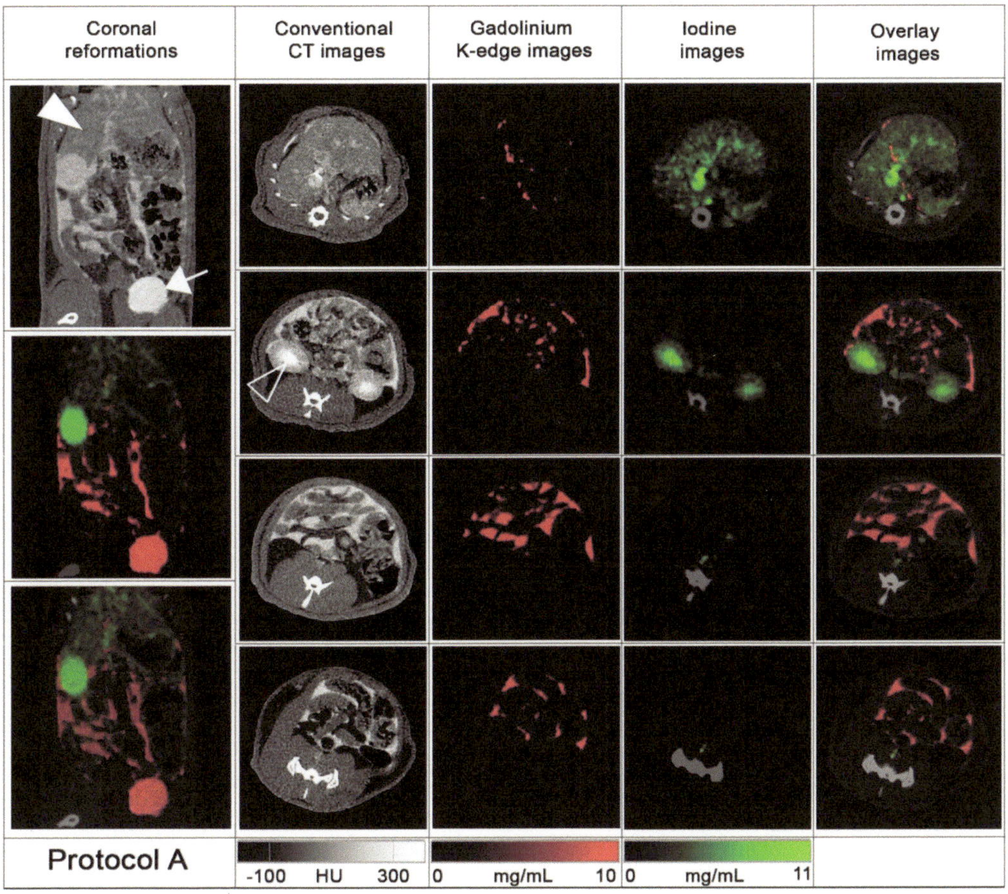

FIGURE 6.12 SPCCT images of a dual-contrast peritoneal protocol taking benefit from an intraperitoneal contrast agent and an intravenous contrast agent in a rat (44). The contrast material maps demonstrated a clear separation of the contrast agents (in red: gadolinated contrast agent, in green: iodinated contrast agent, in gray: bone segmentation). On the gadolinium K-edge map, only the signal arising from gadolinium was seen with the benefit of removal of all the other structures, such as bone and soft tissue. While on the iodine map the signal was preserved in the structures enhanced, without discrimination of the bone signal. These findings were seen in both protocols, and the peritoneal opacification scores were similar between conventional and material maps.

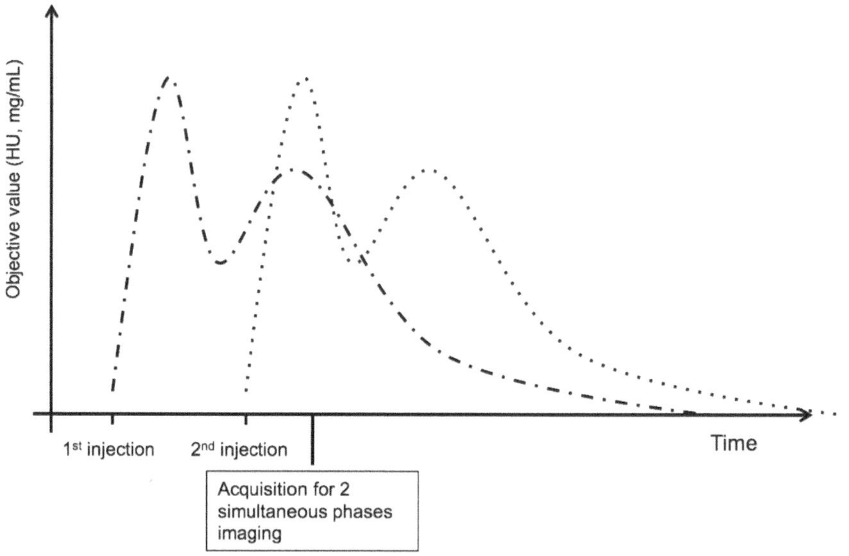

FIGURE 6.13 Graph depicting the SPCCT multiphase imaging per acquisition using dual contrast discrimination that allows, with delayed injection of two contrast agents (first contrast agent: thick dotted line, second contrast agent: thin dotted line), simultaneous organ arterial and portal phase imaging (scan at time T2).

catch two phases of organ enhancement (Figure 6.13). These types of protocol, tuned for each organ specificities, would allow a decrease of number of acquisitions with the benefit of reducing the radiation dose; but also to provide perfect spatial registration of the enhancement phases useful in particular for diagnosing small lesions. Good applications are CT urography and CT liver imaging where multiphase acquisition protocol is mandatory for diagnostic imaging. CT urography is defined as a diagnostic examination optimized for imaging the kidneys, ureters, and bladder and involves the use of multidetector CT with thin-slice imaging, intravenous administration of a contrast medium, and imaging in the excretory phase (CTU Working Group definition) (51). The CT protocol necessitates a single-bolus contrast medium injection technique with three CT acquisitions during the unenhanced, nephrographic, and excretory phases. As a consequence, the high-radiation exposure is one of the major issues of CT urography. Therefore, SPCCT has the potential to overcome this limitation via the use of two contrast agents injected at a different time for two enhancement phases imaging, as demonstrated by us (52) (Figure 6.14). The same applies for the diagnostic imaging of liver lesions such as the hepatocellular carcinome. In a recent study, the authors demonstrated that SPCCT allows *in-vivo* dual contrast qualitative and quantitative multi-phase liver imaging in a single acquisition in rabbits, confirming the potential of multicontrast imaging (53).

6.2.5 Contrast Agent Imaging

SPCCT is expected to require less contrast material to be administered to patients than the currently used amounts due to a better contrast-to-noise ratio (particular at low-current dose) (6, 54). Importantly, SPCCT provides additional energy information and will allow enhanced contrast of different materials in the body due to material mapping as in current DECT imaging, but with improved signal to noise ratio thanks to the multiple energy bins and less noise, and also potential good accuracy quantification of materials (48). Contrast agents reported for SPCCT imaging have been based on heavy elements such as the lanthanides (e.g., gadolinium), gold, ytterbium, bismuth, and tantalum, whose K-edges lie within the range of 40-140 keV (5, 6, 54–59). For example, a first proof of principle measurement using a prototype SPCCT has been performed on a phantom made of Delrin (PTFE, d = 1.4 mg/mL, diameter = 15 cm) containing

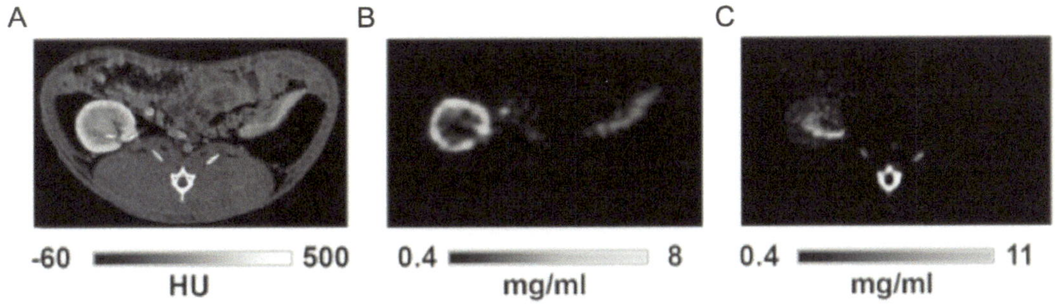

FIGURE 6.14 Simultaneous urinary SPCCT protocol using a single acquisition and two contrast agents injection for differentiation of the nephrographic phase using a gadolinated contrast agent (B) and the urinary excretory phase using an iodinated contrast agent (C) (52). Only the contrast material maps (B,C) allow for a clear differentiation between the enhancement phases conversely to the conventional images (A). Additional advantage of the contrast material maps is the higher contrast-to-noise ratios of the enhanced structures.

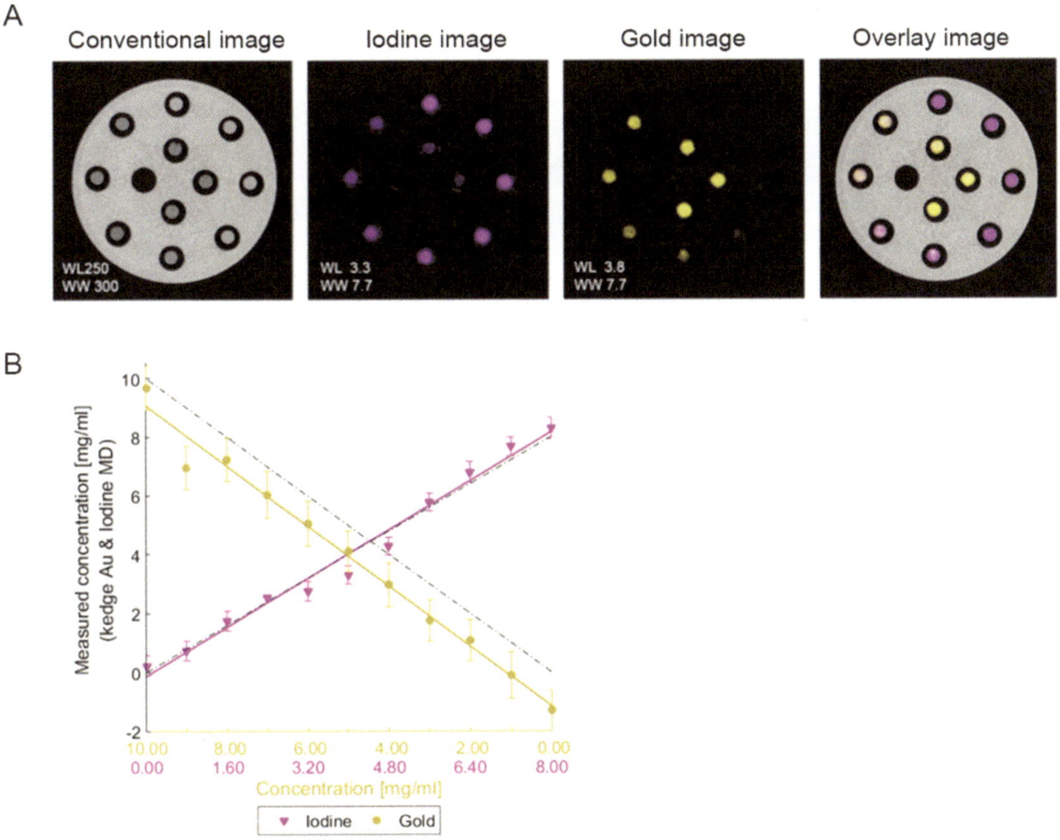

FIGURE 6.15 In-vitro qualitative and quantitative SPCCT discrimination of gold and iodine based contrast agents. Only the contrast material maps allowed the differentiation between the two contrast agents with the additional value to be quantitatively accurate as demonstrated by the linear regression between the prepared and the measured concentrations of the contrast agents. Notably, the measured concentrations in tubes varied inversely between the two mixed contrast agents, as expected. The black dashed lines represent perfect fits i.e. slope of 1 and offset of 0.

multiple test tubes with different dilutions of iodine contrast agent (Iomeron, 400 mg/mL, Bracco) and gold nanoparticles (custom made, 65 mg/mL, University of Pennsylvania) and phosphate buffered saline mixtures (Figure 6.15). Note that the concentrations of contrast agents in each tube were estimated such as they provided the same attenuation level (~250 HU). As expected, the conventional image did not allow either the determination of a material or the discrimination of the iodine from the gold. On the contrary, the iodine material decomposition image and the gold K-edge image successfully show only the specific materials, with signal intensity in proportion to the agents' absolute concentrations, and with the capability for quantification of the concentrations. There was a suppression of the background in the specific images, for example, the plastic phantom, improving drastically the signal to background ratio. This stems from the fact that the specific information about the presence of contrast is obtained by a measured difference in attenuation above and below the K-edge feature of the element, for example, 80.7 keV for gold.

6.2.6 Molecular Imaging

Iodinated and gadolinated contrast agents are in clinical use since more than two decades in CT and MRI, respectively. The commercially available contrast media can be used in both preclinical and clinical angiography and perfusion SPCCT experiments without any specific restriction. However, there is room for contrast agent's development via the specificity of the K-edge imaging and the

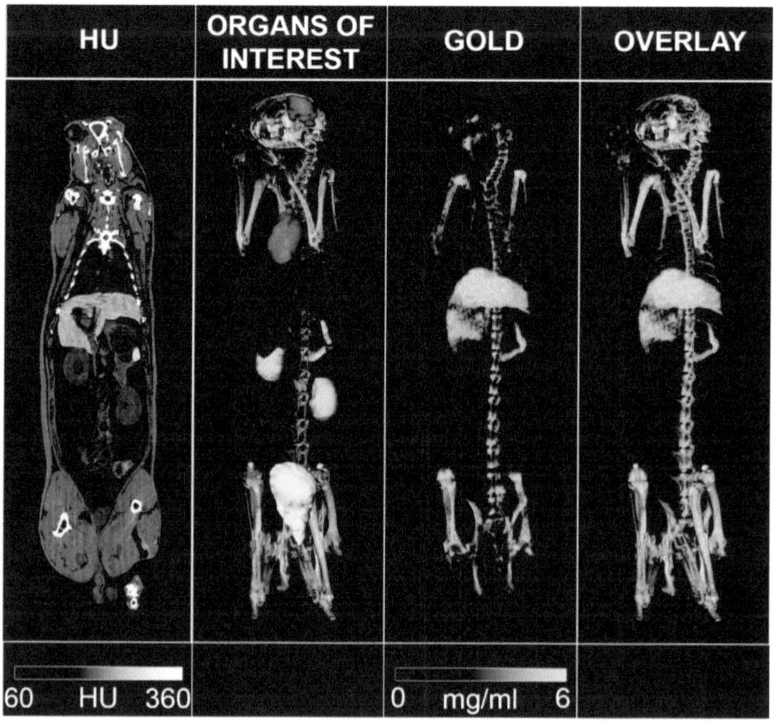

FIGURE 6.16 SPCCT images (conventional, gadolinium K-edge and overlay images) of a rabbit 6 months after injection of pegylated gold nanoparticles. Conventional image did not allow to depict the uptake of the gold nanoparticles. Conversely, K-edge image of gold revealed an excellent depiction of the uptake in the mononuclear phagocyte system, and with a remarkable visualization in the bone marrow, which has been confirmed by ex vivo analysis (47). These findings emphasize the potential of SPCCT for mapping specific tissues due to their uptake of a contrast agent within a clinically significant range of sensitivity and detection threshold (1 mg mL–1) (48) in the scope of future molecular imaging.

combined high-spatial resolution in the perspective of molecular imaging. This explains the recent development of new contrast agents tuned for SPCCT imaging such as targeted nanoparticles containing heavy metals (gold) (5). One of their purposes would be to reach locally high concentrations of heavy atoms for SPCCT detection. However, the challenge of this relies on the possibility, thanks to the exploitation of K-edge detection, to visualize different epitopes in the same anatomical region upon using properly functionalized nanoparticles.

A starting point of this is represented by an in-vivo study (47) on rabbits that demonstrated the specific biodistribution of pegylated gold nanoparticles in the macrophages of the reticuloendothelial system (Figure 6.16). In this study the authors have demonstrated the potential of a SPCCT imaging system for noninvasive quantitative determination of pegylated gold nanoparticle biodistribution in-vivo over time, giving confidence about the impact of SPCCT in the field of molecular imaging.

6.3 CONCLUSION

In conclusion, spectral photon-counting CT imaging represents an emerging field of CT, already existing for clinical use with the DECT systems, and being investigated with the photon-counting CT systems. Preliminary results show the spectral possibilities that the photon-counting technology offers, demonstrating potentially very compelling applications for CVD, organ perfusion, and molecular imaging. Moreover, these findings point to preclinical and clinical applications using multiple types of contrast agents, and also for multiphase imaging in a single scan. In addition, it highlights the need to develop SPCCT specific contrast agents, which could expand the field of CT-based molecular imaging and create new paradigms in diagnostic imaging. This will prepare the evolution of this technology toward non-radioactive intrinsically simultaneous anatomo-molecular imaging with CT in humans as a cost effective and safe new imaging modality.

Acknowledgments: We thank all the participants of the H2020 program, the employees of CERMEP who helped with the experiments, Dr. Philippe Coulon, Dr. Yoad Yagil, Dr. Ewald Roessl, Dr. Klaus Erhard, Dr. David Cormode, Daniel Bar-Ness, Dr. Monica Sigovan, Dr. Pratap Naha, Dr. Ira Blevis, Dr. Felix Kopp, Dr Peter Noel, and Dr. Sara Boccalini.

Funding sources: This project has received funding from the EU's H2020 research and innovation program under the grant agreement No. 633937.

REFERENCES

1. Lehmann LA, Alvarez RE, Macovski A, Brody WR, Pelc NJ, Riederer SJ, et al. Generalized image combinations in dual KvP digital radiography. *Med Phys.* 1981;8(5):659–667.
2. Brody WR, Cassel DM, Sommer FG, Lehmann LA, Macovski A, Alvarez RE, et al. Dual-energy projection radiography: Initial clinical experience. *AJR Am J Roentgenol.* 1981;137(2):201–205.
3. Alvarez RE, Macovski A. Energy-selective reconstructions in x-ray computerized tomography. *Phys Med Biol.* 1976;21(5):733–744.
4. Taguchi K, Frey EC, Wang X, Iwanczyk JS, Barber WC. An analytical model of the effects of pulse pileup on the energy spectrum recorded by energy resolved photon counting x-ray detectors. *Med Phys.* 2010;37(8):3957–3969.
5. Cormode DP, Roessl E, Thran A, Skajaa T, Gordon RE, Schlomka J-P, et al. Atherosclerotic plaque composition: Analysis with multicolor CT and targeted gold nanoparticles. *Radiology.* 2010;256(3):774–782.
6. Taguchi K, Iwanczyk JS. Vision 20/20: Single photon counting x-ray detectors in medical imaging. *Med Phys.* 2013;40(10):100901.
7. Schmitzberger FF, Fallenberg EM, Lawaczeck R, Hemmendorff M, Moa E, Danielsson M, et al. Development of low-dose photon-counting contrast-enhanced tomosynthesis with spectral imaging. *Radiology.* 2011;259(2):558–564.
8. Liu X, Persson M, Bornefalk H, Karlsson S, Xu C, Danielsson M, et al. Spectral response model for a multibin photon-counting spectral computed tomography detector and its applications. *J Med Imaging Bellingham Wash.* 2015;2(3):033502.

9. Shikhaliev PM. Energy-resolved computed tomography: First experimental results. *Phys Med Biol.* 2008;53(20):5595–5613.
10. McCollough CH, Chen GH, Kalender W, Leng S, Samei E, Taguchi K, et al. Achieving routine submillisievert CT scanning: Report from the summit on management of radiation dose in CT. *Radiology.* 2012;264(2):567–580.
11. Si-Mohamed S, Bar-Ness D, Sigovan M, Cormode DP, Coulon P, Coche E, et al. Review of an initial experience with an experimental spectral photon-counting computed tomography system. *Nucl Instrum Methods Phys Res.* 2017;873:27–35.
12. Walsh SLF, Hansell DM. High-resolution CT of interstitial lung disease: A continuous evolution. *Semin Respir Crit Care Med.* 2014;35(1):129–144.
13. Pourmorteza A, Symons R, Henning A, Ulzheimer S, Bluemke DA. Dose efficiency of quarter-millimeter photon-counting computed tomography: First-in-human results. *Invest Radiol.* 2018; 53(6):365–372.
14. Kopp FK, Daerr H, Si-Mohamed S, Sauter AP, Ehn S, Fingerle AA, et al. Evaluation of a preclinical photon-counting CT prototype for pulmonary imaging. *Sci Rep.* 2018;8(1):17386.
15. Le Bihan D. Theoretical principles of perfusion imaging. Application to magnetic resonance imaging. *Invest Radiol.* 1992;27(Suppl 2):S6–11.
16. Felloni P, Duhamel A, Faivre J-B, Giordano J, Khung S, Deken V, et al. Regional distribution of pulmonary blood volume with dual-energy computed tomography: Results in 42 subjects. *Acad Radiol.* 2017;24(11):1412–1421.
17. Meinel FG, Graef A, Thieme SF, Bamberg F, Schwarz F, Sommer WH, et al. Assessing pulmonary perfusion in emphysema: Automated quantification of perfused blood volume in dual-energy CTPA. *Invest Radiol.* 2013;48(2):79–85.
18. Ohno Y, Hatabu H, Higashino T, Takenaka D, Watanabe H, Nishimura Y, et al. Dynamic perfusion MRI versus perfusion scintigraphy: Prediction of postoperative lung function in patients with lung cancer. *AJR Am J Roentgenol.* 2004;182(1):73–78.
19. Meinel FG, Graef A, Thierfelder KM, Armbruster M, Schild C, Neurohr C, et al. Automated quantification of pulmonary perfused blood volume by dual-energy CTPA in chronic thromboembolic pulmonary hypertension. *ROFO Fortschr Geb Rontgenstr Nuklearmed.* 2014;186(2):151–156.
20. Nakazawa T, Watanabe Y, Hori Y, Kiso K, Higashi M, Itoh T, et al. Lung perfused blood volume images with dual-energy computed tomography for chronic thromboembolic pulmonary hypertension: Correlation to scintigraphy with single-photon emission computed tomography. *J Comput Assist Tomogr.* 2011;35(5):590–595.
21. Remy-Jardin M, Faivre J-B, Pontana F, Molinari F, Tacelli N, Remy J. Thoracic applications of dual energy. *Semin Respir Crit Care Med.* 2014;35(1):64–73.
22. Hua C-H, Shapira N, Merchant TE, Klahr P, Yagil Y. Accuracy of electron density, effective atomic number, and iodine concentration determination with a dual-layer dual-energy computed tomography system. *Med Phys.* 2018;45(6):2486–2497.
23. Si-Mohamed S, Cormode DP, Sigovan M, Bar-Ness D, Langlois J, Naha PC, et al. Abstract: In vivo quantitative dynamic angiography with gold nanoparticles and spectral photon-counting computed tomography K-edge imaging. RSNA, Chicago, USA. 2016.
24. Si-Mohamed S, Sigovan, S, Digilio S, Silvio, A, Douek P. Abstract: Potential for highly specific perfusion imaging using gadoteridol and K-edge Spectral Photon Counting CT. RSNA, Chicago, USA. 2017.
25. Lemoine S, Papillard M, Belloi A, Rognant N, Fouque D, Laville M, et al. Renal perfusion: Noninvasive measurement with multidetector CT versus fluorescent microspheres in a pig model. *Radiology.* 2011;260(2):414–420.
26. Si-Mohamed, S, Normand G, Lemoine S, Sigovan M, Bar-Ness D, Langlois J-B, et al. Abstract: Dynamic iodine and gadolinium k-edge kidney perfusion imaging using spectral photon-counting ct. RSNA, Chicago, USA. 2017.
27. Libby P. Inflammation in atherosclerosis. *Nature.* 2002;420(6917):868–874.
28. Malek AM, Alper SL, Izumo S. Hemodynamic shear stress and its role in atherosclerosis. *JAMA.* 1999;282(21):2035–2042.
29. Endarterectomy for asymptomatic carotid artery stenosis. Executive committee for the asymptomatic carotid atherosclerosis study. *JAMA.* 1995;273(18):1421–1428.
30. Randomised trial of endarterectomy for recently symptomatic carotid stenosis: Final results of the MRC European Carotid Surgery Trial (ECST). *Lancet Lond Engl.* 1998;351(9113):1379–1387.
31. Si-Mohamed S, Perrier L, Sigovan M, Bar-Ness D, Douek P. Abstract: Potential for coronary K-edge imaging with Spectral Photon Counting CT. RSNA, Chicago, USA. 2017.

32. Boussel L, Coulon P, Thran A, Roessl E, Martens G, Sigovan M, et al. Photon counting spectral CT component analysis of coronary artery atherosclerotic plaque samples. *Br J Radiol.* 2014;87 (1040):20130798.
33. Mahnken AH. CT imaging of coronary stents: Past, present, and future. *ISRN Cardiol.* 2012;2012:139823.
34. Mannil M, Hickethier T, von Spiczak J, Baer M, Henning A, Hertel M, et al. Photon-Counting CT: High-Resolution Imaging of Coronary Stents. *Invest Radiol.* 2018;53(3):143–149.
35. Sigovan M, Si-Mohamed S, Bar-Ness D, Mitchell J, Langlois J-B, Coulon P, et al. Feasibility of improving vascular imaging in the presence of metallic stents using spectral photon counting CT and K-edge imaging. *Sci Rep.* 2019;9(1):19850.
36. Symons R, De Bruecker Y, Roosen J, Van Camp L, Cork TE, Kappler S, et al. Quarter-millimeter spectral coronary stent imaging with photon-counting CT: Initial experience. *J Cardiovasc Comput Tomogr.* 2018;12(6):509–515.
37. Sigovan M, Coulon P, Si-Mohamed S, Douek P. Abstract:Noninvasive evaluation of coronary artery stenosis: in vitro comparison of a Spectral Photon Counting CT and spectral Dual Layer CT. RSNA, Chicago, USA. 2017.
38. Mewton N, Rapacchi S, Augeul L, Ferrera R, Loufouat J, Boussel L, et al. Determination of the myocardial area at risk with pre- versus post-reperfusion imaging techniques in the pig model. *Basic Res Cardiol.* 2011;106(6):1247–1257.
39. Boussel L, Gamondes D, Staat P, Elicker BM, Revel D, Douek P. Acute chest pain with normal coronary angiogram: Role of contrast-enhanced multidetector computed tomography in the differential diagnosis between myocarditis and myocardial infarction. *J Comput Assist Tomogr.* 2008;32(2):228–232.
40. Cormode DP, Si-Mohamed S, Bar-Ness D, Sigovan M, Naha PC, Balegamire J, et al. Multicolor spectral photon-counting computed tomography: In vivo dual contrast imaging with a high count rate scanner. *Sci Rep.* 2017;7(1):4784.
41. Riederer I, Bar-Ness D, Kimm MA, Si-Mohamed S, Noël PB, Rummeny EJ, et al. Liquid embolic agents in spectral x-ray photon-counting computed tomography using tantalum K-edge imaging. *Sci Rep.* 2019;9(1):5268.
42. Riederer I, Si-Mohamed S, Ehn S, Bar-Ness D, Noël PB, Fingerle AA, et al. Differentiation between blood and iodine in a bovine brain-initial experience with Spectral Photon-Counting Computed Tomography (SPCCT). *PloS One.* 2019;14(2):e0212679.
43. Muenzel D, Bar-Ness D, Roessl E, Blevis I, Bartels M, Fingerle AA, et al. Spectral photon-counting CT: Initial experience with dual-contrast agent K-edge colonography. *Radiology.* 2016;160890.
44. Si-Mohamed S, Thivolet A, Bonnot P-E, Bar-Ness D, Képénékian V, Cormode DP, et al. Improved peritoneal cavity and abdominal organ imaging using a biphasic contrast agent protocol and spectral photon counting computed tomography K-edge imaging. *Invest Radiol.* 2018;53(10):629–639.
45. Galper MW, Saung MT, Fuster V, Roessl E, Thran A, Proksa R, et al. Effect of computed tomography scanning parameters on gold nanoparticle and iodine contrast. *Invest Radiol.* 2012;47(8):475–481.
46. Naha PC, Lau KC, Hsu JC, Hajfathalian M, Mian S, Chhour P, et al. Gold Silver Alloy Nanoparticles (GSAN): An imaging probe for breast cancer screening with dual-energy mammography or computed tomography. *Nanoscale.* 2016;8(28):13740–13754.
47. Si-mohamed S, Cormode D, Bar-Ness D, Sigovan M, Naha PC, Coulon P, et al. Evaluation of spectral photon counting computed tomography K-edge imaging for determination of gold nanoparticle biodistribution in vivo. *Nanoscale.* 2017;9(46):18246–18257.
48. Si-Mohamed S, Bar-Ness D, Boussel L, Douek P. Multicolor imaging with SPCCT: An in vitro study. *Eur Radiol Exp.* 2018;2(1):34.
49. Naha PC, Chhour P, Cormode DP. Systematic in vitro toxicological screening of gold nanoparticles designed for nanomedicine applications. *Toxicol Vitro Int J Publ Assoc BIBRA.* 2015;29(7): 1445–1453.
50. Cai Q-Y, Kim SH, Choi KS, Kim SY, Byun SJ, Kim KW, et al. Colloidal gold nanoparticles as a blood-pool contrast agent for x-ray computed tomography in mice. *Invest Radiol.* 2007;42(12):797–806.
51. Van Der Molen AJ, Cowan NC, Mueller-Lisse UG, Nolte-Ernsting CCA, Takahashi S, Cohan RH, et al. CT urography: Definition, indications and techniques. A guideline for clinical practice. *Eur Radiol.* 2008;18(1):4–17.
52. Si-Mohamed S, Sigovan M, Bar-Ness D, Boussel L, Douek P. Abstract: Spectral Photon-Counting CT multi-phase urinary tract imaging using dual contrast. European Congress of Radiology, Vienne. 2018.
53. Si-Mohamed S, Tatard-Leitman V, Laugerette A et al. Spectral Photon-Counting Computed Tomography (SPCCT): in-vivo single-acquisition multi-phase liver imaging with a dual contrast agent protocol. *Sci Rep.* 2019, https://doi.org/10.1038/s41598-019-44821-z

54. Schirra CO, Brendel B, Anastasio MA, Roessl E. Spectral CT: A technology primer for contrast agent development. *Contrast Media Mol Imaging.* 2014;9(1):62–70.
55. McCollough CH, Leng S, Yu L, Fletcher JG. Dual- and multi-energy CT: Principles, technical approaches, and clinical applications. *Radiology.* 2015;276(3):637–653.
56. Caschera L, Lazzara A, Piergallini L, Ricci D, Tuscano B, Vanzulli A. Contrast agents in diagnostic imaging: Present and future. *Pharmacol Res.* 2016;110:65–75.
57. Pan D, Roessl E, Schlomka J-P, Caruthers SD, Senpan A, Scott MJ, et al. Computed tomography in color: NanoK-enhanced spectral CT molecular imaging. *Angew Chem Int Ed Engl.* 2010;49(50):9635–9639.
58. Pan D, Schirra CO, Senpan A, Schmieder AH, Stacy AJ, Roessl E, et al. An early investigation of ytterbium nanocolloids for selective and quantitative "multicolor" spectral CT imaging. *ACS Nano.* 2012;6(4):3364–3370.
59. Roessl E, Proksa R. K-edge imaging in x-ray computed tomography using multi-bin photon counting detectors. *Phys Med Biol.* 2007;52(15):4679.

7 Spectral CT Imaging Using MARS Scanners

Aamir Y. Raja,[1,3] Steven P. Gieseg,[2,3] Sikiru A. Adebileje,[3,5] Steven D. Alexander,[2] Maya R. Amma,[3] Fatemeh Asghariomabad,[3] Ali Atharifard,[1] Benjamin Bamford,[3] Stephen T. Bell,[1] Srinidhi Bheesette,[3,4] Anthony P. H. Butler,[1–5] Philip H. Butler,[1–5] Pierre Carbonez,[3,4] Alexander I. Chernoglazov,[1,5] Shishir Dahal,[3,7,8] Jérôme Damet,[3,4,9] Niels J. A. de Ruiter,[1–3,5] Robert M. N. Doesburg,[1] Brian P. Goulter,[1] Joseph L. Healy,[1] Praveen K. Kanithi,[2,5] Stuart P. Lansley,[1] Chiara Lowe,[3] V. B. H. Mandalika,[1,2,5] Emmanuel Marfo,[3] Aysouda Matanaghi,[3] Mahdieh Moghiseh,[1,3] Raj K. Panta,[1,3] Hannah M. Prebble,[1] Nanette Schleich,[6] Emily Searle,[2] Jereena S. Sheeja,[3] Rayhan Uddin,[2] Lieza Vanden Broeke,[2] Vivek V. S.,[1] E. Peter Walker,[3] Michael F. Walsh,[1] Manoj Wijesooriya[2]

[1]MARS Bioimaging Limited, Christchurch, New Zealand
[2]University of Canterbury, Christchurch, New Zealand
[3]University of Otago, Christchurch, New Zealand
[4]European Organisation for Nuclear Research (CERN), Geneva, Switzerland
[5]Human Interface Technology Laboratory New Zealand, University of Canterbury, Christchurch, New Zealand
[6]University of Otago, Wellington, New Zealand
[7]Ministry of Health, Nepal
[8]National Academy of Medical Sciences, Kathmandu, Nepal
[9]Institute of Radiation Physics, Lausanne University Hospital, Lausanne, Switzerland

CONTENTS

Medical imaging is key to the diagnosis or assessment of disease response in many areas of medicine. Nevertheless, measuring disease activity, host response and the effectiveness of treatment is frequently indirect, slow, and qualitative unless invasive procedures are performed. Since Hounsfield's revolutionary work in 1972, over 100 million x-ray CT scans are performed annually around the world. CT is well known for its highly detailed anatomical images using an energy-weighted property of x-ray linear attenuation coefficients. However, this type of grayscale CT does not differentiate cell types, nor distinguish different contrast agents from each other. Fortunately, by counting photons and measuring their individual energies, spectral molecular CT has the potential to depict and quantify disease burden, biomarkers of disease activity, drug delivery, and host response, all in an interactive 3D color image obtained in a single scan [1-6]. The immediacy and quantifiable nature of such information will help physicians tailor medical care to the individual patient, making personalized medicine an achievable goal for most people.

7.1 SPECTRAL MOLECULAR CT IMAGING: CONCEPT AND BACKGROUND

In conventional CT systems, photons from the wide x-ray spectrum are attenuated to different degrees depending on a material's atomic composition. The attenuations of different materials are encoded by grayscale (Hounsfield Units or CT number). Conventional CT measures the attenuated signal over the entire range of the broad x-ray spectrum. However, different materials within a conventional CT image may have the same CT numbers at certain concentrations and, therefore, cannot be differentiated from each other.

Alvarez proposed the application of multi-energy/dual-energy CT (DECT) in 1976 [7]; however, the first commercial DECT scanner was developed by Siemens in 2006 [8]. In current commercial DECT systems, materials can be differentiated by two different methods of data acquisition: (1) an x-ray source-based system having two x-ray tubes operating at different voltages or one tube quickly switching between voltages; and (2) a dual-layer detection system in which each layer is sensitive to different x-ray photon energies. Data analysis techniques in DECT exploit the two channels of energy information and the differential x-ray attenuation in each channel to improve information about scanned materials. DECT offers a range of applications including bone removal by a post-processing technique [9], discrimination of calcium from iodine contrast material [10], kidney stone analysis such as discrimination between stones containing uric acid and other materials [11], and abdominal imaging [12]. However, these significant advancements, made in the last decade with DECT, are limited by low-precision information about the x-ray attenuation at different energies. This ultimately limits the capability of DECT for resolving to specific materials. In comparison the ubiquitous energy information provided by energy-discriminating photon-counting spectral detectors overcomes this limitation and enables the discrimination of specific materials. Many new applications utilizing this information are emerging as spectral molecular CT imaging is translated from preclinical research to human imaging.

Other current molecular imaging modalities, especially positron-emission tomography (PET), single photon emission computed tomography (SPECT), magnetic resonance imaging (MRI), and optical, have strengths for viewing biological processes at the molecular and cellular levels but are still far from capturing the whole picture in a majority of cases. PET-CT is the principal spectroscopic imaging modality in current use. It has an exquisite sensitivity (ng/mL) due to the radioactive isotopes used, but in general is not chemically or tissue specific; the nature of the tissue identified has to be inferred from an anatomical or clinical context. MRI has excellent soft tissue contrast but is slow, has poor spatial resolution, and cannot be used for patients with either claustrophobia or metallic implants. Optical molecular imaging is sensitive and specific but its limited penetration depth prevents it from being translated for most clinical tasks.

In consideration, an ideal molecular imaging device would measure multiple intrinsic biomarkers at biological concentrations and measure introduced biomarker labels at the lowest possible concentration anywhere in the body, all in the same image.

Spectral Molecular CT Imaging is the imaging of cellular and molecular targets. The spatial dimensions of these targets are significantly smaller than the intrinsic spatial resolution typically available in standard CT systems. MARS imaging exploits high spatial and energy resolution to identify spectral signatures of targeted materials and tissues at typical spatial resolutions of 50–100 μm depending on the application. This capability has been made possible by the advent of the energy-discriminating photon-counting detector [13], which has opened the door to radically new approaches to medical investigation and monitoring. Analogous to a prism splitting white light into a rainbow of colors; a spectral detector simultaneously captures x-ray attenuation information across multiple energy ranges in a single exposure. The photon-counting nature of these detectors eliminates so-called dark current noise in the intensity domain, significantly improving overall imaging performance at low x-ray exposure levels. These capabilities allow spectral molecular CT imaging to characterize and quantify multiple tissues and materials such as extrinsic biomarkers of biological processes at the tissue, cellular and molecular levels.

The energy-resolving capability of these detectors is a key aspect of the technology. The detector has a semiconductor x-ray sensor layer and electronics [13]. When x-ray photons interact with the sensor layer, the charge generated by each photon interaction is proportional to its energy. The detector electronics process these photon interactions to collect the charge and count the number of photons arriving at the detector in a series of energy bands. This provides the energy-dependent x-ray attenuation information used to identify and quantify scanned materials. Photon-processing detectors with high-atomic number (Z) sensor materials, such as CdTe and CdZnTe, have a high efficiency of photon detection and energy conversion, well above that available in conventional CT, thus radiation dose to the patient will be considerably less than for conventional CT.

At energies relevant to human diagnostic imaging (20–140 keV), x-rays interact predominantly by a combination of the photoelectric (approximately proportional to Z^3/E^3) and Compton effects (approximately proportional to $1/E$) [14]. In general, the linear attenuation coefficient (LAC) decreases with increasing photon energy, except at absorption edges such as the K-edge, and the photon energy of these absorption edges increases with increasing Z. The K-edges of elements between iodine ($Z = 53$) and bismuth ($Z = 83$) lie within the human diagnostic range for spectral molecular CT imaging.

Counting photons and measuring their individual energies can generate a spectral CT image in full-3D color. Different tissue components and contrast agents (lipid, calcium, intravenous high-Z contrast agents, specific cell types, or biomarkers tagged with high-Z metal nanoparticles) can be portrayed in different colors and the concentration of each component denoted by the shade or hue of the color. Each component or element has a unique energy absorption profile. Essentially, the spectral detector measures the energy of each photon to identify it and counts the number of photons with that energy to establish the concentration or quantity, regardless of the anatomic or physiological context.

At present, up to eight different materials have been identified from a single scan using a cutting-edge spectral detector, the Medipix3RX, developed by European Organization for Nuclear Research (CERN) [15]. This detector has a pixel pitch of 110 μm and is capable of separating adjacent elements on the periodic table. As photon-processing detector development progresses, it is expected that the number of simultaneously distinguishable materials per voxel will increase. In effect, spectral molecular CT is the imaging equivalent of combining multiple specific stains used in histology, except that the spectral image is of living tissue *in situ* within the body.

Laboratory and preclinical spectral molecular CT results have been very encouraging, but the question of how spectral molecular CT imaging will be used in clinical practice still remains. The fact is we cannot predict the particular clinical application that will drive the adoption of this disruptive technology. The ability of spectral CT to measure drug delivery, quantify inflammatory response, and characterize tissue components has potential application across a wide range of diseases. Currently, preclinical spectral CT imaging research is focusing on atherosclerosis [16-19], cancer [20-23], and bone [14, 24-26] and cartilage [5, 27] diseases as patients with these pathologies are likely to benefit from an imaging modality that simultaneously quantifies disease activity, disease burden, drug delivery, and response to treatment.

This chapter focuses on the state-of-the-art preclinical MARS scanner and its applications. The scanner is designed and produced by MARS Bioimaging Ltd. in collaboration with the University of

Canterbury (School of Physical and Chemical Sciences and the HITLab NZ) and the University of Otago, Christchurch (Department of Radiology and Centre for Bioengineering), both in New Zealand.

7.2 MARS SCANNER

The MARS scanner is a desk-sized, self-standing spectral molecular CT scanner built around the Medipix detector family of photon-counting detectors. The current version of the MARS spectral scanner is designed for biomedical research users and is suitable for preclinical spectral imaging of small animal models and human samples of diseased tissue. The self-standing cabinet provides a stand-alone turnkey spectral molecular CT imaging system and contains a rotating gantry, MARS camera, cabinet controller, x-ray source, computer hardware and software as shown in Figure 7.1. Separate computer systems are provided for the scanner control and image processing (reconstruction and material analysis).

The camera consists of three main components: (1) an array of MARS fingerboards, on which the ASIC (Medipix3RX) and high-Z sensor layer (typically cadmium zinc telluride, CZT) assembly is mounted; (2) an array of readout boards that provide a 1GbE connection between each ASIC and the control computer, and (3) a bias voltage board, which provides a programmable bias voltage to the sensor layer used for charge collection, and settable from (negative) 50 V to 800 V. The modular design of the MARS camera allows the camera to be supplied with different sensor array configurations depending on user requirements; for example, arrays of $1 \times N$ or $2 \times N$. The MARS camera readout system using Medipix3RX has been described elsewhere [28].

Standard calibration modules are provided. *Threshold equalization* with respect to the noise floor and energy calibration of the detector is performed during initial camera setup, and periodic maintenance. Threshold equalization involves per-pixel calibration to reduce the intrinsic variations in the threshold levels associated with each counter and provides a consistent individual pixel response to a uniform x-ray flux [29]. *Energy calibration* is performed to characterize the energy response of the detector with respect to reference energies such as x-ray fluorescence (XRF) emitted from metallic foils (Mo and Pb) and γ-rays emitted from an Am-241 radioisotope [30].

The gantry of the MARS scanner supports a full-scan with a microfocus poly-energetic x-ray source (Source-Ray SB-120-350 x-ray tube; Source-Ray Inc., Ronkonkoma, NY, USA) and a MARS camera assembly under precise control around a specimen or animal up to 100 mm in diameter and 300 mm in length.

The raw data in DICOM format is transferred from the scanner's server to the scanner's inbuilt picture archive and communication system (PACS), where automated image processing is

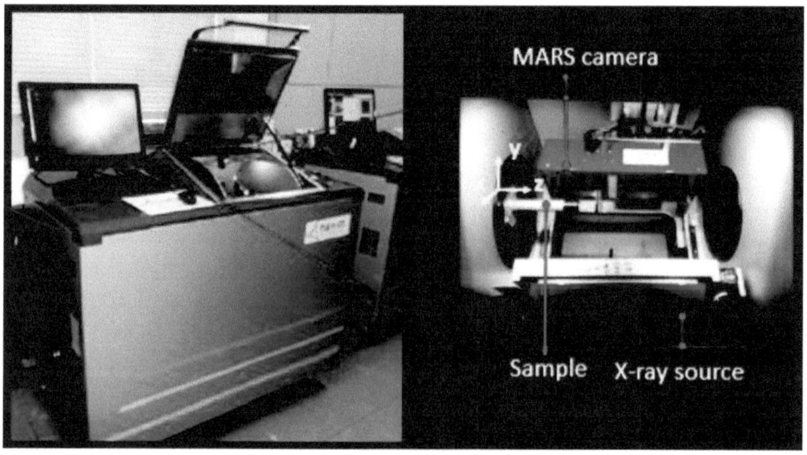

FIGURE 7.1 MARS scanner. Inside view shows x-ray source, camera, phantom sample placed between the MARS camera and x-ray source, and geometry.

performed. The image processing has three stages: pre-reconstruction processing, reconstruction into attenuation volumes, and decomposition into material volumes.

The pre-reconstruction processing consists of three steps: the first step is pixel masking to remove any bad pixels; the second step is flat field correction [31, 32]; and the final step is ring filtration. The ring filter is based on the work by Jan Sijbers and Andrei Postnov [33], but applied to the projection data and adapted into 3D to exploit more information provided by the detector (x, y, and theta). The reconstruction uses a low-resolution version of the polychromatic form of the Beer-Lambert Law. This means that the overlapping, low-threshold counters that measure the data are processed simultaneously to produce attenuation volumes representing non-overlapping energy bins across the measured spectrum. For example, four counters representing the energy ranges 30–120, 45–120, 60–120, and 78–120 keV would simultaneously produce four attenuation volumes representing the energy ranges 30–45, 45–60, 60–78, and 78–120 keV.

Processing the counters simultaneously exploits all photons available in the scan. Consider the attenuation volume for 78–120 keV. All four counters contribute to this volume. The counter for 60–120 keV provides specific information about the energy range but has fewer photons (higher statistical noise). The counter for 30–120 keV is less specific but contains all the photons in the scan (lower statistical noise). Given that the counter measurements are acquired simultaneously, we know each counter maps the same structures. This reconstruction process uses all photons available in the wider counters to reconstruct clean boundaries and structures while using the narrower counters to guarantee that the correct energy response is obtained.

The reconstruction algorithm itself is a statistical iterative technique. It uses multiplicative correction terms similar to OSEM [34], or MART [35]. The statistical element is introduced by weighting the corrections to the volume by a normalized Poisson distribution to slow down convergence when approaching the solution, thereby reducing noise. The reconstruction algorithm also adopts a multi-stage approach where it initially reconstructs voxels that are eight times larger than requested. Later on, this is repeatedly subdivided for a total of four stages until the requested voxel size is reached [36]. This approach allows for the reconstruction to proceed quickly. It is also a weak form of a sparsity constraint as a large voxel is the same as a set of small voxels with the same value. Lastly, the larger the voxel, the more pixels from the projection images will contribute to it. This reduces the effect of dead regions. This is particularly useful during the initial reconstruction stages where the effects of dead regions are the most significant.

The quantitative diagnostic information (decomposed volume) about the material composition of the sample is extracted by applying material decomposition (MARS-MD) at high spatial resolution (<100 microns). Material decomposition is the process of converting spectral attenuation (energy information) into information about the constituent materials contributing to that attenuation. This typically involves obtaining material properties inverting the mass attenuation equation for one of its variants (i.e., volume fraction [37], Compton-photoelectric [7], or ρZ [38, 39]). The weighted average x-ray attenuation of a compound or mixture of the constituent materials is given by

$$\mu_E = \sum_{i=1}^{m} \rho_m \left(\frac{\mu}{\rho}\right)_{mE} \tag{7.1}$$

In this equation, μ_E is the linear attenuation of some composite material for a given energy range E. The material properties desired are the densities of the constituent materials (indexed by m). These are proportionally connected to the linear attenuation through the mass attenuation of the respective materials $(\mu / \rho)_{mE}$ for the given energy ranges. Since attenuation varies differently with energy for different materials, such material properties can be deduced when using multiple energies.

The MARS scanner image processing chain incorporates MARS-MD for converting reconstructed energy bins into sparse material images [40, 41]. This heuristic image space algorithm follows a three-step process for assigning materials to each voxel: (1) each voxel classified as either high, low, or insignificantly attenuating; (2) a calculation of uniquely constrained least squares decomposition for each feasible pair of materials falling into the respective attenuation category; and (3) a classification of the result which has the smallest regression error. The output of this process is that every voxel is assigned the 1 or 2 materials with the most significant contribution to the voxel's attenuation. The algorithm is calibrated using mass attenuation coefficients estimated from reconstructed phantom data. For more details on this algorithm, we direct the reader to our paper [42]. To measure the amount of misidentification between different materials, a metric is generated for quantitative evaluation of post-MD volumes of the calibration phantom that provides sensitivity (true positive rate) and specificity (true negative rate) for correct material identification at various material concentrations [43].

7.3 PRECLINICAL APPLICATIONS OF MARS IMAGING

7.3.1 Bone Health – Osteoporosis

Bone strength comprises bone mineral density (BMD), bone quality, and bone composition [44]. Current methods to measure bone strength or quality are limited to plain x-ray for assessing fractures, and dual x-ray absorptiometry (DXA) for assessing BMD.

The DXA definition of osteoporosis is population-based and does not provide an actual risk assessment for the individual. A clinical assessment of fracture risk (FRAX, the WHO risk assessment tool) has been developed to try and fill this gap, but it is not enough. Fracture risk is related to physical and structural deficiencies at high-risk bone sites. Neither DXA nor FRAX assesses the bone strength or bone quality at these sites in individuals [45] and without this knowledge the development of novel therapeutic agents and improved clinical management is constrained.

At present, bone turnover is measured using serum markers. A synchrotron can perform the required bone quality assessment; however, this football field size device is not convenient for human imaging. Trabecular and cortical bone are metabolically different, and therefore should be measured separately. High-resolution peripheral quantitative CT (HR-pQCT) is a research tool using standard CT detectors that can measure both bone strength and load-bearing properties but its relatively small size restricts analysis to peripheral sites (distal tibia and radius), and the most common osteoporotic fracture sites (such as the hip and spine) cannot be directly assessed [46, 47]. Effective bone quality/strength assessment techniques need to be able to be translated from the research laboratory to clinical practice. Simultaneous assessment of bone density and structure in 3D images will help toward the development of treatment for people with bone and joint diseases, reducing burden and improving quality of life.

Bone density and structure of both normal and osteoporotic bone have been assessed using the MARS scanner. Preliminary research has identified that the MARS scanner, incorporating CZT-Medipix3RX detectors, can provide material-based quantitative assessment for bone strength that combines the measurement of bone microarchitecture features (trabecular/cortex at $<70\ \mu m$ scale) and BMD (by measuring calcium hydroxyapatite (HA) concentration in mg/mL) in a way that can translate to human imaging. Figure 7.2 shows the simultaneous measurement of bone density and thickness in the cortex and trabeculae of human femoral neck samples, which compare favorably to HR-pQCT and DXA [27, 48].

7.3.2 Cartilage Health – Osteoarthritis

Osteoarthritis (OA) is a chronic degenerative joint disease characterized mainly by the degeneration of the articular cartilage, which in turn leads to loss of mobility and pain. It is considered as the underlying cause of nearly all knee and hip joint replacements [49]. This is the most common type of arthritis leading to joint arthroplasty worldwide [50]. It occurs as a result of the mechanical breakdown of the articular cartilage and underlying subchondral bone. Several factors contribute to OA including obesity, injury or overuse and genes, and it has a higher prevalence in women and people over the age of 60 [51].

Sulfated glycosaminoglycans (GAG or sGAG), negatively charged proteins that aid cartilage in resisting compressive loads, are sensitive markers of cartilage degradation and loss of joint function in early OA [52]. GAG is zonally distributed through the depth of articular cartilage, with the

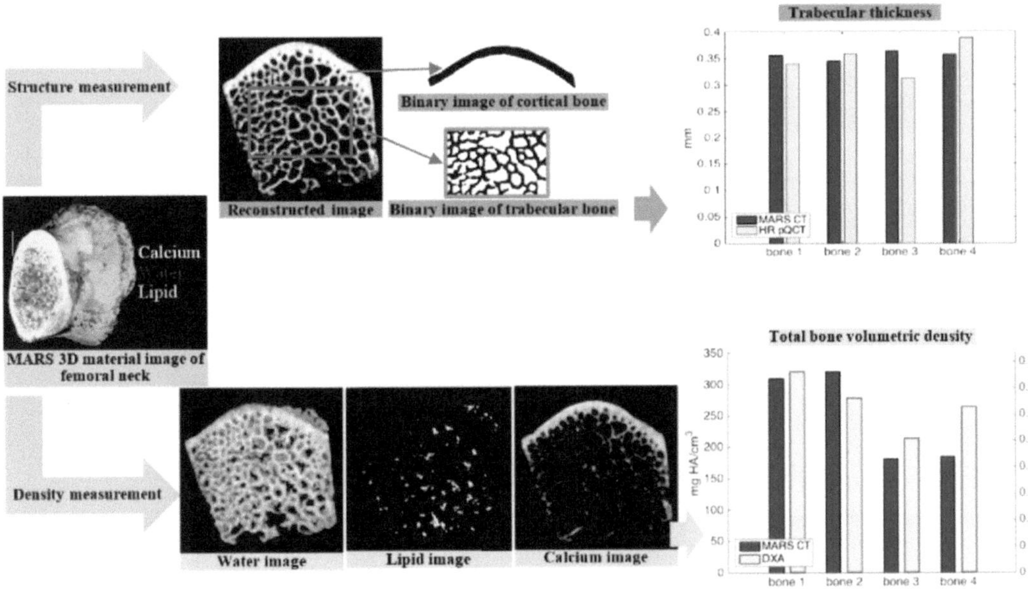

FIGURE 7.2 Simultaneous measurement of bone microstructure and bone mineral density by a MARS scanner. The two graphs show that the MARS results are favorably comparable to HR-pQCT and DXA.

superficial layer containing less GAG relative to the deep layer [53-55]. This zonal distribution of GAG is traditionally measured by destructive techniques such as histology [56] or biochemical methods [57]. In OA, the GAG level in the superficial zone is further deteriorated [51].

Current research methods for determining GAG content include histological staining with Safranin O or Toluidine blue [56] or quantified by 1,9-dimethylmethylate blue (DMMB) colorimetric assay [57]. All these methods are destructive to the sample, such that the sample can no longer be studied, limiting their usefulness for studying changes in GAG over time. Non-destructive methods for determining GAG content are thus particularly valuable, not only for clinical use for detecting early OA changes and thus allowing prompt treatment but also for research purposes, enabling measurement of GAG content over time for studying OA pathogenesis and cartilage response to novel treatment modalities.

The main diagnostic imaging technique used for OA is plain radiographs, from which it is not possible to directly visualize the cartilage. Instead, the thickness is estimated by looking at the joint space width, which is narrowed in OA due to the wearing away of the cartilage [58]. Other radiographic features include sclerosis, osteophytosis and subchondral cysts [59], all of which are late-stage changes, and by the time they are visible, permanent joint damage has occurred. MRI and standard CT imaging have shown some promise for detecting early OA and assessment of cartilage treatment, as well as for semi-quantifying the quality of new cartilage repair strategies [60, 61]. However, quantitative imaging of an *in situ* biomarker of cartilage health is a more desirable strategy [62].

As mentioned, GAG is negatively charged and thus repels other negatively charged molecules. This gives rise to the phenomenon of Equilibrium Partitioning of an Ionic Contrast (EPIC), whereby the electrostatic interaction between GAG and a charged contrast agent results in a non-uniform distribution of the contrast agent, reflecting the GAG distribution. This is exploited in EPIC micro-CT [56, 63], a technique used preclinically with the Hexabrix contrast agent. However, the x-ray attenuation of bone and Hexabrix-equilibrated soft tissue can overlap, thus limiting its ability to segment between subchondral bone and cartilage.

Preliminary work has shown that the MARS scanner can provide a high-resolution, non-destructive method to quantify iodine-based contrast agent (Hexabrix) uptake in articular cartilage (as shown in Figure 7.3) as a marker of GAG (through an inverse relationship) and relate cartilage health

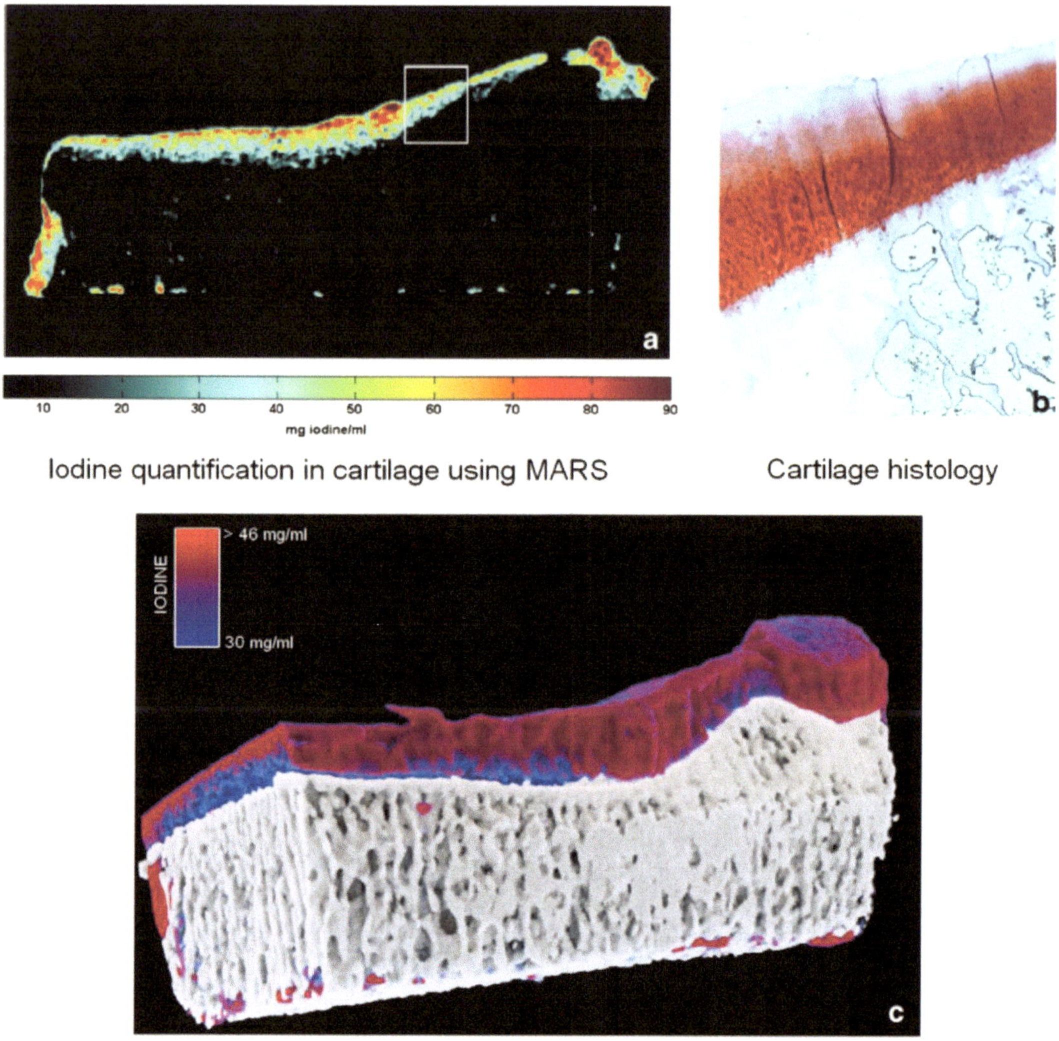

FIGURE 7.3 Quantitative imaging of excised human osteoarthritic cartilage using MARS scanner. Correlation between iodine map (a) and a histological section (b) of the human tibial plateau. The histological section in (b) is the approximate location in the boxed region in (a). An inverse correlation between iodine uptake in the cartilage and GAG density (bright red corresponds to dense GAG in top right image) can be noticed. 3D material decomposed volume of the tibial plateau strip (c) shows the iodine distribution throughout the cartilage. The iodine channel is displayed quantitatively using a blue-red color map. Retrieved with permission from Rajendran et al., *European Radiology*, vol. 27, no. 1, pp. 384–392, Jan 2017.

to the status of subchondral bone. Subsequent to this, discrimination and quantification of GAG using a clinically utilized Gd-based contrast agent in healthy bovine cartilage has also been reported [43].

These preliminary findings show that spectral molecular imaging has the potential to monitor cartilage degradation or repair; however, there are several important milestones yet to be reached before it is ready for clinical practice. These include but are not limited to: determining whether anionic or cationic contrast is the preferred contrast; determining the optimal contrast agent for *in vivo* human cartilage imaging; dosage, timing, and administration method for contrast; characterization of subchondral bone with respect to articular cartilage status; and maturation of cartilage repair strategies. It is believed that overcoming these barriers to clinical translation is achievable and spectral imaging methods have great potential to image and quantify cartilage health.

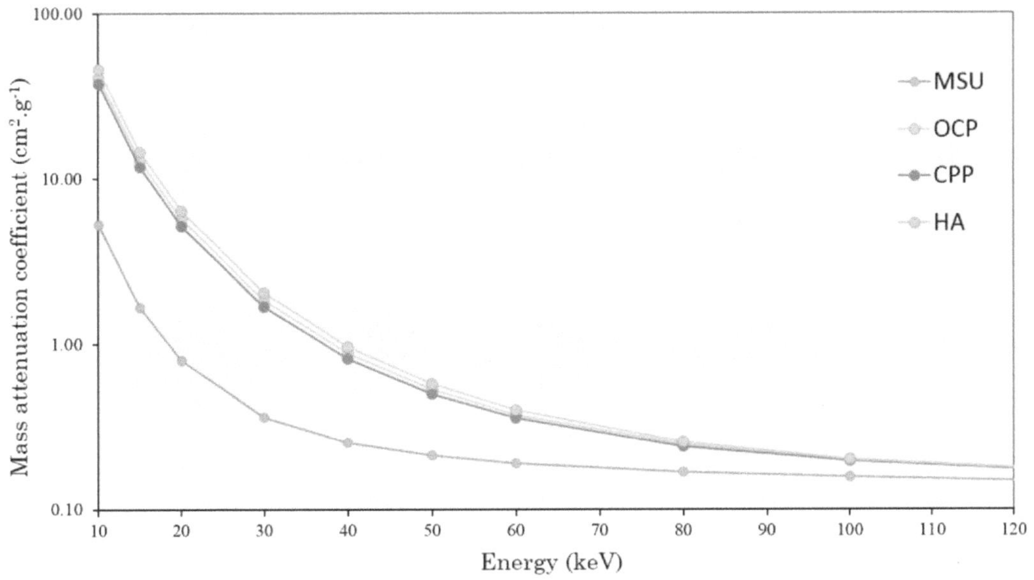

FIGURE 7.4 A logarithmic plot of x-ray mass attenuation of various crystals as a function of photon energy. Monosodium urate (MSU), octacalcium phosphate (OCP), calcium pyrophosphate dihydrate (CPP), and calcium hydroxyapatite (HA). It illustrates that the x-ray attenuation between OCP, CPP, and HA is almost overlapping.

7.3.3 Crystal-Induced Arthropathies

The prevalence of crystal-induced arthropathies (CIA) – gout (monosodium urate, MSU), pseudogout (calcium pyrophosphate dihydrate, CPP), calcium hydroxyapatite (CHA or HA), and octacalcium phosphate (OCP) – is increasing. Distinguishing crystal type, whether MSU or one of the calcium crystal types, is a clinical challenge because diagnosis and treatment depend on the crystal type involved. Therefore, it is clinically relevant to be able to noninvasively distinguish between calcium compounds. Figure 7.4 shows different calcium crystals with almost overlapping x-ray attenuation profiles.

Some of these calcium depositions also pose a diagnostic challenge in breast, cardiovascular, and genitourinary imaging. The K-edge of calcium (4.0 keV) is too low to be used in conventional x-ray imaging and DXA or DECT operating in the human energy range. The reference standard for the diagnosis of crystal arthritis requires aspiration of synovial fluid or tophus and direct visualization of crystals by polarized light microscopy [64]. In the case of gout, MSU crystals appear needle-shaped and negatively birefringent, and CPP crystals are typically monoclinic or triclinic with weak positive or no birefringence. HA and OCP crystals cannot be detected by polarized light microscopy. However, crystal identification is operator dependent and may be suboptimal particularly for crystals other than MSU. Also, aspiration of an acutely inflamed joint is painful and, while rare, joint aspiration may also be associated with complications such as iatrogenic infection.

Other imaging modalities such as ultrasound and DECT are being increasingly used to aid in the diagnosis of gout. A recent study showed that DECT can also detect CPP crystals with a reported sensitivity and specificity of 78% and 94%, respectively [64]. However, the role of these imaging techniques is less well defined in other crystal deposition diseases and cannot easily distinguish between different calcium crystals. The ability to reliably detect and differentiate MSU, CPP, HA, and OCP crystals using noninvasive imaging would be an advancement.

Although similar attenuation coefficients limit the differentiation of different calcium crystals, spectral CT imaging potentially provides a method to overcome this limitation [65, 66]. Using the MARS scanner, differences in LACs between the various crystal suspensions were compared using

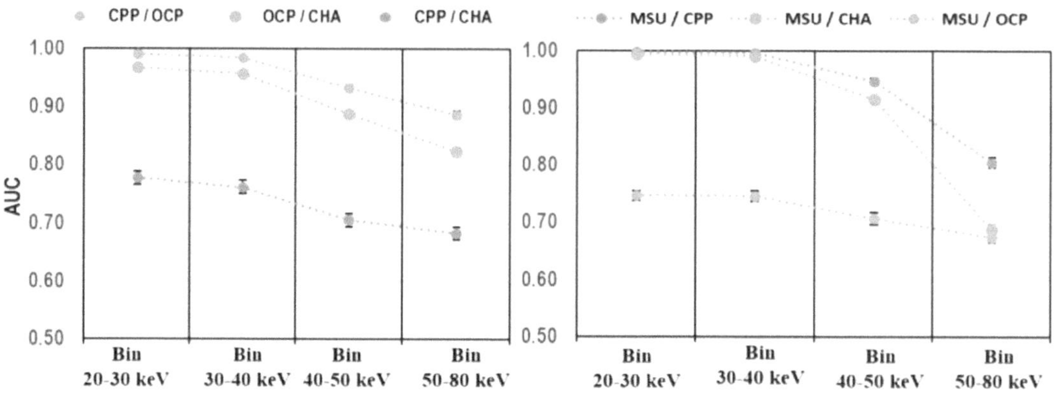

FIGURE 7.5 AUC results as a function of energy bins for all crystal combinations. Error bars represent the 95% confidence interval. Retrieved with permission from Viry et al., Proc. SPIE 10573, *Medical Imaging*, 2018; doi:10.1117/12.2293458.

the receiver operating characteristic (ROC) paradigm. Figure 7.5 shows areas under the ROC curves (AUC) for four crystal types pairwise. Preliminary results indicate that MARS can accurately differentiate MSU from CPP and HA, CPP from OCP, and OCP from HA *in vitro*. The distinction between MSU and OCP, and CPP and HA is more challenging.

7.3.4 Bone Imaging with Metal Implants

Metallic devices (dental implants and joint replacements) are widely used in dentistry and orthopedics. Titanium metallic implants for biological fixation in the form of mesh, plate, screw, or scaffold are becoming increasingly popular for orthopedic and dental applications due to excellent biocompatibility, corrosion resistance, and mechanical strength [67]. Bone tumors, infections, and accidents make bone repair and regeneration a substantial challenge in orthopedics, and therefore surgical procedures such as autografts, allografts, or alloplastic (biomaterials) are usually performed for major bone reconstruction [68].

In implant research, destructive methods, such as histology and scanning electron microscopy, are used for histomorphometric assessment of bone growth/loss around implants. In clinical practice, CT and plain x-ray radiographs are used to assess the bone-metal interface. However, the presence of metallic biomaterial implants leads to metal artefacts in CT imaging due to beam hardening and photon starvation [25].

Beam hardening occurs when low-energy x-ray photons from a polychromatic x-ray spectrum are attenuated more easily, and the remaining high-energy photons are attenuated less easily. Therefore, beam transmission does not follow the simple exponential decrease seen with a monochromatic x-ray beam. Photon starvation is also considered as a byproduct of beam hardening and happens when the detector has low-photon counts due to a severe attenuation of the beam by dense metal implants.

Beam hardening related artefacts appear as bright and dark streaks and also as a cupping effect, affecting the metal and nonmetal regions in the reconstructed image. It is important to highlight that beam hardening occurs in all tissues, but artefacts are most evident in the vicinity of dense materials such as metal, dense bone, and contrast agents. These artefacts severely limit assessment of any tissue adjacent to or within a metal structure such as dental amalgam or tooth implant, orthopedic implants and fixation devices, or metallic foreign bodies. Figure 7.6 shows an example of a cupping effect where a horizontal line profile passing through the center of the metal cylinder reveals the effect of beam hardening.

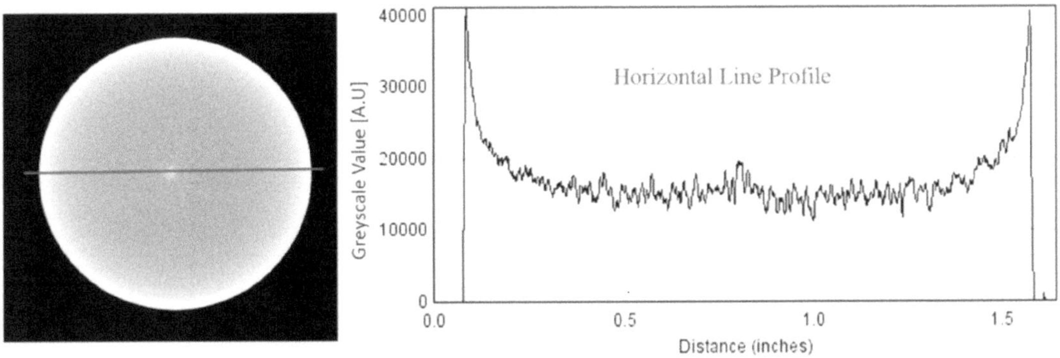

FIGURE 7.6 An example of CT image of the uniform cylindrical phantom (left) and its line profile (right) shows x-rays passing through the middle portion of a phantom are hardened more than those passing through the edges because they are passing through more material.

Hardware filters are commonly used to pre-harden the beam, that is, remove low-energy photons from the beam. However, this process results in poor signal-to-noise ratio, as the soft x-rays provide good contrast information. Mathematical beam hardening corrections are the most commonly used techniques [69]. Dual-energy correction methods [70] image the atomic number dependent photo-electric component and the density-dependent Compton scatter component separately and use them to correct for beam hardening, at the cost of increased exposure.

Photon counting detectors have the unique advantage of capturing information from multiple energy ranges simultaneously. The ability of photon-counting detectors to separate out the high-energy photons (which have least beam-hardening) can be exploited to minimize metal artefacts in spectral CT imaging. This information can be discretely extracted without introducing any major external estimations or corrections within the spectral CT system. Additionally, capturing mid-energy ranges may provide a tradeoff between reduced metal artefacts and high-soft tissue contrast.

Figure 7.7 shows MARS images of a porous 3D lattice structure of titanium (Ti) scaffold (facilitates bone ingrowth into the implant's pores) with 700-μm-thick struts. The bright streaks artefacts around the Ti surface in the lower energy ranges contribute to the increased grayscale values for air due to beam hardening artefacts. The artefacts are less pronounced in higher energies and virtually eliminated at the highest energy bin [25].

Figure 7.8 shows improvement in image quality of a Ti screw in excised sheep bone at higher energies. The image at 20–120 keV exhibits the highest contrast difference (2.44 cm^1) between bone and metal, but the attenuation coefficients along the length of the screw were inhomogeneous due

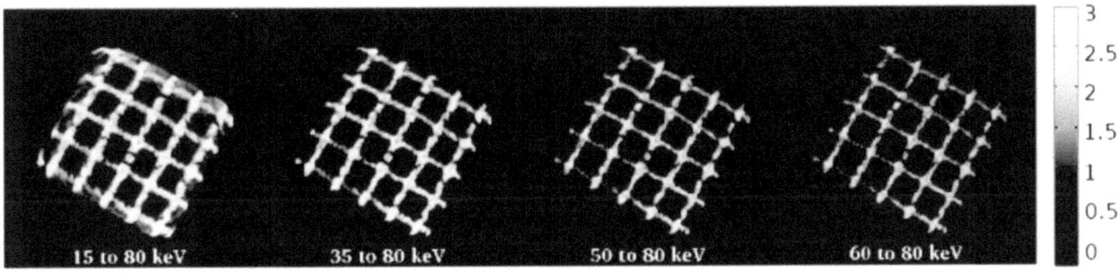

FIGURE 7.7 MARS images of a Ti scaffold sample. Contrast-to-noise ratio (CNR) between metal and air (with bright streaks) in the energy ranges is 4.8, 5.4, 7.9, 8.1, respectively. The color bar represents linear attenuation coefficients (cm^{-1}). Retrieved with permission from K. Rajendran et al., Reducing beam hardening and metal artefacts in spectral CT using Medipix3RX. *Journal of Instrumentation*, vol. 9, P03015, March 2014.

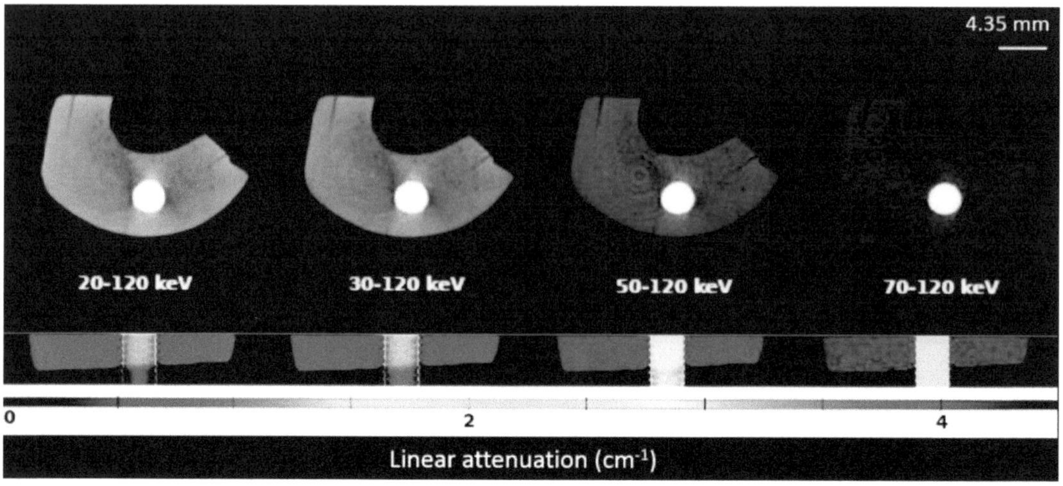

FIGURE 7.8 (Top row) MARS images of a Ti screw in excised sheep bone at multiple energy bins. The streak artefacts at the bone-metal (screw) interface are less pronounced at higher energy bins and virtually eliminated at the highest energy band. The scale bar indicates linear attenuation (cm^{-1}). (Bottom row) The coronal images of a segment of the sample (at the top row) reveal the inconsistency in the metal regions at low-energy bins. The scale bar indicates linear attenuation (cm^{-1}). Retrieved from K. Rajendran, PhD thesis, "MARS spectral CT for orthopaedic applications," Department of Radiology and Centre for Bioengineering, University of Otago, Otago School of Medicine, Christchurch, New Zealand, 2016 [71].

to different degrees of beam hardening by the surrounding bone and air. The image at 70–120 keV shows homogeneous attenuation by the screw as a result of less beam hardening but the metal-bone contrast difference was reduced to 1.56 cm^1. Although a significant amount of work is required, these preliminary results from the MARS scanner pave the way to produce novel imaging methods for dental and orthopedic implant characterization, and for imaging of tissues/scaffolds used in regenerative medicine.

7.3.5 Cancer Imaging with Nanoparticles

Cancers can have variable biomarker expression between primary and metastasis, and over time [72-74]. The small sample obtained at biopsy may not always reflect this variation, and this limits the effectiveness of targeted treatments. Cancer therapies that specifically target markers on or in cancer cells are highly preferred for advancing personalized cancer treatment [75]. Diagnosis, therefore, needs a new approach for noninvasively and specifically identifying biomarkers relevant to treatment strategies and showing how they vary between tumor sites and over time.

Nano-contrast agents can be targeted to a specific cancer biomarker. Inorganic metal nanoparticles can be surface-coated so that they conjugate to the desired cell or molecule, and are made safe to travel in the bloodstream (biocompatibility). These coated nanoparticles are then known as functionalized nanoparticles. Functionalization can be affected using ligands, peptides, antibodies, micelles, liposomes, or nanorods. By attaching antibodies, proteins or other ligands, nanoparticles are used for tumor cell targeting.

We, and others, have exploited the use of the K-edge in spectral molecular CT imaging of gold nanoparticles (AuNPs) tagged to *in situ* biomarkers [20, 76-78]. We have tested MARS with a range of iodine, gadolinium, and gold concentrations and, currently, our system is able to detect concentrations below 1 μg/μL with high sensitivity as shown in Figure 7.9 [79].

The uptake of different sizes of AuNPs (18, 40, 60, and 80 nm) and concentrations (6.4, 12.8, 25.6, and 38.5 μg Au/mL) in SKOV3 and OVCAR5 ovarian cancer cells is studied. The aim was

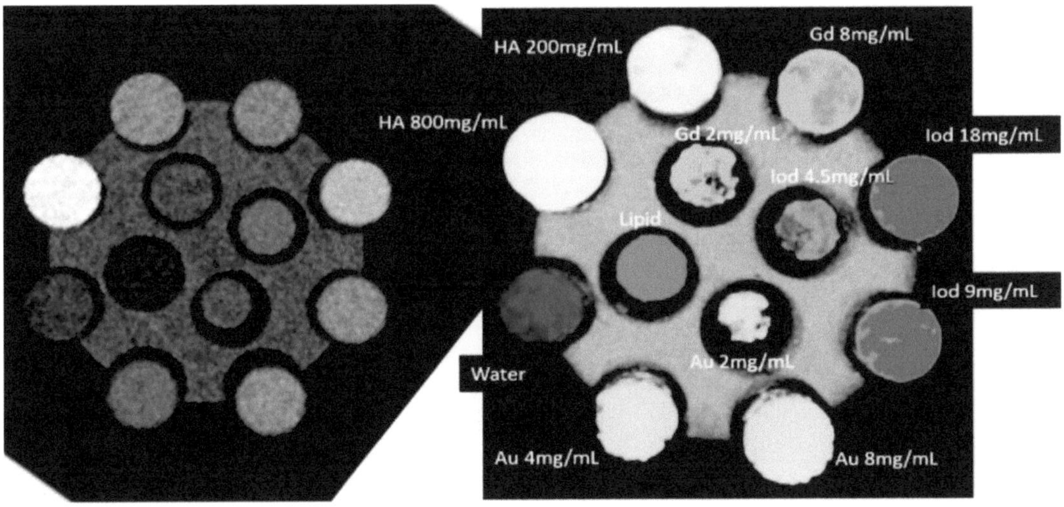

FIGURE 7.9 Identification of MARS image into individual elements. Left: MARS image with one of the energy bins (18–30 keV). Right: Screen shot of 3D volume rendering of composite materials showing gold (yellow), iodine (red), gadolinium (green), hydroxyapatite (white), lipid (magenta), and water (blue).

to optimize a system of functionalized nanoparticles that will be preferentially taken up by mouse ovarian cancer cell line *in vitro* [20]. Figure 7.10 shows that when these cell clumps are imaged with MARS, gold can be measured accurately and the uptake of different concentrations and sizes of AuNPs in OVCAR5 and SKOV3 ovarian cancer cells can be measured.

Figure 7.11 shows a proof of concept using a similar methodology as stated above; AuNPs monoclonal antibodies and MARS imaging show *in vitro* proof of principle that spectral molecular CT can measure gold-labeled specific antibodies targeted to specific cancer cells. A crossover study was performed with Raji lymphoma cancer cells and HER2 positive SKBR3 breast cancer cells using

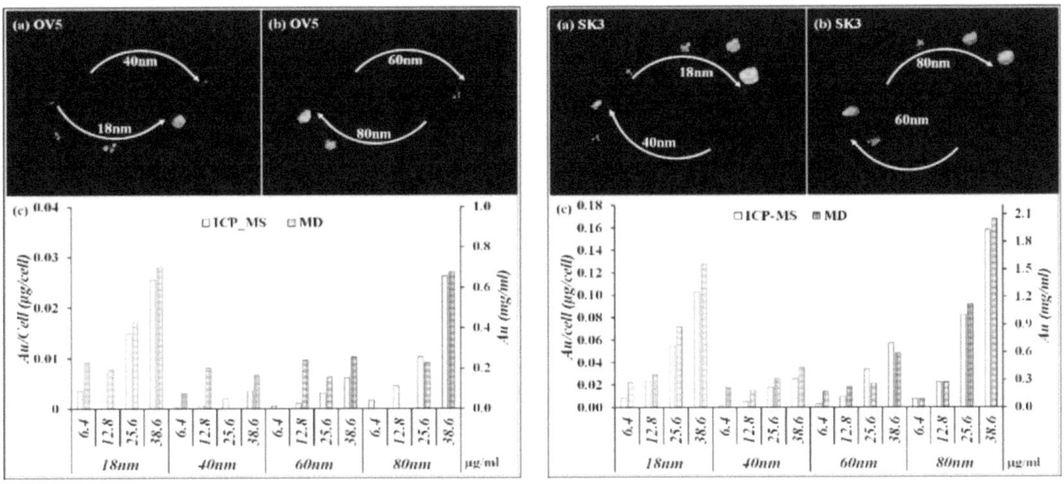

FIGURE 7.10 MARS-MD images of OVCAR5 cells (left) and SKOV3 cells (right) with AuNPs (a & b) and (c) are gold/cell (calculated based on ICP-MS and DNA Quantification) along with quantification of gold by MARS spectral imaging. Arrows direct lower to higher concentration.

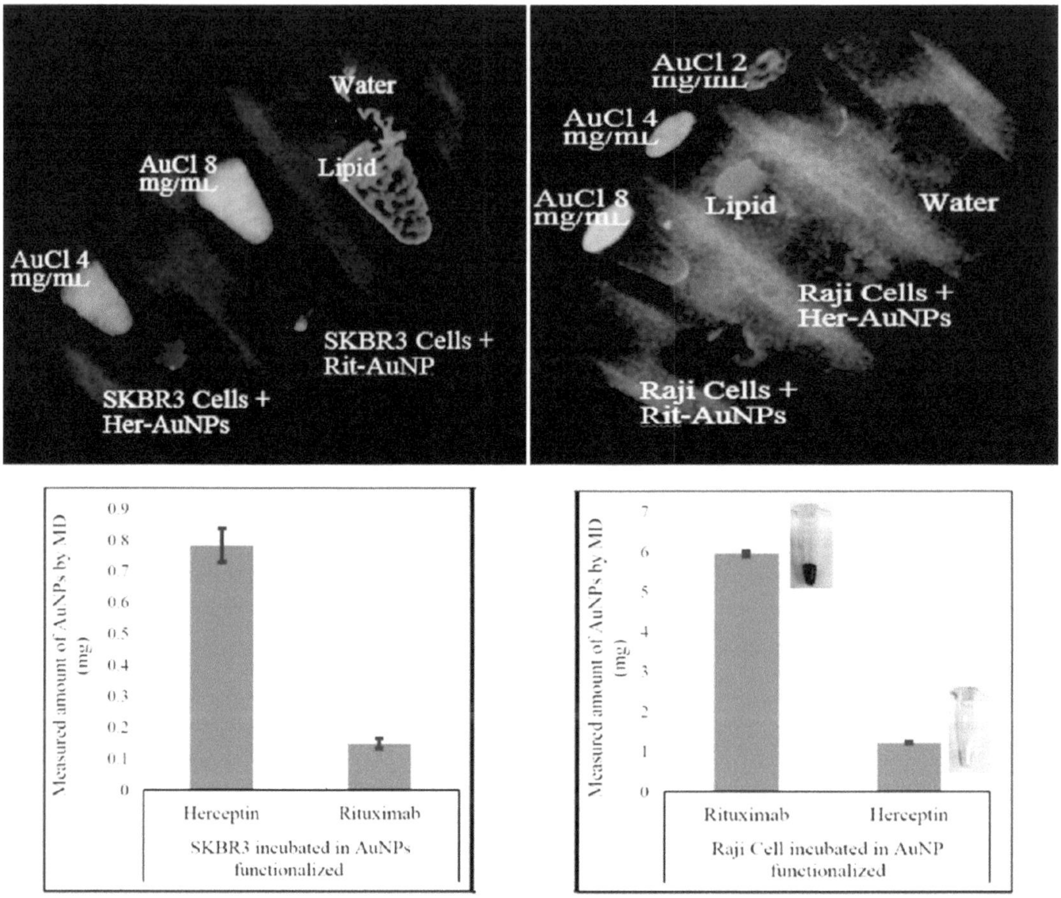

FIGURE 7.11 (left and right) MARS-MD results demonstrate that the scanner is able to detect the relative uptake of functionalized NPs. HER2 positive cells-Herceptin-gold and Raji cells-Rituximab-gold have a measurable gold amount, 0.78 mg and 5.97 mg, respectively. In contrast, both cell lines incubated with gold-labeled control antibodies have less gold attached (0.15 mg and 1.22 mg, respectively).

a MARS scanner. Raji cells were incubated with gold-labeled monoclonal antibody Rituximab (specific antibody that binds to CD20 antigen on human B-cell lymphomas) and Herceptin (as a control). HER2 positive SKBR3 breast cancer cells were incubated with the gold-labeled monoclonal antibody Herceptin (specific antibody to HER2 positive cancer cells) and Rituximab (as a control). For more details on this, we direct the reader to our paper [3]. Figure 7.12 shows *in vivo* imaging of gold in mice with implanted tumor.

The preliminary results suggest that we are able to generate a combined diagnostic imaging and therapeutic agent that can be detected by MARS imaging. It is expected that once spectral CT scanners are available for clinical use, clinicians will be able to monitor the heterogeneity status of all sites of cancer in an individual, detect how and where this status changes, monitor drug delivery and disease response, and adjust treatment to keep pace with these biological changes in various cancer types, that is, be able to detect and respond to tumor heterogeneity.

7.3.6 Cardiovascular Disease and Atheroma Imaging

Cardiovascular disease is a progressive inflammatory disease characterized by the development of atherosclerotic plaques within the walls of arteries [80]. In the advanced stages of the disease the

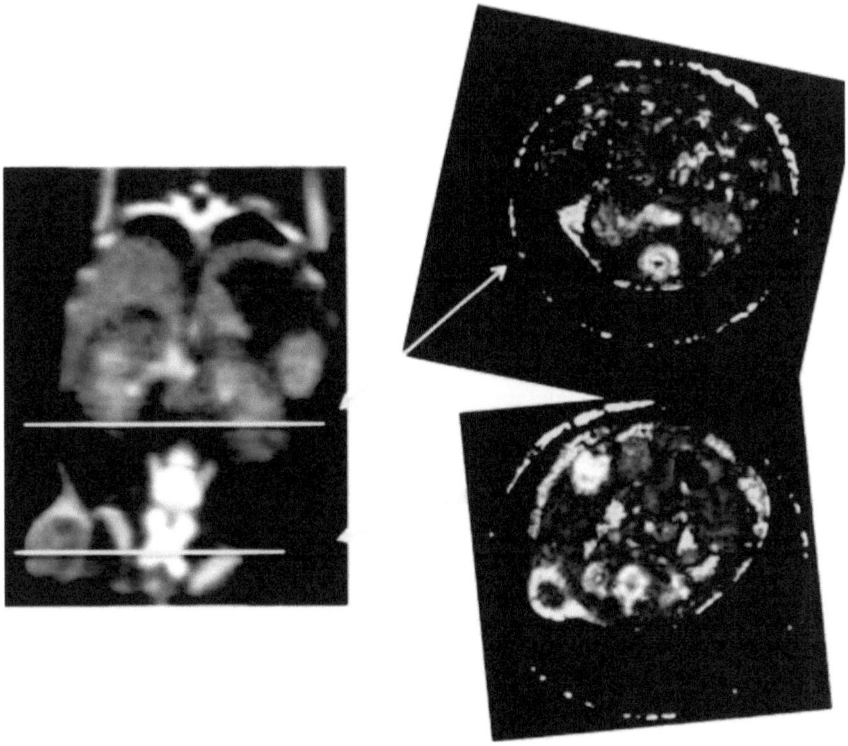

FIGURE 7.12 Non-functionalized AuNPs in Lewis lung tumor in a mouse. The AuNPs were injected into a tail vein, then the mouse was euthanized at 24 hours. Left: Broad spectrum grayscale coronal image of the mouse showing gold in kidneys, liver, spleen, and tumor. Gold is intravascular except for the tumor, liver, and spleen. Top right: The gold (yellow) in the kidneys differentiated from bone (white). Bottom right: The gold (yellow) in the vicinity of the tumor is distinguishable from the bone (white), fat (blue), and soft tissue (gray).

rupture of a plaque, often called an atheroma, triggers blood clots to form, which will block the downstream sections of the artery. This is the basis of heart attacks and strokes where the occlusion of the artery by blood clots causes the tissue to die through a lack of blood supply.

Cardiovascular disease is very much an inflammatory disease that is aggravated by elevated levels of cholesterol ester-carrying low-density lipoproteins (LDLs) in the blood [81]. The LDLs passing through the artery wall appear to become altered, either through oxidation or aggregation to become a form of "high-uptake LDL" that is rapidly taken up by inflammatory macrophage cells recruited into the plaques [82, 83]. These cholesterol-filled macrophages make up a significant part of the atheroma mass, along with T-cells and cholesterol-filled smooth muscle cells. As part of the inflammatory response, these cells release additional oxidants, so exacerbating the process by making more oxidized LDL. In advanced plaques, which typically start forming in late to middle aged patients, the cholesterol filled macrophages start to die through a necrotic process. The dying cells lyse open releasing the cellular contents into the extracellular space of the plaque. The resulting necrotic core region is rich in cholesterol esters and is usually covered by covered by a fibrous cap of proteins and connective tissue cells. If this complex structure is ruptured, usually due to thinning of the fibrous cap, the exposed plaque contents cause blood clotting within the artery.

The inflammatory process driving the disease is relatively slow and silent, with patients showing no signs of the disease until a clinical event occurs triggered by the rupture of the plaque. As the disease is driven by inflammation, it is difficult to detect using inflammatory markers because these do not distinguish from other inflammatory processes, such as muscle strains or a viral infection. The use of high-sensitivity C-reactive protein, IL-1β, and potentially neopterin/7,8-dihydroneopterin has shown some promise of providing some measure of cardiovascular disease progression [18, 84-86]. Lipid profiling to measure cholesterol distribution in the blood only serves to identify at risk persons but fails to provide an actual diagnosis of plaque formation, growth, or instability.

Current noninvasive imaging modalities lack either the resolution or molecular discernment to detect subclinical atherosclerotic plaques as the majority of the plaques are less than 2 mm thick [87-89]. Only in advanced plaques is arterial calcification observed to a level that it can be imaged by standard x-ray CT. Even in the advanced stages where growth of the plaque into the artery is affecting the flow of blood, detection is usually only possible by imaging the blood flow by contrast enhanced CT or Doppler ultrasound [90]. Possibly through the action of the macrophage cells advanced plaques often contain calcium deposits that can be imaged by x-ray CT or ultrasound. The majority of the plaque tissue, though, appears to have the same density under ultrasound or x-ray imaging as the surrounding tissues.

The result of these challenges is that cardiovascular disease is usually only diagnosed at an advanced level – potentially at a stage where treatments are less effective than at an earlier stage. Treatment is often based on lowering risk factors, such as plasma cholesterol monitoring for statin treatment. The effect of treatment on the plaque stability or size is not generally possible. Any effective imaging system, therefore, needs to be able to detect the key features of a plaque that make it likely to cause a serious problem. On histological examination, so-called vulnerable plaques show extensive necrotic core regions, ulceration in the artery wall, often with areas of hemolysis and haem deposition, thinning fibrous cap over the core region and often extensive calcification [91].

Patients with advanced unstable plaques identified following a stroke are often treated by carotid endarterectomy, a surgical procedure where the carotid artery is cut open and the plaque tissue is peeled off the artery muscle layer. This surgery has a significant risk associated with it, so surgeons prefer to operate only when there is a clear risk to the patient from further rupture events. The current imaging techniques, though, provide only limited indications of the plaque stability with much of the decision based on level of stenosis, calcification, and the patient's general health for surgery. MARS imaging of excised atheroma, under typical clinical x-ray dose and energy levels, has shown that the key features of these vulnerable plaques can be clearly seen [6, 18, 92, 93].

The atheroma shown in Figure 7.13A was taken from a 74-year-old non-diabetic male smoker treated following a stroke. The level of stenosis was measured by U.S. to be 70%. The plaque was relatively large with some browning around the bifurcation as seen in the light photographic image taken before MARS imaging (Figure 7.13A). The large vertical cut seen in the image is from where the surgeon opened the carotid artery.

This unfrozen plaque was imaged for lipid, water, iron, and calcium using a MARS scanner. The MARS material decomposition images showed extensive lipid deposition and calcification (Figure 7.13B). Digital subtraction of the lipid, water, and calcium allows the presence of extensive iron deposition, most likely intra-plaque hemorrhage, to be seen (Figure 7.13C). Inter-plaque hemorrhage occurs when the plaque cap has partially eroded and blood has become trapped within the plaque tissue where it has clot with the subsequent lysis of the red blood cells. The contraction of the clot causes the concentrating of the iron as seen in the MARS image.

Sectioning of the plaque with a scalpel showed extensive hemolysis and potential lipid deposition with in the plaque, as seen in the normal light photograph (Figure 7.15A). A cross-sectional MARS image (Figure 7.15B) along the white-dotted line in Figure 7.14A shows extensive lipid and calcium deposition, a very thinned cap and iron deposition.

Clinically these MARS images show that this plaque was highly unstable and warranted the risk involved with surgical removal from the patient's carotid artery. These MARS scans of the excised plaque show that it is feasible to gain significant clinical data to assist in the assessment of advanced vulnerable plaques.

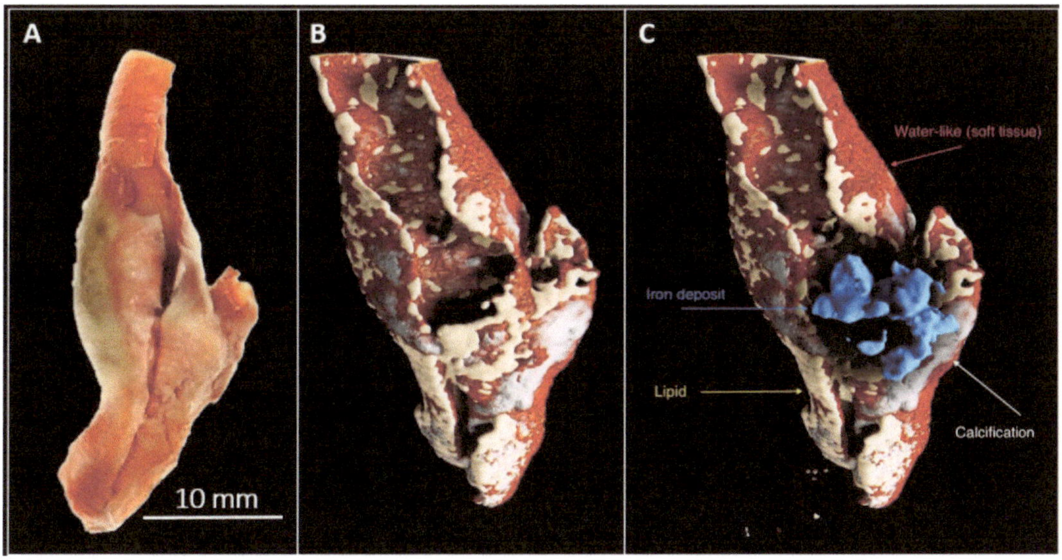

FIGURE 7.13 A surgically removed carotid plaque taken from a 74-year-old non-diabetic male smoker treated following a stroke. The plaque was photographed under white light using a macro-lens (A) before MARS imaging was performed as described in the text to generate image of the plaque's surface (B). Calcium-rich regions are shown in white, lipid-rich are in yellow/white, and water-dominated tissue in red. Subtraction of the water, lipid, and calcium channels allows the iron rich region to be visualized showing the extent of the intra-plaque hemorrhage (C).

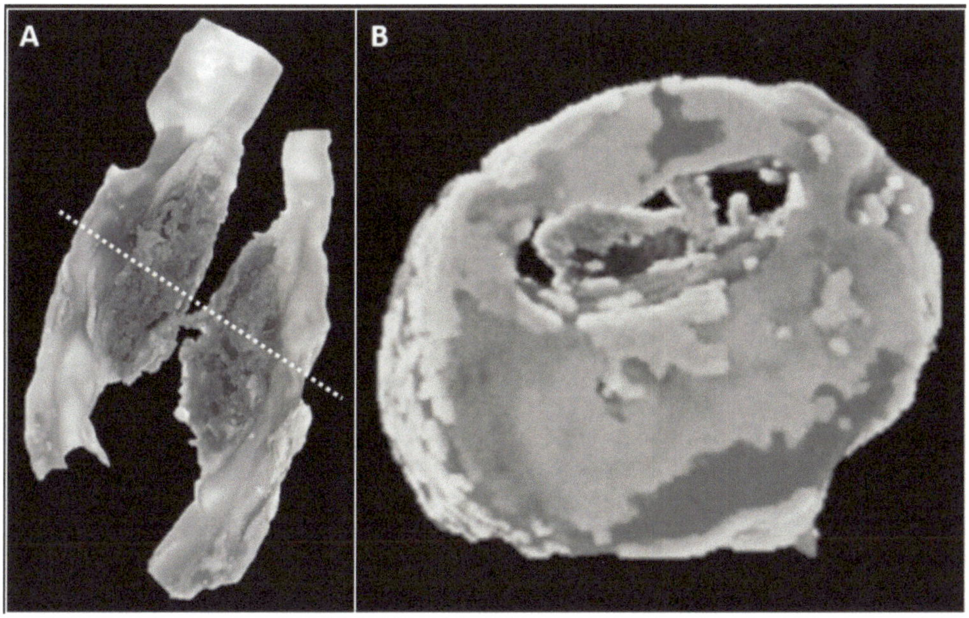

FIGURE 7.14 The plaque from Figure 7.13 was cut horizontally to show the extensive hemorrhage and calcification as photographed under white light (A). The dotted line shows where the cross-sectional MARS image (B) was generated from. The yellow regions are lipid rich, white are calcium rich and the red is iron rich showing the intra-plaque hemorrhage.

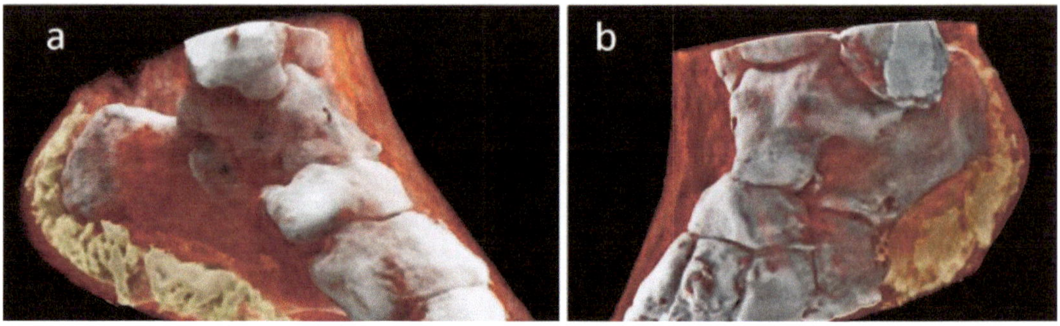

FIGURE 7.15 3D MARS images of an ankle viewed from two sides (a and b) where the soft tissue (colored in red) has been made translucent to show the bones (white) and lipid-like material (yellow) inside the heel (retrieved from https://www.marsbioimaging.com/mars/media-pack/).

7.4 RECENT ADVANCEMENTS

The first living human images from a MARS scanner (Figure 7.15) were released in July 2018. These images have featured in notable technical forums and media agencies such as AuntMinnie.com, The New York Times, BBC World Services, Physics World, Physics.org, Yahoo, Fox News, Forbes, and over 33 other media platforms [94]. *Nature* republished these images as one of their best science images of the month (July 2018 best science images; doi: 10.1038/d41586-018-05858-8).

All these advancements are evidence that MARS spectral technology is translatable to human imaging. The MARS research group has recently obtained ethical approval to undertake further studies in human subjects to evaluate MARS spectral images of hand, wrist, foot, and ankle. And, we are evaluating other applications such cancer-related clinical trials, which are currently at a preliminary planning stage.

REFERENCES

1. N. G. Anderson and A. P. Butler, "Clinical applications of spectral molecular imaging: potential and challenges," (in eng), *Contrast Media Mol Imaging*, vol. 9, no. 1, pp. 3–12, Jan 2014.
2. L. K. Stamp *et al.*, "Clinical utility of multi-energy spectral photon-counting CT in crystal arthritis," *Arthritis & Rheumatology*, 2019.
3. M. Moghiseh *et al.*, "Spectral photon-counting molecular imaging for quantification of monoclonal antibody-conjugated gold nanoparticles targeted to lymphoma and breast cancer: an in vitro study," *Contrast Media & Molecular Imaging*, vol. 2018, p. 9, 2018, Art. no. 2136840.
4. A. Viry *et al.*, "Multi-energy spectral photon-counting CT in crystal-related arthropathies: initial experience and diagnostic performance in vitro," *SPIE Medical Imaging*, 2018, vol. 10573, p. 7: SPIE.
5. K. Rajendran *et al.*, "Quantitative imaging of excised osteoarthritic cartilage using spectral CT," *European Radiology*, pp. 1–9, 2016.
6. R. Zainon *et al.*, "Spectral CT of carotid atherosclerotic plaque: comparison with histology," (in eng), *European Radiology*, vol. 22, no. 12, pp. 2581–2588, Dec 2012.
7. R. E. Alvarez and A. Macovski, "Energy-selective reconstructions in X-ray computerised tomography," *Physics in Medicine and Biology*, vol. 21, no. 5, p. 733, 1976.
8. T. Flohr *et al.*, "First performance evaluation of a dual-source CT (DSCT) system," *European Radiology*, vol. 16, no. 6, pp. 1405–1405, 2006.
9. S. Yamamoto *et al.*, "Dual-energy CT angiography of pelvic and lower extremity arteries: dual-energy bone subtraction versus manual bone subtraction," *Clinical Radiology*, vol. 64, no. 11, pp. 1088–1096, 2009.
10. D. N. Tran, M. Straka, J. E. Roos, S. Napel, and D. Fleischmann, "Dual-energy CT discrimination of iodine and calcium: experimental results and implications for lower extremity CT angiography," *Academic Radiology*, vol. 16, no. 2, pp. 160–171, 2009.

11. P. Stolzmann *et al.*, "Dual-energy computed tomography for the differentiation of uric acid stones: ex vivo performance evaluation," *Urological Research*, vol. 36, no. 3, pp. 133–138, 2008.
12. A. Graser, T. C. Johnson, H. Chandarana, and M. Macari, "Dual energy CT: preliminary observations and potential clinical applications in the abdomen," *European Radiology*, vol. 19, no. 1, pp. 13–23, 2009.
13. K. Taguchi and J. S. Iwanczyk, "Vision 20/20: single photon counting x-ray detectors in medical imaging," (in eng), *Med Phys*, Research Support, N.I.H., Extramural vol. 40, no. 10, p. 100901, Oct 2013.
14. R. Aamir *et al.*, "MARS spectral molecular imaging of lamb tissue: data collection and image analysis," *Journal of Instrumentation*, vol. 9, no. 02, p. P02005, 2014.
15. Ballabriga R. A.J., Blaj G., Campbell M., Fiederle M., Frojdh E., L. X. Heijne EHM., Pichotka M., Procz S., Tlustos L., Wong W., "The Medipix3RX: a high resolution, zero dead-time pixel detector readout chip allowing spectroscopic imaging," *Journal of Instrumentation 8 C02016 doi:10.1088/1748-0221/8/02/C02016,* 2013.
16. P. Baturin, Y. Alivov, and S. Molloi, "Spectral CT imaging of vulnerable plaque with two independent biomarkers," (in eng), *Physics in Medicine and Biology*, vol. 57, no. 13, pp. 4117–4138, Jul 7 2012.
17. D. P. Cormode *et al.*, "Atherosclerotic plaque composition: analysis with multicolor CT and targeted gold nanoparticles," *Radiology*, vol. 256, no. 3, pp. 774–782, 2010.
18. H. Prebble *et al.*, "Induced macrophage activation in live excised atherosclerotic plaque," *Immunobiology*, vol 223, no. 8-9, pp. 526–535, 2018.
19. R. Zainon *et al.*, "Spectral CT of carotid atherosclerotic plaque: comparison with histology," *European Radiology*, pp. 1–8, 2012.
20. A. Raja, M. Moghiseh, D. Kumar, P. Sykes, A. Butler, and N. Anderson, "Effect of size and concentration of gold nanoparticles on spectral CT imaging of cancer cells," *presented at the 8th International conference on advanced materials and nanotechnology Queenstown*, 12–16 Feb, 2017.
21. C. Lowe, M. Moghiseh, J. Lewis, A. Butler, R. Aamir, and N. Anderson, "Spectral photon-counting CT imaging of gold labelled monoclonal antibody drug delivery to Raji and HER2 positive beast cancer cells – a phantom study," presented at the Society for Biomaterials Annual Meeting, Atlanta, GA, April 11–14, 2018.
22. R. Popovtzer *et al.*, "Targeted sold nanoparticles enable molecular CT imaging of cancer," *Nano Letters*, vol. 8, no. 12, pp. 4593–4596, 2008, 2012/09/21.
23. T. Reuveni, M. Motiei, Z. Romman, A. Popovtzer, and R. Popovtzer, "Targeted gold nanoparticles enable molecular CT imaging of cancer: an in vivo study," *International Journal of Nanomedicine*, Journal Article p. 6, Published online 2011 November 11 2011.
24. M. R. Amma *et al.*, "Optimisation of parameters for imaging bone-metal interface using spectral photon-counting computed tomography," *Journal of Medical Radiation Sciences*, vol. 65, no. S1, pp. 114–117, 2018.
25. K. Rajendran *et al.*, "Reducing beam hardening effects and metal artefacts in spectral CT using Medipix3RX," *Journal of Instrumentation*, vol. 9, no. 03, p. P03015, 2014.
26. M. Ramyar, C. Leary, R. Aamir, A. P. H. Butler, T. B. F. Woodfield, and N. G. Anderson, "Establishing a method to measure bone structure using spectral CT," *SPIE International Symposium on Medical Imaging 2017: Physics of Medical Imaging, vol.10132*, pp. 101323I–101323I-9, 2017.
27. M. Ramyar, "MARS spectral CT technology for simultaneous assessment of articular cartilage and bone," Thesis for the Degree of Doctor of Philosophy at University if Otago, Christchurch, New Zealand, 2017.
28. J. P. Ronaldson *et al.*, "Characterization of Medipix3 with the MARS readout and software," *Journal of Instrumentation*, vol. 6, no. 01, p. C01056, 2011.
29. M. F. Walsh, "Spectral computed tomography development," *PhD, Department of Radiology, Centre for Bioengineering and Nanomedicine*, University of Otago, Christchurch, New Zealand, 2014.
30. R. K. Panta, M. F. Walsh, S. T. Bell, N. G. Anderson, A. P. Butler, and P. H. Butler, "Energy calibration of the pixels of spectral x-ray detectors," *IEEE Transactions on Medical Imaging*, vol. 34, no. 3, pp. 697–706, 2015.
31. J. Jakubek, "Semiconductor pixel detectors and their applications in life sciences," *Journal of Instrumentation*, vol. 4, no. 03, p. P03013, 2009.
32. R. Aamir *et al.*, "Pixel sensitivity variations in a CdTe-Medipix2 detector using poly-energetic x-rays," *Journal of Instrumentation*, vol. 6, no. 01, p. C01059, 2011.
33. S. Jan and P. Andrei, "Reduction of ring artefacts in high resolution micro-CT reconstructions," *Physics in Medicine & Biology*, vol. 49, no. 14, p. N247, 2004.
34. H. M. Hudson and R. S. Larkin, "Accelerated image reconstruction using ordered subsets of projection data," *IEEE Transactions on Medical Imaging*, vol. 13, no. 4, pp. 601–609, 1994.

35. R. Gordon, R. Bender, and G. T. Herman, "Algebraic reconstruction techniques (ART) for three-dimensional electron microscopy and X-ray photography," *Journal of Theoretical Biology*, vol. 29, no. 3, pp. 471–481, 1970, 12/01/1970.
36. N. Ruiter, P. H. Butler, A. P. H. Butler, S. T. Bell, A. I. Chernoglazov, and M. F. Walsh, "MARS imaging and reconstruction challenges," *The 14th International Meeting on Fully Three-Dimensional Image Reconstruction in Radiology and Nuclear Medicine*, Xi'an, vol. 14, pp. 852–857, 2017, Xi'an: Fully3D Community, 2017.
37. X. Liu, L. Yu, A. N. Primak, and C. H. McCollough, "Quantitative imaging of element composition and mass fraction using dual-energy CT: three-material decomposition," (in eng), *Medical Physics*, vol. 36, no. 5, pp. 1602–9, May 2009.
38. D. R. White, "An analysis of the Z-dependence of photon and electron interactions," *Physics in Medicine & Biology*, vol. 22, no. 2, p. 219, 1977.
39. B. J. Heismann, J. Leppert, and K. Stierstorfer, "Density and atomic number measurements with spectral x-ray attenuation method," *Journal of Applied Physics*, vol. 94, no. 3, pp. 2073–2079, 2003.
40. C. J. Bateman *et al.*, "Segmentation enhances material analysis in multi-energy CT: A simulation study," in *2013 28th International Conference on Image and Vision Computing New Zealand (IVCNZ 2013)*, pp. 190–195, 2013.
41. C. J. Bateman, "Methods for material discrimination in MARS multi-energy CT," *PhD, Department of Radiology, Centre for Bioengineering*, University of Otago, Christchurch, New Zealand, 2015.
42. C. J. Bateman *et al.*, "MARS-MD: rejection based image domain material decomposition," *Journal of Instrumentation*, vol. 13, no. 05, p. P05020, 2018.
43. A. Raja *et al.*, "Measuring identification and quantification errors in spectral CT material decomposition," *Applied Sciences*, vol. 8, no. 3, p. 467, 2018.
44. T. Sözen, L. Özışık, and N. Ç. Başaran, "An overview and management of osteoporosis," *European Journal of Rheumatology*, vol. 4, no. 1, pp. 46–56, 2017, 08/08/2017.
45. A. A. Licata, "Bone density, bone quality, and FRAX: changing concepts in osteoporosis management," *American Journal of Obstetrics and Gynecology*, vol. 208, no. 2, pp. 92–96, 2013, 02/01/2013.
46. S. L. Manske, Y. Zhu, C. Sandino, and S. K. Boyd, "Human trabecular bone microarchitecture can be assessed independently of density with second generation HR-pQCT," *Bone*, vol. 79, pp. 213–221, 2015, 10/01/2015.
47. A. J. Burghardt *et al.*, "Quantitative in vivo HR-pQCT imaging of 3D wrist and metacarpophalangeal joint space width in rheumatoid arthritis," *Annals of Biomedical Engineering*, vol. 41, no. 12, 2013, 07/26/2013.
48. M. Ramyar *et al.*, "Establishing a method to measure bone structure using spectral CT," *Medical Imaging 2017: Physics of Medical Imaging*, 2017, vol. 10132, p. 101323I: International Society for Optics and Photonics.
49. A. J. Carr *et al.*, "Knee replacement," *Lancet*, vol. 379, no. 9823, pp. 1331–1340, Apr 7 2012.
50. "Osteoarthritis: National Clinical Guideline for Care and Management in Adults," The National Collaborating Center for Chronic Conditions (UK). 2008.
51. P. Kumar and M. Clark, Eds. *Kumar and Clark's Clinical Medicine*, 9th ed. Elsevier, 2016.
52. J. Martel-Pelletier, C. Boileau, J.-P. Pelletier, and P. J. Roughley, "Cartilage in normal and osteoarthritis conditions," *Best Practice & Research Clinical Rheumatology*, vol. 22, no. 2, pp. 351–384, 2008.
53. J. A. Buckwalter, V. C. Mow, and A. Ratcliffe, "Restoration of injured or degenerated articular cartilage," *Journal of the American Academy of Orthopaedic Surgeons*, vol. 2, no. 4, pp. 192–201, 1994.
54. S. R. Frenkel *et al.*, "Regeneration of articular cartilage – evaluation of osteochondral defect repair in the rabbit using multiphasic implants," *Osteoarthritis and Cartilage*, vol. 13, no. 9, pp. 798–807, 2005.
55. T. Woodfield, C. Van Blitterswijk, J. De Wijn, T. Sims, A. Hollander, and J. Riesle, "Polymer scaffolds fabricated with pore-size gradients as a model for studying the zonal organization within tissue-engineered cartilage constructs," *Tissue Engineering*, vol. 11, no. 9-10, pp. 1297–311, 2005.
56. K. E. M. Benders *et al.*, "Formalin fixation affects equilibrium partitioning of an ionic contrast agent-microcomputed tomography (EPIC-μCT) imaging of osteochondral samples," *Osteoarthritis and Cartilage*, vol. 18, no. 12, pp. 1586–1591, 2010.
57. R. W. Farndale, D. J. Buttle, and A. J. Barrett, "Improved quantitation and discrimination of sulphated glycosaminoglycans by use of dimethylmethylene blue," *Biochimica et Biophysica Acta (BBA) – General Subjects*, vol. 883, no. 2, pp. 173–177, 1986, 09/04/1986.
58. A. J. Palmer *et al.*, "Non-invasive imaging of cartilage in early osteoarthritis," *The Bone and Joint Journal*, vol. 95-B, no. 6, pp. 738–46, Jun 2013.

59. D. J. Hunter, "Osteoarthritis," *Best Practice & Research Clinical Rheumatology*, vol. 25, no. 6, pp. 801–814, 2011.
60. S. Trattnig, S. A. Millington, P. Szomolanyi, and S. Marlovits, "MR imaging of osteochondral grafts and autologous chondrocyte implantation," *European Radiology*, vol. 17, no. 1, pp. 103–118, Jan 2007.
61. H. S. Vasiliadis and J. Wasiak, "Autologous chondrocyte implantation for full thickness articular cartilage defects of the knee," *Cochrane Database of Systematic Reviews,* no. 10. doi: 10.1002/14651858.CD003323.pub3 Available: http://onlinelibrary.wiley.com/doi/10.1002/14651858.CD003323.pub3/abstract
62. E. H. Oei, J. van Tiel, W. H. Robinson, and G. E. Gold, "Quantitative radiological imaging techniques for articular cartilage composition: towards early diagnosis and development of disease-modifying therapeutics for osteoarthritis," *Arthritis Care & Research (Hoboken)*, Feb 27 2014.
63. L. Xie, A. S. Lin, R. E. Guldberg, and M. E. Levenston, "Nondestructive assessment of sGAG content and distribution in normal and degraded rat articular cartilage via EPIC-microCT," *Osteoarthritis Cartilage*, vol. 18, no. 1, pp. 65–72, Jan 2010.
64. T. Neogi *et al.*, "2015 Gout classification criteria. An American College of Rheumatology/European League Against Rheumatism Collaborative Initiative," *Annal of the Rheumatic Diseases,* vol. 74, no. 10, pp. 1789–1798, 2015.
65. T. E. Kirkbride, A. Y. Raja, K. Müller, C. J. Bateman, F. Becce, and N. G. Anderson, "Discrimination between calcium hydroxyapatite and calcium oxalate using multienergy spectral photon-counting CT," *American Journal of Roentgenology*, vol. 209, no. 5, pp. 1088–1092, 2017.
66. A. Viry *et al.*, "Multi-energy spectral photon-counting CT in crystal-related arthropathies: initial experience and diagnostic performance in vitro," *Medical Imaging 2018: Physics of Medical Imaging*, vol. 10573, p. 1057351, 2018, International Society for Optics and Photonics.
67. G. Li *et al.*, "In vitro and in vivo study of additive manufactured porous Ti6Al4V scaffolds for repairing bone defects," *Scientific Reports*, vol. 6, p. 34072, 2016, 09/26/2016 online.
68. P. V. Giannoudis, H. Dinopoulos, and E. Tsiridis, "Bone substitutes: an update," *Injury*, vol. 36, no. 3, pp. S20–S27, 2005.
69. P. Stradiotti, A. Curti, G. Castellazzi, and A. Zerbi, "Metal-related artefacts in instrumented spine. Techniques for reducing artefacts in CT and MRI: state of the art," *European Spine Journal*, vol. 18, no. 1, pp. 102–108, June 01 2009.
70. J. D. Silkwood, K. L. Matthews, P. M. Shikhaliev. "Photon counting spectral breast CT: effect of adaptive filtration on CT numbers, noise, and contrast to noise ratio," *Medical Physics*, vol. 40, no. 5, p. 051905.
71. K. Rajendran, "MARS spectral CT for orthopaedic applications," *PhD, Department of Radiology and Centre for Bioengineering*, University of Otago, Otago School of Medicine, Christchurch, New Zealand, 2016.
72. R.-F. Chang, H.-H. Chen, Y.-C. Chang, C.-S. Huang, J.-H. Chen, and C.-M. Lo, "Quantification of breast tumor heterogeneity for ER status, HER2 status, and TN molecular subtype evaluation on DCE-MRI," *Magnetic Resonance Imaging*, vol. 34, no. 6, pp. 809–819, 2016, 07/01/2016.
73. I. Dagogo-Jack and A. T. Shaw, "Tumour heterogeneity and resistance to cancer therapies," *Nature Reviews Clinical Oncology*, vol. 15, no. 2, pp. 81–94, 2017, 11/08/2017 online.
74. B. Ganeshan and K. A. Miles, "Quantifying tumour heterogeneity with CT," *Cancer Imaging*, vol. 13, no. 1, pp. 140–149, 2013, 02/04/2013.
75. ASTM E1695-95, *"Standard Test Method for Measurement of Computed Tomography (CT) System Performance,"* Ed. West Conshohocken, PA: ASTM International, 2006.
76. R. Aamir, "Using MARS spectral CT for identifying biomedical nanoparticles.," Ph.D Thesis Ph.D, Department of Physics & Astronomy, University of Canterbury, Christchurch, 2013.
77. J. R. Ashton, J. L. West, and C. T. Badea, "In vivo small animal micro-CT using nanoparticle contrast agents," (in English), *Frontiers in Pharmacology*, vol. 6, 2015-November-4 2015.
78. D. P. Cormode *et al.*, "Multicolor spectral photon-counting computed tomography: in vivo dual contrast imaging with a high count rate scanner," *Scientific Reports*, vol. 7, no. 1, p. 4784, 2017, 07/06 2017.
79. M. Moghiseh *et al.*, "Discrimination of multiple high-Z materials by multi-energy spectral CT – a phantom study," *JSM Biomed Imaging Data Paper*, vol. 3, no. 1, 2016.
80. P. Libby, P. M. Ridker, and A. Maseri, "Inflammation and atherosclerosis," *Circulation*, vol. 105, no. 9, pp. 1135–1143, 2002.
81. I. Levitan, S. Volkov, and P. V. Subbaiah, "Oxidized LDL: diversity, patterns of recognition, and pathophysiology," (in English), *Antioxidants & Redox Signaling*, vol. 13, no. 1, pp. 39–75, Jul 2010.

82. S. P. Gieseg, E. Crone, and Z. Amit, "Oxidised low density lipoprotein cytotoxicity and vascular disease," *Endogenous Toxins: Diet, Genetics, Disease And Treatment*, vol. Chapter 25, P. J. O'Brien and W. R. Bruce, Eds. Weinheim: Wiley-VCH, 2010, pp. 620–645.
83. X.-H. Yu, Y.-C. Fu, D.-W. Zhang, K. Yin, and C.-K. Tang, "Foam cells in atherosclerosis," *Clinica Chimica Acta*, vol. 424, no. 0, pp. 245–252, 2013, 9/23/2013.
84. P. M. Ridker *et al.*, "Rosuvastatin to prevent vascular events in men and women with wlevated C-reactive protein," *New England Journal of Medicine*, vol. 359, no. 21, pp. 2195–2207, 2008.
85. P. M. Ridker *et al.*, "Relationship of C-reactive protein reduction to cardiovascular event reduction following treatment with canakinumab: a secondary analysis from the CANTOS randomised controlled trial," *The Lancet*, vol. 391, no. 10118, pp. 319–328, 2017.
86. V. K. Patel, H. Williams, S. C. H. Li, J. P. Fletcher, and H. J. Medbury, "Monocyte inflammatory profile is specific for individuals and associated with altered blood lipid levels," (in English), *Atherosclerosis*, vol. 263, pp. 15–23, Aug 2017.
87. J. M. Tarkin *et al.*, "Imaging atherosclerosis," *Circulation Research,* vol. 118, no. 4, pp. 750–769, 2016.
88. N. Maldonado, A. Kelly-Arnold, D. Laudier, S. Weinbaum, and L. Cardoso, "Imaging and analysis of microcalcifications and lipid/necrotic core calcification in fibrous cap atheroma," *International Journal of Cardiovascular Imaging,* vol. 31, no. 5, pp. 1079–1087, Jun 2015.
89. S. Divakaran *et al.*, "Use of cardiac CT and calcium scoring for detecting coronary plaque: implications on prognosis and patient management," *The British Journal of Radiology*, vol. 88, no. 1046, pp. 20140594-20140594, 2015.
90. R. S. Cires-Drouet, M. Mozafarian, A. Ali, S. Sikdar, and B. K. Lal, "Imaging of high-risk carotid plaques: ultrasound," *Seminars in Vascular Surgery*, vol. 30, no. 1, pp. 44–53, 2017, 03/01/2017.
91. J. S. Marques and F. J. Pinto, "The vulnerable plaque: current concepts and future perspectives on coronary morphology, composition and wall stress imaging," *Revista Portuguesa De Cardiologia*, vol. 33, no. 2, pp. 101–110, Feb 2014.
92. R. Zainon *et al.*, "High resolution spectral micro-CT imaging of atherosclerotic plaque," *2014 IEEE Region 10 Symposium* New York: IEEE, 2014, pp. 568–571.
93. J. P. Ronaldson *et al.*, "Toward quantifying the composition of soft tissues by spectral CT with Medipix3," *Medical Physics*, vol. 39, no. 11, pp. 6847–6857, 2012.
94. M. B. Ltd. (2018). *First in human MARS 3D colour x-rays.* Available: https://www.marsbioimaging.com/mars/wp-content/uploads/2018/08/Report-on-MBI-publicity-updated.pdf

8 Advances in and Uses of Contrast Agents for Spectral Photon Counting Computed Tomography

Johoon Kim,[1,2] Pratap C. Naha,[1] Peter B. Noël,[1] and David P. Cormode[1,2,3]

[1]Department of Radiology, University of Pennsylvania, Philadelphia, Pennsylvania, USA

[2]Department of Bioengineering, University of Pennsylvania, Philadelphia, Pennsylvania, USA

[3]Department of Cardiology, University of Pennsylvania, Philadelphia, Pennsylvania, USA

CONTENTS

8.1 INTRODUCTION

Computed tomography (CT) is an X-ray based medical imaging technique that was first brought into clinical use in the 1970s.[1] CT now sees broad clinical use, with approximately 80 million scans being performed per year in the USA alone and many more being done abroad.[2] CT imaging is used to diagnose and monitor many conditions such as trauma, cancer, cardiovascular diseases, and gastrointestinal disorders. Its quick image acquisition time and wide clinical availability also allows it to be extensively used in emergency medicine. Although this technique is now well-established, it is undergoing a period of rapid innovation. More powerful algorithms such as iterative reconstruction and model-based iterative reconstruction have been developed for improved image quality.[3–7] The speed of image acquisition has increased and new innovations such as dual energy systems that can provide spectral information in the image have also become available.

CT imaging is frequently done by rotating an X-ray source around a subject, thereby exposing the subject to X-rays from all angles. Detector systems located on the opposite side of the subject absorb transmitted photons, those that are not absorbed or scattered by the subject. This information is used to reconstruct images. The loss of X-ray beam intensity after passing through the patient, also known as X-ray attenuation, is predominantly caused by the photoelectric effect and Compton scattering in the diagnostic X-ray energy range (~25–150 keV). The photoelectric effect describes the phenomena in which incident X-rays collide with the inner shell electrons (K-shell or L-shell) of atoms that constitute the subject. As a result, the energy of the incident X-ray is transferred to the inner shell electron, ejecting it from the atom. An outer shell electron possessing higher energy fills the vacancy and releases some of its energy as a photon, a particle whose energy is characteristic of the atom. In the phenomena of Compton scattering, the incident X-ray interacts with outer shell electrons, which causes it to lose some of its energy and be deflected from its path.

In conventional CT systems, once the X-ray beam reaches the detectors, most of the scattered X-ray photons are absorbed in the collimator in front of the detector and X-ray radiation of diagnostic value is absorbed and converted to light in scintillators. The converted light energy in each pixel of the scintillator is then converted into electronic current, which is transmitted as digital output data. These conventional CT scanner detectors are known as energy-integrating detectors (EIDs) since all of the energy deposited in each pixel is summed and is transmitted as a single signal, omitting any energy-dependent information on individual X-ray photons. This also leads to the heavier weighting of higher energy photons, which carry less information on soft tissue contrast.

EIDs provide attenuation information that is dependent on the mass density and atomic number of the material. Hence, materials of different elemental compositions and varying concentrations can produce identical CT attenuation values, making differentiation of such materials extremely difficult. A clinical scenario that could benefit from material differentiation is separation of calcified plaques from the lumen of iodine-filled blood vessels. Calcium deposits within vulnerable atherosclerotic plaques and bones near plaque sites not only obscure the lumen anatomy but can also generate similar CT attenuation as iodine-filled blood vessels to hinder clear visualization of the plaques. This can lead to incorrect diagnoses. Material differentiation imaging methods that can resolve such issues are highly attractive.

One method that allows material differentiation is dual energy CT (DECT) imaging. The principle of DECT is to acquire two sets of CT data using two different energy spectra. This idea was first introduced and demonstrated in the 1970s, although the speed of image acquisition at that time was not sufficient for clinical implementation. Since then, multiple approaches have been developed for clinical use, such as slow kVp switching, rapid kVp switching, and using multilayer detectors or dual X-ray sources.[8] DECT techniques are FDA approved, and clinical CT scanners with two energy spectra are commercially available.[9] Many clinical applications of DECT also have been studied, including virtual monoenergetic imaging for optimal contrast-to-noise ratio (CNR) of iodine, bone removal in CT angiography, and virtual non-contrast enhanced images.[8,10] However, DECT techniques still have several limitations including susceptibility to motion that can lead to image misregistration, high overlap of energy spectra, and high noise levels in low-energy data. All of these restraints can cause degradation in image quality and inaccurate material differentiation. Moreover, in some forms of DECT, there is increased radiation dose to the patient, since two X-ray tubes are used to scan.

Spectral photon counting CT (SPCCT) is a rapidly emerging imaging modality that is currently under extensive investigation for its clinical feasibility. Since its first evaluation in preclinical CT systems about a decade ago, the latest prototypes of SPCCT scanners have evolved to be based on modified clinical CT systems.[11] SPCCT uses a standard polychromatic X-ray source and photon-counting detectors (PCDs) that can potentially provide more accurate material decomposition (Figure 8.1).

PCDs are composed of semiconductor materials such as cadmium zinc telluride or silicon. When an X-ray photon is absorbed by these detectors, electron hole pairs are formed, resulting in a charge cloud and current pulse whose magnitude is proportional to the photon energy. The magnitude of each current pulse is measured by the electronics and each X-ray photon event is recorded in one of several energy bins. The number of bins and their energy thresholds can be adjusted for user-specific applications (e.g., near the K-edge of the material of interest) (Figure 8.1).[13] These data sets are then

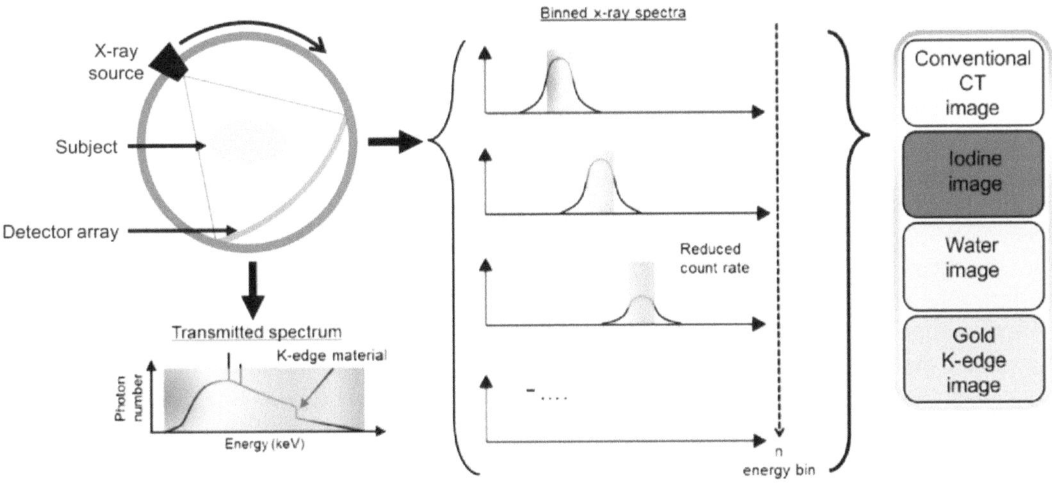

FIGURE 8.1 Schematic depiction of an SPCCT system. The binned data may be used to generate different types of image sets such as those listed (i.e., synthesized conventional CT images and iodine, water, and gold material specific images) or other sets of images. Figure adapted with permission from reference.[12]

processed together to provide a set of images, which typically include a conventional image and material-specific images (e.g., water, iodine, and gold) (Figure 8.1). SPCCT systems have several benefits, such as lower noise levels, improved CNR and spectral separation, higher spatial resolution, fewer image artifacts, and increased geometric and dose efficiency.[14–16] Another benefit of SPCCT imaging is that they can provide absolute quantification of exogeneous contrast agents *in vivo*, which can be utilized in targeted or molecular imaging.[11] Recent studies have demonstrated the feasibility of differentiating multiple materials in both small and large animals.[17–19] In addition, the clinical emergence of SPCCT technology has been embraced by multiple studies demonstrating comparable image quality between conventional CT and SPCCT scanners in terms of noise levels and CNR.[20–23]

Many aspects of SPCCT systems, such as image reconstruction methods and detector models, are being further improved to provide better images. One area in SPCCT imaging that can also significantly contribute to the improvement of diagnostic quality of SPCCT images is development of SPCCT-specific contrast agents. Currently, the only clinically approved CT contrast agents are small-molecule based tri-iodinated benzene rings for blood pool imaging and barium sulfate for gastrointestinal imaging. Approximately half of CT scans are performed with intravenous injection of iodinated contrast agents. While these iodine-based contrast agents provide sufficient contrast in both single energy CT and DECT, there are concerns over allergic reactions to these agents and renal toxicity, particularly in patients with renal insufficiency.[24,25] Iodine-based contrast agents also suffer from low contrast at the higher X-ray tube potentials that are needed for large adults (e.g., 140 kVp). Moreover, they do not take full advantage of the robust material decomposition capabilities of SPCCT imaging because of iodine's low K-edge energy of 33.2 keV. Most photons are absorbed by the patient at the energy level lower than and near the K-edge energy of iodine. For this reason, there are not enough photons in transmitted X-ray spectra below iodine's K-edge energy to allow K-edge imaging of this element. Despite the disadvantages of iodinated contrast agents, there has not been a new CT contrast agent clinically approved for over 20 years. Therefore, considerable research interest has been garnered in the development of novel heavy element contrast agents whose K-edge energies are higher.[11,12,26–28] New studies have demonstrated that heavy metal elements, such as gadolinium, ytterbium, tantalum, gold, and bismuth, perform well in both conventional CT imaging and K-edge imaging with SPCCT, demonstrating the feasibility of these elements for possible clinical use in the future. A number of studies have evaluated the capacity of SPCCT imaging when using nanoparticle-based contrast agents made from the aforementioned heavy metal elements.[11,12,26–29] These nanoparticles can be designed to have variable circulation times, target specificity and to deliver high payloads to regions of interest. They are also less likely to extravasate than small-molecule based contrast agents, improving targeted to background ratios in blood vessel imaging.

In the development of a novel SPCCT contrast agent, some important factors need to be considered. The first and most crucial consideration is the toxicity profile of the element or the compounds into which it can be formed. Although future advances in CT technology are expected to reduce needed doses, the low sensitivity of CT imaging requires significantly higher doses of contrast agents when compared to other imaging modalities, such as MRI.[30] Thus, any new contrast agents will need to be made of an element or a compound that causes minimal adverse effects in patients. Another important consideration is the manufacturing cost and availability of the element. To meet the global demand of contrast-enhanced CT scans, the new contrast agent will need to be made of an element that has plenty of reserves on Earth and is reasonably low in cost. Lastly, the K-edge of the element should be in a region where there are adequate numbers of photons both below and above the K-edge to enable effective K-edge imaging. The ratio of photon numbers below and above the K-edge is also an important parameter as Kim et al. recently demonstrated its correlation with CNR.[31] In the same paper, the authors also considered heavy elements' safety, radioactivity, K-edge energy, salt price, availability, as well as previous studies in nanoparticle synthesis and *in vivo* X-ray imaging in order to select a number of candidate elements with strong potential to be used as nanoparticle-based SPCCT-specific contrast agents (Figure 8.2). The elements that were chosen for further investigation were gadolinium, ytterbium, tantalum, tungsten, gold, and bismuth. This list is in agreement with a review paper published by Yeh et al.[9] whose focus was to discuss and identify practical elements for SPCCT contrast agent development based on literature review.

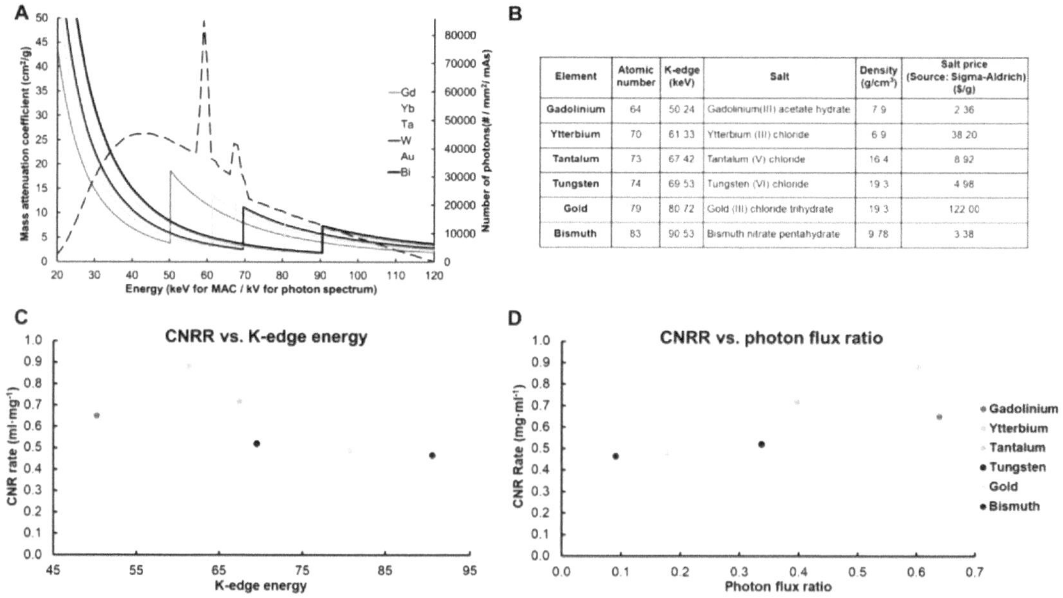

Element	Atomic number	K-edge (keV)	Salt	Density (g/cm³)	Salt price (Source: Sigma-Aldrich) ($/g)
Gadolinium	64	50.24	Gadolinium(III) acetate hydrate	7.9	2.36
Ytterbium	70	61.33	Ytterbium (III) chloride	6.9	38.20
Tantalum	73	67.42	Tantalum (V) chloride	16.4	8.92
Tungsten	74	69.53	Tungsten (VI) chloride	19.3	4.98
Gold	79	80.72	Gold (III) chloride trihydrate	19.3	122.00
Bismuth	83	90.53	Bismuth nitrate pentahydrate	9.78	3.38

FIGURE 8.2 (A) X-ray photon energy spectrum at tube voltage of 120 kVp and mass attenuation coefficients of gadolinium, ytterbium, tantalum, tungsten, gold, and bismuth. (B) Characteristics of the six elements in Figure 8.2A. Figure adapted with permission from reference.[31] (C) The contrast-to-noise ratio rate of the six elements listed in Figure 8.2A compared with their K-edge energies. (D) The contrast-to-noise ratio of the elements compared to the ratio of the number of photons below and above their K-edge energy based on the spectrum in Figure 8.2A. The key is the same in (C) and (D).

TABLE 8.1
Summary of the Properties and the Potential for SPCCT Contrast Agent Development of All Elements Covered in This Chapter

Element	Atomic number	K-edge (keV)	Density (g/cm³)	Element price ($/g) Source: Sigma-Aldrich	Pro/con	Development status	Degree of studies for CT contrast agent
Iodine	53	33.17	4.9	8.40	**Pro:** Clinically approved for contrast-enhanced CT imaging; excellent safety profile **Con:** Concern over renal damage and allergic reactions; low K-edge for photon-counting CT imaging; sharp decrease in attenuation generation in higher tube potentials	Iodinated contrast agents are clinically available	Well-studied in human subjects; commonly used as a control for contrast enhanced CT imaging
Gadolinium	64	50.24	7.9	10.40	**Pro:** K-edge close to mean photon energy in clinical X-ray spectra; chelates are FDA approved for clinical MRI imaging. **Con:** Toxicity concern over nephrogenic systemic fibrosis and accumulation in the bones, brain and kidneys	Gadolinium chelates are clinically available for MRI imaging; are under clinical trial for CT imaging with low dose	Well-studied for MRI imaging; studies in CT imaging and SPCCT imaging.
Ytterbium	70	61.33	6.9	23.00	**Pro:** K-edge close to mean photon energy in clinical X-ray spectra **Con:** Unknown safety profile and efficacy in *in vivo* CT imaging	Preclinical CT and SPCCT imaging with small animals	Several studies in CT imaging and SPCCT imaging in preclinical stage
Hafnium	72	65.35	13.3	4.50	**Pro:** K-edge close to mean photon energy in clinical X-ray spectra **Con:** Unknown safety profile and yet unexplored for bioapplication	Preclinical SPCCT imaging with small animals	One experimental study in SPCCT imaging
Tantalum	73	67.42	16.4	6.20	**Pro:** K-edge close to mean photon energy in clinical X-ray spectra; well-studied for CT imaging; chemically inert; biocompatible; high elemental density **Con:** Unknown toxicity and safety profile in human patients	Preclinical CT and SPCCT imaging with small animals	Several studies for CT imaging and SPCCT imaging in preclinical stage
Gold	79	80.72	19.3	298.00	**Pro:** K-edge close to mean photon energy in high clinical X-ray spectra; high density; high biocompatible; highly bioinert; easy synthesis and size and shape control; very well-studied in the field of nanomedicine **Con:** Expensive	Preclinical CT and SPCCT imaging with small animals	Most well-studied and characterized for CT and SPCCT contrast agent at experimental and preclinical stage
Bismuth	83	90.53	9.8	0.48	**Pro:** Fairly biocompatible (currently used in gastrointestinal treatments); cheap; effective attenuation generation at higher tube potentials **Con:** low density compared to other high Z metals	Preclinical CT and SPCCT imaging with small animals	Numerous studies for CT and SPCCT imaging in preclinical stage

In support of these findings, a majority of the studies that have investigated SPCCT-specific contrast agent development have focused on the six aforementioned elements – gadolinium, ytterbium, tantalum, tungsten, gold, and bismuth.[12,19,26,27,31,32] Other elements that have also been explored include iodine, due to its broad use in conventional CT and DECT imaging, and hafnium for its appropriate K-edge energy in the clinical X-ray energy spectra, despite its largely unknown safety profile.[28,33] This chapter has summarized the characteristics and previous studies of these elements in X-ray imaging and has highlighted the studies that have explored these elements for SPCCT contrast agent development. Table 8.1 briefly summarizes the properties (e.g., atomic number, K-edge, density) and the potential for SPCCT contrast agent development (e.g., pro/con, development status, and degree of studies for CT and SPCCT contrast agent) of the elements that are covered in this chapter.

In the following sections, we first focus on studies that use gold as the element for SPCCT-specific contrast agent development, since it is the most widely studied element for this application. Subsequently, studies that use other elements are introduced in order of the atomic numbers of the elements.

8.2 GOLD

Nanoparticle formulations of gold, commonly known as gold nanoparticles (AuNP), have been proposed for numerous biomedical applications, such as photoacoustic imaging, photothermal ablation, optical imaging, and cell tracking.[34–37] AuNP also has been by far the most extensively studied experimental CT contrast agent due to its excellent safety profile, colloidal stability, ease of control over their size, morphology and surface chemistry, and its high atomic number (Z = 79) and density (d = 19.3 g/cm^3).[38–40]

The K-edge of gold at 80.7 keV is advantageous, as it provides strong contrast, especially when higher clinical X-ray tube potentials of 100–140 kVp are used.[41] This is due to the fact that the mass attenuation coefficient of gold is about 2.7 times greater than that of iodine in the range of 80–120 keV as a result of the increase of gold's coefficient after its K-edge. The findings from studies comparing contrast production between AuNP and iodine confirm the excellent contrast generation of AuNP at higher tube potential. In a study from Jackson et al., AuNP displays up to 65%, 111%, and 140% greater attenuation than iopromide at tube potentials of 100 kVp, 120 kVp, and 140 kVp, respectively.[42] Galper et al. also shows that only a minor degradation in attenuation rate is observed from AuNP going from 80 kVp to 140 kVp, whereas the attenuation of iodine is severely reduced at higher tube potentials.[41] These higher tube potentials are expected to be used more frequently in clinics due to an increasing number of obese patients in the populations of many countries, supporting the future need for contrast agents based on heavier elements.

Apart from the intrinsic characteristics of gold as a strong CT contrast generating element, the ease of control over the size and surface chemistry of AuNP bolsters the potential use of AuNP in SPCCT imaging, since it is expected to benefit from targeted molecular imaging and multiphase imaging with dual or multiple contrast agents.[19,26,43] While small AuNP (< 5 nm) can be synthesized in order to have short blood circulation times and efficient bioelimination from swift renal excretion, larger AuNP can be formulated for efficient uptake by phagocytic cells for CT cell tracking applications and for prolonged blood circulation, which can enhance tumor accumulation.[38,44,45] The surface of AuNP also can be readily modified to attach targeting moieties that allow active targeting in coronary diseases and certain types of cancer.[19,46]

The earliest study that combined targeted molecular imaging and SPCCT imaging was reported by Cormode et al.[19] In this study, small AuNP (~ 3 nm) were encapsulated in a coating derived from high-density lipoprotein and were termed Au-HDL (Figure 8.3A,B). The coating promoted uptake of these nanoparticles by macrophages, a cell type connected with risk of cardiovascular events in atherosclerosis. In their artery phantom experiments, contrast arising from Au-HDL, iodine, and calcium phosphate in the field of view could be correctly differentiated, and the concentrations of Au-HDL and iodine were accurately calculated. *In vivo* imaging with an atherosclerosis-prone, apolipoprotein E-deficient knock-out (apo E-KO) mouse model of atherosclerosis readily detected the accumulation of Au-HDL in their aortas (Figure 8.3C,D). An iodinated contrast agent and the calcium-rich tissues were also clearly distinguished to visualize the vasculature lumen and the bones in mice, demonstrating the feasibility of SPCCT targeted molecular imaging against macrophage burden in the arteries and simultaneous material decomposition between gold, iodine, and calcium phosphate (Figure 8.3D).

In another study, AuNP-encapsulating low-density lipoprotein (Au-LDL) was formulated to promote tumor accumulation and detection with SPCCT.[43] In SPCCT imaging of B16-F10 melanoma tumor bearing mice (a tumor type that overexpresses the LDL receptor), accumulation of Au-LDL at the rim of tumor was clearly visualized. Another example of targeted molecular imaging with SPCCT was reported by Schirra et al.[29] The authors synthesized AuNP-loaded carriers that they called gold nanobeacons (GNB) by encapsulating payloads of small AuNP within a polysorbate core and stabilizing it by a phospholipid layer. GNB was biotinylated to target *in vitro* fibrin-rich clots that were incubated with biotinylated anti-fibrin monoclonal antibodies and subsequently with avidin to promote targeting via biotin-avidin coupling. *In vitro* SPCCT phantom imaging of the aforementioned fibrin-rich clots readily detected GNB that were bound on the periphery of the fibrin-rich clot.

One of the main advantages of SPCCT imaging is its ability to perform multiphase imaging via simultaneous material decomposition of dual contrast agents without the need of pre-injection scans. For instance, different contrast agents can be injected in the blood at different time points

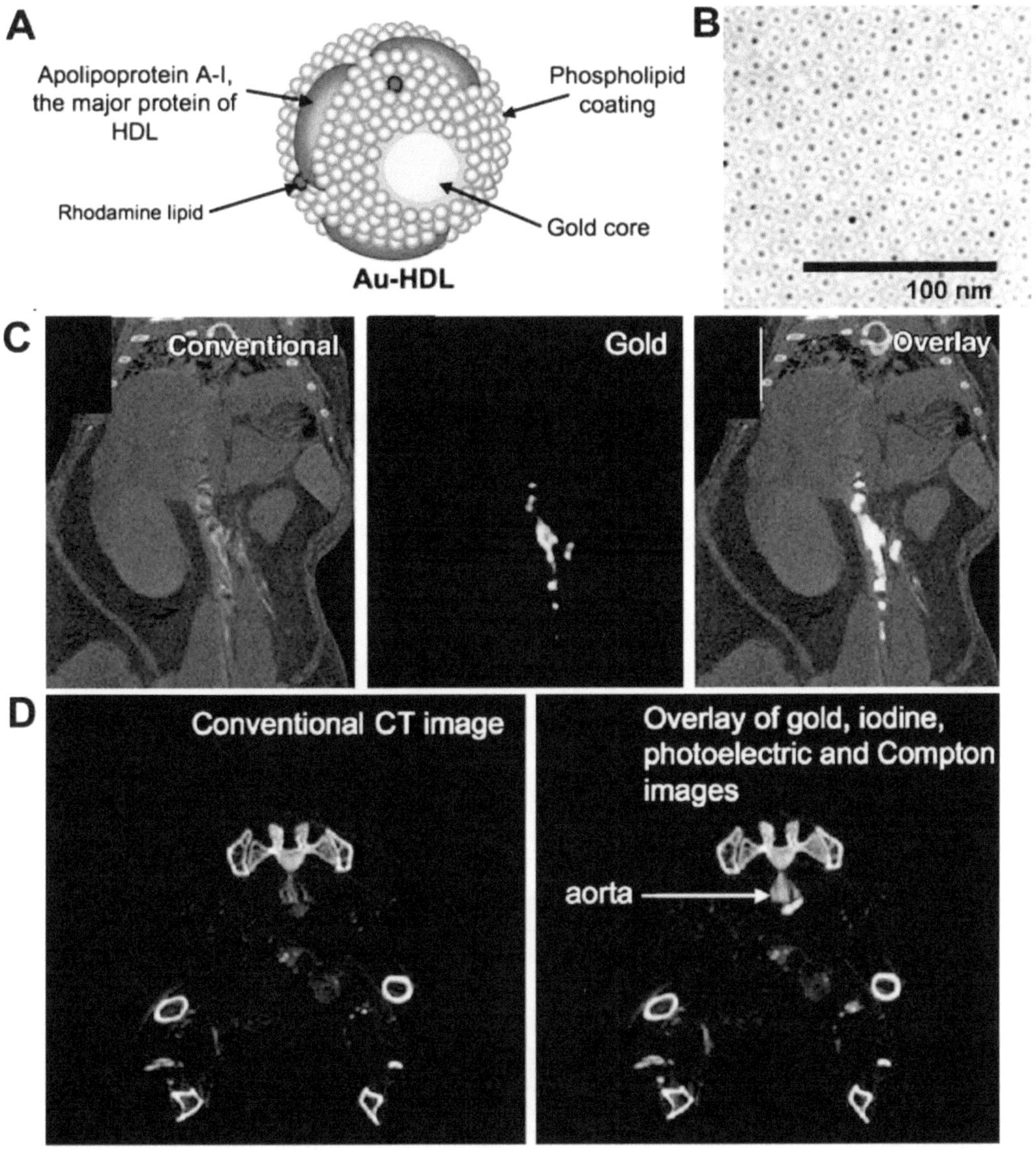

FIGURE 8.3 (A) Schematic depiction of Au-HDL. (B) Transmission electron microscopy (TEM) of Au-HDL. (C) Conventional CT-like image (left), gold-based image (middle) and overlay image (right) from SPCCT imaging of thorax and abdomen in apo E-KO mouse. (D) SPCCT images of apo E-KO mouse injected with both Au-HDL and an iodinated contrast agent.

and the uptake in certain tissues or organs of interest can be visualized and quantified in multiple phases.[11,47] Cormode et al. recently investigated the feasibility of dual contrast agent imaging using polyethylene glycol-coated AuNP that are 18 nm in average hydrodynamic diameter and an iodinated contrast agent with a prototype SPCCT scanner that was based on a modified clinical CT system (Figure 8.4A,B).[12] Accurate discrimination and quantification of AuNP and iodine was confirmed in a phantom study with mixed solutions of the two contrast agents.

After the phantom study, *in vivo* dual contrast agent imaging was performed in New Zealand White rabbits. The rabbits were injected with AuNP and an iodinated agent and imaged at several time points (T0: pre-injection, T1: 10 min after AuNP injection, T2: 1 min after iodinated contrast agent injection and 25 min after the AuNP injection, T3: 15 min after iodinated contrast agent injection). At all time points, material specific images clearly differentiated AuNP and iodine in the chest (Figure 8.4C) and abdomen. Concentrations of the two contrast agents in major organs could also be quantified. The quantification results matched the expected pharmacokinetics of the two agents – swift excretion of iodinated agent from T2 to T3 and prolonged residence of AuNP in the blood vessels of the major organs. As shown in Figure 8.4C, the conventional images were only able to display changes in attenuation, but material specific images could identify the distributions of both the gold and iodine agents. The authors highlighted that the clinically relevant scan time of the scanner used in this study allowed observation of pharmacokinetics from multiple repeated scans, hinting at the broadening applications of SPCCT imaging.

Until a study published in 2017 by Si-Mohamed et al., the accuracy of material quantification from SPCCT K-edge imaging had only been assessed in phantoms or in *ex vivo* imaging. Si-Mohamed et al. studied the capability of a clinical-scale prototype SPCCT system to quantify the *in vivo* biodistribution of polyethylene glycol-coated AuNP that are 18 nm in average hydrodynamic diameter

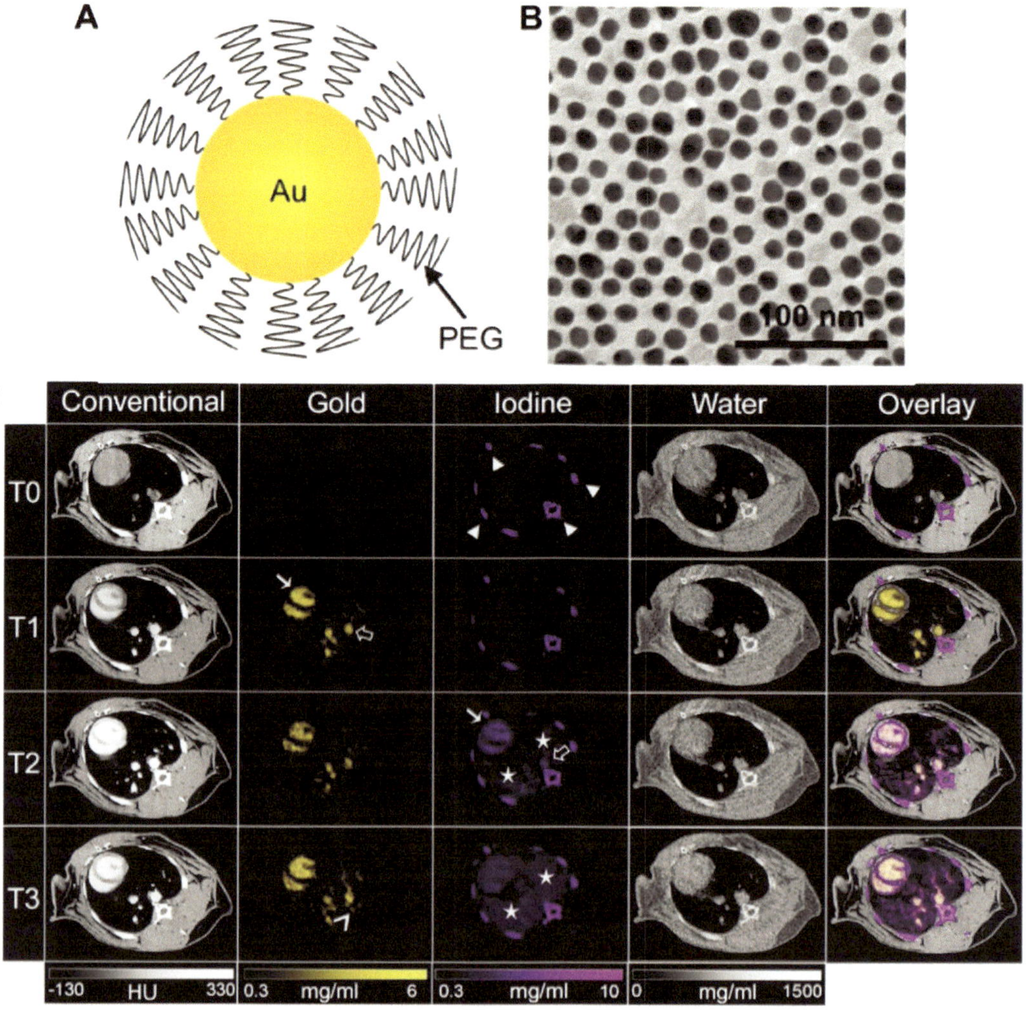

FIGURE 8.4 (A) Schematic depiction of AuNP in this study. (B) TEM of the AuNP. (C) SPCCT images of the chest of a rabbit. Figure adapted with permission from reference.[12]

via longitudinal imaging of New Zealand White rabbits.[48] A phantom study was first performed to establish a good linear relationship between concentrations measured from SPCCT imaging and actual concentrations of AuNP. During the *in vivo* experiment, images were taken at 40 seconds, 8 minutes, 1 week, 1 month and 6 months after the injection to visualize and quantify the AuNP amount in different organs. The quantification results showed high concentrations of AuNP in the blood up to the 8-minute time point and negligible concentrations at 1 week and thereafter. Gold content was persistent throughout the duration of the study in liver, spleen, and bone marrow. At 1 week, 1 month, and 6 months, animals were sacrificed, and their major organs were harvested for ICP-OES (inductively coupled plasma atomic emission spectroscopy) measurements. Comparing the measurements from SPCCT imaging and ICP-OES, good linear correlation ($R^2 = 0.93$) was observed between the two measures. Bland-Altman plots demonstrated that the two measurements were in good agreement with a bias of 0.11. This study underscored the ability of SPCCT to provide accurate quantification of exogenous contrast agents *in vivo.*

8.3 IODINE

Small-molecule based iodinated contrast agents are currently the only clinically approved CT contrast agents for intravascular administration. Although there are concerns over renal damage and allergic reactions in subpopulations of patients, the safety of iodinated contrast agents is well-established. In addition, the chemical structures of these iodinated contrast agents can be modified to achieve desired viscosity and osmolarity.[49] Despite possible modifications to achieve desired physicochemical properties, the small sizes of these iodinated contrast agents lead to very short circulation times in the blood and rapid extravasation, which in turn leads to a very short time window in which post-injection blood vessel images can be acquired. To resolve this issue, iodine payloads have been formulated into larger dendrimers, emulsions, micelles, and liposomes.[50] These nanoparticle-based contrast agents can also be used for targeted molecular CT imaging. Gaikwad et al. recently developed iodinated nanoscale activity-based probes which consist of iodine-loaded spherical nanostructures made of polymeric dendrimers.[51] These contrast agents contain short targeting peptides as well as acyloxymethyl ketones to target and covalently bind to cysteine cathepsins that are overexpressed in cancer. These formulations lead to increased tumor accumulation in mice due to active targeting and prolonged blood circulation, allowing signal detection in tumors at a low dose of 20 mg/kg.

These recent advances in formulations have made iodine more desirable as a contrast generating payload for CT imaging. However, iodine still suffers substantially reduced contrast production at high tube potentials. When using a conventional CT scanner at 140 kVp approximately only half the contrast is generated compared to when using 80 kVp, since the K-edge energy of iodine is at 33.2 keV, which is well below the mean energy of X-ray spectra of clinically used tube potentials.[52] Yeh et al. recently demonstrated that iodine is the lowest contrast generating element compared to barium, gadolinium, ytterbium, tantalum, gold, and bismuth when using tube potentials of 100–140 kVp (that are practical for scanning medium and larger adults).[52] Even at lower tube potentials, iodine yields less contrast than gadolinium and ytterbium.

The reduction of iodine's contrast when using high-tube potential is a disadvantage in conventional CT. However, this effect makes iodine a favorable contrast material for DECT imaging since DECT imaging quantifies iodine by differentiating high energy X-ray photons from low-energy photons. For this reason, iodine has been well studied in DECT imaging.[53–55] Some studies have demonstrated that it would be feasible to discriminate iodine-based nanoparticles from other elements such as gold and gadolinium.[11,53] In addition, the quantification of iodine can be performed without the need of a pre-scan. This can provide valuable information such as tissue perfusion rate without additional radiation exposure to the patient. Furthermore, virtual monoenergetic images can be reconstructed from DECT imaging, which can lead to a decreased beam hardening effect and an increased iodine signal for better detection of lesions even at lower iodine dose injection.[56,57]

However, DECT imaging still cannot accurately discriminate between iodine and calcium. Because of the similarity in mass attenuation coefficient between iodine and calcium, iodine is challenging to specifically distinguish in K-edge imaging using SPCCT systems as well. Panta et al. and Moghiseh et al., however, have demonstrated that material decomposition between iodine and calcium can be done with a preclinical SPCCT scanner in a plastic phantom.[58,59] The usefulness of iodine in SPCCT has also been endorsed in a study by Leng et al. that has demonstrated accurate iodine quantification in iodine mapping done in a clinical scale SPCCT scanner.[60] Symon et al. also investigated the feasibility of quantifying iodine concentration with a similar SPCCT scanner. The results show good accuracy and reproducibility in the quantification of iodine samples placed underneath a canine model during the scan.[18]

The feasibility of iodine imaging in SPCCT has perhaps been best demonstrated by de Vries et al.[33] In this study, a preclinical SPCCT scanner was used to visualize and quantify the concentration of iodine-based nanoparticle contrast agents in mice. The preclinical SPCCT scanner used a beam of 70 kVp and six energy bins whose thresholds were set at 25, 34, 39, 44, 49, and 55 keV. The iodinated nanoparticle was synthesized by stabilizing iodinated oil with an amphiphilic diblock polymer of DOTA-PBD-PEO, resulting in emulsions with a mean hydrodynamic radius of 95 nm (Figure 8.5A). The polymer also was labeled with ^{111}In to allow SPECT imaging for comparison. Phantom imaging was performed to demonstrate quantification accuracy and iodine decomposition for this agent. The iodine images of the phantom only showed the vials containing iodine and did not contain any signal from the highly concentrated calcium solution (Figure 8.5B), which is possible due to low shielding and high number of low-energy photons in the beam used in this small animal system. In *ex vivo* mouse imaging, even blood vessels that go through bone structures could be successfully delineated from the bone by combining information from the photoelectric and

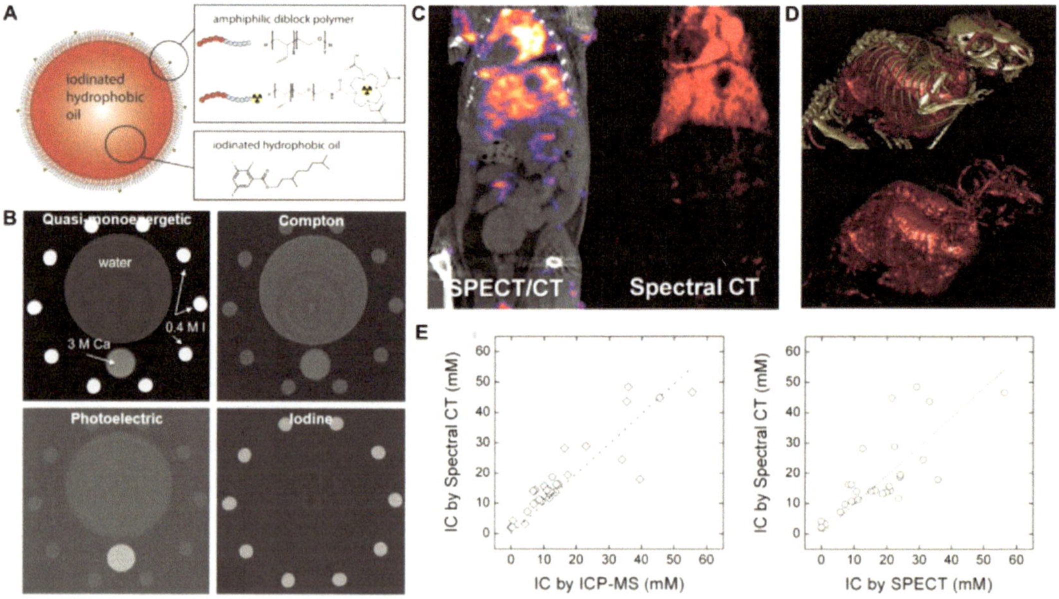

FIGURE 8.5 (A) Schematic depiction of the iodinated emulsion. (B) SPCCT images of a phantom with water, 0.4 M of iodine solution, and 3 M calcium chloride solution. Quasi-monoenergetic image at 40 keV (top left), Compton imaging (top right), photoelectric image (bottom left), and iodine-based image (bottom right). (C) *Ex vivo* SPECT/CT (left) and SPCCT images (right) of iodinated emulsion-injected mice. (D) Attenuation derived discrimination of iodine and bone from SPCCT scan: iodine and bone (top right) and iodine only (bottom right). (E) Correlation between SPCCT, ICP-MS, and SPECT. Figure adapted with permission from reference.[33]

iodine images (Figure 8.5C,D). Similar biodistribution patterns for the iodine-based contrast agents were observed between SPECT and SPCCT images, with high concentrations of agent found in the blood vessels, heart, liver, and spleen with both modalities. The iodine concentrations in different volumes of interest were measured and compared to ICP-MS (inductively coupled plasma mass spectroscopy) measurements (Figure 8.5E). The results showed good correlation between SPCCT and ICP-MS, especially at lower iodine concentrations (< 18 mM), demonstrating that it is feasible to quantify iodine concentration *in vivo* with SPCCT imaging.

Iodine seems to benefit from the inherent noise reduction and increased CNR of SPCCT imaging as demonstrated by Pourmorteza et al. in human patients and Gutjahr et al. in human cadavers.[20,22] While iodine is useful for multiphase imaging and dual contrast imaging accompanied by the injection of other heavy metal contrast agents, material decomposition of iodine from calcium is going to be challenging in clinical settings due to photon starvation at its low K-edge energy. This is due to the fact that a large number of low-energy photons are absorbed in the patient before reaching the detector. To fully appreciate the capabilities of SPCCT imaging in material differentiation, elements with higher K-edge energies continue to be explored for their development into SPCCT contrast agents.

8.4 GADOLINIUM

Gadolinium has the highest paramagnetism of any element, which has led to its development into several widely used MRI contrast agents. Because of the toxicity of free gadolinium ions, gadolinium-based contrast agents consist of gadolinium ions that are complexed with chelator molecules that reduce the bioavailability of gadolinium enormously. Since the first FDA approval of gadolinium chelate $[Gd(DTPA)(H_2O)]_2$ in 1988, a number of other gadolinium-based contrast agents such as gadobenate (MultiHance), gadobutrol (Gadavist), and gadodiamide (Omniscan) have been approved for clinical use.[61]

Beyond its wide use in MRI, gadolinium has potential to be developed into a SPCCT contrast agent due to its K-edge energy of 50.2 keV, which is very close to the mean photon energy in clinical X-ray spectra. In addition, gadolinium has excellent contrast generation especially at lower X-ray tube potentials in conventional CT imaging.[52] Moreover, since its linear attenuation coefficient is sufficiently different from that of calcium, gadolinium-based contrast agents will be particularly beneficial in the intravascular imaging of coronary disease diagnoses in which differentiation between the vasculature structure, calcified plaques, and metal stents is crucial. Feuerlein et al. demonstrated the feasibility of differentiating a gadolinium-based contrast agent from calcified plaque and stent material using a preclinical SPCCT scanner.[62] K-edge imaging of gadolinium in a phantom that contained a gadolinium chelate-filled blood vessel with partial occlusion in the stent revealed clear differentiation of gadolinium-filled area from the occlusion and the stent material. In conventional CT images, the low density calcified plaque in the occlusion and the gadolinium-filled lumen exhibited the same level of attenuation and could not be distinguished.

The K-edge energy of gadolinium is also well-separated from K-edge energy of iodine, which can allow dual contrast imaging of gadolinium and iodine. Dangelmaier et al. investigated the feasibility of differentiating endoleaks from intra-aneurysmatic calcifications after repair in a single CT scan.[63] In their phantom model, a stent-lined compartment that represented an aortic aneurysm was filled with both gadolinium chelate (gadopentetic acid dimeglumine) and iodine. Several compartments adjacent to the first were filled with either iodine representing an endoleak in the arterial phase, gadolinium representing a leak in the venous or delayed phase, or calcium chloride representing calcifications. These different compartments of similar attenuation values could be easily differentiated in the material-specific images of gadolinium, iodine, and calcium that were generated in the study.

Dual contrast agent imaging with SPCCT systems can also lead to successful detection of liver lesions as demonstrated by Muenzel et al. This study once again utilized a gadolinium-based contrast agent to image its distribution in portal venous phase and an iodine-based contrast agent to image its distribution in arterial phase.[64] Using a specialized algorithm, liver lesions of four different types were successfully detected and classified in a liver phantom by the material specific imaging of gadolinium and iodine. In a related study, Muenzel et al. demonstrated that it was possible to differentiate gadolinium-filled polyps from iodine-filled colon and quantify concentration of each contrast agent.[65]

The studies that demonstrated the potential uses of gadolinium-based contrast agents in SPCCT imaging were mostly evaluated with either preclinical SPCCT scanners or custom-designed phantoms. As whole-body imaging CT scanners have lower spatial resolution and *in vivo* environment has much more complex anatomical structure, more studies need to be carried out to fully validate the feasibility of using gadolinium-based contrast agents in clinical SPCCT imaging.

A recent study by Si-Mohamed et al. endeavored to understand the feasibility of gadolinium differentiation in clinical settings by imaging rats with a whole-body prototype SPCCT scanner.[32] The authors confirmed that it is possible to differentiate between gadolinium chelate and iodine-based contrast agent and quantify the concentrations of both materials via *in vitro* phantom imaging. They then injected two groups of rats with a gadolinium chelate and an iodinated contrast agent by either (1) intraperitoneal injection of gadolinium chelate and intravenous injection of iodine or (2) intraperitoneal injection of iodine and intravenous injection of gadolinium chelate. The image quality and ease of differentiation between gadolinium and iodine were evaluated (Figure 8.6A,B). SPCCT images were of higher spatial resolution than conventional CT images, which provided better imaging of small structures (Figure 8.6A). Material-specific images clearly visualized and separated the two contrast agents (Figure 8.6B), allowing complete assessment of the peritoneal cavity, as reported by independent radiologist analysis.

For many years, gadolinium chelates were believed to be safe; however, multiple studies that emerged about a decade ago reported a correlation between the administration of gadolinium-based contrast agents and nephrogenic systemic fibrosis in patients with severe renal insufficiency.[66,67] Newer reports found that gadolinium chelates also accumulated in the bones, brains, and the kidneys of patients with no renal impairment.[68,69] Since the estimated required dose of gadolinium-based contrast agents for CT imaging is higher than that of MRI, the potential safety of using gadolinium-based contrast agents for SPCCT imaging is a prominent concern.

Nanoparticle contrast agents that contain gadolinium have safety concerns due to the likely long-lasting retention of gadolinium in these organs. Nevertheless, they continue to be explored as contrast agents for conventional CT and SPCCT. For example, in a study conducted by Roeder et al., gadolinium oxide nanoparticles were clearly distinguished from bone, water, and soft tissue in mice carcasses via material-specific imaging with a preclinical SPCCT system.[70]

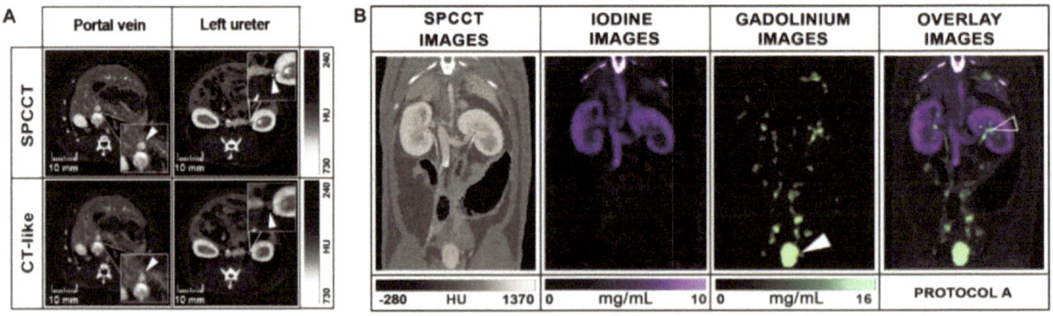

FIGURE 8.6 (A) SPCCT and CT-like images of different levels in a rat injected with both gadolinium chelate and iodinated contrast agent at early IV and IP phase. (B) Coronal oblique SPCCT images and the corresponding material-specific images for iodine and gadolinium. Figure adapted with permission from reference.[32]

8.5 YTTERBIUM

The K-edge energy of ytterbium (61.3 keV) sits near the middle of the X-ray tube energy spectra typically used in SPCCT and is close to the characteristic radiation energy of the anode material, tungsten, at which a large increase in photon flux is observed. Since K-edge imaging is mainly affected by the characteristics of the energy bin that contains the K-edge of the element, having a high number of photons near its K-edge energy can result in low noise and high CNR.[31] For this reason, ytterbium is a very promising element for SPCCT contrast agent development. However, not much is known about ytterbium in terms of its safety in humans and its utility in X-ray imaging. Only a few studies have used ytterbium-based nanoparticles for multimodal imaging and X-ray CT imaging so far.[71,72]

A study by Pan et al. examined ytterbium's potential for use in SPCCT imaging and its relative safety profile in rodents using a ytterbium complex-based nanoparticle as a contrast agent for SPCCT imaging.[27] These nanocolloids were synthesized by suspending a commercially available trivalent ytterbium complex called ytterbium (III) 2,4-pentanedionate in polysorbates and then encapsulating the resulting hydrophobic core in a phospholipid monolayer (Figure 8.7A). The ytterbium nanocolloids incorporated a substantial payload of ytterbium atoms (> 500,000 per nanoparticle) into a stable nanoparticle. In phantom imaging with a prototype SPCCT system, the signal intensity of ytterbium nanocolloids in ytterbium images was linearly correlated with ytterbium concentration (Figure 8.7B). K-edge imaging of ytterbium with iterative reconstruction was able to detect the ytterbium nanoparticles *in vivo* even at low doses (Figure 8.7C). The ytterbium nanocolloids exhibited excellent bioelimination with approximately 90% of the injected dose eliminated within 7 days. The remaining ytterbium largely accumulated in the liver.

8.6 HAFNIUM

Hafnium (Z = 72) has similar CT contrast generation as ytterbium (Z = 70) since they are very close in atomic number. There have been a few studies in recent years that have reported different approaches to synthesizing hafnium oxide nanoparticles (HfO_2 NP).[73,74] The safety profiles and

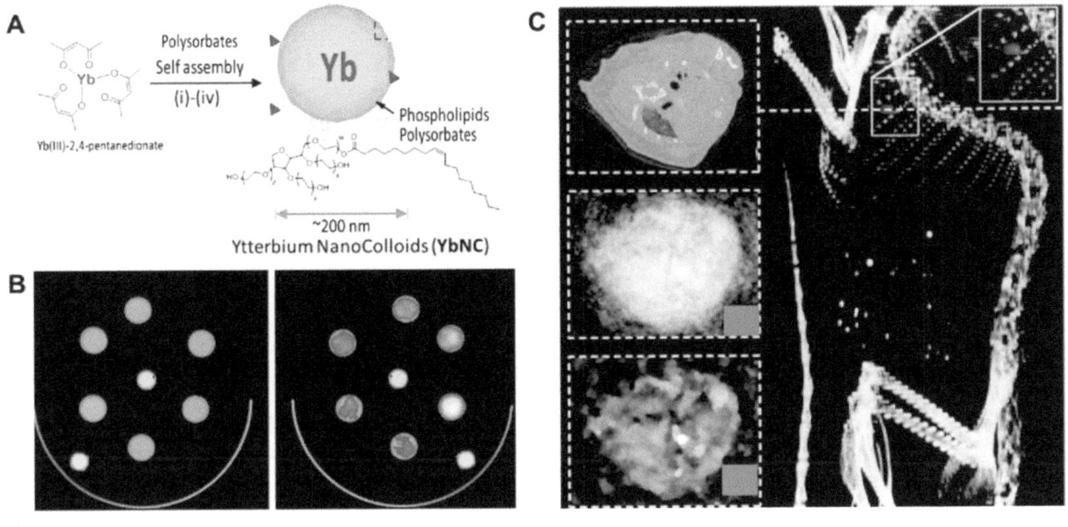

FIGURE 8.7 (A) Schematic depiction of ytterbium nanocolloid design. (B) Conventional CT-like image (left) and the same image overlaid with ytterbium-specific K-edge images (right). C) SPCCT image of mouse with signal from ytterbium in the heart shown in the boxed inset (right). Conventional CT-like image (top left), ytterbium-specific images after one (middle left), and twenty iterations (bottom left) in iterative image reconstruction. Figure adapted with permission from reference.[27]

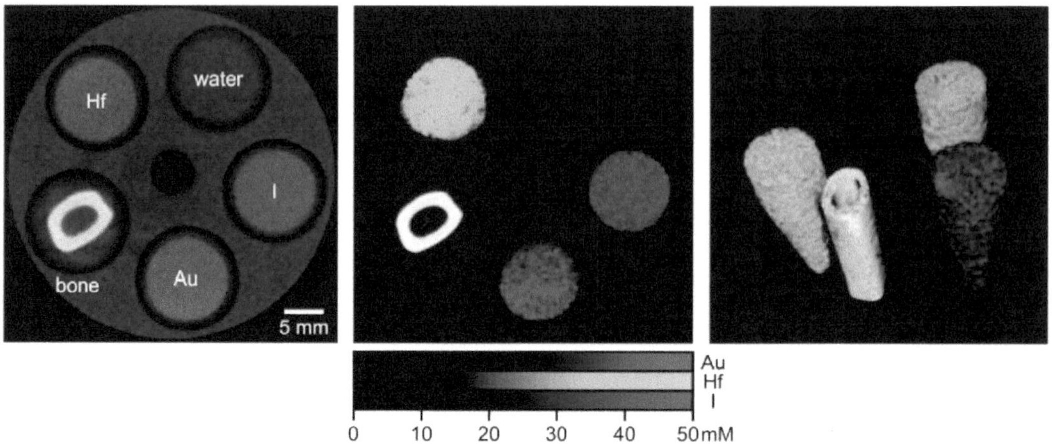

FIGURE 8.8 A 2D conventional CT image (left), a post-processed, overlay 2D SPCCT image of AuNP, HfO_2 NP, iodine, bone, and water images (middle), and a post-processed 3D-reconstructed SPCCT image of the phantom containing HfO_2 NP, AuNP, iodine, bone, and water. Figure adapted with permission from reference.[28]

possible biomedical applications of these nanoparticles are largely unknown and are under investigation.[75–77] HfO_2 NP are being explored for photodynamic therapy agents for cancer treatment, with one formulation already seeing use in clinical trials in Europe.[76,78]

Another possible bioapplication of HfO_2 NP is development into X-ray CT or SPCCT contrast agent as explored by McGinnity et al.[28] In phantom imaging with a conventional clinical CT system, polyvinylpyrrolidone-functionalized HfO_2 NP generated higher CT attenuation when compared with gold nanoparticles and iodine at tube potentials of 100 kVp, 120 kVp, and 140 kVp. In SPCCT imaging with a preclinical system, HfO_2 NP, gold nanoparticles, and iodine contrast agents were all successfully delineated and quantified simultaneously (Figure 8.8).

8.7 TANTALUM

Similar to ytterbium and hafnium, the K-edge of tantalum (67.3 keV) is near the mean photon energies of the types of X-ray spectra typically used in SPCCT. Aside from its K-edge, tantalum has other favorable properties that make it a candidate element for development into a CT or SPCCT contrast agent. It has high-elemental density of 16.4 g/cm^3 that can allow high payloads to be delivered to a target, and it is much more affordable than other high-performing elements that are being experimentally considered for CT contrast agents (approximately 13-fold cheaper than gold and 4-fold cheaper than ytterbium). Due to these advantages, tantalum has been among the most widely studied elements for use in CT contrast agents in the past decade, together with gold and bismuth.

Among different tantalum compounds, tantalum oxide has been the focus of CT contrast agent studies due to its well established chemical inertness and biocompatibility.[79,80] Tantalum oxide has been formulated into nanoparticles with various coatings to make it water-soluble, which is necessary for use as a CT blood pool agent. Bonitatibus et al. developed zwitterionic tantalum oxide nanoparticles that are smaller than 6 nm in diameter to promote renal clearance, hence bolstering bioelimination and long-term safety. Both of these factors are important considerations for experimental nanoparticle-based contrast agents.[80] Through several papers, the group has shown that tantalum oxide nanoparticles have good biocompatibility, desirable physicochemical properties, excellent bioelimination, and exceptional contrast enhancement in CT imaging.[80–82] In conventional CT imaging of rats, the authors also demonstrated that tantalum has better contrast enhancement than clinically approved iodine-based contrast agents while boasting a comparable safety profile and similar bioelimination.[81] The efficacy of tantalum for CT imaging was further supported by Oh et al. who were able to synthesize tantalum oxide nanoparticles on a large scale with good uniformity in size via a microemulsion technique.[83]

Kim et al. has recently demonstrated that tantalum oxide nanoparticles also have good potential as SPCCT contrast agents.[31] In their phantom study performed at 120 kVp with a clinical scale prototype SPCCT scanner, tantalum generated superior CNR over tungsten, gold, and bismuth. The authors also demonstrated the feasibility of differentiating TaONP from iodine. K-edge imaging of tantalum accurately determined its location and clearly distinguished tantalum oxide nanoparticles from both iodine and calcium phosphate with the detection limit of tantalum oxide nanoparticles being as low as 1 mg/mL.

8.8 BISMUTH

Bismuth is the highest atomic number ($Z = 83$) element that can be considered to potentially form SPCCT contrast agents due to the radioactivity of higher atomic number elements (e.g., polonium ($Z = 84$), astatine ($Z = 85$), radon ($Z = 86$), etc.). Therefore, bismuth has the highest K-edge energy (91 keV) of all the potential elements. Bismuth produces similar contrast at varying tube potentials from 80 kVp to 140 kVp, and the contrast it generates is comparable to that of other highly contrast generating elements, such as ytterbium and tantalum at 140 kVp, making it an appealing element for CT contrast agent development especially when imaging at high-tube potentials.[52,84] Bismuth is also considered to be a fairly biocompatible element.[85,86] Bismuth has long been used for treatment of gastrointestinal ailments, thus bismuth seems to be the most feasible for use as enteric contrast material via oral administration.[87] In addition, bismuth-based nanoparticles have been synthesized into promising blood pool agents by coating nanoparticle surfaces with safe materials in order to promote chemical inertness and biocompatibility.

Bismuth may also be considered as a strong candidate for a CT or SPCCT contrast agent because it is much cheaper than gold. The feasibility of using bismuth for SPCCT contrast agent has been demonstrated by Symons et al. who successfully distinguished orally administered bismuth subsalicylate from intravenously injected gadolinium chelate and iodinated contrast agent via SPCCT imaging of canine model.[18] However, the density of bismuth (9.78 g/cm^3) is less than half the density of gold, and its nanoparticle synthesis methods often require incorporation of other ions such as sulfur and oxygen, making the delivery of high bismuth payloads challenging.[88–90]

To explore the feasibility of imaging intravascular thrombi via SPCCT imaging, Pan et al. synthesized a nanoparticle that they termed NanoK.[26] Similarly to the ytterbium- and gold-based nanoparticles introduced earlier, the bismuth payload, bismuth n-decanoate, was encapsulated in polysorbates and stabilized by a phospholipid layer. Anti-fibrin monoclonal antibodies were attached to the surface via biotinylated phospholipids to allow imaging of fibrin-rich clots, *in vitro* and *in vivo*.

The delineation of NanoK from calcium and the linear relationship between the attenuation and concentration of NanoK were first established by imaging a phantom containing different concentrations of NanoK. In another phantom study, the possibility of fibrin targeting with NanoK and its detection in K-edge imaging were investigated with the imaging of a human carotid artery endarterectomy specimen of unstable human atherosclerotic vascular tissue (Figure 8.9A). Once again, NanoK and calcium were successfully distinguished by K-edge imaging, and NanoK signals were found in fibrin-rich areas of microthrombi in the specimen. After the confirmation of NanoK detection in these phantom studies, NanoK and its biodistribution were examined by incubating the NanoK particles with the thrombus between snares *in situ* for 30 min then restoring the blood circulation for 90 min. There was immediate contrast in the blood after the intravenous injection, although no contrast could be detected after 30 min. Post mortem images displayed intra-arterial thrombus via K-edge imaging of bismuth that was clearly distinguished from bone (Figure 8.9B).

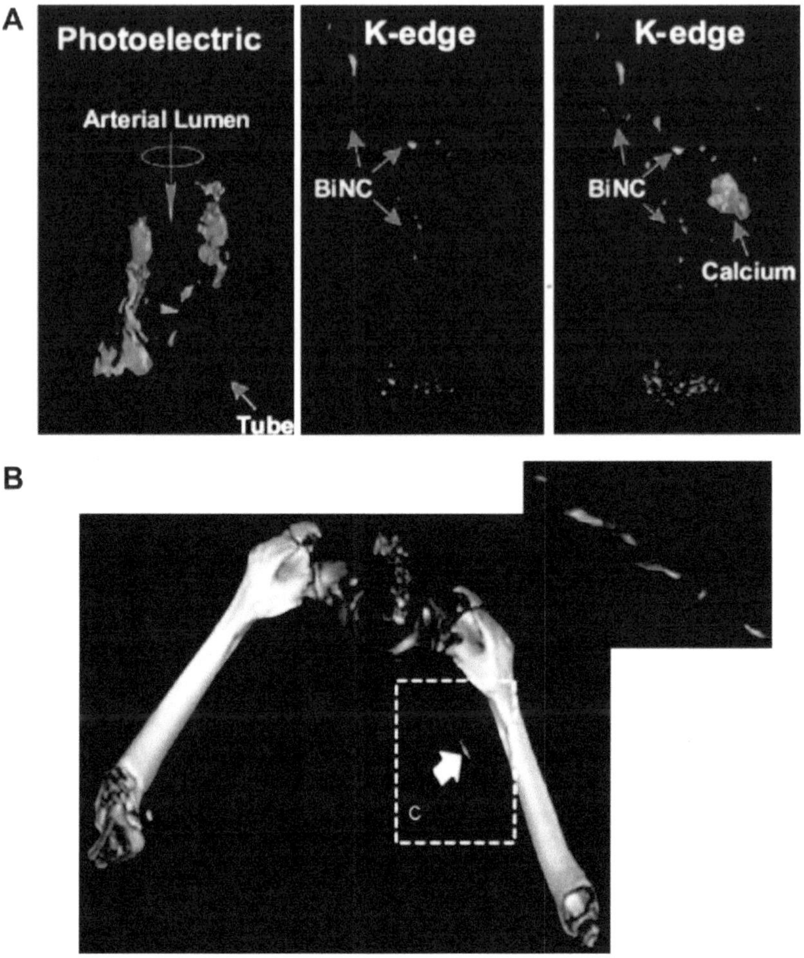

FIGURE 8.9 (A) Photoelectric effect image (left), bismuth-specific image (middle), and overlay of the two images (right) of human atherosclerotic vascular tissue that had been incubated with 100 mL of 200 μg/mL NanoK particles for 1 hour at 37°C. (B) SPCCT image of rabbit with bismuth signal from an *in situ* clot indicated by the white arrow (left), enlarged image of the dotted area (top right). Figure adapted with permission from reference.[26]

8.9 DISCUSSION

Over the last decade, SPCCT imaging has witnessed rapid advances in prototype scanners, which have evolved from preclinical micro-CT-based scanners to whole-body clinical CT-modified scanners, as well as improvements in spectral and K-edge image reconstruction methods.[13,91–95] Moreover, the advantages of SPCCT imaging in noise reduction, high contrast generation, and multiple material decomposition have been assessed in human subjects in recent years.[21–23,96] However, for the short term, any clinical use of SPCCT systems will be confined to using iodinated or barium-based contrast agents due to the fact that they are the only clinically approved agents. Though iodinated contrast agents can be effective in conventional CT imaging, as described above, recent studies have identified other experimental contrast agents made of heavy metal elements that can produce higher CNR and provide clearer material decomposition from the underlying tissue (e.g., bones) in SPCCT imaging. Although it may be a long process for them to get to FDA approval, these experimental contrast agents would benefit SPCCT imaging by taking advantage of its full potential for K-edge imaging. For this to happen, more comprehensive studies will first to be completed in order to evaluate the long-term safety of novel agents.

The most promising elements for the development of SPCCT-specific contrast agents are gold, tantalum, ytterbium, bismuth, and gadolinium. Gold has been the most extensively studied element for its use as a nanoparticle-based SPCCT contrast agent, and its biocompatibility and high-contrast generation have already been demonstrated in small animals. However, its high cost could limit its potential uses. Tantalum and ytterbium both have K-edge energies near the mean photon energy spectrum, which can lead to higher CNR production.[31] The efficacy in X-ray CT imaging and the biocompatibility of nanoparticle formulations that are based on these two elements have also been demonstrated in several studies. However, the safety profiles of agents based on both of these elements are still poorly understood and more comprehensive studies are needed in order to consider clinical use. Bismuth's high K-edge energy is considerably greater than the mean photon energy of spectra typically used, which is a disadvantage when considering its use as a SPCCT contrast agent. Yet, because of its chemical inertness and affordability, it may continue to gather significant interest. Gadolinium has been broadly studied for its delineation from other elements in phantom imaging due to the fact that its chelates are already FDA approved for MRI. Because of this, gadolinium chelates have potential to be used for SPCCT imaging applications as well, although recent findings of their retention in brains and other organs raise a concern.[66]

Potentially the most attractive novel SPCCT agent for clinical translation would be a vascular agent that is based on a higher Z element than iodine (to allow its detection via K-edge imaging and to allow it to be distinguished from iodine agents, so that both iodine and the novel agent can be simultaneously imaged). In addition, an agent that has somewhat different pharmacokinetics to iodine would be preferable, that is, somewhat longer lasting vascular contrast. This property would address a shortcoming of the currently FDA-approved iodinated agents, that is, very rapid blood clearance and therefore very narrow imaging window. Moreover, a longer blood residence time might allow for additional diagnostic properties compared to the iodinated agents. Last, the agent should be excreted within a reasonably short timeframe, that is, within a few days. The agent design that might fulfill these criteria could be nanoparticles or other types of structures in the 1–5 nm size range that are based on elements whose K-edge is in the range of 40–100 keV (i.e., the region of the spectrum where there are typically high numbers of photons). Structures in the 1–5 nm size range should have longer circulation times than iodine-based molecules due to less extravasation, but are still small enough for rapid renal clearance.[97,98] Structures larger than 5 nm that are injected intravenously are typically retained for months.[11] An alternative clinically translatable composition is a structure that is larger than 5 nm, but can be degraded into sub-5 nm components.[99,100] By analogy with iron oxide nanoparticles, a new agent of such characteristics could potentially be used for cell tracking or for targeted imaging as well, if suitably modified.[101] Of the currently published agents, certain types of tantalum oxide nanoparticles and gold nanoparticles best fulfill the above criteria, although there is no bar in principle to the development of such agents based on other elements.

In conclusion, there are several elements that are currently being considered and investigated for their feasibility to be developed as SPCCT-specific contrast agents. In the past decade, the studies that have explored these experimental contrast agents have moved into use with larger animal models and imaging with prototype scanners that are modified from clinical CT scanners, increasing their potential clinical relevance. More comprehensive studies that validate contrast agents' safety profiles and superior effectiveness in SPCCT imaging will continue to bring them closer to clinical approval and help unravel the full capabilities of SPCCT imaging.

ACKNOWLEDGMENTS

This work was supported in part by the NIH (R01 HL131557) and the American Heart Association (18PRE34030383). We acknowledge the assistance of Portia Maidment in preparing this manuscript.

REFERENCES

1. Hounsfield, G. N., Computerized transverse axial scanning (tomography). 1. Description of system. *Br J Radiol* 1973, *46*(552), 1016–1022.
2. Health equipment—Computed tomography (CT) scanners—OECD Data [Internet]. The OECD. [cited 2018 May 30]. Available from: ⟨http://data.oecd.org/healtheqt/computed-tomography-ct-scanners.htm⟩.
3. Bernstein, A. L.; Dhanantwari, A.; Jurcova, M.; Cheheltani, R.; Naha, P. C.; Ivanc, T.; Shefer, E.; Cormode, D. P., Effect of iterative model-based reconstruction on the sensitivity of computed tomography towards iodine and gold nanoparticle contrast agents. *Sci Rep* 2016, *6*, 26177.
4. Noel, P. B.; Renger, B.; Fiebich, M.; Munzel, D.; Fingerle, A. A.; Rummeny, E. J.; Dobritz, M., Does iterative reconstruction lower CT radiation dose: Evaluation of 15,000 examinations. *PloS one* 2013, *8*(11), e81141.
5. Willemink, M. J.; de Jong, P. A.; Leiner, T.; de Heer, L. M.; Nievelstein, R. A.; Budde, R. P.; Schilham, A. M., Iterative reconstruction techniques for computed tomography part 1: Technical principles. *Eur Radiol* 2013, *23*(6), 1623–1631.
6. Willemink, M. J.; Leiner, T.; de Jong, P. A.; de Heer, L. M.; Nievelstein, R. A.; Schilham, A. M.; Budde, R. P., Iterative reconstruction techniques for computed tomography part 2: Initial results in dose reduction and image quality. *Eur Radiol* 2013, *23*(6), 1632–1642.
7. Marin, D.; Nelson, R. C.; Schindera, S. T.; Richard, S.; Youngblood, R. S.; Yoshizumi, T. T.; Samei, E., Low-tube-voltage, high-tube-current multidetector abdominal CT: Improved image quality and decreased radiation dose with adaptive statistical iterative reconstruction algorithm–initial clinical experience. *Radiology* 2010, *254*(1), 145–153.
8. McCollough, C. H.; Leng, S.; Yu, L.; Fletcher, J. G., Dual- and multi-energy CT: Principles, technical approaches, and clinical applications. *Radiology* 2015, *276*(3), 637–653.
9. Yeh, B. M.; FitzGerald, P. F.; Edic, P. M.; Lambert, J. W.; Colborn, R. E.; Marino, M. E.; Evans, P. M.; Roberts, J. C.; Wang, Z. J.; Wong, M. J.; Bonitatibus, P. J., Jr., Opportunities for new CT contrast agents to maximize the diagnostic potential of emerging spectral CT technologies. *Adv Drug Deliv Rev* 2017, *113*, 201–222.
10. Leithner, D.; Wichmann, J. L.; Vogl, T. J.; Trommer, J.; Martin, S. S.; Scholtz, J. E.; Bodelle, B.; De Cecco, C. N.; Duguay, T.; Nance, J. W., Jr.; Schoepf, U. J.; Albrecht, M. H., Virtual monoenergetic imaging and iodine perfusion maps improve diagnostic accuracy of dual-energy computed tomography pulmonary angiography with suboptimal contrast attenuation. *Invest Radiol* 2017, *52*(11), 659–665.
11. Si-Mohamed, S.; Bar-Ness, D.; Sigovan, M.; Cormode, D. P.; Coulon, P.; Coche, E.; Vlassenbroek, A.; Normand, G.; Boussel, L.; Douek, P., Review of an initial experience with an experimental spectral photon-counting computed tomography system. *Nuc Instr Meth Phys Res* 2017, *873*(21), 27–35.
12. Cormode, D. P.; Si-Mohamed, S.; Bar-Ness, D.; Sigovan, M.; Naha, P. C.; Balegamire, J.; Lavenne, F.; Coulon, P.; Roessl, E.; Bartels, M.; Rokni, M.; Blevis, I.; Boussel, L.; Douek, P., Multicolor spectral photon-counting computed tomography: In vivo dual contrast imaging with a high count rate scanner. *Sci Rep* 2017, *7*(1), 4784.
13. Roessl, E.; Herrmann, C., Cramer-Rao lower bound of basis image noise in multiple-energy x-ray imaging. *Phys Med Biol* 2009, *54*(5), 1307–1318.
14. Boussel, L.; Coulon, P.; Thran, A.; Roessl, E.; Martens, G.; Sigovan, M.; Douek, P., Photon counting spectral CT component analysis of coronary artery atherosclerotic plaque samples. *Br J Radiol* 2014, *87*(1040), 20130798.
15. Leng, S.; Yu, Z.; Halaweish, A.; Kappler, S.; Hahn, K.; Henning, A.; Li, Z.; Lane, J.; Levin, D. L.; Jorgensen, S.; Ritman, E.; McCollough, C., Dose-efficient ultrahigh-resolution scan mode using a photon counting detector computed tomography system. *J Med Imaging* 2016, *3*(4), 043504.
16. Taguchi, K.; Iwanczyk, J. S., Vision 20/20: Single photon counting x-ray detectors in medical imaging. *Med Phys* 2013, *40*(10), 100901.

17. Symons, R.; Cork, T. E.; Lakshmanan, M. N.; Evers, R.; Davies-Venn, C.; Rice, K. A.; Thomas, M. L.; Liu, C. Y.; Kappler, S.; Ulzheimer, S.; Sandfort, V.; Bluemke, D. A.; Pourmorteza, A., Dual-contrast agent photon-counting computed tomography of the heart: Initial experience. *JACC Cardiovasc Imaging* 2017, *33*(8), 1253–1261.
18. Symons, R.; Krauss, B.; Sahbaee, P.; Cork, T. E.; Lakshmanan, M. N.; Bluemke, D. A.; Pourmorteza, A., Photon-counting CT for simultaneous imaging of multiple contrast agents in the abdomen: An in vivo study. *Med Phys* 2017, *44*(10), 5120–5127.
19. Cormode, D. P.; Roessl, E.; Thran, A.; Skajaa, T.; Gordon, R. E.; Schlomka, J. P.; Fuster, V.; Fisher, E. A.; Mulder, W. J.; Proksa, R.; Fayad, Z. A., Atherosclerotic plaque composition: Analysis with multicolor CT and targeted gold nanoparticles. *Radiology* 2010, *256*(3), 774–782.
20. Gutjahr, R.; Halaweish, A. F.; Yu, Z.; Leng, S.; Yu, L.; Li, Z.; Jorgensen, S. M.; Ritman, E. L.; Kappler, S.; McCollough, C. H., Human imaging with photon counting-based computed tomography at clinical dose levels: Contrast-to-noise ratio and cadaver studies. *Invest Radiol* 2016, *51*(7), 421–429.
21. Pourmorteza, A.; Symons, R.; Reich, D. S.; Bagheri, M.; Cork, T. E.; Kappler, S.; Ulzheimer, S.; Bluemke, D. A., Photon-counting CT of the brain: In vivo human results and image-quality assessment. *AJNR Am J Neuroradiol* 2017, *38*(12), 2257–2263.
22. Pourmorteza, A.; Symons, R.; Sandfort, V.; Mallek, M.; Fuld, M. K.; Henderson, G.; Jones, E. C.; Malayeri, A. A.; Folio, L. R.; Bluemke, D. A., Abdominal imaging with contrast-enhanced photon-counting CT: First human experience. *Radiology* 2016, *279*(1), 239–245.
23. Symons, R.; Reich, D. S.; Bagheri, M.; Cork, T. E.; Krauss, B.; Ulzheimer, S.; Kappler, S.; Bluemke, D. A.; Pourmorteza, A., Photon-counting computed tomography for vascular imaging of the head and neck: First in vivo human results. *Invest Radiol* 2018, *53*(3), 135–142.
24. Tepel, M.; Aspelin, P.; Lameire, N., Contrast-induced nephropathy: A clinical and evidence-based approach. *Circulation* 2006, *113*(14), 1799–1806.
25. Solomon, R.; Dumouchel, W., Contrast media and nephropathy: Findings from systematic analysis and food and drug administration reports of adverse effects. *Invest Radiol* 2006, *41*(8), 651–660.
26. Pan, D.; Roessl, E.; Schlomka, J. P.; Caruthers, S. D.; Senpan, A.; Scott, M. J.; Allen, J. S.; Zhang, H.; Hu, G.; Gaffney, P. J.; Choi, E. T.; Rasche, V.; Wickline, S. A.; Proksa, R.; Lanza, G. M., Computed tomography in color: NanoK-enhanced spectral CT molecular imaging. *Angew Chem Int Ed* 2010, *49*(50), 9635–9639.
27. Pan, D.; Schirra, C. O.; Senpan, A.; Schmieder, A. H.; Stacy, A. J.; Roessl, E.; Thran, A.; Wickline, S. A.; Proska, R.; Lanza, G. M., An early investigation of ytterbium nanocolloids for selective and quantitative "multicolor" spectral CT imaging. *ACS Nano* 2012, *6*(4), 3364–3370.
28. McGinnity, T. L.; Dominguez, O.; Curtis, T. E.; Nallathamby, P. D.; Hoffman, A. J.; Roeder, R. K., Hafnia (HfO2) nanoparticles as an x-ray contrast agent and mid-infrared biosensor. *Nanoscale* 2016, *8*(28), 13627–13637.
29. Schirra, C. O.; Senpan, A.; Roessl, E.; Thran, A.; Stacy, A. J.; Wu, L.; Proska, R.; Pan, D., Second generation gold nanobeacons for robust K-edge imaging with multi-energy CT. *J Mater Chem* 2012, *22*(43), 23071–23077.
30. Chinen, A. B.; Guan, C. M.; Ferrer, J. R.; Barnaby, S. N.; Merkel, T. J.; Mirkin, C. A., Nanoparticle probes for the detection of cancer biomarkers, cells, and tissues by fluorescence. *Chem Rev* 2015, *115*(19), 10530–10574.
31. Kim, J.; Bar-Ness, D.; Si-Mohamed, S.; Coulon, P.; Blevis, I.; Douek, P.; Cormode, D. P., Assessment of candidate elements for development of spectral photon-counting CT specific contrast agents. In press.
32. Si-Mohamed, S.; Thivolet, A.; Bonnot, P. E.; Bar-Ness, D.; Kepenekian, V.; Cormode, D. P.; Douek, P.; Rousset, P., Improved peritoneal cavity and abdominal organ imaging using a biphasic contrast agent protocol and spectral photon counting computed tomography K-edge imaging. *Invest Radiol.* 2018, *53*(10), 629–639.
33. de Vries, A.; Roessl, E.; Kneepkens, E.; Thran, A.; Brendel, B.; Martens, G.; Proska, R.; Nicolay, K.; Grull, H., Quantitative spectral K-edge imaging in preclinical photon-counting x-ray computed tomography. *Invest Radiol* 2015, *50*(4), 297–304.
34. Chhour, P.; Naha, P. C.; O'Neill, S. M.; Litt, H. I.; Reilly, M. P.; Ferrari, V. A.; Cormode, D. P., Labeling monocytes with gold nanoparticles to track their recruitment in atherosclerosis with computed tomography. *Biomaterials* 2016, *87*, 93–103.
35. Li, W.; Chen, X., Gold nanoparticles for photoacoustic imaging. *Nanomedicine* 2015, *10*(2), 299–320.
36. Mieszawska, A. J.; Mulder, W. J.; Fayad, Z. A.; Cormode, D. P., Multifunctional gold nanoparticles for diagnosis and therapy of disease. *Mol Pharm* 2013, *10*(3), 831–847.

37. von Maltzahn, G.; Park, J. H.; Agrawal, A.; Bandaru, N. K.; Das, S. K.; Sailor, M. J.; Bhatia, S. N., Computationally guided photothermal tumor therapy using long-circulating gold nanorod antennas. *Cancer Res* 2009, *69*(9), 3892–3900.
38. Chhour, P.; Kim, J.; Benardo, B.; Tovar, A.; Mian, S.; Litt, H. I.; Ferrari, V. A.; Cormode, D. P., Effect of gold nanoparticle size and coating on labeling monocytes for CT tracking. *Bioconjug Chem* 2017, *28*(1), 260–269.
39. Kim, J.; Chhour, P.; Hsu, J.; Litt, H. I.; Ferrari, V. A.; Popovtzer, R.; Cormode, D. P., Use of nanoparticle contrast agents for cell tracking with computed tomography. *Bioconjug Chem* 2017, *28*(6), 1581–1597.
40. Pan, D.; Schirra, C. O.; Wickline, S. A.; Lanza, G. M., Multicolor computed tomographic molecular imaging with noncrystalline high-metal-density nanobeacons. *Contrast Media Mol Imaging* 2014, *9*(1), 13–25.
41. Galper, M. W.; Saung, M. T.; Fuster, V.; Roessl, E.; Thran, A.; Proksa, R.; Fayad, Z. A.; Cormode, D. P., Effect of computed tomography scanning parameters on gold nanoparticle and iodine contrast. *Invest Radiol* 2012, *47*(8), 475–481.
42. Jackson, P. A.; Rahman, W. N.; Wong, C. J.; Ackerly, T.; Geso, M., Potential dependent superiority of gold nanoparticles in comparison to iodinated contrast agents. *Eur J Radiol* 2010, *75*(1), 104–109.
43. Allijn, I. E.; Leong, W.; Tang, J.; Gianella, A.; Mieszawska, A. J.; Fay, F.; Ma, G.; Russell, S.; Callo, C. B.; Gordon, R. E.; Korkmaz, E.; Post, J. A.; Zhao, Y.; Gerritsen, H. C.; Thran, A.; Proksa, R.; Daerr, H.; Storm, G.; Fuster, V.; Fisher, E. A.; Fayad, Z. A.; Mulder, W. J.Cormode, D. P., Gold nanocrystal labeling allows low-density lipoprotein imaging from the subcellular to macroscopic level. *ACS Nano* 2013, *7*(11), 9761–9770.
44. Chen, F.; Goel, S.; Hernandez, R.; Graves, S. A.; Shi, S.; Nickles, R. J.; Cai, W., Dynamic positron emission tomography imaging of renal clearable gold nanoparticles. *Small* 2016, *12*(20), 2775–2782.
45. Perrault, S. D.; Walkey, C.; Jennings, T.; Fischer, H. C.; Chan, W. C., Mediating tumor targeting efficiency of nanoparticles through design. *Nano Lett* 2009, *9*(5), 1909–1915.
46. Jiao, P. F.; Zhou, H. Y.; Chen, L. X.; Yan, B., Cancer-targeting multifunctionalized gold nanoparticles in imaging and therapy. *Curr Med Chem* 2011, *18*(14), 2086–2102.
47. Mullner, M.; Schlattl, H.; Hoeschen, C.; Dietrich, O., Feasibility of spectral CT imaging for the detection of liver lesions with gold-based contrast agents - A simulation study. *Phys Med* 2015, *31*(8), 875–881.
48. Si-Mohamed, S.; Cormode, D. P.; Bar-Ness, D.; Sigovan, M.; Naha, P. C.; Langlois, J. B.; Chalabreysse, L.; Coulon, P.; Blevis, I.; Roessl, E.; Erhard, K.; Boussel, L.; Douek, P., Evaluation of spectral photon counting computed tomography K-edge imaging for determination of gold nanoparticle biodistribution in vivo. *Nanoscale* 2017, *9*(46), 18246–18257.
49. Bourin, M.; Jolliet, P.; Ballereau, F., An overview of the clinical pharmacokinetics of x-ray contrast media. *Clin Pharmacokinet* 1997, *32*(3), 180–193.
50. Cormode, D. P.; Naha, P. C.; Fayad, Z. A., Nanoparticle contrast agents for computed tomography: A focus on micelles. *Contrast Media Mol Imaging* 2014, *9*(1), 37–52.
51. Gaikwad, H. K.; Tsvirkun, D.; Ben-Nun, Y.; Merquiol, E.; Popovtzer, R.; Blum, G., Molecular imaging of cancer using x-ray computed tomography with protease targeted iodinated activity-based probes. *Nano Lett* 2018, *18*(3), 1582–1591.
52. FitzGerald, P. F.; Colborn, R. E.; Edic, P. M.; Lambert, J. W.; Torres, A. S.; Bonitatibus, P. J., Jr.; Yeh, B. M., CT image contrast of high-Z elements: Phantom imaging studies and clinical implications. *Radiology* 2016, *278*(3), 723–733.
53. Ashton, J. R.; Clark, D. P.; Moding, E. J.; Ghaghada, K.; Kirsch, D. G.; West, J. L.; Badea, C. T., Dual-energy micro-CT functional imaging of primary lung cancer in mice using gold and iodine nanoparticle contrast agents: A validation study. *PloS One* 2014, *9*(2), e88129.
54. Badea, C. T.; Guo, X.; Clark, D.; Johnston, S. M.; Marshall, C.; Piantadosi, C., Lung imaging in rodents using dual energy micro-CT. *Proc SPIE Int Soc Opt Eng* 2012, *8317*.
55. Ferda, J.; Ferdova, E.; Mirka, H.; Baxa, J.; Bednarova, A.; Flohr, T.; Schmidt, B.; Matejovic, M.; Kreuzberg, B., Pulmonary imaging using dual-energy CT, a role of the assessment of iodine and air distribution. *Eur J Radiol* 2011, *77*(2), 287–293.
56. Hanson, G. J.; Michalak, G. J.; Childs, R.; McCollough, B.; Kurup, A. N.; Hough, D. M.; Frye, J. M.; Fidler, J. L.; Venkatesh, S. K.; Leng, S.; Yu, L.; Halaweish, A. F.; Harmsen, W. S.; McCollough, C. H.; Fletcher, J. G., Low kV versus dual-energy virtual monoenergetic CT imaging for proven liver lesions: What are the advantages and trade-offs in conspicuity and image quality? A pilot study. *Abdom Radiol* 2018, *43*(6), 1404–1412.

57. Sellerer, T.; Noel, P. B.; Patino, M.; Parakh, A.; Ehn, S.; Zeiter, S.; Holz, J. A.; Hammel, J.; Fingerle, A. A.; Pfeiffer, F.; Maintz, D.; Rummeny, E. J.; Muenzel, D.; Sahani, D. V., Dual-energy CT: A phantom comparison of different platforms for abdominal imaging. *Eur Radiol* 2018, *28*(7), 2745–2755.
58. Moghiseh, M.; Aamir, R.; Panta, R. K.; de Ruiter, N.; Chernoglazov, A.; Healy, J. L.; Butler, A. P. H.; Anderson, N. G., Discrimination of multiple high-Z materials by multi-energy spectral CT – A phantom study. *JSM Biomedical Imaging Data Papers* 2016.
59. Panta, R. K.; Bell, S. T.; Healy, J. L.; Aamir, R.; Bateman, C. J.; Moghiseh, M.; Butler, A. P. H.; Anderson, N. G., Element-specific spectral imaging of multiple contrast agents: A phantom study. *J Instrum* 2018, *13*.
60. Leng, S.; Zhou, W.; Yu, Z.; Halaweish, A.; Krauss, B.; Schmidt, B.; Yu, L.; Kappler, S.; McCollough, C., Spectral performance of a whole-body research photon counting detector CT: Quantitative accuracy in derived image sets. *Phys Med Biol* 2017, *62*(17), 7216–7232.
61. Caravan, P.; Ellison, J. J.; McMurry, T. J.; Lauffer, R. B., Gadolinium(III) chelates as MRI contrast agents: Structure, dynamics, and applications. *Chem Rev* 1999, *99*(9), 2293–2352.
62. Feuerlein, S.; Roessl, E.; Proksa, R.; Martens, G.; Klass, O.; Jeltsch, M.; Rasche, V.; Brambs, H. J.; Hoffmann, M. H.; Schlomka, J. P., Multienergy photon-counting K-edge imaging: Potential for improved luminal depiction in vascular imaging. *Radiology* 2008, *249*(3), 1010–1016.
63. Dangelmaier, J.; Bar-Ness, D.; Daerr, H.; Muenzel, D.; Si-Mohamed, S.; Ehn, S.; Fingerle, A. A.; Kimm, M. A.; Kopp, F. K.; Boussel, L.; Roessl, E.; Pfeiffer, F.; Rummeny, E. J.; Proksa, R.; Douek, P.; Noel, P. B., Experimental feasibility of spectral photon-counting computed tomography with two contrast agents for the detection of endoleaks following endovascular aortic repair. *Eur Radiol* 2018, *28*(8), 3318–3325.
64. Muenzel, D.; Daerr, H.; Proksa, R.; Fingerle, A. A.; Kopp, F. K.; Douek, P.; Herzen, J.; Pfeiffer, F.; Rummeny, E. J.; Noel, P. B., Simultaneous dual-contrast multi-phase liver imaging using spectral photon-counting computed tomography: A proof-of-concept study. *Eur Radiol Exp* 2017, *1*(1), 25.
65. Muenzel, D.; Bar-Ness, D.; Roessl, E.; Blevis, I.; Bartels, M.; Fingerle, A. A.; Ruschke, S.; Coulon, P.; Daerr, H.; Kopp, F. K.; Brendel, B.; Thran, A.; Rokni, M.; Herzen, J.; Boussel, L.; Pfeiffer, F.; Proksa, R.; Rummeny, E. J.; Douek, P.; Noel, P. B., Spectral photon-counting CT: Initial experience with dual-contrast agent K-edge colonography. *Radiology* 2017, *283*(3), 723–728.
66. Rogosnitzky, M.; Branch, S., Gadolinium-based contrast agent toxicity: A review of known and proposed mechanisms. *Biometals* 2016, *29*(3), 365–376.
67. Tsushima, Y.; Kanal, E.; Thomsen, H. S., Nephrogenic systemic fibrosis: Risk factors suggested from Japanese published cases. *Br J Radiol* 2010, *83*(991), 590–595.
68. Murata, N.; Gonzalez-Cuyar, L. F.; Murata, K.; Fligner, C.; Dills, R.; Hippe, D.; Maravilla, K. R., Macrocyclic and other non-Group 1 gadolinium contrast agents deposit low levels of gadolinium in brain and bone tissue: Preliminary results from 9 patients with normal renal function. *Invest Radiol* 2016, *51*(7), 447–453.
69. McDonald, R. J.; McDonald, J. S.; Kallmes, D. F.; Jentoft, M. E.; Paolini, M. A.; Murray, D. L.; Williamson, E. E.; Eckel, L. J., Gadolinium deposition in human brain tissues after contrast-enhanced MR imaging in adult patients without intracranial abnormalities. *Radiology* 2017, *285*(2), 546–554.
70. Roeder, R. K.; Curtis, T. E.; Nallathamby, P. D.; Irimata, L. E.; McGinnity, T. L.; Cole, L. E.; Vargo-Gogola, T.; Cowden, D. K., Nanoparticle imaging probes for molecular imaging with computed tomography and application to cancer imaging. *J Med Imaging* 2017, *10132*.
71. Liu, Y.; Ai, K.; Liu, J.; Yuan, Q.; He, Y.; Lu, L., A high-performance ytterbium-based nanoparticulate contrast agent for in vivo x-ray computed tomography imaging. *Angew Chem Int Ed* 2012, *51*(6), 1437–1442.
72. Zeng, S.; Tsang, M. K.; Chan, C. F.; Wong, K. L.; Hao, J., PEG modified BaGdF(5): Yb/Er nanoprobes for multi-modal upconversion fluorescent, in vivo x-ray computed tomography and biomagnetic imaging. *Biomaterials* 2012, *33*(36), 9232–9238.
73. Ramadoss, A.; Krishnamoorthy, K.; Kim, S. J., Novel synthesis of hafnium oxide nanoparticles by precipitation method and its characterization. *Mater Res Bull* 2012, *47*(9), 2680–2684.
74. Ramadoss, A.; Krishnamoorthy, K.; Kim, S. J., Facile synthesis of hafnium oxide nanoparticles via precipitation method. *Mater Lett* 2012, *75*, 215–217.
75. Field, J. A.; Luna-Velasco, A.; Boitano, S. A.; Shadman, F.; Ratner, B. D.; Barnes, C.; Sierra-Alvarez, R., Cytotoxicity and physicochemical properties of hafnium oxide nanoparticles. *Chemosphere* 2011, *84*(10), 1401–1407.
76. Maggiorella, L.; Barouch, G.; Devaux, C.; Pottier, A.; Deutsch, E.; Bourhis, J.; Borghi, E.; Levy, L., Nanoscale radiotherapy with hafnium oxide nanoparticles. *Future Oncol* 2012, *8*(9), 1167–1181.

77. Marill, J.; Anesary, N. M.; Zhang, P.; Vivet, S.; Borghi, E.; Levy, L.; Pottier, A., Hafnium oxide nanoparticles: Toward an in vitro predictive biological effect? *Radiat Oncol* 2014, *9*, 150.
78. Bonvalot, S.; Le Pechoux, C.; De Baere, T.; Kantor, G.; Buy, X.; Stoeckle, E.; Terrier, P.; Sargos, P.; Coindre, J. M.; Lassau, N.; Ait Sarkouh, R.; Dimitriu, M.; Borghi, E.; Levy, L.; Deutsch, E.; Soria, J. C., First-in-human study testing a new radioenhancer using nanoparticles (NBTXR3) activated by radiation therapy in patients with locally advanced soft tissue sarcomas. *Clin Cancer Res* 2017, *23*(4), 908–917.
79. Wang, N.; Li, H.; Wang, J.; Chen, S.; Ma, Y.; Zhang, Z., Study on the anticorrosion, biocompatibility, and osteoinductivity of tantalum decorated with tantalum oxide nanotube array films. *ACS App Mater Interfaces* 2012, *4*(9), 4516–4523.
80. Bonitatibus, P. J., Jr.; Torres, A. S.; Goddard, G. D.; FitzGerald, P. F.; Kulkarni, A. M., Synthesis, characterization, and computed tomography imaging of a tantalum oxide nanoparticle imaging agent. *Chem Commun (Camb)* 2010, *46*(47), 8956–8958.
81. FitzGerald, P. F.; Butts, M. D.; Roberts, J. C.; Colborn, R. E.; Torres, A. S.; Lee, B. D.; Yeh, B. M.; Bonitatibus, P. J., Jr., A proposed computed tomography contrast agent using carboxybetaine zwitterionic tantalum oxide nanoparticles: Imaging, biological, and physicochemical performance. *Invest Radiol* 2016, *51*(12), 786–796.
82. Bonitatibus, P. J., Jr.; Torres, A. S.; Kandapallil, B.; Lee, B. D.; Goddard, G. D.; Colborn, R. E.; Marino, M. E., Preclinical assessment of a zwitterionic tantalum oxide nanoparticle x-ray contrast agent. *ACS Nano* 2012, *6*(8), 6650–6658.
83. Oh, M. H.; Lee, N.; Kim, H.; Park, S. P.; Piao, Y.; Lee, J.; Jun, S. W.; Moon, W. K.; Choi, S. H.; Hyeon, T., Large-scale synthesis of bioinert tantalum oxide nanoparticles for x-ray computed tomography imaging and bimodal image-guided sentinel lymph node mapping. *J Am Chem Soc* 2011, *133*(14), 5508–5515.
84. Brown, A. L.; Naha, P. C.; Benavides-Montes, V.; Litt, H. I.; Goforth, A. M.; Cormode, D. P., Synthesis, x-ray opacity, and biological compatibility of ultra-high payload elemental bismuth nanoparticle x-ray contrast agents. *Chem Mater* 2014, *26*(7), 2266–2274.
85. Bradley, B.; Singleton, M.; Lin Wan Po, A., Bismuth toxicity–A reassessment. *J Clin Pharm Ther* 1989, *14*(6), 423–441.
86. Luo, Y.; Wang, C.; Qiao, Y.; Hossain, M.; Ma, L.; Su, M., In vitro cytotoxicity of surface modified bismuth nanoparticles. *J Mater Sci Mater* 2012, *23*(10), 2563–2573.
87. Gorbach, S. L., Bismuth therapy in gastrointestinal diseases. *Gastroenterology* 1990, *99*(3), 863–875.
88. Ai, K.; Liu, Y.; Liu, J.; Yuan, Q.; He, Y.; Lu, L., Large-scale synthesis of Bi(2)S(3) nanodots as a contrast agent for in vivo x-ray computed tomography imaging. *Adv Mater* 2011, *23*(42), 4886–4891.
89. Andres-Verges, M.; del Puerto Morales, M.; Veintemillas-Verdaguer, S.; Palomares F. J.; Serna, C. J., Core/shell magnetite/bismuth oxide nanocrystals with tunable size, colloidal, and magnetic properties. *Chem Mater* 2012, *24*(2), 319–324.
90. Kinsella, J. M.; Jimenez, R. E.; Karmali, P. P.; Rush, A. M.; Kotamraju, V. R.; Gianneschi, N. C.; Ruoslahti, E.; Stupack, D.; Sailor, M. J., X-ray computed tomography imaging of breast cancer by using targeted peptide-labeled bismuth sulfide nanoparticles. *Angew Chem Int Ed* 2011, *50*(51), 12308–12311.
91. Mechlem, K.; Ehn, S.; Sellerer, T.; Braig, E.; Munzel, D.; Pfeiffer, F.; Noel, P. B., Joint statistical iterative material image reconstruction for spectral computed tomography using a semi-empirical forward model. *IEEE Trans Med Imaging* 2018, *37*(1), 68–80.
92. Roessl, E.; Brendel, B.; Engel, K. J.; Schlomka, J. P.; Thran, A.; Proksa, R., Sensitivity of photon-counting based K-edge imaging in x-ray computed tomography. *IEEE Trans Med Imaging* 2011, *30*(9), 1678–1690.
93. Foygel Barber, R.; Sidky, E. Y.; Gilat Schmidt, T.; Pan, X., An algorithm for constrained one-step inversion of spectral CT data. *Phys Med Biol* 2016, *61*(10), 3784–3818.
94. Cai, C.; Rodet, T.; Legoupil, S.; Mohammad-Djafari, A., A full-spectral Bayesian reconstruction approach based on the material decomposition model applied in dual-energy computed tomography. *Med Phys* 2013, *40*(11), 111916.
95. Long, Y.; Fessler, J. A., Multi-material decomposition using statistical image reconstruction for spectral CT. *IEEE Trans Med Imaging* 2014, *33*(8), 1614–1626.
96. Symons, R.; Pourmorteza, A.; Sandfort, V.; Ahlman, M. A.; Cropper, T.; Mallek, M.; Kappler, S.; Ulzheimer, S.; Mahesh, M.; Jones, E. C.; Malayeri, A. A.; Folio, L. R.; Bluemke, D. A., Feasibility of dose-reduced chest CT with photon-counting detectors: Initial results in humans. *Radiology* 2017, *285*(3), 980–989.

97. Hainfeld, J. F.; Smilowitz, H. M.; O'Connor, M. J.; Dilmanian, F. A.; Slatkin, D. N., Gold nanoparticle imaging and radiotherapy of brain tumors in mice. *Nanomedicine* 2013, *8*(10), 1601–1609.
98. Choi, H. S.; Liu, W.; Misra, P.; Tanaka, E.; Zimmer, J. P.; Itty Ipe, B.; Bawendi, M. G.; Frangioni, J. V., Renal clearance of quantum dots. *Nature Biotechnol* 2007, *25*(10), 1165–1170.
99. Cheheltani, R.; Ezzibdeh, R. M.; Chhour, P.; Pulaparthi, K.; Kim, J.; Jurcova, M.; Hsu, J. C.; Blundell, C.; Litt, H. I.; Ferrari, V. A.; Allcock, H. R.; Sehgal, C. M.; Cormode, D. P., Tunable, biodegradable gold nanoparticles as contrast agents for computed tomography and photoacoustic imaging. *Biomaterials* 2016, *102*, 87–97.
100. Mukundan, S., Jr.; Ghaghada, K. B.; Badea, C. T.; Kao, C. Y.; Hedlund, L. W.; Provenzale, J. M.; Johnson, G. A.; Chen, E.; Bellamkonda, R. V.; Annapragada, A., A liposomal nanoscale contrast agent for preclinical CT in mice. *Am J Roentgenol* 2006, *186*(2), 300–307.
101. Tassa, C.; Shaw, S. Y.; Weissleder, R., Dextran-coated iron oxide nanoparticles: A versatile platform for targeted molecular imaging, molecular diagnostics, and therapy. *Acc Chem Res* 2011, *44*(10), 842–852.

9 Clinical Applications of Spectral Computed Tomography

Enabling Technique for Novel Contrast Development and Targeting Imaging

Thorsten Fleiter
Department of Diagnostic Imaging, University of Maryland School of Medicine, Shock Trauma Center, Baltimore, Maryland, USA

CONTENTS

9.1 INTRODUCTION

The development of computed tomography (CT) technologies during the last three decades was focused on ever-increasing acquisition speed, improved spatial resolution, and radiation dose efficiency. The new spectral photon counting CT (SPCCT) technology will advance the material decomposition compared to the current state-of-the-art dual-energy CT (DECT) variants, will improve the signal to noise ratio and therefore the detection of smaller attenuation differences, it will improve the spatial resolution and it will reduce the radiation dose necessary to acquire diagnostic images. But the introduction of this new technique into clinical practice will be certainly more complex and complicated compared to DECT more than a decade ago – which is still not used to the fullest potential in most places. Every new CT scanner generation added new capabilities to the portfolio of available diagnostic procedures and those new features were often quickly explored primarily by radiologists in the large academic centers but took considerable time to be considered outside of these centers. It could be argued that DECT did not achieve a general acceptance until this day and that the added complexity of the scanners might have caused this development. Additional settings were necessary to utilize for instance the flexible mixture between the high and low energy signals or to make use of completely new features like the virtual monochromatic images. Every change of the scanning parameters required additional evaluation to ensure that the intended effect was achieved. The new scanner technology lead also to alterations of the iv contrast injection protocols and allowed for the first-time basic material decomposition leading to improvements like renal stone analysis or the generation of iodine uptake maps of entire organ regions like the lungs. But it spurred also secondary and less expected developments like the bone marrow edema visualization to better analyze osseous lesions and fractures. SPCCT will add another level of complication compared to DECT and several aspects of these new systems beyond the detector technology must be address for a successful introduction into routine clinical practice:

a. Detector technology and signal processing will continue to evolve.
b. Task specific configuration and separation of energy bins must be developed.
c. Energy-, organ- and task-specific image reconstruction methods need to be developed and tested.
d. Multi-energy optimized dose regulation methods must be further developed.
e. Task specific protocols including x-ray settings, filtering, energy-bin selection, dose regulation, scan speed and relative table speed (pitch), reconstruction method, and distribution and relative mixture of the available energy bins will be more complex compared to DECT and useful combinations must be created and tested.
f. Contrast injection protocol optimization for SPCCT including contrast density, volume, and dynamics must be altered to compliment the higher sensitivity and detection capabilities of SPCCT.
g. Alternative contrast media including multimodality and targeting variants with consecutive necessary alteration of the scan timing after contrast injection might be developed parallel to these developments.

The intention of this overview is to highlight short- and long-term goals for the clinical application of the SPCCT.

It is certain that the new CT scanner technology will alter but not overcome the principle limitation of any CT scan: the often minimal or not existing attenuation differences between normal and pathologic tissues within the same organ. The new scanner technology will therefore not eliminate the need for contrast enhancement – which has been an integral part of CT imaging since the introduction of the first systems into clinical practice in 1974 for head scans and 1976 for body scans. But it will change what amount and concentration of contrast media will be used and it will initiate the development of new contrast injection protocols.

9.2 SPCCT CONTRAST MEDIA REQUIREMENTS

The new more efficient detector technology will change the contrast media use in routine clinical work but it will not alter the principle requirements for any diagnostic iv contrast application:

1. The contrast must increase the attenuation and therefore the detectability of the structure or tissue of interest significantly. The differences attributed by the contrast must be significant enough to overcome the signal to noise limitation of the imaging system.
2. The increased attenuation caused by the contrast must last for the length of the scanning procedure and should be as homogenous as possible during the scan to enable acquisitions throughout the body in the same contrast phase.
3. The contrast material itself must be stable and all its components must be non-toxic. Ideally it should not interact with the body or change physiological processes. The

contrast media should not alter cell structures or cause persistent changes on molecular level – such as DNA alterations.
4. The contrast material should be completely cleared from the body within a reasonable time. A clearance within 24 hours or shorter is the accepted reference for the currently available contrast media.
5. The contrast material should not generate long-term effects to any tissue in the human body.
6. The contrast media must be efficient enough to be applied in as small quantities as possible and it should ideally not alter the fluid distribution and balance in a human body.
7. The contrast media must be available in required quantities and must be cost effective.

The currently available and FDA approved CT contrast media are fulfilling these basic requirements and will continue to be used for all types of CT – be it conventional, true mono-energetic synchrotron based, dual-energy or photon counting. Additional specialized and probably targeting structures might be added to the spectrum of available contrast media but will require significant investment into research and testing before they might become available. But the main hurdle for the development of a new iv contrast medium is that every alteration of the formula or the composition of the molecules requires a re-evaluation by the FDA – regardless if completely new formulations or combinations of existing and well-known components are used. This process is expensive and does only make commercial sense if the development offers clinically significant advantages compared to already available contrast materials.

9.3 SPCCT AND CONTRAST MEDIA

The SPCCT acquisition with multiple energy bins is promising to deliver a better approximation of the attenuation curve of any given material in a human body and therefore enabling a more precise and complex material decomposition. This advantage will not only improve the differentiation between the multiple tissue types in a human body, but also the detection of currently used iodine-based contrast agents. However, sampling close to the K-edge of the iodine (33.2 KeV) component of the classic contrast media as one of the added possibilities for SPCCT will be limited by the size and composition of the scanned body parts and the useable portion of the x-ray spectrum in clinical practice. The trade-off between radiation dose and achievable signal to noise ratio will be altered but not eliminated. The filtering of the low energies out of the polychromatic x-ray beams will remain necessary to avoid unnecessary radiation of the patients (1). It can be assumed that the projected increased sensitivity of SPCCT will not eliminate the need to perform multiphase or "dynamic" contrast enhanced scans to capture the often only in a very distinctive time window existing contrast enhancement differences between normal and pathologic tissue. Repeated scans during the arterial and venous/excretory phase will remain to be the standard option for many applications and derived virtual unenhanced and monochromatic/bin specific reconstructed images will likely provide additional information that radiologists must learn to interpret. SPCCT will all but certain enable significant reductions of the contrast volume and concentration being used for standard applications but the limits for this reduction must be evaluated for every single clinical application.

9.4 SPCCT AND IODINE BASED CONTRAST AGENTS

Iodine was among the first elements to be tested for the potential use as contrast for x-ray imaging. The main advantage is the relatively high atomic number compared to regular tissue in a human body ($Z = 53$) and the relative low toxicity if bound into the now commonly used contrast molecules.

The currently FDA approved iodinated contrast media (ICM) are listed in Figure 9.1.

There were in general two different types of these contrast media "ionic" – most commonly negative charged – and the "non-ionic" variants. The latter have become the standard in most clinical applications because the "ionic" version exhibited a variety of problematic characteristics that lead

Generic name	Brand name(s)
diatrizoate meglumine	Cystografin , Cystografin Dilute
diatrizoate meglumine and diatrizoate sodium	MD-76R
iodipamide meglumine	Cholografin Meglumine
Iodixanol	Visipaque 270, 320
Iohexol	Omnipaque 140, 180, 240, 300, 350
Iopamidol	Isovue-200, 250, 300, 370 Isovue-M 200, 300 Scanlux-300, 370
Iopromide	Ultravist 150, 240, 300, 370
iothalamate meglumine	Conray 30, 43
Ioversol	Optiray 240, 300, 320, 350
ioxaglate meglumine and ioxaglate sodium	Hexabrix
Ioxilan	Oxilan-300, 350

Source: www.FDA.gov

FIGURE 9.1 Currently FDA approved computed tomography contrast media.

to increased complication rates for instance through interaction with cell membranes or through physical effects due to the high osmolality of the commonly used preparations – resulting in significant water retention which could cause acute pulmonary hypertension and edema and even acute cardiac failure in predisposed patients. These negative side effects have been evaluated in numerous studies and been described in multiple publications (2).

The "non-ionic" contrast variants were developed to lower the osmolality and to reduce these negative side effects that occurred especially by intravascular administration. Additional variations of the molecule structures improved the water solubility and further reduced the fluid retention and direct effects on cell membranes. One of the disadvantages in clinical practice is that higher concentrations of the contrast agents are favorable to achieve the maximum contrast per injected volume but lead to a higher viscosity that directly effects the distribution of the contrast into peripheral vessels and tissues. It took literally decades and numerous iterations and variants of basically the same contrast media type to establish the now available products that exhibit vastly decreased side effects, less biochemical interaction with human tissues, and decreased production costs compared to the early years of the x-ray contrast development.

The structure, concentration, and viscosity of these contrast agents contribute to distribution and washout or clearance times differences that are used to optimize the contrast injection and scanning parameters to further enhance the attenuation differences between normal tissues and actual pathologies. The CT and contrast injection protocols vary therefore between institutions and the available scanner technology and the clinical requests – indicating that there is no standard solution that would fulfill all clinical requirements. The intention for all contrast developments and alterations of the injection and scanning protocols is however the same for most users: to improve the pathology detection with the least-possible interaction and harm to the human body. Not only the anatomical appearance of a pathology, but also the contrast uptake and washout dynamics are used to further differentiate between benign and malignant lesions and tumors. Dynamic and even perfusion scans with repeated acquisitions of the same body parts at different delays after the contrast injection are utilized to further enhance the differentiation of pathologies and for instance tumor types. Dynamic scans are for instance improving the detection of perfusion deficits between normal brain tissue and portions of the brain distal to vascular occlusions in acute stroke patients but they are also used in numerous other applications including the differentiation between benign lesions like for instance a liver hemangioma from a primary tumor or metastasis. These scanning methods and contrast injection protocols are part of what could be described as "anatomical imaging" and are fundamentally different from imaging the activities on molecular level that remains to be the domain of nuclear medicine and increasingly MRI.

The most commonly used small molecule iodinated contrast agents share some main characteristics:

a. fast clearance from the body through renal excretion. Renal malfunction is therefore a limiting factor for the use of ICM.
b. ubiquitous and non-specific distribution of the contrast agent in a human body.
c. fast exchange between intravascular and extravascular compartments that force rapid imaging to detect contrast differences that exist only during a short period before the contrast is evenly distributed on a capillary level.
d. residual toxicity, allergic, and adverse reactions still exist but the incidence has vastly improved compared to the early stages of CT contrast development (3).

These characteristics are forcing compromises and should be remembered that an ideal contrast material would target the structure of interest – as for instance a tumor – and accumulate only in that structure. This would require developing a particle or molecule that interacts with parts of cells, binding areas, enzymes, etc. or might even be integrated into the structural elements of cells. Such a contrast media would be used to achieve the exact opposite of the current contrast CT contrast media: interaction with the human body on a molecular level. Significantly more sensitive imaging systems than a conventional CT scanner are necessary to detect the very small amounts of a contrast agent that would be accumulating in a targeted structure. Even the newest CT detector technologies are magnitudes less sensitive compared to standard nuclear medicine methods. This might explain why truly targeting CT contrast techniques never found their way into common clinical routine. Only a few semi-targeting contrast media like Iodipamide were developed and the excretion of this material into the bile ducts was more frequently used to detect obstructions or masses in these bile ducts during the early days of CT (4). Less invasive and clinical more relevant examinations like the magnetic resonance cholangiopancreatography (MRCP) have meanwhile replaced these special CT techniques.

9.5 SPCCT POTENTIAL FOR SELECTIVE IMAGING

The potential advantages of photon counting compared to the standard energy integrating x-ray detectors were already described early on and promised to provide the reconstruction of CT images freed of spectral artifacts and with significantly reduced noise levels compared to the energy integrating detectors (5). New techniques for K-edge imaging and therefore selective detection of specifically designed contrast media for this scanner type were discussed early on (6) and sparked the development of numerous experimental contrast agents and molecules. Especially the use of nanoparticle contrast agents for cell tracking and labeling gained immediate attention. But it is important to remember that any potential alternative contrast must pass the rigorous testing and approval process defined by the FDA (7) and variants specifically be designed for the new scanner technique will therefore become available only years after the introduction of SPCCT and it remains to be seen for which applications.

9.6 SPCCT AND NANOSCALE CONTRAST AGENTS

Nanoscale particles that contain a contrast core are an often discussed potential alternative to conventional CT contrast media promising a shift from "anatomical" to "molecular" imaging. The contrast agent can be as simple as a nanosuspension or nano-emulsion but also as complex as polymeric particles with more than one contrast agent and multiple functional groups attached to them to target specific "docking" areas that are characteristic for certain tissue type or for instance tumor masses. One step further is the combination of a targeting molecule or particle that contains not only the contrast agent but also delivers a therapeutic agent at the same time. The contrast accumulation in the targeted structure can then be used to monitor the delivery of that therapeutic agent to a tumor or other specified lesions. Liposomal delivery systems have recently gained attention among the nanostructures for that reason. They are used to improve the transport of therapeutic payloads into the targeted tissues (8).

There are in general two different types of CT contrast containing nanoscale structures:

1. particles that contain conventional contrast agents like iodine or gadolinium
2. particles that contain alternative high-Z materials that are suitable for K-edge detection using SPCCT like for instance Gold (Au) or Bismuth (Bi)

9.7 LIPOSOMAL CONTRAST AGENTS

Liposomes are spherical structures consisting of layered lipids with an internal cavity that were originally developed to improve drug delivery to malignant tumors. Liposomes containing a therapeutic drug are more successful than simple iv application of the same drug due to their prolonged circulation time in the blood pool and a higher probability to accumulate in tissues with increased vascularization and perfusion rate – which is the case for most malignant tumors. This delivery system is using the greater permeability of the vasculature in tumor tissues to reach the target and to release the load once they are dismantled within the target (Figure 9.2).

The dual layer liposomes can carry both hydrophobic and hydrophilic drugs that either are attached to the lipid layers or remain in the cavity (Figure 9.3).

There are already numerous released therapeutic products using this technique. The first successful such delivery system was approved and introduced into clinical practice in 1995 for the treatment of ovarian cancer as doxorubicin (Doxil®, Lipodox®) (9) and shortly thereafter followed by

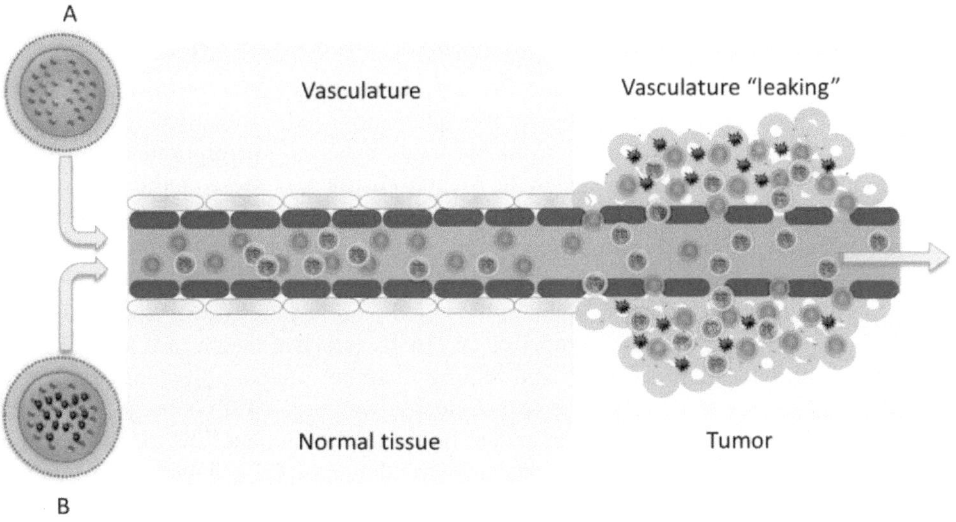

FIGURE 9.2 Liposomal transport of a contrast agent (A) and a contrast agent and therapeutic drug (B) into a tumorous structure using the extended blood-pool time of the liposomes and the greater permeability of the pathologic tumor vasculature to deploy the load into the tumor tissue – enhancing the local accumulation and therefore improving the effectivity of the drug and decrease the systemic side effects. The potentially added contrast agent can be used to monitor the therapy.

liposomal daunorubicin (DaunoXome®) to fight the HIV/AIDS related Karposi sarcoma. Numerous variants and sizes of this nanoscale delivery system have been developed in the meantime and are already approved and used in daily clinical practice primarily for cancer treatment.

The advantage is not only a more efficient delivery of therapeutic drugs into the target structure but more so the reduction of the negative side effects for the patients: a smaller percentage of the toxic drugs carried within the liposomes is released into the blood pool – reducing the interaction with organs that are not the target of the therapy. Adding a contrast agent is a logic addition to this concept to monitor the distribution and delivery of the therapeutic drug itself. Adding a contrast

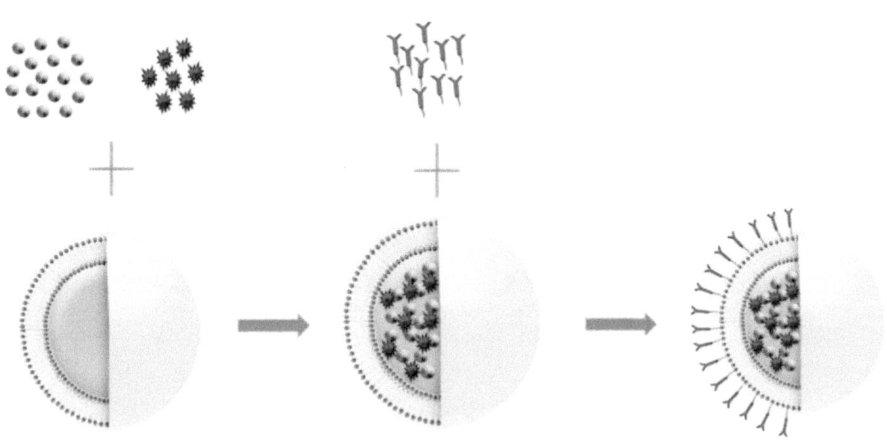

FIGURE 9.3 Potential utilization of liposomal delivery and targeting systems for SPCCT consisting of the contrast agent (spheres), a chemotherapy (stars) targeting ligands (Y-shapes).

media like Gold or comparable would additionally take advantage of the SPCCT capabilities to detect the specific K-edge attenuation changes. Recently developed thermosensitive variants of these delivery system that are based on the same transport principles are designed to release their payload enhanced by a induced temperature increase in the target area for instance with focused ultrasound (10). There is no technical limitation to add nano-sized CT contrast agents to any of the liposomal delivery systems but currently available solutions usually incorporate agents for nuclear medicine and MRI imaging – simply due to the higher sensitivity of those methods and the lacking specificity of the current CT generations to differentiate contrast materials from tissue attenuation. Early experiments to monitor the liposomal drug delivery could demonstrate the feasibility CT for this purpose but also highlighted the challenges imposed by the complex pharmacokinetics of prolonged circulation of the delivery system in the blood-pool and the correct timing of the control scans (11–13). The size, weight, and number of eventually attached ligands are all influencing the blood pool time of these nanostructures and require therefore imaging protocols adjustments for every single variant of these. But there are also obvious advantages of CT contrast loaded liposomal nanostructures that could be utilized independent from tumor treatment. The increased circulation time is broadening the time window for arterial and vascular phase CT acquisitions. Adding SPCCT detectable K-edge contrast materials could potentially further improve the achievable contrast enhancement without causing additional problems due to consecutive increased toxicity or immune reaction to the contrast material (13). SPCCT could be the key technology needed to translate such techniques from the experimental stage into clinical practice. The next logic development is to add more than one high-Z elements with K-edge attenuation changes at different KeVs to better utilize the capabilities of SPCCT and further reduce the contrast volume to achieve a comparable attenuation compared to conventional CT (14).

Additional variants of delivery systems have been developed to further prolong the release of the transported drugs. These consist of multivesicular liposomes carrying the drugs contained in small aqueous chambers that are arranged in a honeycomb like structure (Figure 9.4). This solution is capable to release the drugs over a longer period between 1–30 days and can be adjusted to the therapeutic need (DepoFoam®, Parcira Pharmaceuticals Inc., Parsippany, NJ, USA). Using such a transport system for contrast agents could be helpful for instance to monitor the results of a local chemoembolization (15) with multiple follow-up scans without the need of repeated iv contrast injection.

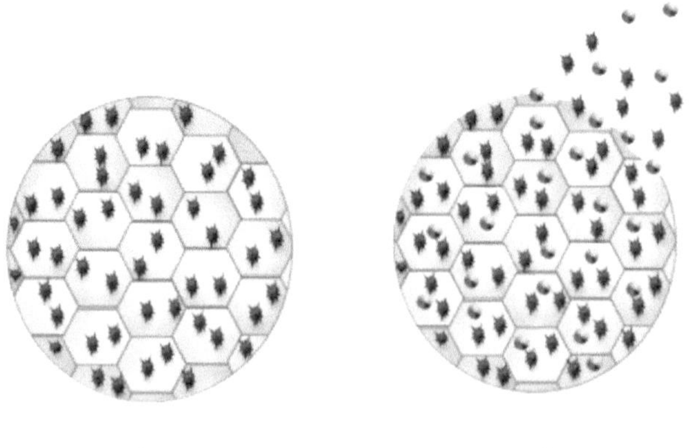

FIGURE 9.4 A variation of the liposomal delivery systems are spheroids (A) there were developed to achieve a sustained delivery of chemotherapy into tumor tissues. Adding a K-edge detectable contrast (spheres) could be used to monitor the efficiency of this delivery by measuring the accumulation in the target structure (B).

9.8 MICELLES

Micelles are consisting of a monolayer of surfactants compared to the bilayer of phospholipids that define liposomes. They are therefore significant smaller (2–20 nm) compared to liposomes that can vary in size (20 nm–3 μm) and tend to have a hydrophobic core enabling the transport hydrophobic molecules in a hydrophilic environment compared to liposomes that can transport hydrophobic materials in between the two layers of the phospholipids and hydrophilic drugs in their core or cavity. Micelles occur naturally in the digestive tract and help to resorb otherwise non-soluble molecules. They are therefore attractive for alternative ways of drug or potential contrast agent delivery – including oral application. One of the main advantages is the relative simple and cost effective production of this nanoscale-delivery system. They have already been used for the delivery of alternative contrast agents like Bismuth into targeted structures and the resulting enhancement could be reliable detected in actual tumor tissues (16).

9.9 SPCCT AND TARGETING NANOPARTICLES

The relative low sensitivity of CT to detect small attenuation differences is significantly limiting the capabilities to detect small amounts of contrast materials in human tissues and is the main reason why truly targeting contrast media combinations never progressed from the experimental state into clinical routine. The prospect of the photon counting CT has certainly fueled the hope that it might alter these limitations and has sparked the development of numerous truly targeting contrast containing molecules. SPCCT is promising to enable molecular imaging with a simple and fast imaging technique that might be capable to compete for certain applications with traditional nuclear medicine methods. The intention for truly targeting structures is to significantly improve the accumulation of the contrast agent in the structure of interest without causing critical new unintended effects from increased toxicity to decreased or incomplete elimination of the agent through the reticuloendothelial/macrophage system (RES) or renal clearance. This process is complex and must include every potential side effect from allergic reactions to potential vascular complications caused by the unintended activation of the coagulation cascade or aggregate buildup of the nanoparticles and molecules that are sticking together and could lead to vascular occlusion. Potential candidates for the imaging marker of targeting nanostructures include the classic x-ray iodine, barium, and gadolinium but also alternatives like gold, bismuth, and more exotic materials including tungsten, ytterbium, or platinum. These elements are responsible for the x-ray attenuation and are usually at the core of the nanoparticle – often coated to increase the solubility, biocompatibility, and to improve the attachment of ligands to these cores to interact with the targeted structure. They can be used for pure diagnostic purposes or the tracking and control of the delivery of therapeutic materials. A combination of multiple contrast agents in one molecule can be used to enable multimodality imaging with the same nanoparticle. These particles are in most cases competing with natural occurring cell structures, transmitters, and enzymes for the same binding area and have an equal or higher affinity to the target to successfully compete with these. They maintain the competitive "binding" capabilities to that target is therefore one of the main goals to improve the specificity of these targeting structures. The size and number of attached ligands are not only affecting the binding capabilities, but also the biocompatibility of the structure. The clearance of the nanostructure is another concern and must be considered and verified like for any other contrast media in diagnostic imaging. But the main challenge is unchanged regardless of the recently achieved progress: generating a sufficient contrast agent concentration in the target to overcome the intrinsic detection threshold the available CT technology – which is mainly defined by the signal to noise level. Additional complicating is the fact that some of the factors that are defining the detection probability of a targeting nanoparticle for CT usage are directly opposing each other and are forcing compromises. The binding capabilities with the targeted structure are for instance decreasing with the size and weight of the particle which is increasing with the concentration of contrast materials incorporated into the nanostructure. But a higher contrast concentration in the target would improve the detection of this contrast accumulation at the same time. To find the best compromise is part of the corresponding research.

9.10 GOLD CONTAINING TARGETING NANOPARTICLES

Colloidal gold is one example of elements exhibiting a significant K-edge attenuation change well within the clinical useable x-ray spectrum, provides a higher attenuation (2.7 × > iodine) and the biocompatibility, toxicity and pharmacodynamics are well known. The renal excretion is of gold nanoparticles (AuNP) is dependent on the size of particle. Larger AuNP are more likely to be retained. It is therefore important to control the size and size tolerances during the AuNP synthesis using well-established methods. The most attractive aspect of AuNP as imaging marker that surface modification and coupling with various targeting molecules can be relative easily achieved and controlled. The synthesis of such molecules has already been evaluated in numerous applications and the development targeting variants for CT use is taking advantage of the already existing knowledge. Consequently, AuNP based new contrast materials were the first commercially available for research purposes (AuroVist®, Nanoprobes, Inc. Yaphank, NY, USA) are meanwhile multiple variants with stable gold core sizes and prefabricated coatings that can be easily assembled with the preferred ligands into targeting nanoparticles that are suitable for CT detection (17, 18).

The combination of multiple imaging markers into one targeting nanostructure promises even more tracking and application capabilities using more than one imaging technique (Figure 9.5). A popular combination is the integration of AuNP and gadolinium into one nanostructure. Both the gold and gadolinium are effective CT contrast agents and the gadolinium portion itself ensures the detection with MRI which can have advantages for cell tracking for instances in tumorous tissues (19–22).

But the nanoparticles can also be used for more than imaging purposes. The accumulation in the target tissue can increase the local thermo-conductivity and therefore amplify the effects of thermotherapies or ablation techniques (23, 24).

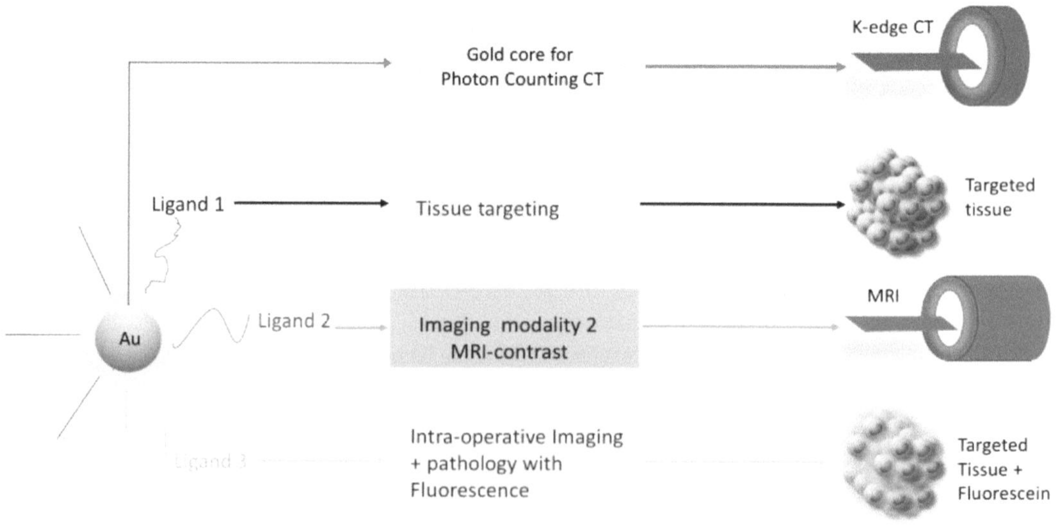

FIGURE 9.5 Multimodality targeting molecule with nano-gold core and ligands for tissue targeting, MRI imaging and fluorescence ligand for intraoperative and pathology imaging of the targeted tissue.

There are numerous studies evaluating the systematic effects of the AuNP and their different preparations demonstrating the potential but also the numerous challenges that must be addressed before the nanoparticles will be available in clinical routine (25, 26). The capability of CT to detect any changes (up to 10^{-3} mol/L) caused by a contrast agent in a human tissue is significantly lower compared to MRI (up to 10^{-5} mol/L) and especially nuclear medicine techniques (up to 10^{-10} mol/L). This principle disadvantage will be altered with the arrival of SPCCT but the sensitivity differences between these diagnostic imaging methods will not significantly change (27). The signal to noise level will improve – probably the most important progress together with improved spatial resolution and energy discrimination specifically for the detection of particles like AuNPs. But it remains to be seen if scanner technology changes are sufficient to establish new scanning protocols that are using targeting nanoparticles/molecules clinical practice and if SPCCT will become the alternative to established molecular imaging for selected applications.

9.11 SPCCT AND ALTERNATIVE CONTRAST MEDIA APPLICATIONS

The capabilities of SPCCT might lead to the development of the above described advanced contrast media but will all but certain have direct impact on scans with conventional iodinated contrast agents. The new detector technology will be used to decrease the amount of contrast used while maintaining or improving the contrast enhancement compared to current standard or dual energy method scans. The K-edge detection capabilities could also be relative easily converted from the research phase into clinical practice to differentiate between oral or rectal and intravenous contrast media – opening a pathway to simplified scanning protocols for instance to detect colon cancer converting previously explored methods for positron emission tomography (PET)-CT (28). The use of K-edge attenuation differences will be relatively simple if used for these large volumes of highly concentrated contrast – in opposite to the potential liposomal or targeting nanostructures. The sensitivity to detect those is not only depending on the concentration of the contrast material itself but also the type and size of the surrounding tissues, the object thickness and the still existing x-ray artifacts like beam hardening and photon starvation.

9.12 SPCCT CHALLENGES

Finding the optimal combination of KVp, mAs, rotation time and pitch, slice thickness, and reconstruction parameters for the individual patient and the purpose of a CT examination is already a challenge for modern dual-energy scanners and SPCCT is going to add more variables to this problem. Selecting the optimal energy bin thresholds and position within the spectrum for any given examination will add a new layer of complication to the already complex current dual-energy protocols. Finding the right combination that warrants the highest sensitivity and specificity to detect pathologies while using the lowest amount of conventional contrast agents, the lowest reasonable patient radiation dose and the best combination of image reconstruction techniques will already be a challenge but will be significantly more complex if new contrast media with significantly different pharmacokinetics will be added to a routine scan procedure. Injection protocols that were developed since the introduction of CT will be of little use for these new materials and must therefore be redeveloped. The enhancement pattern of any of the discussed nanoparticles differs significantly from any of the contrast media currently used in clinical routine and the optimal delay between the injection and the diagnostic scans must be redefined and tested for every single particle and application (29). The fact that simple dynamic monitoring scans that are now used to adjust the scan start to the physiological conditions of the individual patients by varying the delay based on the iv-contrast enhancement will be of little value for the new contrast agents and will further complicate the scanning procedure. Finding the optimal combination of contrast volume, concentration, injection protocols, scan delays, and acquisition and image reconstruction parameters will likely require years' worth of research and clinical trials.

9.13 SUMMARY

The development and introduction of SPCCT into clinical practice will primarily be driven by image quality improvements, decreased radiation exposure, and improved detection of conventional contrast media. It seems to be mandatory that the new scanner generation will match conventional single- or dual-energy machines in acquisition and reconstruction speed to succeed in clinical practice. A parallel development of SPCCT specific contrast agents will continue and probably lead to the initial steps toward molecular imaging using targeting agents designed for SPCCT. But there are challenges that are beyond the new scanner and nanoparticle technologies that will have direct influence on the development. Every aspect from the logistic challenges to coordinate the application of a targeting K-edge detectable nanoparticle with the actual scan – which might vary from minutes to days depending on the targeted structure – to the regulatory hurdles and the substantial costs for the development and commercialization of any new contrast agent will influence the progress. This process will take years or even decades if the historic development of the currently used CT contrast agents can be taken as reference. But it is also safe to predict that photon counting CT scanners will improve the current status quo from day 1 of clinical introduction and benefit patients with less radiation dose, improved sensitivity and spatial resolution, improved contrast agent detection with the potential to reduce the used contrast volume and concentration – which will help to further reduce significant side effects like the contrast induced nephropathy or even enable contrast enhanced scans for patients that are now not eligible due to borderline renal function of limited cardiac capacity. The reduction of contrast use will help to justify repeat enhanced scans for follow-up and therapy monitoring but might potentially also contribute to the cost effectiveness of SPCCT. The clinical introduction of the new scanner technology will enable the search for the most sensitive and specific combination of SPCCT specific contrast media but it will take years before the results of the corresponding research will become part of the clinical routine.

REFERENCES

1. Roessl E, Proksa R. K-edge imaging in x-ray computed tomography using multi-bin photon counting detectors. *Phys Med Biol.* 2007;52(15), IOP Publishing Ltd.
2. Singh J, Daftary A. Iodinated contrast and their adverse reactions. *J Nucl Med Technol.* 2008;36(2):69–74.
3. Bottinor W, Polkampally P, Jovin I. Adverse reactions to iodinated contrast media. *Int J Angiol.* 2013;22(3):149–154. doi:10.1055/s-0033-1348885.
4. Van Beers BE, Lacrosse M, Trigaux J-P, de Canniere L, De Ronde T, Pringot J. Noninvasive imaging of the biliary tree before or after laparascopic cholecystectomy: Use of three-dimensional spiral CT cholangiography. *AJR.* 1994;162:1331–1335.
5. Johns PC, Dubeau J, Gobbi DG, Li M, Dixit MS. Photon-counting detectors for digital radiography and x-ray computed tomography. *SPIE TD01.* 2002;367–369.
6. Schlomka JP, Roessl E, Dorscheid R, Dill S, Martens G, Istel T, Baeumer C, Hermann C, Steadman R, Zeitler G, Livne A, Proska R. Experimental feasibility of multi-energy photon-counting K-edge imaging in pre-clinical computed tomography. *Phys Med Biol.* 2008;53(15):4031–4047.
7. Nanotechnology Guidance Documents, https://www.fda.gov/ScienceResearch/SpecialTopics/Nanotechnology/ucm602536.htm.
8. Cormode DP, Naha PC, Fayad ZA. Nanoparticle contrast agents for computed tomography: A focus on micelles. *Contrast Media Mol Imaging.* 2014;9(1):37–52. doi:10.1002/cmmi.1551.
9. Doxil, Barenholz YC. Doxil®—The first FDA-approved nano-drug: Lessons learned. *J Control Release.* 2012;160:117–134.
10. Kim HR, You DG, Park SJ, Choi KS, Um W, Kim JH, Park JH, Kim YS. MRI monitoring of tumor-selective anticancer drug delivery with stable thermosensitive liposomes triggered by high-intensity focused ultrasound. *Mol Pharm.* 2016;13(5):1528–39. doi: 10.1021/acs.molpharmaceut.6b00013. Epub 2016 Mar 29. PMID:26998616.
11. Zheng J, Perkins G, Kirilova A, Allen C, Jaffray DA. Multimodal contrast agent for combined computed tomography and magnetic resonance imaging applications. *Invest Radiol.* 2006;41(3):339–348.

12. Zheng J, Jaffray D, Allen C. Quantitative CT imaging of the spatial and temporal distribution of liposomes in a rabbit tumor model. *Mol Pharm.* 2009;6(2):571–580.
13. Kao CY, Hoffman EA, Beck KC, Bellamkonda RV, Annapragada AV. Long-residence-time nano-scale liposomal iohexol for x-ray-based blood pool imaging. *Acad Radiol.* 2003;10(5):475–483.
14. Liu Y, Ai K, Lu L. Nanoparticulate x-ray computed tomography contrast agents: From design validation to in vivo applications. *Acc Chem Res.* 2012;45(10):1817–1827.
15. Bulbake U, Doppalapudi S, Kommineni N, Khan W. Liposomal formulations in clinical use: An updated review. *Pharmaceutics.* 2017;9(2).
16. Kinsella JM, Jimenez RE, Karmali PP, Rush AM, Kotamraju VR, Gianneschi NC, Ruoslahti E, Stupack D, Sailor MJ. X-ray computed tomography imaging of breast cancer by using targeted peptide-labeled bismuth sulfide nanoparticles. *Angew Chem Int Ed.* 2011;50(51):12308–12311.
17. Ghann WE, Aras O, Fleiter T, Daniel MC. Syntheses and characterization of lisinopril-coated gold nanoparticles as highly stable targeted CT contrast agents in cardiovascular diseases. *Langmuir.* 2012;28(28):10398–10408.
18. Cole LE, Ross RD, Tilley JM, Vargo-Gogola T, Roeder RK. Gold nanoparticles as contrast agents in x-ray imaging and computed tomography. *Nanomedicine (Lond).* 2015;10(2):321–341.
19. Alric C, Taleb J, Le Duc G, Mandon C, Billotey C, Le Meur-Herland A, Brochard T, Vocanson F, Janier M, Perriat P, Roux S, Tillement O. Gadolinium chelate coated gold nanoparticles as contrast agents for both x-ray computed tomography and magnetic resonance imaging. *J Am Chem Soc.* 2008;130(18):5908–5915.
20. Tan G, Onur MA. Cellular localization and biological effects of 20 nm-gold nanoparticles. *J Biomed Mater Res A.* 2018;106(6):1708–1721.
21. Chhour P, Kim J, Benardo B, Tovar A, Mian S, Litt HI, Ferrari VA, Cormode DP. Effect of gold nanoparticle size and coating on labeling monocytes for CT tracking. *Bioconjug Chem.* 2017;28(1):260–269.
22. Nicholls FJ, Rotz MW, Ghuman H, MacRenaris KW, Meade TJ, Modo M. DNA-gadolinium-gold nanoparticles for in vivo T1 MR imaging of transplanted human neural stem cells. *Biomaterials.* 2016;77:291–306.
23. Kolovskaya OS, Zamay TN, Belyanina IV, Karlova E, Garanzha I, Aleksandrovsky AS, Kirichenko A, Dubynina AV, Sokolov AE, Zamay GS, Glazyrin YE, Zamay S, Ivanchenko T, Chanchikova N, Tokarev N, Shepelevich N, Ozerskaya A, Badrin E, Belugin K, Belkin S, Zabluda V, Gargaun A, Berezovski MV, Kichkailo AS. Aptamer-targeted plasmonic photothermal therapy of cancer. *Mol Ther Nucleic Acids.* 2017;9:12–21.
24. Chandrasekaran R, Lee AS, Yap LW, Jans DA, Wagstaff KM, Cheng W. Tumor cell-specific photothermal killing by SELEX-derived DNA aptamer-targeted gold nanorods. *Nanoscale.* 2016;8(1):187–196.
25. Cancino-Bernardi J, Marangoni VS, Besson JCF, Cancino MEC, Natali MRM, Zucolotto V. Gold-based nanospheres and nanorods particles used as theranostic agents: An in vitro and in vivo toxicology studies. *Chemosphere.* 2018;213:41–52.
26. Cheng YH, Riviere JE, Monteiro-Riviere NA, Lin Z. Probabilistic risk assessment of gold nanoparticles after intravenous administration by integrating in vitro and in vivo toxicity with physiologically based pharmacokinetic modeling. *Nanotoxicology.* 2018;12(5):453–469.
27. Schirra CO, Brendel B, Anastasio MA, Roessl E. Spectral CT: A technology primer for contrast agent development. *Contrast Media Mol Imaging.* 2014;9(1):62–70.
28. Antoch G, Freudenberg LS, Stattaus J, Jentzen W, Mueller SP, Debatin JF, Bockisch A. Whole-body positron emission tomography-CT: Optimized CT using oral and IV contrast materials. *AJR Am J Roentgenol.* 2002;179(6):1555–1560.
29. Park YS, Kasuya A, Dmytruk A, Yasuto N, Takeda M, Ohuchi N, Sato Y, Tohji K, Uo M, Watari F. Concentrated colloids of silica-encapsulated gold nanoparticles: Colloidal stability, cytotoxicity, and x-ray absorption. *J Nanosci Nanotechnol.* 2007;7(8):2690–2695.

Part III

Photon-Counting Detectors for Spectral CT

10 X-Ray Detectors for Spectral Photon Counting CT

Ira Blevis
Philips Healthcare, Haifa, Israel

CONTENTS

10.1 INTRODUCTION

Room Temperature Semiconductor Detectors (RTSCD) absorb and detect x-ray imaging photons by generating individually detectable and measurable electric current pulses without the intermediary step of production and detection of visible light photons. In principle the elimination of an intermediary step can reduce the total entropy of signal conversions and in practice these detectors now provide increased and more precise information for medical imaging. Since the signals are immediately available on the back of the detectors, they are sensed with close fitting miniature electronics that significantly reduce sources of noise and expensive infrastructure and overhead. The extra and new kinds of information also allow algorithm development to extract the relevant imaging parameters. Thus the technique with the vertical integration as it occurs in medical imaging is called photon counting (PC).

The RTSCD began to replace optical detectors and older gas detectors in radiology in the 1990s. The goal was to further improve CT which itself was having revolutionary impact in the field of medicine. In the CT application, RTSCD were capable of individual photon detection and energy measurement, which in turn could fully exploit the newest dimension in clinical CT, that of more detailed material identification in the body, as well as delivering a significant step in spatial resolution. Extended material identification would be immediately useful for example to separately image injected iodine contrast agent and calcium in coronary arteries, or even ultimately, show pathological and physiological native ion distributions and biochemical processes in tissues and organs of the body. The spatial resolution improvement possible with electrostatic collection of signal quanta was also expected to break the limiting tradeoff in scintillators of narrow collimated collection versus full acceptance collection.

But candidate RTSCD's for CT had insufficient stability that got worse at the high and continuously increasing x-ray fluxes (needed to reduce motion artifacts…) used in clinical practice. Some classes of detectors, like amorphous-Selenium for example, found early commercial applications in low-energy imaging like mammography [ZHA97], while higher energy, but still low-rate applications like SPECT, [BOC10] later could adopt crystalline Cadmium-Zinc-Teluride (CZT). The new detectors extended the range of medical imaging, permitting metabolic cancer imaging in the breast (again) for example, improved the image quality and convenience in dedicated cardiac systems, a growing niche, and segued into the infrastructure of digital imaging. Thus a sure and effective cycle of development was indeed leading toward mainstream clinical (general purpose) CT with its ever increasing reach and importance.

In 2005/6 CZT and cadmium telluride (CdTe) were used in CT prototypes with limited scope [BEN08, ZAF12] and then again in 2008 [SCH08] to iterate toward the goal. In 2015, two commercial research groups [BLE15, ROE15, KAP15] were reporting feasibility of full flux, full scale prototypes based on new generations of detector technologies and the CT application came visibly into reach.

In this chapter, we will first review direct conversion CT detectors from CZT, their principles of operation, and first attempts to overcome the main barrier, namely polarization or accumulation of bulk electric charge that changed or extinguished the response to incoming photon fluxes. Then we will discuss signal formation, the small pixel effect, and systematic variables: E-field, risetime, split charge, pixel geometry, and interaction depth. The full detector physics has been simulated in computers using these effects and variables, and the performance parameters of detective quantum efficiency (DQE), spectral response, and the capability for CT material decomposition (identification in the body) will be estimated and reported.

Disclosure: The learnings from these studies are now incorporated in a spectral photon counting CT (SPCCT) prototype built for a European Union H2020 funded project starting in 2016, directed by University of Claude Bernard at Lyon [EUR16], and for which the author of this article is collaborator. Publications of the performance of the prototype with phantoms and with medium animals are published [SIM17, COR17] and examples are shown in Chapter 6 of this publication. Clinical studies with humans are in progress at the time of this writing.

10.2 DIRECT CONVERSION

10.2.1 Absorption

Direct conversion semiconductor materials should have high atomic number, high density, low-dark current, and good electric carrier transport, that is, high mobilities, μ, and high lifetimes before trapping, τ, for both electrons e^-, and holes, h^+. (Of course these materials should also be easy to fabricate or manufacture.)

The main materials being considered for PC CT include $Cd_{1-x}(Zn_x)Te$, denoted CZT for $0<x<0.2$, CdTe, GaAs, and Si. Each has its advantages and challenges. The first challenge is the requirement for and availability of detector grade materials. Figure 10.1 shows how quickly 90% absorption (dose utilization) is reached for quantities of the top candidates. CdTe and CZT are the same and seen to sustain 90% absorption for a 2-mm thick layer even up to ~100 keV [NIS04].

10.2.2 Semiconductor Dark Current

Considering CZT and CdTe further then, CZT has the higher band gap (BG) and lower leakage current than CdTe, but is newer and the reproducibility of the $\mu\tau$s are less assured. The BG of CdZnTe may be only a few percent higher for example, but the thermal carrier density which depends on exp(-kT/BG) is reduced by 95% for a 5% change in BG near 1.5 eV; this is an effective reduction on the dark current over intrinsic CdTe. Then the problem of controlling τ and maybe μ

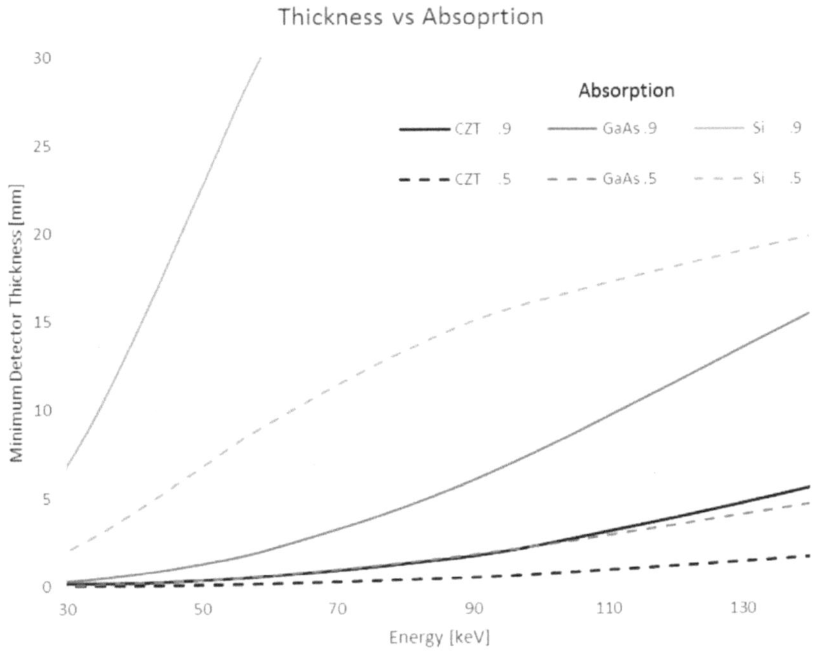

FIGURE 10.1 Thickness requirements for 50% and 90% absorption for candidate RTSCD materials.

also is the industrial problem of pure and coordinated crystal growth with minimal contaminants and BG defect states. Without the Zn, other strategies have developed to reduce dark current in CdTe including p-doping to replace fast carriers by slow ones and p-blocking to prevent this then dominant carrier from injection at the anode. A possible problem with this strategy arises under high bias when the depletion current of the free carriers leads to a negative lattice space charge and a non-uniform electric field, shown in Figure 10.2. A first fast and then long continuing slow-depletion current from the spectrum of dopant charge will lead to reduced and changing field throughout the bulk, while the anode field remains high; this is manifest as diminishing peak count rate without a peak shift (as opposed to a peak shift to low energy for reduced anode field as will be discussed below).

This electric field increases near the anode, which may speed up signal risetimes and facilitate high-electronic count rates, as will be shown further below in connection with the small pixel effect, but the low-electric field produced at the cathode results in reduced clearance of holes from the bulk and thus dynamic buildup of holes and a consequent instability under high flux [e.g., COL99, HAG95]. These phenomena and lessons carry over to CZT where n-type and p-type and injecting and blocking

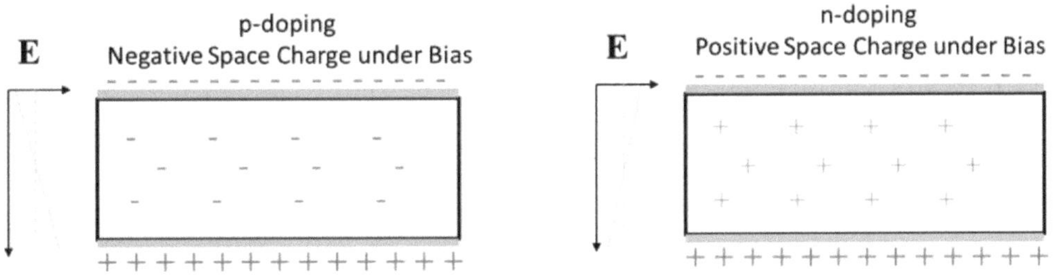

FIGURE 10.2 Electric field changes (from uniform field as dotted line) for lattice charge left after the bias has depleted the bulk semiconductor for p- and n-doping.

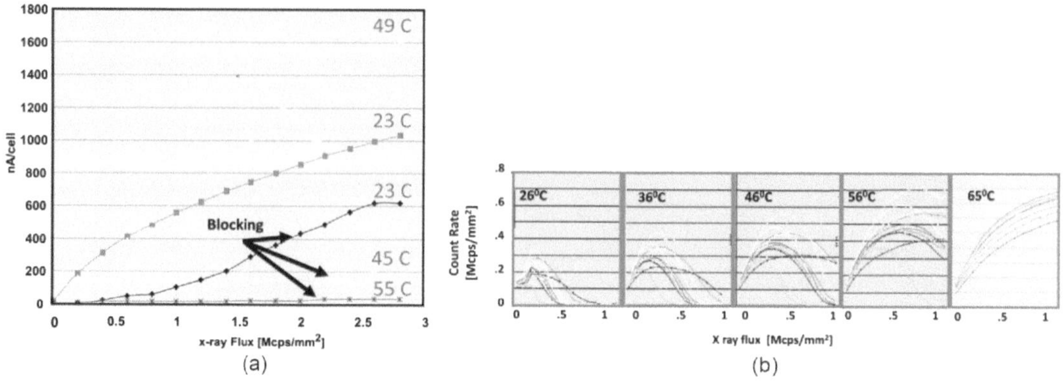

FIGURE 10.3 (a) Detector current is high, increases with flux and further increases with temperature for Ohmic contacts, and decreases for blocking contacts. (b) At the same time the count rate for the blocking contact increases with temperature. Increased current with flux is the expected behavior for E-field collapse to the cathode at high flux for both cases without heating, whereas heating reduces the current for blocking contacts because of the reduction of dynamic hole accumulation.

contacts have all been tried. The best strategy may be intrinsic material, with a high BG and the least thermal carrier concentration[1] and a balanced tradeoff of electron rise time and hole dwell time.

10.2.3 Dynamic Polarization

The clearance of holes was the barrier to overcome in the CZT prototype of 2005 [ZAF12] mentioned above and is still an instructive study. Some conventional wisdom at the time taught that the holes could be cancelled by electron injection at the cathode using a so-called Ohmic contact. Careful measurement of the detector current showed that even when the injection current was growing exponentially the E-field and output count rate (OCR) was in fact collapsing due to the increasing bulk hole concentration. The test of the failure mechanism was to reverse it by heating the CZT to detrap the holes (with a lab blower at first, and then a dedicated heating strip installed in contact with the whole CZT array). Quite dramatically the detector current reduced and the OCR recovered, both to expected levels. [BLE05]

Figure 10.3a shows the detector current for Ohmic and blocking CZT versus flux and temperature. The OCR for blocking is also displayed showing that at higher temperature the OCR recovers from a flux-induced polarization, whereas Figure 10.3b shows that the CZT current decreases, and even decreases to the calculated photocurrent. The explanation for the higher currents at lower T when polarization is occurring is that the extremely high E-field that occurs at the cathode causes an increased Field Assisted Thermionic Emission (FATE, or Richardson effect). In the case of Ohmic contacts with even higher currents it was estimated that the high fluctuations of the high-current emulated pulses of a real OCR, but the pulses were not individually correlated to incident photons. A simulation of the dynamic equilibrium of holes production from the ICR and holes clearance under the E-field was performed [BLEV08]. The small pixel effect of the electron pulses was taken into account and the red shift of the energy response of the CZT was seen. By fitting the OCR (above fixed counting thresholds) to the ICR of the flux, the temperature dependence of μ_h was obtained. The temperature dependence was fitted to a Boltzman model using $\mu_{eff} \sim e^{-BE/kT}$ and the binding energy of the hole traps was determined to be BE = 0.7 keV ≈Band Gap/2 for that first generation CZT-CT experiment. Figure 10.4 shows how the model emulates both the buildup of the Electric field at high flux and low temperature and the CZT detector response function shift to lower energies at a fixed high flux and several temperatures.

[1] The equilibrium concentration of electron and holes in a semiconductor is $n_n \times n_p = N^2$ (see KAS96). The minimum of $n_n + n_p$ is therefore $n_n = n_p = N$, i.e., no doping.

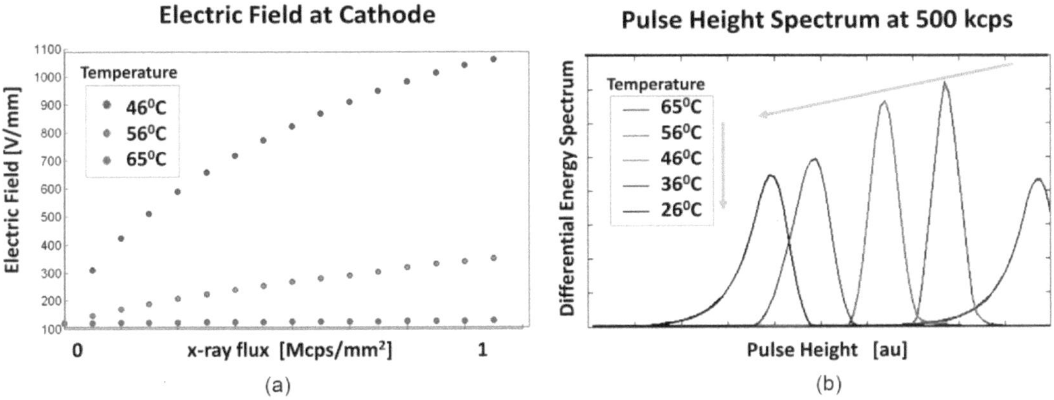

FIGURE 10.4 Simulation of dynamic hole accumulation. At high flux, low temperature, and high-hole accumulation the Electric field at the cathode is high (a) and the pulse height is low (b). At high temperature the Electric field at the cathode is constant and low up to high flux (a) and the pulse height remains high (b).

10.3 SIGNAL FORMATION

10.3.1 Charge Cloud Formation

In CT the incident photon energy is in the range of 30–140 keV. Such photons are absorbed in detector materials by the photoelectric effect, the Compton effect, or a small cascade of both resulting in one or more energetic free 'photo' electrons. The photoelectrons travel through the semiconductor by multiple scattering, producing primary ionization by atomic scattering and secondary ionization from the energetic primaries, finally dissipating their energy into a cloud of electron hole pairs (ehp). The amount of charge produced is accurately determined by the ionization energy in the semiconductor material, which is 4.5 eV in CZT in accordance with the Klein relation (Band Gap ~ 1.6 eV). [KLE68] Thus a 100 KeV x-ray photon produces 3.5 fC of e^{-}s and h^{+}s.

The initial size of the cloud is a few microns across, as shown in Figure 10.5, but with the applied electric field the electrons and holes separate from each other into two clouds traveling to

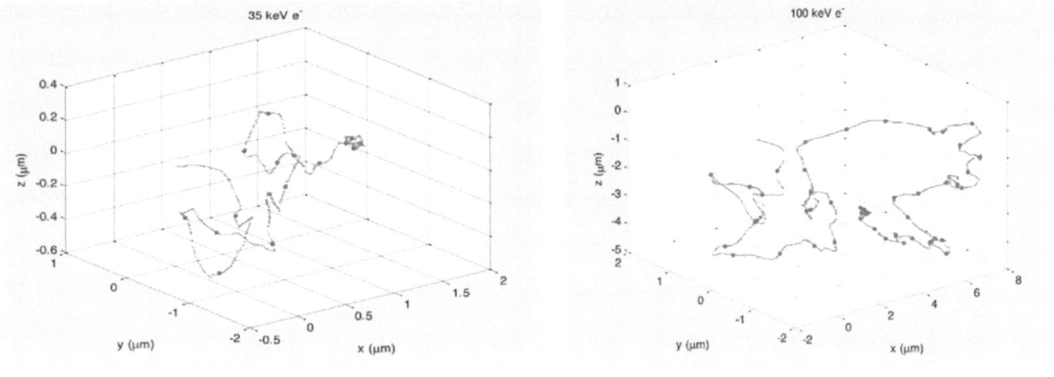

FIGURE 10.5 Photoelectron trajectory and initial ionization in CZT using GEANT. A blue dot marks points of cumulative 2 keV E loss. The dots cluster at the end of the trajectory in accordance with the Bragg peak. The overall E loss is ~5 eV/nm. The initial size of the cloud of ionization is less than 10 microns across for a 100-keV photoelectron and 2 microns for a 35-keV photoelectron.

opposite electrodes. The electric field E is $E = V/t$, where V is an applied bias voltage and t is the distance between electrodes, that is, the thickness of the semiconductor slab. Once separated, the two charge clouds each undergo self-repulsive Coulomb explosions and each inflate an order of magnitude in size during the transit time to the collecting electrodes (all charges separating uniformly as in a Hubble expansion!). The final size is of order 50–100 μm, discussed further below. This final size is important because it determines limits to the spatial and energy resolution of the detection process.

10.3.2 Charge Collection

Blocks of semiconductor material are coated with metal electrodes on facing sides to which a 'bias' voltage (V) is applied, producing an electric field throughout the interior bulk of the material. If the BG > ~1.5 eV, there are few free e^-s or h^+s at room temperature and thus negligible dark current-Id. The low Id allows signal sensing and readout using miniature application-specific integrated circuit (ASIC) electronics, possibly without the need for bulky capacitive coupling or active current compensation.

Blocks of semiconductor, in particular CZT, are made into radiation detectors by depositing and configuring thin metal electrodes on a pair of facing surfaces. The electrodes are biased as cathode and anode with voltage to give electric fields E in the bulk material up to 100's V/mm, but usually less than 500 V/mm simply to reduce the high-voltage (HV) engineering requirements. The flux of the charge clouds toward the biased electrodes induces current on the electrodes that can be detected with an amplifier circuit. With sufficiently high μ_e and τ_e from the RTSCD, and velocity $v = \mu \cdot V/t$ from the applied V, then the time structure of the electron current is comprised of pulses and allows the detection and counting of individual photons by external electronics, even from deep within thick detectors. Electronics for detection, measurement, and scaling of the current pulses are presented in companion chapters of the current text.

The depth of interaction profile for x-rays is exponential and given by the Beer-Lambert law. The mean depth is about .2 mm for 60 keV photons (~1 mm for 100 keV). Since electrons have higher μ than holes by about 10× due to reduced shallow traps [KAR18, JAM95], the magnitude of the current pulse can be increased and the duration decreased, by illumination of the cathode instead of the anode, thereby allowing the electrons to have the longer trajectories. This is illustrated in Figure 10.6a showing the induced current I and integrated charge Q signals for two photons, one absorbed near the cathode and one absorbed near the anode. The total Q collected is the same in both cases since the same total charge is neutralized by the external circuit; however, a representative time for thickness 2 mm, $\mu = 1000\ cm^2/Vs$ and E = 1000 V is also included and the dramatic effect on event duration and limiting count rates in electronic stages is apparent.

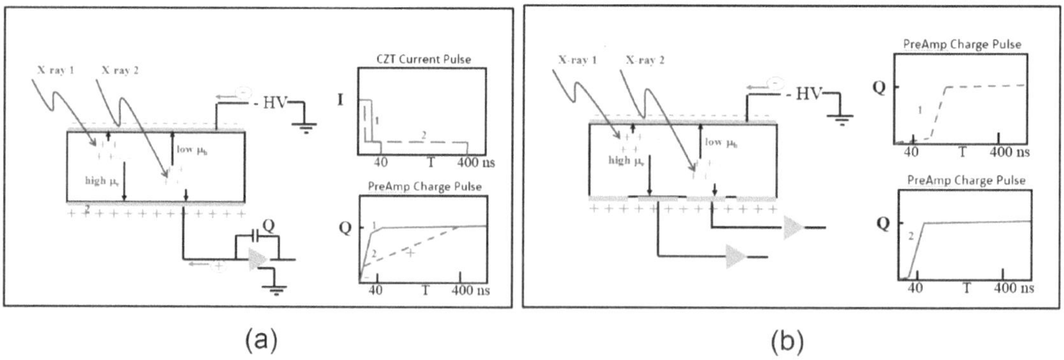

FIGURE 10.6 (a) Signal formation for continuous anodes showing large induction pulse shape differences for different depths of interaction. (b) Subdividing the anode in order to make image pixels has the welcome effect of making the induced pulses dramatically faster and more uniform for high-count rate applications.

10.3.3 Image Pixels and Small Pixel Effect

To achieve (medical) imaging of the subject the anode is subdivided to pixels. The applied bias collects the holes to the cathode and the electrons to the pixelated anode. The pixels which are of size ¼ mm to 1 mm in practice are still large compared to the electron charge clouds of 50–100 μm described above. The electron charge cloud usually arrives at a single anode pixel because of its size, but sometimes is split between two neighboring pixels.

One main purpose of the pixels is to detect the location of the conversion charge above the anode plane, but in addition it is found that the induced charge on the pixels for both holes and electrons is subdivided amongst all the nearby pixels. While the conversion charge is still in the middle of the CZT volume many almost equidistant pixels participate in the induced charge. As the electron charge approaches a single final pixel on the anode the induction diminishes on the further pixels and increases on the final pixel (it can be described as 'moving' because the total induction is preserved). The signal on the final pixel increases slowly until the electron cloud is close and then it increases quickly as the total induction is concentrated by this geometric effect. The holes on the other hand move toward the cathode and their induction on the particular final hit pixel of the electron starts small and then further diminishes. The final amplitude of the signal on the hit pixel is almost independent of the depth of the interaction as shown in Figure 10.6b. It also has a delayed but faster rise that is important to limit overlap or pileup at high-count rates as found in PC CT. The total effect is called the small pixel effect [BAR95, HE00] and also sometimes called an 'electron only' signal. Figure 10.7 shows the Q signal (the integral of the current pulse for an incident x-ray photon) for a selection of Electric fields resulting from different CZT doping, either accidental or intentional; the simulation was performed as the Coulomb induction due to a suspended (and moving) charge above a grounded pixel plane as described above. For this figure the cathode plane and the hole motion was neglected. The

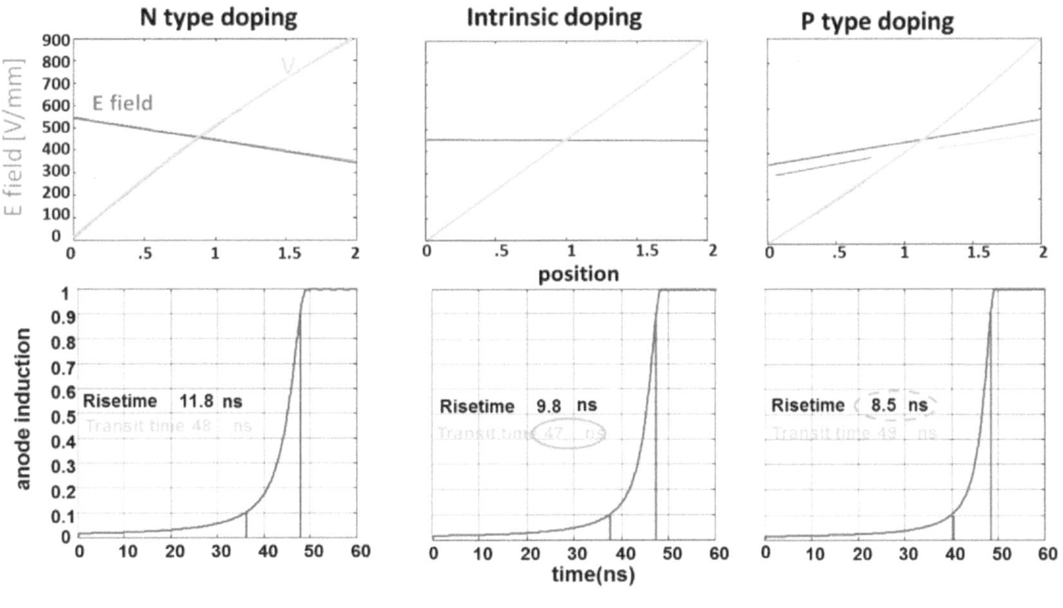

FIGURE 10.7 shows the Q signal (the integral of the current pulse for an incident x-ray photon) for a selection of Electric fields resulting from different CZT doping, either accidental or intentional; the simulation was performed as the Coulomb induction due to a suspended (and moving) charge above a grounded pixel plane.

risetime for 10–90% of the signal and the transit time is shown as well. It is apparent that p-type doping gives the fastest risetimes, but the weakest hole clearance and thus greatest risk of dynamic polarization; n-type doping would give better hole clearance but significantly slower signal risetimes. Intrinsic-type gives a compromise risetime and notably the least dwell time for deeply generated holes or anode injected holes that have to clear via the cathode. Taking into account the time constant for the depletion current and therefore the E-field stabilization, it may be suggested that intrinsic is a better strategy.

10.3.4 E-Field Focusing

A second type of small pixel effect is often described where small pixel pads, compared to the pixel pitch, are expected to cause E-field focusing in the region of the pixel pad and then accelerating electrons and a faster risetime. To ensure this effect it is conjectured that a perfect insulating passivation from a deposited material or even air on the anode plane would ensure that the interpad region charges up and causes the focused field lines. The counter argument is that the CZT is always a good conductor for charge, even in contact with this nonconductive passivation layer, and will never charge up in the anode plane, just as it is impossible to charge the surface of an insulator (say wood or plastic) in contact with a grounded aluminum sheet. The Al, like the CZT, will drain the charge to an available ground connection. The experiment has been tried several times over the years because of the search for that perfect passivation layer. A recent result is shown in Figure 10.8. It shows a test structure with four regions of pixels with the same pitch and different anode pads. The map image shows count rate above 115 keV for Co57. The larger pixels show higher peak count rate in both the map image (there is also some dome effect visible from the proximity of the source) and in the regional spectra (spectra normalized to the same peak height). This higher rate for the larger pads is consistent with non-focusing E-field and inconsistent with a focusing E-field.

10.3.5 Split Charge

Small pixels do produce faster induction signals facilitating high count rates as noted above; however, they also cause a significant occurrence of split charge clouds and a transfer from peak to tail in the spectral response. Now we also know that the field lines in CZT are straight from cathode to anode without focusing because of the measurements of the last section. With this we can build a simple geometrical model of the split charges, fit it to experimental data, and extract some characteristic physical parameters. Figure 10.9 shows the basic model of a spherical charge cloud of uniform density (from the 'Hubble' expansion discussed above) that is split to parts inside and outside the

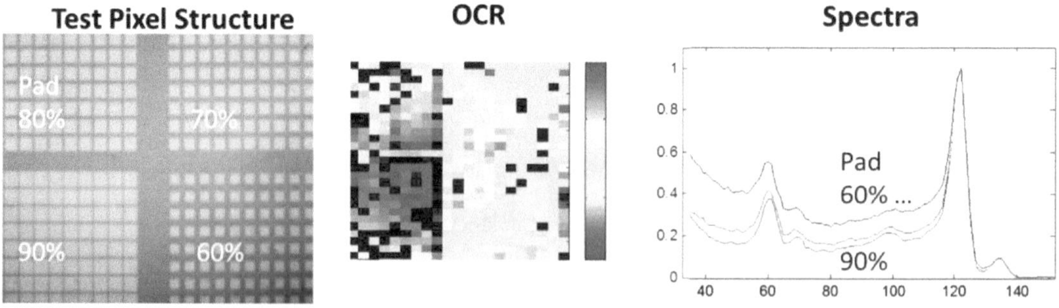

FIGURE 10.8 A test structure with four regions of pixels with the same pitch and different anode pads. The map image shows count rate above 115 keV for Co57. The larger pixels show higher peak count rate in the map image and in the regional spectra (spectra normalized to the same peak height).

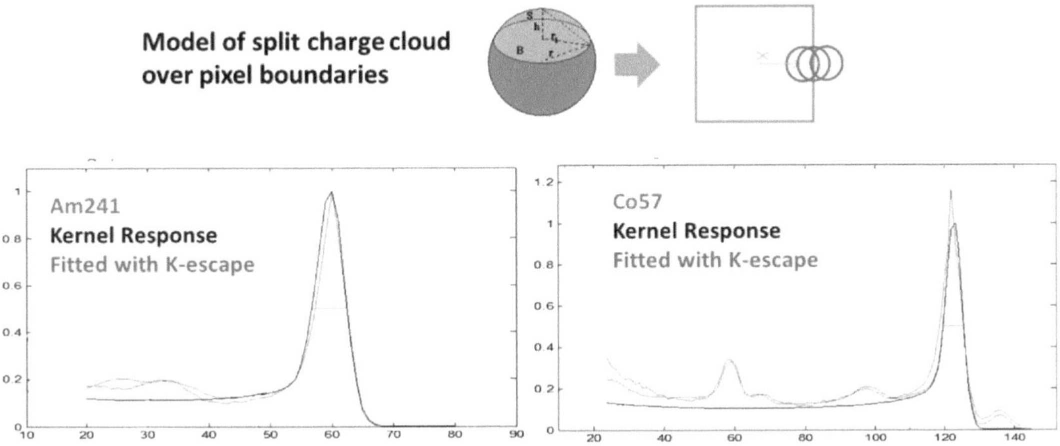

FIGURE 10.9 The basic model of a spherical charge cloud of uniform density that is split to parts inside and outside the pixel. Simulating a uniform flux on the pixel and adjusting the only free parameter, the cloud radius, to fit spectra of 60 keV and 122 keV from Am241 and Co57 allows determination of the cloud size versus energy.

pixel. A uniform flux on the pixel was simulated and the projections of spheres entirely contained in the pixel contributed to the spectral peak and partial projection volumes contained in the pixels contributed to the spectral tail. The peaks (and tails although they don't change) were convoluted with the measured amplifier noise. Then the only free parameter, the cloud radius, was adjusted to fit the peak to tail ratio of 60 keV and 122 keV measured spectra from Am241 and Co57, thereby allowing determination of the cloud size vs Energy. (Note that the Co57 spectra shows a sharp peak processing artifact that was ignored in the fitting). The result is that the cloud radius varies from 50 to 75 um over this range. The model can be augmented with the depth of interaction and time of expansion for 2 mm thickness and 900 V to estimate sizes for other detector configurations. This result is an important ingredient for simulations of PC involving polychromatic spectra as below.

10.3.6 Simulation of Combined Effects

The effects described above, namely the Beer-Lambert deposition profile, the charge cloud size, the E-field collection, the pixel geometry and the split charge clouds, have been combined in simulations to help guide the development of the SPCCT photon counting CT mentioned in the introduction and elsewhere in this volume. The simulation was first used to examine the fidelity of the detector response function and the degradation resulting from different Anti-scatter grid (ASG) design capabilities. A realistic x-ray tube spectrum with correct filtration was used as input. The simulated x-ray photons were passed through a 30-cm water phantom, then through the ASG to land on the detector array varying with the configuration and alignment of the ASG. Then depending on the energy and the location in the pixel the correct pixel and energy according to the split charge model with E-field was calculated. Figure 10.10 shows resultant spectra for the case of (a) no ASG, (b) an ASG fully aligned to the pixels, and (c to e) three values of misalignment, and finally (d) a coarse ASG with septa only for every other pixel (of double height). The misidentification of photons into the tail of the spectrum is apparently quite strong for the case (a). Cases (b to d) show that the ASG is very effective to remove these confounding photons and that some level of misalignment may even be acceptable. Case (d) shows that the coarse ASG would still give substantial 'flowdown' to the lower energy in the detected spectrum.

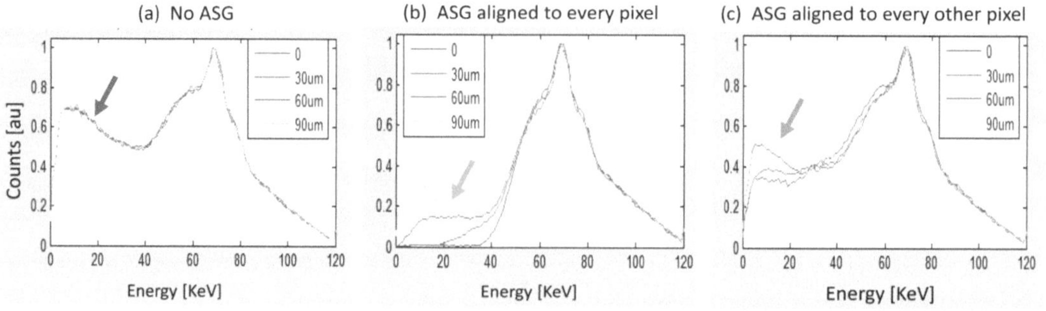

FIGURE 10.10 Simulation of x-ray tube, 30 cm water, ASG designs and alignments, split charge model and E-field collection. Resultant spectra are shown for the case of (a) no ASG, (b) an ASG aligned to the pixels, and (c to e) misalignment by 30, 60 or 90μm, and (c) a coarse ASG with septa only for every other pixel (of double height). The misidentification of photons into the tail of the spectrum is apparently strong for the case (a). Case (b) shows that the ASG is very effective to remove these confounding photons and that some level of misalignment may even be acceptable. Case (c) shows that the coarse ASG would still give substantial 'flow-down' to lower energy in the detected spectrum.

Using the known original energies (called 'preimage') of the photons that are detected in the final simulated spectra (called 'bin'), a figure of merit (FOM) can be defined measuring the capability of the system for correct material decomposition.

$$\mathrm{FOM} = (< E_{\mathrm{preimage\ bin\ 1}} > - (< E_{\mathrm{preimage\ bin\ 2}} >) / \mathrm{sqrt}\left(1 / n_{\mathrm{preimage\ bin\ 1}} + 1 / n_{\mathrm{preimage\ bin\ 2}}\right)$$

This FOM increases if the energy separation of the preimage photons increases and if the statistics of that preimage energy bin is increased. Thus we can first scan the placement of thresholds in the output spectrum to find an optimum of the FOM; then for any design configuration we can re-find the optimum and compare the relative values of the FOM to optimize between design choices. Figure 10.11 shows output response spectra for different pixel sizes with 3 E bins in the top row and

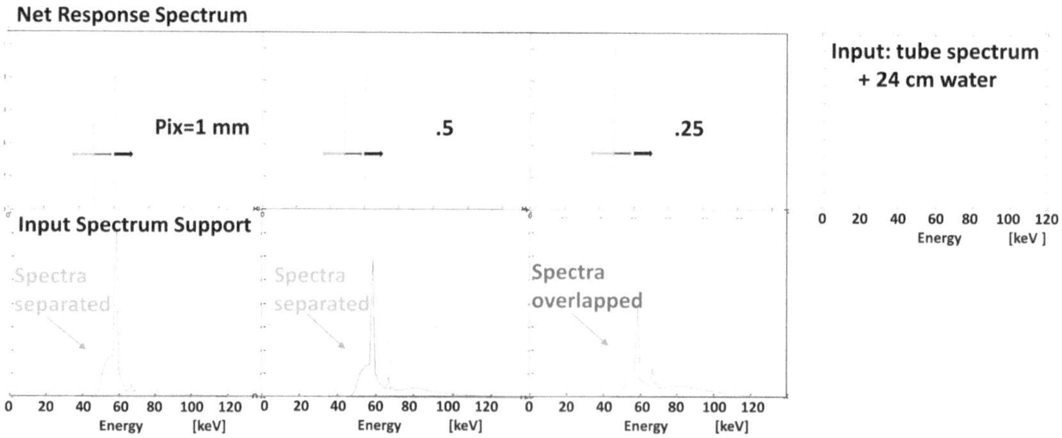

FIGURE 10.11 The output response spectra for different pixel sizes is shown with 3 E bins in the top row and then the three true energies distributions contributing to the 3 E bins that would be measured by the system counting electronics in the bottom row. The quickly increasing overlap of the preimage spectra for small pixels is apparent.

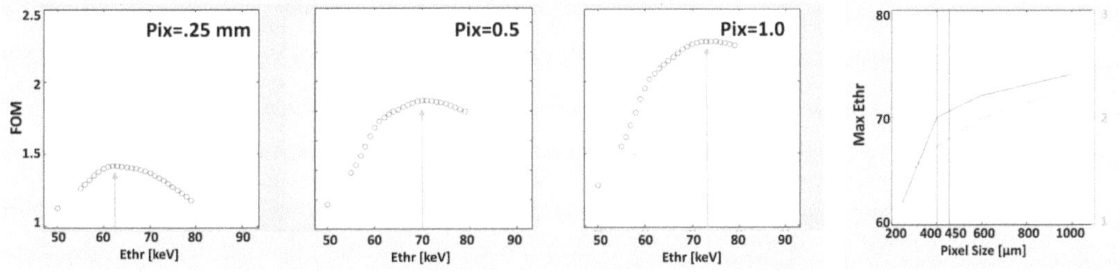

FIGURE 10.12 The optimization of the FOM by scanning over the possible E threshold choices is shown for each pixel size separately. The position and value of the optimum is plotted at the right showing a significant increase in FOM for larger pixels and a region of diminishing benefits of increased pixel size.

then the three true energies distributions contributing to the 3 E bins that would be measured by the system counting electronics in the bottom row. Already the quickly increasing overlap of the preimage spectra for small pixels is apparent.

Figure 10.12 shows the optimization of the FOM by scanning over the possible E threshold choices for each pixel size separately. The best E threshold value in the measured spectrum is not the same for all pixel sizes. Choosing the best value from the scan and comparing the FOM value that results for the different pixel sizes show a significant increase in FOM for larger pixels. The graph at the far right tracks the increase in FOM value for the pixel size and shows a knee, that is, the beginning of diminishing benefits of increased pixel size. The position of the knee is a consideration in the balance of count rate capability versus E bin separation for material separation of a PC design.

10.3.7 Small Pixels

Small pixels have been shown in a few cases to severely degrade the performance parameters needed for good material decomposition in PC. However, small pixels are an advantage for subdividing the imaging surface to reduce the count rate at any given pixel to be handled better by realistic counting electronics. The degree of reduction is still a parameter optimized by various research and commercial groups differently. One strategy to get the best of both worlds is to be able to combine energy measurements from different small pixels to counteract the increased frequency of splits charges that results. However, this has so far proved to be problematic in that the processing time cost of this operation counteracts the benefits hoped for. So far a winning strategy has been to optimize the pixel size, the ASG, and the risetime simultaneously using the above described researches.

REFERENCES

BAR95 H.H. Barrett, J.D. Eskin, H.B. Barber, Charge transport in arrays of semiconductor gamma-ray detectors. *Phys Rev Lett.* 1995 July;75(1):156–159.

BEN08 O. Benjaminov, E. Perlow, Z. Romman, R. Levinson, B. Bashara, M. Cohen, A. Zelikovsky, Novel Energy-Discriminating Photon Counting CT System (EDCT): First Clinical Evaluation—CT Angiography: Carotid Artery Stenosis. Radiological Society of North America 2008 Scientific Assembly and Annual Meeting; Chicago IL. 2008.

BLE05 I.M. Blevis, Method and apparatus for reducing polarization within an imaging device, US Patent US7312458B2.

BLEV08 I.M. Blevis, J.P. Bouhnik, A. Cohen, Measurements of Dark Current in CZT with Variable Flux IEEE Room Temperature Semiconductor Detectors, Dresden, 2008.

BLE15 I.M. Blevis, A. Altman, Y. Berman, R. Levinson, A. Livne, M. Rokni, Y. Younes, O. Zarchin, C. Herrmann, R. Steadman, Introduction of Philips Preclinical Photon Counting Scanner and Detector Technology Development, IEEE Medical Imaging Conference, M4D2-1, San Diego, Nov 2015.

BOC10 M. Bocher, I.M. Blevis, L. Tsukerman, Y. Shrem, G. Kovalski, L. Volokh, A fast cardiac gamma camera with dynamic SPECT capabilities: Design, system validation and future potential. *E J Nuc Med.* 2010;37(10):1887–1902.

COL99 A. Cola, I. Farella, The polarization mechanism in CdTe Schottky detectors. *Appl. Phys. Lett.* 2009;94:102113.

COR17 David P. Cormode, Salim Si-Mohamed, Daniel Bar-Ness, Monica Sigovan, Pratap C. Nahal, Joelle Balegamire, Franck Lavenne, Philippe Coulon, Ewald Roessl, Matthias Bartels, Michal Rokni, Ira Blevis, Loic Boussel, Philippe Douek, Multicolor spectral photon counting computed tomography: In vivo dual contrast imaging with a high count rate scanner. *Sci Rep.* 2017 July 6;7(1):4784.

EUR16 European Union's Horizon 2020 research and innovation program grant agreement No 668142.

HAG95 M. Hage-Ali, P. Siffert, CdTe nuclear detectors and applications. *In Semiconductors for Room Temperature Nuclear Detector Applications*; Schlesinger T.E., James R.B., Eds.; Academic Press: San Diego, CA, USA, 1995; Vol. 43, pp. 291–331.

HE00 Z. He, Review of the Shockley–Ramo theorem and its application in semiconductor gamma-ray detectors. *Nucl Instrum Methods Phys Res A.* 2001;463:250–267.

JAM95 R.B James, T.E. Schelsinger, J.C. Lund, M. Scheiber, Cd1-xZnxTe spectrometers for gamma and x-ray applications. *In Semiconductors for Room Temperature Nuclear Detector Applications*; Schlesinger T.E., James R.B., Eds.; Academic Press: San Diego, CA, USA, 1995; Vol. 43, pp. 336–378.

KAP15 S. Kappler, K. Hahn, A. Henning, E. Göderer, B. Kreisler, K. Stadlthanner, P. Sievers, S. Ulzheimer, Towards high-resolution multi-energy CT: Recent results from our wholebody prototype scanner with high-flux capable photon counting detector. 3rd Workshop on Medical Applications for Spectroscopic X-ray Detectors CERN, April 2015.

KAR18 P. Karasyuk, Y. Shepelytskyi, O. Semeniu k, O. Bubon, G. Juska, I. Blevis, A. Reznik, Investigation of photoconductivity and electric field distribution in CZT detectors by time-of-flight (TOF) and charge extraction by linearly increasing voltage (CELIV). *J Mater Sci Mater Electron.* 2018;29(16):13941–13951.

KAS96 Principles of Electrical Materials and Devices, Safa O. Kasap Irwin (1996).

KLE68 A. Claude. Klein bandgap dependence and related features of radiation ionization energies in semiconductors. *J Appl Phys.* 1968;39:2029.

NIS04 NIST-Ray Mass Attenuation Coefficients Standard Reference Database 126 https://www.nist.gov/pml/x-ray-mass-attenuation-coefficients. July 2004.

ROE15 E. Roessl, M. Bartels, B. Brendel, H. Daerr, K.-J. Engel, C. Herrmann, R. Levinson, A. Livne, M. Rokni, D. Rubin, R. Steadman, A. Thran, Y. Younes, R. Proksa, A. Altman, O. Zarchin, I. Blevis. Imaging Performance of a Photon-Counting Computed Tomography Prototype 3rd Workshop on Medical Applications for Spectroscopic X-ray Detectors CERN, April 2015.

SCH08 J. P. Schlomka, E. Roessl, R. Dorscheid, S. Dill, G. Martens, T. Istel, C. Baumer, C. Herrmann, R. Steadman, G. Zeitler, A. Livne, Experimental feasibility of multi-energy photon-counting K-edge imaging in pre-clinical computed tomography R Proksa1. *Phys Med Biol.* 2008;53:4031–4047.

SIM17 Salim Si-Mohamed, Daniel Bar-Ness, Monica Sigovan, David P. Cormode, Philippe Coulon, Emmanuel Coche, Alain Vlassenbroek, Gabrielle Normand, Loic Boussel, Philippe Douek, Review of an initial experience with an experimental spectral photon-counting computed tomography system. *Nucl Instrum Methods Phys Res A.* 2017;873:27–35.

ZAF12 Nili Zafrir, Gigeon Shafir, Gil Kovalski, Israel Mats, Jean-Paul Bouhnik, Alexander Battler, Alejandro Solodky, Yield of a novel ultra-low-dose computed tomography device. *J Nucl Cardiol.* 2012 Apr;19(2):303–310.

ZHA97 W. Zhao, I. Blevis, S. Germann, J.A. Rowlands, D. Waechter, Z. Huang, Digital radiology using active matrix readout of amorphous selenium: Construction and evaluation of a prototype real-time detector. *Med Phys.* 1997 Dec;24(12):1834–1843.

11 Spectral Performance of Photon-Counting X-Ray Detectors

How Well Can We Capture the Rainbow?

Peter Trueb, Pietro Zambon, and Christian Broennimann
Dectris Ltd., Taefernweg, Baden-Dättwil, Switzerland

CONTENTS

11.1 INTRODUCTION

Assessing and understanding the performance of photon-counting X-ray detectors is an essential prerequisite for successfully applying them to Spectral Computed Tomography. After a short overview of the technology, the detector response function is introduced as a characteristic spectral property of photon-counting detectors from which many performance parameters can be extracted.

Subsequently we discuss how different physical effects like charge sharing between pixels or pulse pile-up at high photon fluxes affect this detector response function. In a second part several figures of merit are presented for a quantitative comparison of photon-counting detectors. The definition, measurement, interpretation, and limitations of quantities like the energy resolution, quantum, and spectral efficiency are discussed. The last part reviews different approaches to improve the spectral response of photon-counting detectors. Fast pulse shaping, charge-sharing, and pile-up rejection, or charge summing mechanisms help to clean the measured spectrum. We analyze their advantages and disadvantages with respect to improving the detector response function. It is the hope of the authors that the reader will gain a good understanding about the assessment of the spectral performance of photon-counting detectors as well as about the current state of the technology.

11.2 PHOTON-COUNTING X-RAY DETECTORS

Photon-counting X-ray detectors (PCDs) have the capability of providing spectral information about the incoming radiation by individually analyzing the energy of every photon. Their main components are an X-ray sensitive semiconductor sensor and an Application Specific Integrated Circuit (ASIC) for processing the signal of the detected photons (see Figure 11.1). Each pixel of the semiconductor sensor is electrically connected to one pixel of the ASIC by a small solder bump bond. Different semiconductor materials like Si, GaAs, CdTe, or CdZnTe with a thickness ranging from hundreds of micrometers to few millimeters are used to absorb the X-rays. High-grade single crystal materials are the key elements for highly efficient detectors that provide good contrast even at low doses. Since the semiconductor directly converts the X-ray photons into an electrical signal, this measuring method falls into the category of *direct detection*. In contrast, *indirect detection* methods first convert the X-rays into visible light before transforming the energy into an electrical signal. By omitting the conversion into visible light, the direct detection method avoids the blurring associated with this step and therefore profits from a better spatial resolution.

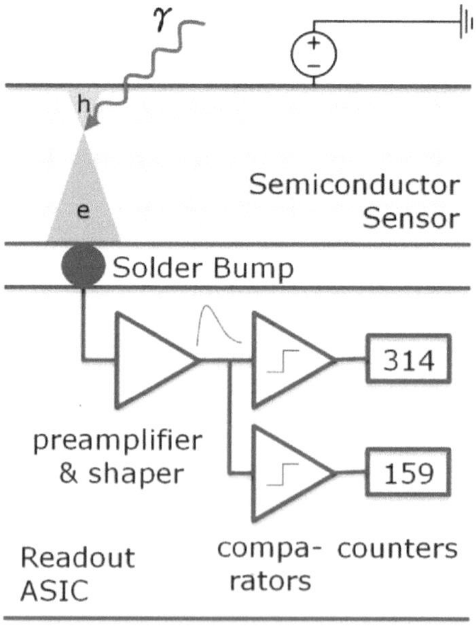

FIGURE 11.1 Schematic overview of one pixel of a photon-counting detector. X-rays are directly converted into electron-hole pairs in the semiconductor sensor. The readout ASIC amplifies the collected charge and compares the pulse height to predefined energy thresholds. The counters are increased every time a pulse exceeds the energy threshold.

The semiconductor sensor has an unstructured entrance side where a bias voltage is applied and a pixelated side with readout electrodes for every pixel. If a photon is absorbed by the photoelectric effect, its energy is transferred to an electron (known as photoelectron). This electron loses its energy by scattering with other electrons in the semiconductor sensor. Along its track the photoelectron thereby creates a large number of electron-hole pairs, which start to drift under the influence of the applied bias voltage. The generated amount of charge is proportional to the energy deposited in the sensor. In CdTe on average, one electron-hole pair is created per 4.4 eV. For a negative bias voltage the electrons are collected at the pixel electrode, while the holes drift to the unstructured side of the sensor.

The first block in the readout ASIC consists of a charge sensitive preamplifier, which generates a voltage pulse for every charge packet collected at its input. These pulses can be further amplified and filtered by a shaper stage. The amplitude of each pulse, which is proportional to the amount of collected charge, is subsequently compared to the different threshold levels of multiple comparators [1]. In the simplest case, the value of a corresponding downstream counter is increased whenever a pulse exceeds the threshold level of one of the comparators. The number of counts therefore yields the X-ray intensity above certain photon energy. The values of all the counters are read out at the end of an acquisition time window. The number of photons in an energy interval $[E_1, E_2]$ can be obtained by subtracting the value of a counter with energy threshold E_2 from the value of a counter with threshold $E_1 < E_2$. The number of implemented energy thresholds varies for different ASICs. The spectral information obtained in this way makes it possible to explore new imaging modalities like multi-material decomposition.

Photon-counting detectors have many advantages. The usage of energy thresholds effectively removes any contribution of dark currents to the measured signal. The digital processing offers a very high dynamic range with single photon resolution and avoids the readout noise present in integrating detectors. Altogether, this leads to images free of any noise hits as long as the energy thresholds are set sufficiently high above the noise level of the detector. Since the digitization of the measured intensities takes place in each pixel of the ASIC, photon-counting detectors can be read out very fast. Frame rates of several kHz as required by CT applications are possible without any degradation of the data quality. Thanks to the fast signal processing in the ASIC, counting detectors can finally deliver spectral information up to X-ray fluxes of several hundred millions of photons per second and square millimeter.

11.3 DISSECTING THE DETECTOR RESPONSE FUNCTION

11.3.1 Detector Response Function

Ideally, all photons with a specific energy generate pulses of equal amplitude. Unfortunately in practice, this is not the case, mainly due to electronic noise and due to charge sharing and atomic fluorescence within the sensor. This has the consequence that the observed number of counts changes with the threshold level of the comparators even if it is set significantly below the energy of uniform and monochromatic radiation. While this behavior is not desirable, it is at least helpful to characterize the detector. Many performance parameters can be retrieved by measuring the number of counts as a function of the threshold energy, which yields a fingerprint of the examined photon-counting detector. If the recorded counts are derived with respect to the threshold energy, the energy spectrum as seen by the comparator is obtained. This function is called *differential pulse height spectrum* [2] or *detector response function* [3] since it describes how the detector responds to X-ray photons of a given energy. Formally, we can define the detector response (*DR*) as:

$$DR\left(E_\gamma, E\right) = \frac{\frac{d}{dE_t} N_c(E_t)(E_t = E)}{N_\gamma}, \tag{11.1}$$

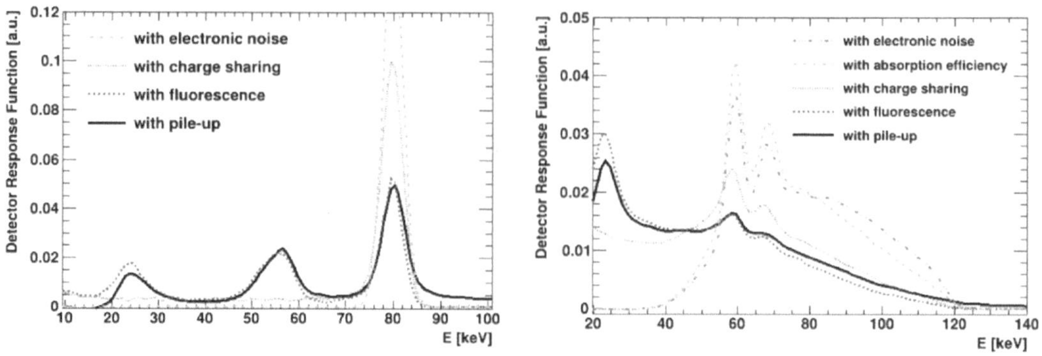

FIGURE 11.2 Examples of simulated detector response functions for mono- (left) and polychromatic (right) radiation. The different lines show the response functions after enabling additional effects in the simulation (including all previous effects). The simulation parameters were chosen to highlight the impact of the different physical effects on the detector response function: (left) 80 keV photon energy, 2 mm thick CdTe sensor, 150 μm pixel size, 2 keV ENC, 200 Mph/s/mm^2, (right) RQA9 spectrum, 1 mm thick CdTe sensor, 150 μm pixel size, 1 keV ENC, 50 Mph/s/mm^2.

where E_γ is the photon energy and E the energy with which an event is detected by a pixel of the detector. $N_C(E_t)$ is the number of counts above a threshold energy E_t and N_γ the number of incoming photons [4]. Examples of detector response functions are shown in Figure 11.2.

Different approaches have been used for modeling the detector response function. Analytical models can precisely describe the detector response as a function of a few key parameters like pixel size, charge cloud size, and electronic noise [5–8]. However, in general they are limited to low photon fluxes and energies below the K-edges of Cadmium and Tellurium. To model the more complex phenomena of pulse pile-up and fluorescence effects, Monte-Carlo methods are used [4, 9]. They are well suited to deal with these stochastic processes but tend to be very time consuming. Independent of the chosen approach, detector models are useful tools to characterize and optimize the behavior of photon counting X-ray detectors. The following sections discuss the detector response and its dependency on different detector parameters.

11.3.2 Noise in the Sensor and Readout ASIC

The response function of an ideal detector for a monochromatic radiation is a delta function peaking at the photon energy. In practice, the delta function is smeared out by the noise of the detector system as shown in Figure 11.2. The resulting shape is well described by a Gaussian function and is called the *photo peak*. The electronic noise is conventionally specified in terms of an *equivalent noise charge (ENC)*. It is defined as the charge which would generate the same voltage variation at the output of the analog processing chain as the root mean square of the noise fluctuation. Typical ENC values for existing pixelated photon counting ASICs range from a few tens to a few hundreds of electrons.

The main contribution to the peak width originates from the noise of the ASIC and depends on the pixel geometry, front-end topology, fabrication technology, and operative settings. A detailed description of the underlying device-level physical mechanisms and of the signal processing techniques can be found in dedicated in-depth studies like [10–14]. Another minor source of statistical noise is called *Fano* noise. It is related to the statistical uncertainty involved in the generation of the electron-hole pairs in the sensor material [2], but is usually negligible with respect to the contribution of the electronic noise of the front-end circuitry.

If the energy threshold is set lower than about five times the ENC, a counting detector starts to register noise hits even in the absence of X-ray photons. This would show up as a strong increase of the detector response function at low energies (not shown in Figure 11.2). For higher energy thresholds photon-counting detectors are free of noise hits, which is a big advantage with respect to integrating detectors. The minimization of the ENC is an important aspect in the development of a readout ASIC, but it has to be balanced with other conflicting requirements such as high radiation tolerance, functional versatility, robustness and simplicity, limited power budget, and fast shaping time.

11.3.3 Charge Sharing Between Neighboring Pixels

Each photon absorbed in the sensor material creates a charge cloud, which drifts toward the readout electrodes under the influence of the bias voltage applied across the sensor. If the absorption takes place close to the border of neighboring pixels, the charge cloud is split across several pixels. Consequently, multiple pixels capture a fraction of the total charge. This effect is known as charge sharing. Depending on the programmed energy threshold, the photon is counted by none, one or multiple pixels. In the worst case of a hit close to a pixel corner, one photon can be counted up to four times. Due to the effect of charge sharing, hits with a fractional energy show up in the detector response function. This leads to an approximately constant background below the photo peak as shown in Figure 11.2.

The amount of charge sharing strongly depends on the pixel size and the sensor thickness. For large pixels, the probability for a photon to hit the sensor close to a pixel border is significantly smaller. To a lesser degree, the amount of charge sharing is also influenced by the size of the charge cloud when it arrives at the pixel electrodes. During its drift to the electrodes, the charge cloud grows due to thermal diffusion and electrostatic repulsion. Therefore, the size correlates with the drift time in the semiconductor sensor. Low-energetic photons penetrate less into the sensor material and therefore, they have a longer drift time and are more subject to charge sharing. To some extent, the drift time and thus the amount of charge sharing can be reduced by increasing the applied bias voltage. However, the velocity of the charge carriers cannot be increased beyond a saturation value specific for a given type of sensor material. At high photon energies also the average track of the photoelectron is longer, which leads to a somewhat larger initial charge cloud and therefore to an increased amount of charge sharing.

The size of the charge cloud typically ranges from 10 to 20 micrometers. Its value can for example be measured by scanning a pencil beam over a pixel edge while monitoring the pixel response [15]. Alternatively, the response function can be fitted with a detector model describing the charge sharing process, yielding an estimate for the charge cloud size [16, 17].

11.3.4 Fluorescence Effects in High-Z Semiconductors

When a photon is absorbed in the sensor material by the photoelectric effect, its energy is transferred to the photoelectron, which escapes the atom and leaves it in an excited state. The atom subsequently relaxes to its ground state either by emission of a fluorescence photon with a characteristic energy or by non-radiative processes like the emission of an Auger electron. The probabilities for a radiative relaxation are given by the fluorescence yields of the chemical elements, which increase with the atomic number and for shells closer to the nucleus. For Cd and Te, the fluorescence yields for the K-shell amount to 84% and 87% [18]. This means that for photon energies above the corresponding K-edges (26.7 and 31.8 keV for Cd and Te), the absorption is very often followed by the emission of a fluorescence photon. Unfortunately, the absorption distances of these photons are quite large (128 μm for Cd and 68 μm for Te fluorescence photons) so that they are likely to be either reabsorbed in a different pixel or to leave the sensor volume completely. In the first case, events with characteristic energies of 23.2 and 27.5 keV show up in the detector response function. The resulting peaks are known as *fluorescence peaks*. In both cases, the corresponding energy is missing in the pixel of the primary interaction. As a consequence two additional *escape peaks* appear 23.2 and

27.5 keV below the photo peak as shown in Figure 11.2. In Cd(Zn)Te sensors, the response function is further distorted by secondary Cd fluorescence photons that were created from the reabsorption of Te fluorescence photons.

11.3.5 Pulse Pile-Up at High Photon Fluxes

In order to reliably detect the relatively small number of electron-hole pairs generated in the sensor, the signal has to be amplified in the readout ASIC before its amplitude is evaluated by the comparator. The time duration of the amplified signal is mainly determined by the chosen bandwidth of the front-end electronics and normally ranges in between 20–100 ns [19]. If a second X-ray quantum hits the pixel during this period, the two pulses overlap and the signal at the comparator input is the superposition of the two corresponding pulse shapes. If the signals overlap only little in time, the comparator still registers two counts, but the energy of the second pulse is slightly overestimated. For larger overlaps, the comparator counts only one hit, but with an energy which can be as high as the sum of the energies of the individual photons. To reduce pulse pile-up, the pulse width after the amplification stage has to be minimized as much as possible while keeping the ENC as low as possible. A lower limit on the viable pulse width is given by the finite charge collection time of the sensor pixel and by the possible difference in drift time between events generated by atomic fluorescence.

While describing the effect of pulse pile-up on the detector response function is quite intricate [20, 21], the loss of counts above a given energy threshold is usually well depicted by the paralyzable detector model. This analytical model relates the observed count rate N_O to the rate of the absorbed photons N_p by the equation $N_O = N_p \exp(-\tau N_p)$, where τ is the detector dead time. The dead time is directly related to the pulse width of the amplified signal.

The effect of pulse pile-up on the detector response is shown in Figure 11.2. The presence of superposed pulses leads to a decrease of counts at low energies and to an increase at high energies. All peaks are thus slightly shifted to higher energies. However, the most prominent effect is the appearance of counts above the photo peak, where basically no events are present at low fluxes. For CT applications with fluxes up to 10^9 photons/s/mm^2, pulse pile-up can severely degrade the spectral performance. Since for a given photon flux the count rate per pixel is proportional to the pixel area, smaller pixels help to mitigate the effects of pulse pile-up.

11.3.6 Recombination and Trapping in the Semiconductor Sensor

Crystal defects and impurities contained in the sensor material can give rise to recombination and trapping effects during the drift of the charge carriers to the readout electrodes. Recombination between photo-generated electron-hole pairs mainly occurs through defects with levels close to the middle of the band gap. The amount of collected charge is thereby reduced and a low-energy tail can show up below the photo peak in the detector response function. Trapping delays the collection of electron and holes and leads to reduced amplitude of the measured signal. This applies for deep level defects with a trapping time longer than the peaking time of the preamplifier. However, even shallow level defects can delay the charge collection significantly if their concentration is high enough to trap the carriers many times during their drift time. A low concentration of any crystal defects is therefore essential for a clean detector response.

As stated by Ramo's theorem [22], the current signal induced at the pixel read-out electrode is determined by the motion of both charge carriers – electrons and holes, drifting in opposing directions according to the electric field distribution within the sensor volume. But for small pixels the signal induced to the pixel results *almost* completely from the carriers drifting toward the pixel during the fraction of drift time spent in its neighborhood. This effect, known as *the small pixel effect* [23], also shortens the induced signal duration with respect to the total charge collection time. In principle, any loss of carriers during their drift to the corresponding electrodes leads to a reduction of the induced electric signal and therefore to an underestimation of the energy of the absorbed photon. The severity of this effect is proportional to the amount of charge loss and also related to the weighting potential at the position where the charge loss occurs. In particular, the loss of carriers drifting away from the pixel electrodes will result in stronger effects if the trapping occurs in high weighting field regions. The opposite holds for the carriers drifting toward the pixel electrodes [12]. Since the absorption depth of photons impinging on the sensor follows a decreasing exponential probability distribution – with mean value depending on the energy – the overall effect on the energy spectra is a peculiar broadening of the low-energy side of the energy peaks that takes the name of *tailing* [24–27].

In Cd(Zn)Te sensors, holes have a much shorter mean free path than electrons and are therefore more prone to recombination and trapping. Electrons are thus the preferred collected carrier type, even though there are examples of CdTe sensors operated in hole-collection mode [28]. The mean free path is both proportional to carrier mobility μ and the carrier life time τ. For CdTe the corresponding $\mu\tau$ products are $\mu_e\tau_e = 10^{-3}$ cm^2/V and $\mu_h\tau_h = 10^{-4}$ cm^2/V and for CdZnTe $\mu_e\tau_e = 10^{-3}$–10^{-2} cm^2/V and $\mu_h\tau_h = 10^{-5}$–10^{-4} cm^2/V [29, 30]. At normal operating conditions, electrons are fully collected with charge *collection efficiency* close to 100%. The tailing is mainly due to the residual effect of holes trapping during their drift toward the high-voltage electrode.

11.3.7 Compton Scattering in the Sensor Material

At high X-ray energies, Compton scattering in the sensor material may affect the detector response function. Incoming photons can inelastically scatter off electrons with a fraction of their energy being transferred to the electron. In this process, the photon changes its direction and potentially passes to a neighboring pixel or escapes the sensor. Fortunately, the differential scattering cross section has a minimum for orthogonal scattering. Furthermore, for high-Z sensor materials, Compton scattering only dominates over the photoelectric effects for photon energies above 260 keV. Compared to other effects, the impact on the detector response function is therefore often negligible. For silicon however, Compton scattering already starts to dominate at 60 keV. If present, Compton scattering leads to additional events at low energies due to photon escape and a tail below the photo peak due to scattered photons entering from neighboring pixels. These events are flanked by small peaks at $E_\gamma - E_{\text{Compton}}$ and E_{Compton} corresponding to the maximum energy transfer E_{Compton} for a given photon energy [31].

11.3.8 Polarization in High-Z Sensor Materials

The *polarization* effect in semiconductor sensors leads to time and flux dependent degradations of the overall performance. The microscopic mechanism at the basis of polarization consists of slow (with a time scale from seconds to hours) charge trapping phenomena that distort the electric field profile in the sensor volume. This leads to potential-suppressed regions where signal charges are easily trapped, resulting in a reduced charge collection efficiency [32, 33]. In contrast to the *static* charge trapping effects described above, polarization is more difficult to account due to its time and flux dependence. The impact of the polarization effect depends on many variables such as the sensor material, the growing technique, the nature of the electrode contacts, the operating temperature, and bias voltage and is therefore difficult to quantify or predict. However, as a qualitative behavior, the polarization causes a shift of the detector response function to lower energies and an increase of the signal dispersion, *that is*, reduced energy resolution [34–36].

11.3.9 Absorption Efficiency of the Semiconductor Sensor

So far, we only considered the response of photon-counting detectors to monochromatic radiation and discussed its usefulness for detector characterization. However, the detector response function can also be obtained for a polychromatic X-ray spectrum. The polychromatic response is a weighted sum of the monochromatic detector responses, with the weights given by the energy spectrum Φ of the incoming X-rays:

$$DR(\Phi, E) \propto \int_0^{\infty} DR(E_\gamma, E)\Phi(E_\gamma)dE_\gamma. \tag{11.2}$$

The detector response function as defined in Eq. (11.1) implicitly depends on the absorption efficiency of the semiconductor sensor. The smaller the absorption efficiency the smaller the monochromatic detector response function and therefore its contribution to the polychromatic response function $DR(\Phi, E)$. The absorption efficiency is a function of photon energy, but also depends on the sensor thickness and absorption coefficient of the material. The latter is composed of different contributions from photoelectric absorption, elastic Rayleigh, and inelastic Compton scattering. For CdTe and photon energies below 260 keV, the dominant contribution originates from the photoelectric absorption, which scales as Z^n (with n between 4 and 5) with the atomic number Z [37]. Therefore, sensor materials with heavier elements have much higher absorption efficiencies. The lower absorption efficiency at high photon energies shifts the average recorded photon energy to lower energies as shown in Figure 11.2.

11.4 DETECTOR HEALTH TRACKING

11.4.1 Energy Resolution

The precision of a detection system in discerning the energy of the incoming radiation is expressed by its *energy resolution*. This figure of merit quantifies the statistical dispersion of the photon energy measurement. Usually it is reported in terms of the *full width at half maximum (FWHM)* of the photo peak in the response function to monochromatic radiation.

The energy resolving capabilities of hybrid photon-counting detectors using high-Z sensor materials are limited by several factors. The first and usually most important – regardless of the sensor material – is the random electronic noise affecting the analog signal as given by the ENC. Besides the electronic noise, the spectral distortion effects discussed in the previous section – charge sharing, atomic fluorescence, recombination and trapping, Compton scattering and polarization – lead to an artificial increase of low-energy events in the detector response function and thus to a broadening of the low-energy side of the photo peak. This effect not only degrades the energy resolution but also shifts the photo peak position to slightly lower energies. At high fluxes, the energy resolution is further degraded by pile-up effects.

The energy resolution of a detection system is typically obtained from pulse height spectra recorded under monochromatic beam conditions. To fulfill this requirement, synchrotron light, radioactive sources, or fluorescence light from elemental target are customarily used. The photon flux is usually kept low enough not to incur in additional distorting effects due to pile-up. Examples of measured values for CdTe/CdZnTe sensors bonded to different ASICs are summarized in Table 11.1. The table should not be interpreted as a direct performance comparison as the sensor parameters (geometry, contact nature) and the experimental conditions differ considerably between the references.

Considering a pixel neighborhood area, an additional source of uncertainty originates from pixel-to-pixel variations of the energy threshold. Due to unavoidable variations in the microelectronics

TABLE 11.1
Summary of Energy Resolution Values Measured with CdTe/CdZnTe Sensors, for Several Photon-Counting ASICs

ASIC	Photon Energy [keV]	Sensor Type	Pixel Size [μm] Thickness [μm]	Energy Resolution [keV FWHM]
PIXIE II [38]	3–60	CdTe Schottky	Hexagonal, 60 × ~52 650	0.76–1.73
IBEX [7]	10–60 for several chip settings	CdTe Ohmic	75/150/300 750–1000	1.5–3.5
HEXITEC [17]	60	CdTe Schottky	250 1000	1.5–2
MEDIPIX 2 [39]	60	CdTe	110/165 1000	2.2
TIMEPIX [40]	30, 70	CdTe Ohmic	55 1000	7, 9.1
XPAD 3.2 [28]	60	CdTe Ohmic/Schottky	130 500	2.4
ERPC [41]	12-200	CdTe Ohmic	350 1000	3–4
DXMCT (DxRay) [42]	20–120	CdTe	1100 × 1600 1000	2–3.5
ChromAIX 2 (Philips) [43]	60	CZT	500 2000	4.8
GM-I CA 3 [44]	25-60	CdTe	380 × 1600 (ave) 3000	~5-~10
Actaeon (XCounter) [45]	60	CdTe	100 750	12

fabrication process and voltage drops along the power distribution lines, the response of individual pixels may deviate significantly from the average in terms of gain and offset. At the ASIC design level, this issue has been addressed by the implementation of additional in-pixel programmable circuitry. This enables to compensate for offset and/or gain mismatches and to equalize the threshold levels among pixels. However, any threshold calibration algorithm causes residual statistical threshold dispersion, ultimately limited by the digital nature of the compensation circuitry. The total energy dispersion is given by the root sum squared (RSS) of the standard deviation $\sigma_{th.disp}$ of the energy threshold dispersion and the energy resolution of a single pixel. Reported values of $\sigma_{th.disp}$ for ASICs equipped with CdTe sensors range from few hundreds of eV rms [38, 46] to few keV rms. In general, the threshold dispersion is strongly dependent on the energy calibration algorithm and tends to increase with the photon energy, since high energy thresholds are more difficult to calibrate.

Pile-up effects at increasing photon fluxes also contribute to a degradation of the energy resolution. As an example, Figure 11.3 shows the behavior of the energy resolution at the incoming photon energy of 60 keV as a function of photon flux, expressed both per pixel (top) and per unit area (bottom), for the case of 1 mm-thick CdTe sensors with a pixel size of 150 and 300 μm [7]. On one hand, a smaller pixel size clearly allows for a higher photon flux pixel per unit area (bottom figure). On the other hand, it is important to note that for photon fluxes above 10^6 cts/s/pixel (top figure), the 150 μm pixel detector experiences a higher degradation than the 300 μm pixel detector due to more fluorescence photons originating from neighboring pixels.

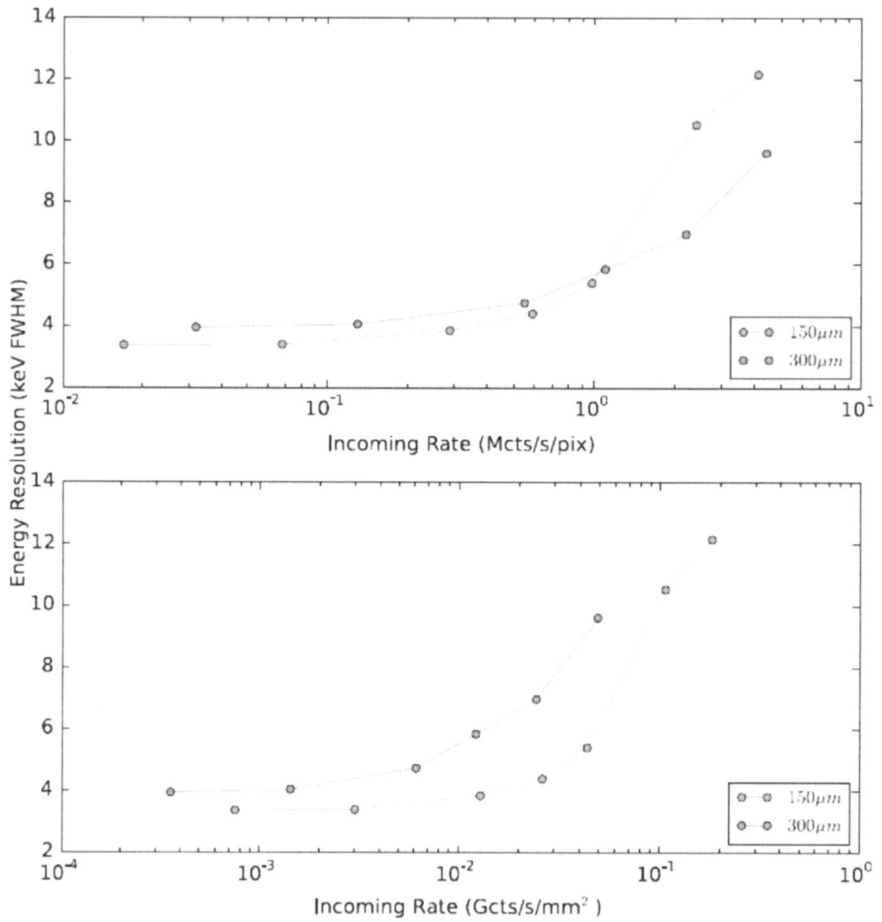

FIGURE 11.3 Energy resolution measured at 60 keV for increasing photon fluxes for the 150 and 300 μm pixel sizes. The incoming rate is expressed both per pixel (top) and per unit area (bottom) [7].

11.4.2 Quantum Efficiency

In an ideal photon-counting detector, every impinging photon gives rise to exactly one count. In reality, the number of detected counts may differ for several reasons, the most important being:

- no absorption of the photons by the sensor as a consequence of the finite sensor thickness.
- no registration of a photon due to a signal amplitude below the configured energy threshold.
- charge sharing, secondary fluorescence or Compton effects can cause partial loss of charge or spurious additional counts in neighboring pixels.

In order to quantify these effects, we can define – without losing general validity – the quantity called quantum efficiency (*QE*) as the ratio between the number of counted events and the number of impinging photons. With the definition of the detector response function *DR* in (1) one obtains:

$$QE\left(E_\gamma, E_{th}\right) = \int_{E_{th}}^{\infty} DR(E_\gamma, E)\mathrm{d}E \tag{11.3}$$

with E_γ the energy of the incoming photons and E_{th} the threshold energy of the detector.

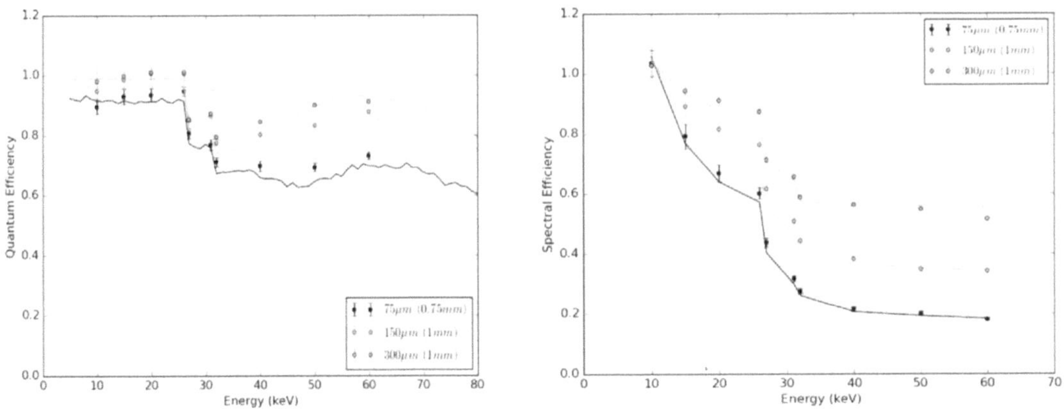

FIGURE 11.4 Experimental (dots) and simulated (continuous lines) quantum (left) and spectral (right) efficiency for CdTe sensors of different pixel sizes and sensor thicknesses combinations as indicated in the legend, as a function of photon energy [7].

The measurement of the QE requires the acquisition of an image at a given energy threshold and the less trivial knowledge of the absolute number of impinging photons. This information can be retrieved through the use of calibrated sensors like Si-PIN diodes as demonstrated for the case of synchrotron radiation by [47].

In case of monochromatic incoming radiation with energy below the K-edges of the sensor material, the threshold energy which maximizes the *QE* while at the same time avoiding shared counts from neighboring pixels is $E_{th} = E_\gamma/2$. Under these conditions, the *QE* at low energies is limited by the fraction of photons hitting the sensor close to pixel corners with their charge being shared between more than two pixels. At high energies, the QE is determined by the absorption efficiency of the sensor material. For smaller pixel sizes, charge-sharing effects are more dominant, which leads to a decrease of the *QE*. This behavior is well visible in Figure 11.4 for energies below 26 keV. The curves represent measured (dots) and simulated (continuous line) values of $QE(E_\gamma, E_{th} = E_\gamma/2)$ for several pixel sizes – 75, 150, and 300 μm (corresponding thickness indicated in the legend) [7]. While for the largest pixel size the *QE* is close to 100%, for the smallest pixel it reduces down to about 90%. For photon energies above the K-edges of the sensor material, *that is*, in presence of significant fluorescence effects, the interpretation of the *QE* is more difficult. The spectra become structured due to the appearance of spurious fluorescence and escape peaks, which, according to their energy relatively to the threshold, are counted or not. This causes an abrupt decrease of the quantum efficiency at the Cd and Te K-edges at 26.72 keV and 31.82 keV as can be seen in Figure 11.4. For further increasing photon energy, the *QE* recovers when the escape peaks, located at a fixed distance from the main peak, are exceeding the threshold energy. Above a local maximum at around 60 keV, the *QE* slowly decreases since the sensor material becomes more and more transparent to the incoming radiation. Consistent results are reported by [48], where simulated *QE* values of CdTe, GaAs, and Ge sensors with a smaller pixel size of 55 μm are investigated.

11.4.3 Spectral Efficiency

The difficulties of interpreting the *QE* for complex response functions and the limitations set by the dependence on the threshold energy lead to the definition of a further quantity called spectral efficiency (*SE*) [4]. The *SE* is defined as the fraction of events counted within a certain energy window $\pm\Delta E$ around the incoming photons energy E_γ, and can be written as:

$$SE\left(E_\gamma,\Delta E\right)=\int_{E_\gamma-\Delta E}^{E_\gamma+\Delta E} DR(E_\gamma,E)\mathrm{d}E. \tag{11.4}$$

For polychromatic radiation, the concept can be defined as the weighted integral over the normalized energy spectrum $\Phi(E_\gamma)$:

$$SE(\Phi,\Delta\mathrm{E})=\int SE\left(E_\gamma,\Delta E\right)\cdot\Phi\left(E_\gamma\right)\mathrm{d}E_\gamma. \tag{11.5}$$

The *SE* provides several advantages with respect to other figures of merit, like the *peak-to-background ratio* and the *intrinsic peak efficiency* as defined in [2] and measured for spectroscopic CdTe, for example, in [49] and for CZT in [50]. First, for smaller pixel sizes the photo peaks smear out to a level where they become hardly identifiable, because of increased charge sharing and atomic fluorescence effects. Second, the definition of the *SE* holds even in case of high photon fluxes, when pulse pile-up effects distort the detector response function. However, also the concept of *SE* becomes difficult to interpret when the recorded spectrum gets severely distorted by pile-up effects, which hampers the correct assessment of the energy of a single event. From an experimental point of view, the *SE* is just slightly more demanding with respect to the *QE*, as it requires the acquisition of at least two images at different thresholds.

Figure 11.4 shows the *SE* in an energy window ΔE of ±6 keV for the same conditions as for the *QE*. For energies below the Cd K-edge, the *SE* is limited by charge sharing. The slight decrease in efficiency toward the K-edge energy is due to a reduced fraction of shared events in the $\pm\Delta E$ energy interval. At 10 keV the *SE* slightly exceeds 100% since for energy thresholds below 50% of the incoming beam energy, some photons will be double counted due to charge sharing. Above the K-edges, the *SE* drops and converges at levels around 18%, 34%, and 51% for the 75, 150, and 300 μm pixel size case, respectively, since no other effects are impairing the main energy peaks integrity.

The study of the *SE* as a function of the incoming photon rate as shown in Figure 11.5 constitutes a powerful analysis tool to evaluate the performance of photon-counting detectors [7]. The *SE* clearly reflects the opposing influences of charge sharing/atomic fluorescence and pile-up effects as a function of the pixel size. Larger pixel sizes reduce the influence of charge sharing/fluorescence effects and thus increase the *SE* in the low-flux regime. On the other hand, smaller pixel sizes reduce the count rate per pixel and thus allow for higher count rates per unit area. The lower plot in Figure 11.5 clearly shows the crossover point, where smaller pixels exhibit superior *SE* than larger pixels. For the 300 μm and 150 μm pixel curves, the crossover point is at 3×10^7 cts/s/mm^2. The expected crossover point for the 150 μm and 75 μm pixel curves is even greater than 10^8 cts/s/mm^2, with a low-flux *SE* limit of 0.18 for the 75 μm pixel. The crossover point obviously depends on the dead time of the readout ASIC.

The knowledge of the *SE* dependence on the pixel size and photon flux can also be used for the optimization of the pixel size for specific applications. Figure 11.6 shows simulated *SE* curves at 60 keV for a 1 mm-thick CdTe sensor as a function of the pixel size and photon flux [4] with an energy window ΔE of ±4 keV. For a pulse width of 44 ns and a flux of 5×10^7 photons/s/mm^2, which is estimated to be the typical flux in a CT system after attenuation by 20 cm of water, the best performance is achieved with a pixel size in the range of 150–300 μm.

11.4.4 Dead Time

Pile-up effects occurring at high photon fluxes degrade the spectral efficiency but also cause count rate losses. It is therefore of common practice to study the behavior of the *measured* count rate as a function of the *incoming* count rate. The measurement in principle relies on the knowledge of the incoming photon flux. However, even if an absolute flux reference is not available, it is often possible

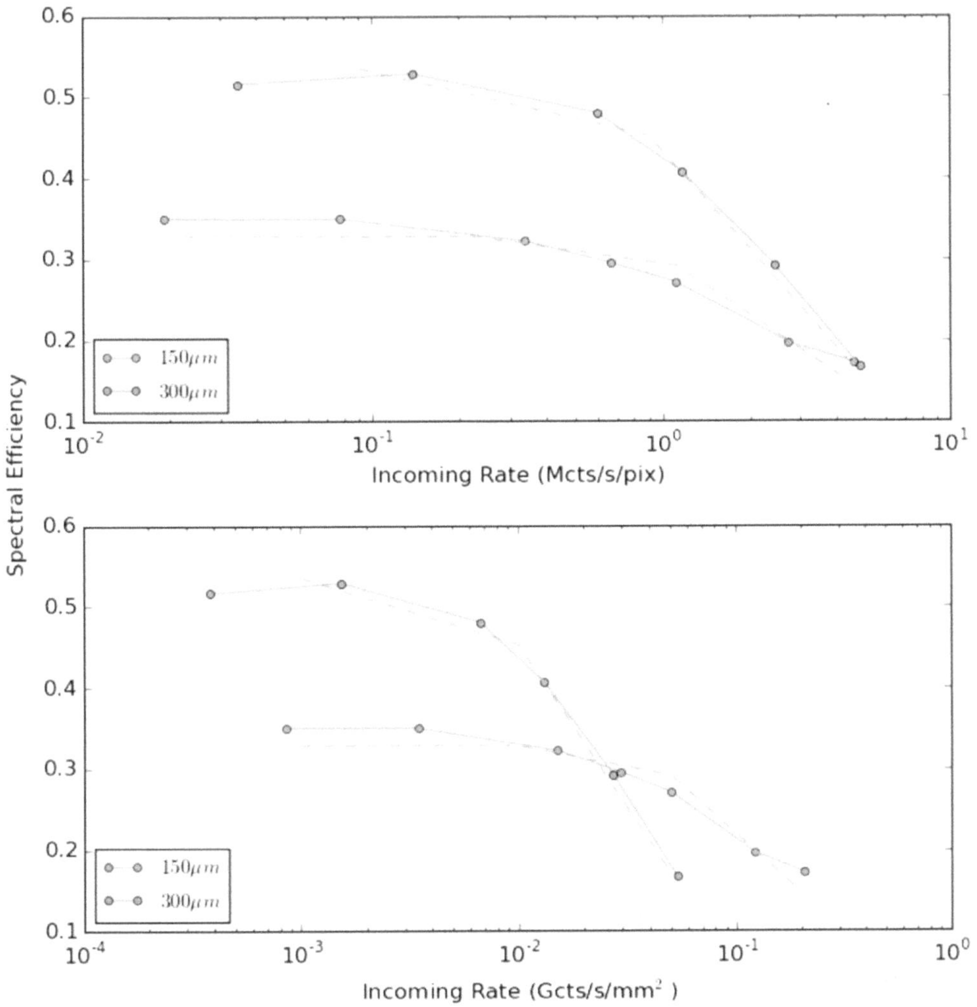

FIGURE 11.5 Measured (continuous) and simulated (dashed) spectral efficiency at 60 keV for increasing photon fluxes for the 150 and 300 μm pixel sizes. The incoming rate is expressed both per pixel (top) and per unit area (bottom) [7].

to estimate it. For example, it can be extracted using low-flux irradiation under the assumption that the counts recorded at low intensity *correspond* to the number of incoming photons. Another approach is to calibrate the transmission of a set of filters at low beam intensity as in [51].

Figure 11.7 shows count rate curves taken with CdTe sensors of different pixel sizes (150 and 300 μm) bonded to an IBEX ASIC. The measurements were performed with a photon energy of 60 keV and with the threshold energy set to half the photon energy [7]. The system was operated in paralyzable counting mode and the measurement time was short enough to avoid polarization effects. The deviation of the two curves at high fluxes is due to the different impact of fluorescence and charge sharing on the pile-up. The different pixel size also plays a role in terms of capacitance, as a bigger input capacitive load has the effect of slowing down the shaping time. The incoming count rates leading to 50% count rate loss are 9.8×10^6 and 6.65×10^6 cts/s/pix, respectively, and the mean signal lengths (at the specified threshold energy) are about 60 ns and 85 ns, respectively. The system dead time tends to be shorter for higher threshold settings as the comparator is paralyzed as long as the signal is above the threshold. It is worth noting how at the "critical" flux of 10^6 cts/s/pixel (see Energy Resolution and Spectral Efficiency), the count rate curves of Figure 11.7 exhibit a count rate loss of only about 10%.

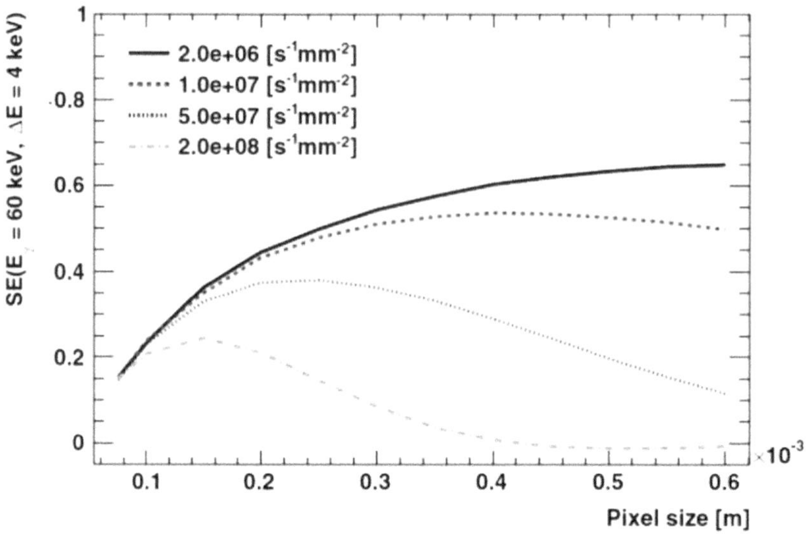

FIGURE 11.6 Simulated spectral efficiency (E_γ = 60 keV, ΔE = ±4 keV) as a function of pixel size and incoming photon flux for a pulse width of 44 ns. For a typical flux of 5 × 10^7 photons/s/mm², the optimal pixel size lies in the range between 150 × 150 μm² and 300 × 300 μm² [4].

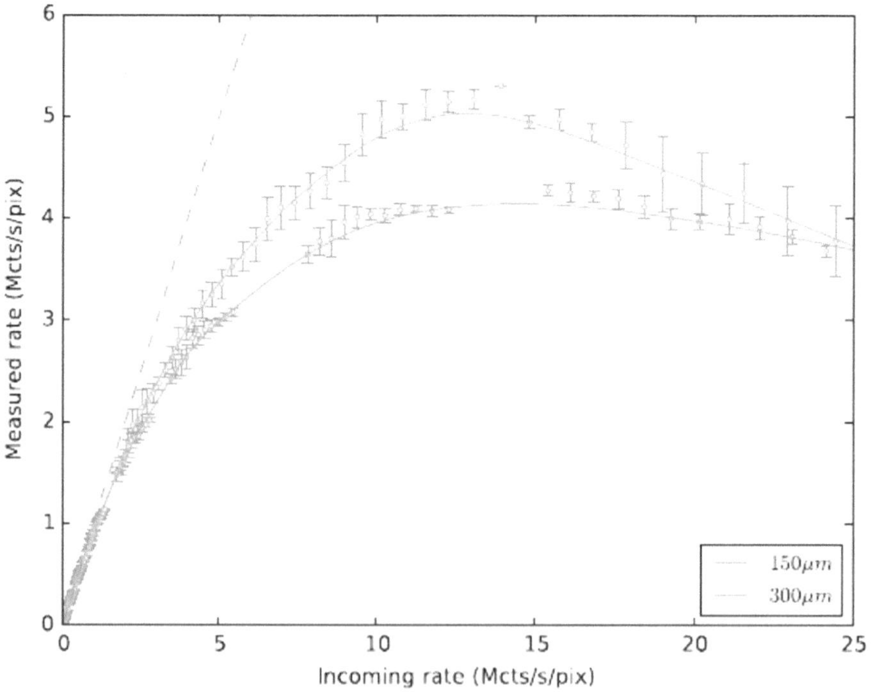

FIGURE 11.7 Unfiltered (markers with error bars) and filtered (continuous lines) count rate curves for CdTe sensors of 150 and 300 μm pixel size, bonded to the IBEX ASIC. The photon energy is 60 keV, and the threshold energy is set to half the photon energy. The dashed line corresponds to an ideal detector without any count loss [7].

11.4.5 Imaging Performance

As a prominent figure of merit in the imaging community, the detective quantum efficiency (*DQE*) also deserves a brief discussion for its non-trivial dependence on the X-ray energy. The *DQE* – not to be confused with the previously described *QE* – quantifies the degradation of the signal-to-noise ratio in the two-dimensional spatial domain (in opposition to the energy or spectral domain) as a result of the measurement process by the imaging system. For convenience, the *DQE* is usually expressed as a function of spatial frequency. The definition of the frequency-dependent *DQE* is:

$$DQE(u,v) = \frac{SNR(u,v)_{out}^2}{SNR(u,v)_{in}^2}, \tag{11.6}$$

where u and v denote the orthogonal spatial frequencies for a two-dimensional imaging system. The *DQE* describes for any given spatial frequency, *how efficiently* the information contained in the incoming radiation is used [52].

According to [53], Eq. (11.6) can be rewritten in order to separate the terms related to signal and noise processing:

$$DQE(u,v) = G^2 MTF(u,v)^2 \frac{NPS(u,v)_{in}}{NPS(u,v)_{out}}, \tag{11.7}$$

where G is the detector gain or conversion factor at zero spatial frequency, *MTF* is the normalized pre-sampling Modulation Transfer Function of the detection system, NPS_{in} is the noise power spectrum of the radiation field at the detector surface, and NPS_{out} is the noise power spectrum at the output of the detection system. The number of incoming photons $N_{ph,in}$ during a given time interval follows a Poisson distribution. Therefore, the magnitude of the associated (white) noise power spectrum $NPS(u,v)_{in}$ only depends on the number of impinging photons $N_{ph,in}$, with $N_{ph,\,in} = \int \Phi(E)dE$ for polychromatic radiation with the spectrum $\Phi(E)$. The measurement of the number of incoming photons requires a calibrated measurement tool (a dosimeter) and the conversion from dose to number of photons (by using tabulated values or results of simulations).

The spatial resolution of an imaging system is quantified by the *MTF*, which is a measure of the attenuation as a function of spatial frequency experienced by a signal in the passage through the detector. The *MTF* is computed as the Fourier transform of the line spread function (*LSF*), which on its turn corresponds to the derivative of the edge spread function (*ESF*):

$$MTF(u,v) = \frac{|\mathcal{F}(LSF)(u,v)|}{|\mathcal{F}(LSF)(u=v=0)|} = \frac{|\mathcal{F}(ESF')(u,v)|}{|\mathcal{F}(ESF')(u=v=0)|}, \tag{11.8}$$

Practical guidelines to measure all the quantities involved in the *DQE* including the *MTF* as well as the NPS_{out} are contained in the IEC 62220-1 international standard, which applies in general to two-dimensional detectors used for imaging applications [54]. According to that, the *MTF* can be retrieved by recording a set of images under uniform X-ray illumination and by using a highly absorbing object with a sharp edge slightly tilted (1–3) with respect to the pixel matrix orientation. This allows for the "oversampling" of the detector response function along one of the two dimensions. By analyzing the edge profile, it is therefore possible to retrieve the oversampled pixel *ESF* and consequently the pixel *LSF*. Incidentally, the *LSF* corresponds to the two-dimensional pixel point spread function (*PSF*) averaged over one of the two coordinates.

Computed in this way, the *MTF* describes the average behavior of the "single-pixel" response. Since the sampling process of the pixel matrix is not taken into account – which can cause a folding of the high-frequency components of the signal to the base frequency range allowed by the Nyquist theorem – this quantity is referred to as *pre-sampling MTF*. The use of the pre-sampled *MTF* in the computation of the *DQE* is motivated by the fact that otherwise the *DQE* would be a quantity dependent on the signal frequency components (because of the aliasing) and on its phase (relative position with respect to the pixel matrix). In addition, the information carried by the *MTF* at frequencies above Nyquist, although physically inaccessible, gives an idea of the magnitude of the possible aliasing effects to be expected.

In the case of an ideal pixel response function, the *MTF* corresponds to the Fourier transform of the geometrical pixel shape. For square pixels of size d, the *MTF* has the shape of a two-dimensional cardinal sine or *sinc* function with nodes at n/d with $n \in \mathbb{Z}_{\neq 0}$. The Nyquist frequency corresponds then to the half of the sampling frequency, that is, $f_{Nyq} = 1/2d$. The value of the ideal *MTF* at the Nyquist frequency is 0.64, and the frequency value at which the ideal *MTF* is 0.1 is $0.91 f_{Nyq}$.

The *MTF* of a photon-counting detector depends on the energy of the incoming photons and on the threshold energy. In case of no atomic fluorescence effects – *that is,* for photon energies below the K-edges of the sensor material – the *MTF* can get very close to the *MTF* of an ideal detector with small deviations due to charge sharing effects. By increasing (decreasing) the position of the threshold energy, shared events occurring at the pixel edges can be excluded (included), which narrows (broadens) the *LSF* and therefore increases (decreases) the *MTF* for increasing frequencies. Note however that the maximum allowed frequency remains constant, fixed by the pixel pitch. In presence of atomic fluorescence effects – *that is,* for photon energies above the K-edges – the *MTF* may significantly degrade because of the bigger spread of the signal, which is in turn dependent on the position of the threshold energy relative to the escape and fluorescence peaks. Figure 11.8 shows

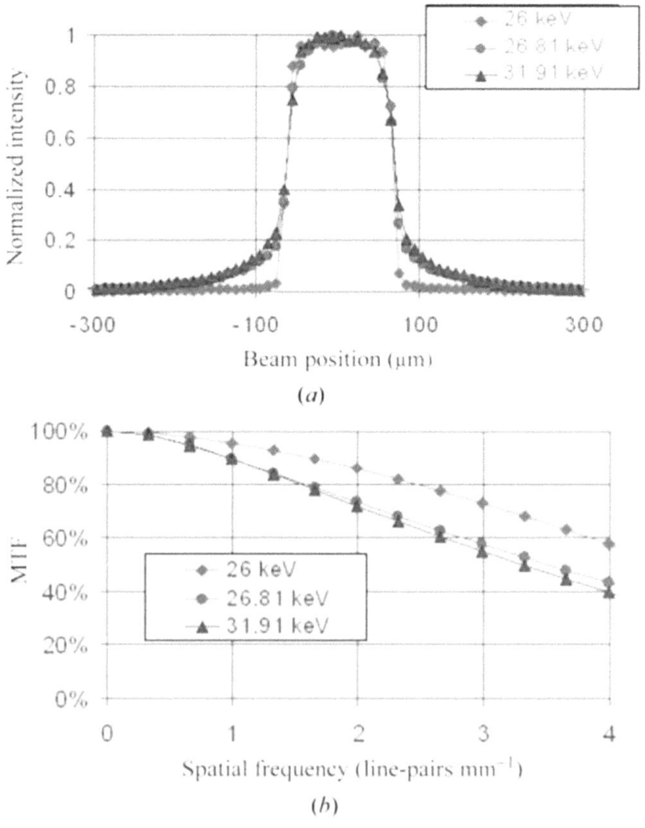

FIGURE 11.8 Example of LSF (a) and MTF (b) measured for a 700-µm thick CdTe sensor with 130-µm pixel size, at threshold energy 14 keV under illumination with monochromatic light below the K-edges (26 keV), above the Cd K-edge but below the Te one (26.81 keV) and above the Te K-edge (31.91 keV). *Reproduced with permission of the International Union of Crystallography* [55].

the *LSF* (a) and *MTF* (b) for a detector with a 700-μm thick CdTe sensor and 130-μm pixel size. The threshold energy is 14 keV and the illumination is a monochromatic beam below the K-edges (26 keV, red curve), above the Cd K-edge but below the Te one (26.81 keV, green curve) and above the Te K-edge (31.91 keV, blue curve) [55]. Above the Cd and the Te K-edges, a large tail at the edges of the LSF, caused by the atomic fluorescence effect, is observed. As a result, the *MTF* at Nyquist frequency decreases from 60% to 40%.

The output noise power spectrum NPS_{out} measures the amount and the composition of the signal variations at the detector output in the spatial frequency domain. The IEC 62220-1 standard defines the procedure for the calculation of the NPS_{out}. According to this standard, the detector has to be uniformly illuminated and the images – corrected for the non-uniformity of the radiation field and for the gain/offset for the individual pixels – have to be subdivided into partially overlapping ROIs of definite size. For each ROI, the two-dimensional square modulus of the Fourier transform is calculated and the average over the ROI set corresponds to the NPS_{out}. A numerically alternative but mathematically equivalent method would be to compute the NPS_{out} as the Fourier transform of the autocorrelation function of the acquired images eventually subdivided as well into proper ROIs.

For the following discussion, it is useful to define the normalized noise power spectrum $NNPS_{out} = NPS_{out}/G^2$. For an ideal detector, the $NNPS_{out}$ equals the NPS_{in} – *that is*, no uncertainty is added to the signal at any frequency by the detection process. In reality, the $NNPS_{out}$ increases due to the imperfect sensor efficiency, which leaves some photons undetected. In addition, charge sharing and atomic fluorescence effects introduce spatial correlations between neighboring pixels, decreasing the magnitude of the high-frequency components of the $NNPS_{out}$. While the sensor efficiency for a given material is mainly dependent on the energy of the incoming radiation, the pixel-to-pixel correlation is mainly due to the relative position of the energy threshold with respect to the incoming photon energy. Increasing thresholds decrease the amount of detected photons and simultaneously decrease the spatial correlation as shared events of lower energies are excluded. An example of the threshold energy dependence of the $NNPS_{out}$ for a silicon microstrip detector is reported in [56]. Figure 11.9 shows the reported behavior of the $NNPS_{out}$ at different threshold energy levels, under uniform illumination with monochromatic X-rays at 17.4 keV (Mo-fluorescence).

How does the DQE depend on the threshold energy? For increasing threshold energies, the *MTF* improves whereas the $NNPS_{out}$ degrades. As the degradation of the $NNPS_{out}$ appears to be dominating, it turns out that lower threshold energies increase the DQE. This effect is clearly visible in Figure 11.10, which shows the DQE measured for a 700-μm thick CdTe sensor with a pixel size of 130 μm, illuminated with the standard IEC mammography RQA3-M spectrum (Mo-target, 30 kV_p plus 2 mm Al filtration) at different dose levels and at different threshold energies [57]. The highest DQE is obtained for the lowest threshold energy in virtue of the higher signal detected. The decrease of the DQE – in principle unexpected – at the highest dose level is justified with the comparison of strong count non-uniformities in the analyzed images especially at low spatial frequencies, probably due to pile-up effects.

In any case, the non-trivial behavior of the *DQE* as a function of the threshold energy – for a given experimental condition – has to be carefully studied in order to determine optimal threshold settings or even a weighted combination of thresholds [58].

11.5 SPECTRAL FACE-LIFTING

11.5.1 Large Pixels with Fast Pulse Shaping

A common approach to optimize the spectral performance of photon-counting detectors is the usage of relatively large pixel pitches in the range of 500–1000 μm, combined with a reduction of the pulse peaking time to its viable minimum. This strategy has many advantages. The large

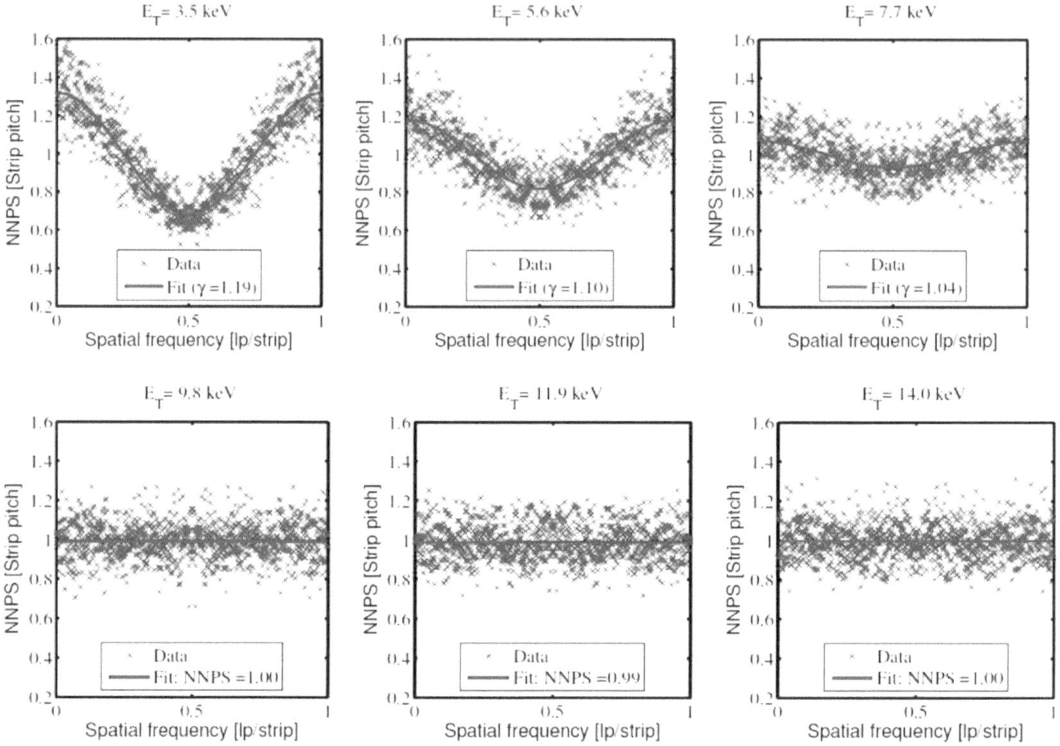

FIGURE 11.9 Example of the threshold energy dependence of the $NNPS_{out}$ for the case of a silicon microstrip detector irradiated with monochromatic X-rays at 17.4 keV (Mo-fluorescence) [56] *© SISSA Medialab Srl. Reproduced by permission of IOP Publishing. All rights reserved.*

pixel area reduces the probability of photon hits close to pixel boundaries as well as the probability of fluorescence photons escaping to adjacent pixels. As a consequence, the spectral efficiency increases because the charge sharing background and the escape and fluorescence peaks in the detector response function are minimized. The relatively large area per pixel also facilitates the implementation of multiple threshold comparators and counters with high dynamic range in the ASIC. The low channel density reduces the amount of data to be read out and thus allows detector operation at high frame rates.

The obvious drawback of large pixels is the increased rate of incoming photons that has to be handled by an individual pixel. As shown in [19], the maximum sustainable X-ray flux decreases with the pixel size. To minimize spectral distortions, the pulse peaking time has to be decreased as much as possible. This is achieved by the implementation of higher order shaping stages, which are usually not used in smaller pixels due to restrictions on the available space and power consumption. ASICs with peaking types as low as 10–20 ns have been presented [19]. A lower limit is imposed by the time that is required to collect most of charge created in the semiconductor sensor. Photons separated by less than the charge collection time cannot be separated since their photo-currents start to overlap. Peaking times shorter than the charge collection time therefore do not help to further reduce the amount of pulse pile-up. Instead they lead to a loss of signal amplitude (known as ballistic deficit), which can have a negative effect on the energy resolution. The situation is exacerbated by the fact that large pixels profit less from the small pixel effect, which reduces the charge collection time. This makes them more susceptible to the slow and incomplete collection of holes. Large pixels also have the disadvantage of an increased capacitance of the sensor pixel, which degrades the achievable energy resolution.

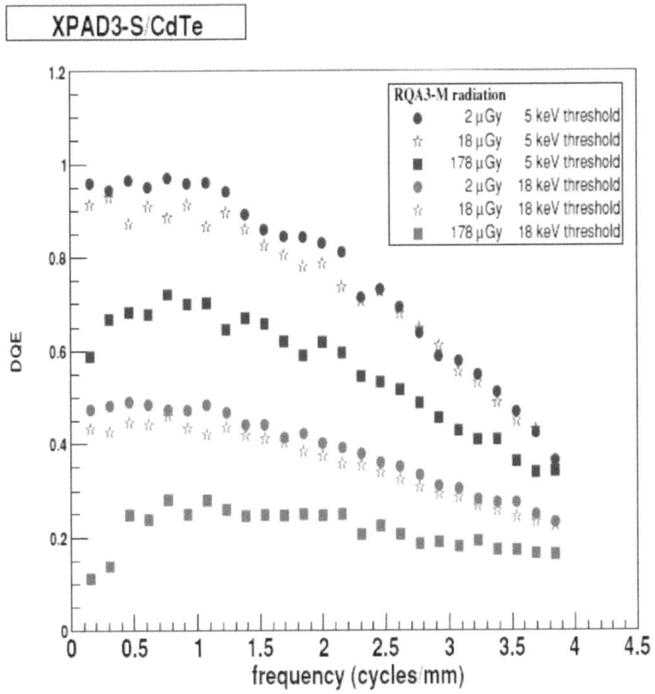

FIGURE 11.10 Measured DQE of a 700-μm thick CdTe sensor with a pixel size of 130 μm, illuminated with a RQA3-M spectrum (Mo-target, 30 kV_p plus 2 mm Al) at different dose levels and at different threshold energies [57] © *Institute of Physics and Engineering in Medicine. Reproduced by permission of IOP Publishing. All rights reserved.*

An example of a spectral CT readout ASIC with a relatively large area of 500 × 500 μm^2 and a very short shaping time is ChromAIX2 [43] as described in a dedicated chapter of this book. Its peaking time is shorter than 10 ns and the dead-time was measured to be about 25 ns as measured with electrical excitations. The output count rate therefore saturates at an incoming flux of 1.6×10^8 photons/s/mm^2, but spectral distortions will start to be perceivable at much lower fluxes. Each pixel has 5 energy thresholds with 16 bit counters allowing for dual contrast applications with the possibility to use the highest threshold for pile-up detection (see next section). An energy resolution of 4.8 keV (FWHM) was measured at an energy of 60 keV.

11.5.2 Charge Sharing and Pile-Up Rejection

Pixie III [59] is a photon counting ASIC with a very small pixel size of 62 μm × 62 μm, which makes it prone to the effects of charge sharing and secondary fluorescence photons. To counteract their detrimental effects on the spectral response, it implements a neighbor pixel inhibit mode. If an event spreads over multiple pixels, only the pixel that collects most of the charge is allowed to increase its counter. This prevents a single event to be counted by more than one pixel. Nonetheless, the event is still counted with a too small energy. The correct energy can be restored by combining this neighbor pixel inhibit mode with a pixel summing mode (see next section). Like charge summing modes (CSM), this feature comes at the cost of an increased ASIC complexity, since additional logic for the inter-pixel communication is needed.

A method to improve the spectral response in presence of pulse pile-up has been proposed by [60]. The so-called pile-up trigger method sets one of the available comparator thresholds slightly above the maximum energy of the incident X-ray radiation. This channel only triggers when two photons arrive more or less simultaneously and therefore paralyzes only at higher photon fluxes than channels with energy thresholds below the maximum photon energy. The information obtained from the high-threshold channel can be combined offline with the output of the other channels by means of a weighted sum. The implementation of an additional energy threshold with a corresponding counter requires additional space in each pixel of the ASIC, which might not be available for systems with small pixel pitches.

Another method to correctly measure the photon energy in presence of pulse pile-up has been presented by [61]. They propose a *cross detection method* in combination with energy *correction logic* to improve the spectral capabilities of photon-counting detectors at high photon fluxes. The cross detection method uses the zero crossings in the derivative of the pulse shape to determine whether pile-up has occurred or not. If pile-up is detected, corrected amplitude is obtained by digitally subtracting the amplitude of the previous pulse. In this way the maximum count rate as well as the spectral response is improved. However, the required logic seems to be rather complex and it is not discussed how well the digital subtraction of the pulse amplitudes works for not-equally spaced energy thresholds.

Furthermore, [62] have implemented an ASIC with an active reset circuit for the shaping filter. After a hit is detected, the pulse is sampled to determine the pulse amplitude. After a fix time interval, the pulse is reset in order to speed up the return to the baseline. This increases the maximum count rate and the dead-time behavior is that of a non-paralyzable detector. A drawback of this solution is an increase in the noise level of the detector.

11.5.3 Charge Summing Architectures

While detectors with large pixels have to deal with a higher count rate per pixel, the spectral response of detectors with small pixels suffers from more charge sharing and the escape of fluorescence photons to adjacent pixels. The MEDIPIX collaboration was the first group to implement a charge summing mechanism in their ASIC to compensate for the corresponding loss in spectral efficiency. Their solution consists of an intricate mechanism, which compares the charge deposited in each pixel to the charge measured in its eight neighboring pixels. If an event is spread over several pixels, an arbitration circuitry makes sure that only the pixel with the maximum charge can increase its counter value. Additionally, in each corner of an ASIC pixel the charges of the four adjacent pixels are summed up, to determine the correct energy of the incoming photon. If the pixel with the maximum charge has a corner with a charge exceeding its programmed threshold level, its counter is increased by one. This charge summing mechanism makes sure that events which do not spread beyond two by two pixels are always reconstructed with their correct energy. The effect on the detector response function is shown in Figure 11.11. The charge sharing background present in the single pixel mode (SPM) is strongly reduced in the CSM.

The effects of a charge summing mechanism on performance parameters like MTF, NPS, and DQE for polychromatic applications are quantitatively studied in [63]. Two XCounter XC225 ASICs bump-bonded to CdTe sensors of different thicknesses have been used to perform the measurements. In the charge correction mode, the total charge of adjacent pixels is attributed to the pixel with the highest charge if the pulses of these pixels coincide in time. The results show how charge summing architectures tend to improve the MTF, NPS, and DQE of photon-counting detectors. In general, the benefits are more pronounced for harder X-ray spectra. For energies below the K-edge energies of Cd and Te, the summing mechanism helps to reduce charge sharing effects; above the K-edge energies they additionally reduce the impact of secondary fluorescence photons. This leads to an improved spatial resolution, and therefore to a higher MTF at high frequencies. The lower probability of events with multiple counts reduces the correlations between adjacent pixels and results in a flatter NPS. Concerning DQE, the CSM of the XC225 ASIC shows a slightly better performance at zero frequency and at Nyquist frequency. At zero frequency, the charge summing helps to detect events spread over several pixels with none of the pixels having enough charge to exceed the threshold

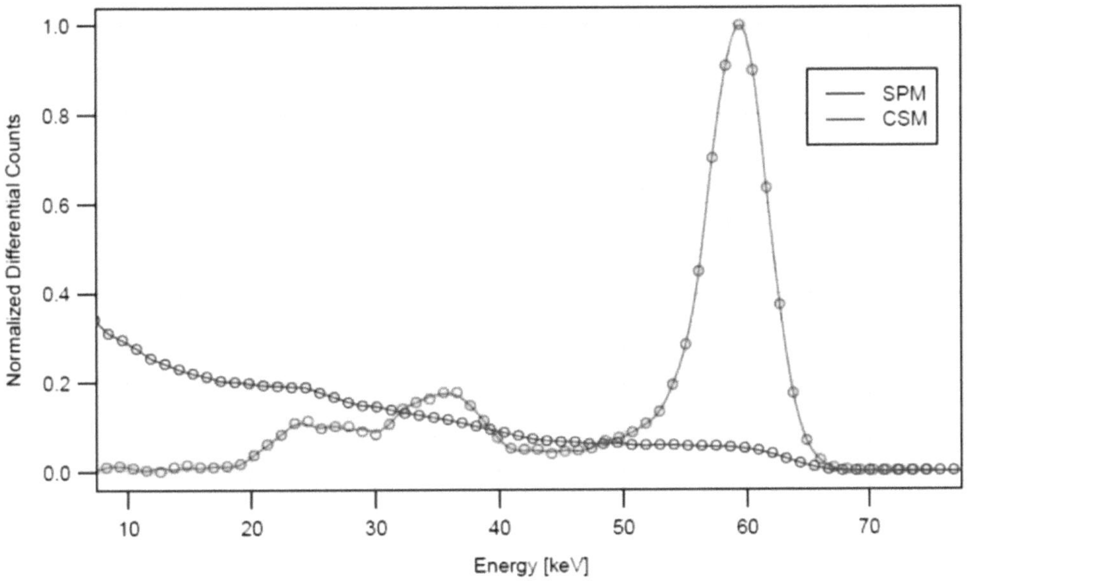

FIGURE 11.11 Detector response function of the MEDIPIX3 ASIC (110 μm pixel size) bump bonded to a 2-mm thick CdZnTe sensor in single pixel mode (SPM) and charge summing mode (CSM) [19].

energy. At frequencies close to the Nyquist frequency, the DQE profits from the higher MTF. At intermediate frequencies, the DQE is slightly worse in summing mode due to a higher NPS.

Charge summing mechanisms affect the energy resolution in two different ways. The reduced charge sharing background slightly reduces the width of the energy peak. However, this advantage is outbalanced by the fact, that the summed signal receives noise contributions from multiple preamplifiers. The summing of the signals from N pixels leads to a $N^{1/2}$ higher noise level. This inherent drawback leads to a typically two times worse energy resolution when summing the signals from four pixels. Nonetheless, the height of the photo peak and the spectral efficiency (given by the area below the peak) are generally larger than in SPM (see Figure 11.11).

Charge summing mechanisms always decrease the sustainable photon flux since each pixel becomes sensitive to photon hits on adjacent pixels while summing the corresponding signals. In addition, the summing circuitry might require additional time for the hit allocation. For the MEDIPIX3 ASIC the peaking time is only about 120 ns, but in charge-summing mode the dead time is slightly above one microsecond [64]. The Chase ASIC [65] shows a comparable increase in dead time from 0.2 μs in SPM to 1.0 μs in CSM. As a consequence, charge summing pixels lose part of their advantage over large pixels with respect to higher sustainable photon fluxes.

Charge summing architectures are still an active field of research. With the first functional ASICs having been presented in 2007 [66], the field is only about 10 years old. With smaller CMOS technologies becoming better affordable and 3D technology improving in maturity level, more and more complex pixel designs become available [67, 68]. One of the main development directions is the search for better compatibility with high photon fluxes. At the moment, charge summing might not yet be ready for the fluxes used in human CT, but they are already well suited for applications which have high demands on spatial resolution and spectral capabilities at the same time.

11.6 SUMMARY

Understanding the strengths and weaknesses of photon-counting detectors is an important prerequisite for their appropriate and successful usage in spectral applications. The main advantage is evidently the capability to register and analyze individual X-ray quanta. This forms the basis of their ability to retrieve information about the energy distribution of the incoming X-ray radiation by measuring the X-ray intensity in multiple energy bins. The presence of energy thresholds also has the benefit of effectively removing any contributions of the dark current from the semiconductor sensor to the measured signal. The digital processing and storage allow for a very high dynamic range and for small readout times. Thanks to the direct detection process, photon-counting detectors also provide high spatial resolution. As often the case, the biggest strength of an approach also constitutes a starting point of its limitations. In the case of photon-counting detectors, the finite amount of time required to analyze each event sets an upper limit on the viable photon flux. For many applications, the capability to process several millions of photons per second and pixel is more than sufficient. However, for spectral CT, where high flux is a strict requirement, the performance at high photon flux needs special attention when assessing the performance of photon-counting detectors. Besides pulse pile-up at high fluxes, the recorded spectrum is also affected by charge-sharing, fluorescence effects, electronic noise, and the absorption efficiency, which depend on the incoming photon energy.

The detector response function constitutes a fingerprint of photon-counting detectors. It is obtained from energy threshold scans and describes the spectrum as recorded by the detector. Its measurement as a function of photon energy is a crucial step in evaluating the spectral performance of counting detectors. Several figures of merit can be used to quantify the performance of photon-counting detectors. An intuitive and useful quantity for spectral applications is the *spectral efficiency*, which denotes the fraction of photons that are measured with their correct energy. Its value as a function of photon energy or photon flux gives a good impression of the spectral capabilities of a photon-counting system. It can also be used for quantitative comparisons of detectors with different sensor materials, different pixel sizes, or different charge summing architectures. Other important figures of merit are the energy resolution, which stands for the width of the photon peak in the detector response function, or the quantum efficiency, which measures the fraction of photons registered above a given threshold energy. The dead time of the readout ASIC indicates at which photon flux pulse pile-up starts to lead to event loss. The spatial resolution is described by the MTF and spatial correlation between noise hits can be studied with the help of the noise power spectrum. Finally, the very important detective quantum efficiency quantifies the degradation of the signal to noise ratio due to the imperfections of the complete detection process. To simplify their interpretation, most quantities are usually determined for monochromatic radiation and then analyzed as a function of photon energy. They have also been studied for application-specific radiation spectra, but this usually goes along with a loss of generality.

An active field is the development of approaches to reduce spectral distortions due to charge sharing, fluorescence effect, or pulse pile-up. While good spectral performance has already been presented at low photon fluxes, obtaining high spectral efficiency at large fluxes is still challenging. Some vendors use large pixels combined with very fast pulse shaping to minimize the effects of pulse pile-up. A competing approach is to work with small pixels and to compensate for charge sharing and fluorescence effects with charge summing architectures. These solutions still have to prove the ability to deliver a high spectral efficiency at high fluxes. If sufficiently robust and fast charge-summing architectures can be implemented, they have the potential to deliver good spectral information at high fluxes combined with spatial resolutions of about one hundred micrometers.

REFERENCES

1. X. Llopart, M. Campbell, R. Dinapoli, D. San Segundo, E. Pernigotti, "Medipix2: A 64-k pixel readout chip with 55-μm square elements working in single photon counting mode", *IEEE Trans. Nucl. Sci.*, vol. 49, n. 5, pp. 2279–2283, 2002.
2. G. F. Knoll, *Radiation Detection and Measurement*, 3rd ed. John Wiley & Sons, Inc., 2000.
3. L. Wielopolski, R. P. Gardener, "Development of the detector response function approach in the least-squares analysis of X-ray fluorescence spectra", *Nucl. Instrum. Meth. A*, vol. 165, n. 2, pp. 297–306, 1979.
4. P. Trueb, P. Zambon, C. Broennimann, "Assessment of the spectral performance of hybrid photon counting X-ray detectors", *Med. Phys.*, vol. 44, n. 9, pp. e207–e214, 2017.

5. J. Marchal, "Theoretical analysis of the effect of charge-sharing on the detective quantum efficiency of single-photon counting segmented silicon detectors", *J. Instrum.*, vol. 5, p. P01004, 2010.
6. P. Kraft, A. Bergamaschi, Ch. Broennimann, R. Dinapoli, E. F. Eikenberry, B. Henrich, I. Johnson, A. Mozzanica, C. M. Schlepuetz, P. R. Willmott, B. Schmit, "Performance of single-photon-counting PILATUS detector modules", *J. Synchr. Rad.*, vol. 16, pp. 368–375, 2009.
7. P. Zambon, V. Radicci, P. Trueb, C. Disch, M. Rissi, T. Sakhelashvili, M. Schneebeli, C. Broennimann, "Spectral response characterization of CdTe sensors of different pixel size with the IBEX ASIC", *Nucl. Instrum. Meth. A*, vol. 892, pp. 106–113, 2018.
8. J. Tanguay, S. Yun, H. K. Kim, I. A. Cunningham, "The detective quantum efficiency of photon-counting X-ray detectors using cascaded systems analyses", *Medical Physics*, vol. 40, p. 041913, 2013.
9. K. Taguchi, C. Polster, O. Lee, K. Stierstorfer, S. Kappler, "Spatio-energetic cross talk in photon counting detectors: Detector model and correlated poisson data generator", *Med. Phys.*, vol. 43, n. 12, 2016.
10. E. Gatti, P. F. Manfredi, "Processing the signals from solid-state detectors in elementary-particle physics", *Rivista Del Nuovo Cimento*, vol. 9, n. 1, 1986.
11. G. Lutz, *Semiconductor Radiation Detectors*, Springer, 2007.
12. V. Radeka, "Low-noise techniques in detectors", *Ann. Rev. Nucl. Part. Sci.*, vol. 38, pp. 217–277, 1988.
13. W. M. C. Sansen, Z. Y. Chang, "Limits of low noise performance of detector readout front ends in CMOS technology", *IEEE Trans. Circ. Syst.*, vol. 37, n. 11, 1990.
14. G. Lioliou n, A.M. Barnett, "Electronic noise in charge sensitive preamplifiers for X-ray spectroscopy and the benefits of a SiC input JFET", *Nucl. Instrum. Meth. A*, vol. 801, pp. 63–72, 2015.
15. E. N. Gimenez, R. Ballabriga, M. Campbell, I. Horswell, X. Llopart, J. Marchal, K. J. S. Sawhney, N. Tartoni, D. Turecek, "Study of charge-sharing in MEDIPIX3 using a micro-focused synchrotron beam", *J. Instrum.*, vol. 6, p. C01031, 2011.
16. P. Zambon, V. Radicci, M. Rissi, C. Broennimann, "A fitting model of the pixel response to monochromatic X-rays in photon counting detectors", *Nucl. Instrum. Meth. A*, vol. 905, pp. 188–192, 2018.
17. M. C. Veale, S. J. Bell, D. D. Duarte, A. Schneider, P. Seller, M. D. Wilson, K. Iniewski, "Measurements of charge sharing in small pixel CdTe detectors", *Nucl. Instrum. Meth. A*, vol. 767, pp. 218–226, 2014.
18. C. Thompson, D. Attwood, E. Gullikson, M. Howells, K. Kim, J. Kirz, J. Kortright, I. Lindau, Y. Liu, P. Panetta, A. Robinson, J. Scofield, J. Underwood, G. Williams, H. Winick, "X-ray data booklet". Center for X-ray optics and Advanced Light Source. *http://xdb.lbl.gov*, 2009.
19. R. Ballabriga, J. Alozy, M. Campbell, E. Frojdh, E.H.M. Heijne, T. Koenig, X. Llopart, J. Marchal, D. Pennicard, T. Poikela, L. Tlustos, P. Valerio, W. Wong, M. Zuber, "Review of hybrid pixel detector readout ASICs for spectroscopic X-ray imaging", *JINST*, vol. 11, p. P01007, 2016.
20. K. Taguchi, M. Zhang, E. C. Frey, X. Wang, "Modeling the performance of a photon counting X-ray detector for CT: Energy response and pulse pileup effects", *Med Phys.*, vol. 38, n. 2, pp. 1089–1102, 2011.
21. E. Frojdh, R. Ballabriga, M. Campbell, M. Fiederle, E. Hamann, T. Koenig, X. Llopart, D. de Paiva Magalhaes, M. Zuberc, "Count rate linearity and spectral response of the Medipix3RX chip coupled to a 300 mm silicon sensor under high flux conditions", *J. Instrum.*, vol. 9, p. C04028, 2014.
22. S. Ramo, "Currents Induced by Electron Motion", *Proceedings of the I.R.E.*, 1939.
23. M. D. Wilson, P. Seller, M. C. Veale, P. J. Sellin, "Investigation of the small pixel effect in CdZnTe detectors", *IEEE 2007 Nuclear Science Symposium Conference Records*, N24E 20, pp. 1255–1259, 2007.
24. A. Kargar, A. C. Brooks, M. J. Harrison, H. Chen, S. Awadalla, G. Bindley, B. Redden, D. S. McGregor, "Uniformity of charge collection efficiency in Frisch collar spectrometer with THM grown CdZnTe crystals", *Proc. of SPIE*, vol. 7449, p. 744908, 2009.
25. D. Kurková, L. Judas, "An analytical X-ray CdTe detector response matrix for incomplete charge collection correction for photon energies up to 300 keV", *Radiation Physics and Chemistry*, vol. 146, pp. 26–33, 2018.
26. E. Guni, J. Durst, B. Kreisler, T. Michel, G. Anton, M. Fiederle, A. Fauler, A. Zwerger, "The Influence of pixel pitch and electrode pad size on the spectroscopic performance of a photon counting pixel detector with CdTe sensor", *IEEE Trans. Nucl. Sci.*, vol. 58, n. 1, 2011.
27. C. Xu, M. Danielsson, H. Bornefalk, "Evaluation of energy loss and charge sharing in cadmium telluride detectors for photon-counting computed tomography", *IEEE Trans. Nucl. Sci*, vol. 58, n. 3, 2011.
28. C. Buton, A. Dawiec, J. Graber-Bolis, K. Arnaud, J. F. Bérar, N. Blanc, N. Boudet, J. C. Clémens, F. Debarbieux, P. Delpierre, B. Dinkespiler, T. Gastaldi, S. Hustache, C. Morel, P. Pangaud, H. Perez-Ponce, E. Vigeolas, "Comparison of three types of XPAD3.2/CdTe single chip hybrids for hard X-ray applications in material science and biomedical imaging", *Nucl. Instrum. Meth. A*, vol. 758, pp. 44–56, 2014.

29. S. Del Sordo, L. Abbene, E. Caroli, A. M. Mancini, A. Zappettini, P. Ubertini, "Progress in the development of CdTe and CdZnTe semiconductor radiation detectors for astrophysical and medical applications" *Sensors*, vol. 9, pp. 3491–3526, 2009.
30. K. Iniewski, "CZT sensors for computed tomography: from crystal growth to image quality", *JINST*, vol. 11, p. C12034, 2016.
31. T. E. Hansen, N. Ahmed, A. Ferber, G. Bouquet, "Edge-on detectors with active edge for X-ray photon counting imaging", *IEEE NSS Conference Record*, pp. 1341–1408, 2011.
32. A. Cola, I. Farella, "The polarization mechanism in CdTe Schottky detectors", *Appl Phys Lett. 2009*; vol. 94, p. 102113, 2009.
33. R. Grill, E. Belas, J. Franc, M. Bugàr, S. Uxa, P. Moravec, P. Höschl, "Polarization study of defect structures of CdTe radiation detectors", *IEEE Trans Nucl Sci.*, vol. 58, n. 6, pp. 3172–3181, 2011.
34. M. Niraula, A. Nakamura, T. Aoki, Y. Tomita, Y. Hatanak, "Stability issues of high-energy resolution diode type CdTe nuclear radiation detectors in a long-term operation", *Nucl. Instrum. Meth. A*, vol. 491, pp. 168–175, 2002.
35. T. Seino, I. Takahashi, T. Ishitsu, K. Yokoi, K. Kobashi, "Suppressing the polarization effect in high temperature conditions for an In/CdTe/Pt detector", 2012 IEEE Nuclear Science Symposium and Medical Imaging Conference Record (NSS/MIC), R08–2, 2012.
36. O. Godet, G. Nasser, J.-L. Atteia, B. Cordier, P. Mandrou, D. Barret, H. Triou, R. Pons, C. Amoros, S. Bordon, O. Gevin, F. Gonzalez, D. Goetz, A. Gros, B, Houret, C. Lachaud, K. Lacombe, W. Marty, K. Mercier, D. Rambaud, P. Ramon, G. Rouaix, S. Schanne, V. Waegebaert, "The X-/Gamma-ray camera ECLAIRs for the Gammay-ray burst mission SVOM", arXiv:1406.7759v1 [physics.ins-det], 2014.
37. L. Rossi, P. Fischer, T. Rohe, N. Wermes, *Pixel Detectors*, Springer, 2006.
38. A. Vincenzi, P. L. d. Ruvo, P. Delogu, R. Bellazzini, A. Brez, M. Minuti, M. Pinchera, G. Spandre, "Energy characterization of Pixirad-1 photon counting detector system", *J. Instrum.*, vol. 10, p. C04010, 2015.
39. T. Koenig, J. Schulze, M. Zuber, K. Rink, J. Butzer, E. Hamann, A. Cecilia, A. Zwerger, A. Fauler, M. Fiederle, U. Oelfke, "Imaging properties of small-pixel spectroscopic X-ray detectors based on cadmium telluride sensors", *Phys. Med. Biol.*, vol. 57, pp. 6743–6759, 2012.
40. M. Ruat, C. Ponchut, "Characterization of a pixelated CdTe X-ray detector using the timepix photon-counting readout chip", *IEEE Trans. Nucl. Sci.*, vol. 59, pp. 2392–2401, 2012.
41. L.-J. Meng, J. W. Tan, K. Spartiotis, T. Schulman, "Preliminary evaluation of a novel energy-resolved photon-counting gamma ray detector", *Nucl. Instrum. Meth. A*, vol. 604, pp. 548–554, 2009.
42. S. Huang, F. Alhassen, A. M. Hernandez, R. G. Gould, Y. Seo, W. C. Barber, J. S. Iwanczyk, N. E. Hartsough, T. Gandhi, J. C. Wessel, "Energy Response of a Room-Temperature Cadmium Telluride (CdTe) Photon-Counting Detector for Simultaneous and Sequential CT and SPECT", *2012 IEEE Nuclear Science Symposium and Medical Imaging Conference Record (NSS/MIC)*, M16–51, 2012.
43. R. Steadman, C. Herrmann, A. Livne, "ChromAIX2: A large area, high count-rate energy-resolving photon counting ASIC for a Spectral CT Prototype", *Nucl. Instrum. Meth. A*, vol. 862, pp. 18–24, 2017.
44. P. Schlomka, E. Roessl, R. Dorscheid, S. Dill, G. Martens, T. Istel, C. Bäumer, C. Herrmann, R. Steadman, G. Zeitler, A. Livne, R. Proksa, "Experimental feasibility of multi-energy photon-counting K-edge imaging in pre-clinical computed tomography", *Phys. Med. Biol.*, vol. 53, pp. 4031–4047, 2008.
45. A. Shankar, J. Krebs, D. R. Bednarek, S. Rudin, "Spectroscopy with a CdTe-based photon-counting imaging detector (PCD) having charge sharing correction capability", *Proc SPIE Int Soc Opt Eng.*, vol. 10573, 2018.
46. K. Medjoub, A. Thompson, J. Berar, J. Clemens, P. Delpierre, P. Da Silva, B. Dinkespiler, R. Fourme, P. Gourhant, B. Guimaraes, S. Hustache, M. Idir, J. Itie, P. Legrand, C. Menneglier, P. Mercere, F. Picca, J. Samama, "Energy resolution of the CdTe-XPAD detector: Calibration and potential for Laue diffraction measurements on protein crystals", *J. Synchr. Rad.*, vol. 19, pp. 323–331, 2012.
47. M. Krumrey, E. Tegeler, "Selfcalibration of semiconductor photodiodes in the soft xray region", *Rev. Sci. Instrum.*, vol 63, pp. 797–801, 1992.
48. D. Pennicard, H. Graafsma, "Simulated performance of high-Z detectors with Medipix3 readout", *J. Instrum.*, vol. 6, p. P06007, 2011.
49. A. Tomal, J. C. Santos, P. R. Costa, A. H. Lopez Gonzales, M. E. Polett, "Monte Carlo simulation of the response functions of CdTe detectors to be applied in X-ray spectroscopy", *Appl. Radiat. Isot.*, vol. 100, pp. 32–37, 2015.
50. S. Miyajima, K. Imagawa, M. Matsumoto, "CdZnTe detector in diagnostic X-ray spectroscopy", *Med. Phys.*, vol. 29, n. 7, pp. 1421–1429, 2002.

51. P. Kraft, A. Bergamaschi, C. Broennimann, R. Dinapoli, E. F. Eikenberry, H. Graafsma, B. Henrich, I. Johnson, M. Kobas, A. Mozzanica, C. M. Schlepuetz, B. Schmitt, "Characterization and calibration of PILATUS detectors", *IEEE Trans. Nucl. Sci.*, vol. 56, pp. 758–764, 2009.
52. M. Bath, "Evaluating imaging systems: practical applications", *Radiation Protection Dosimetry*, vol. 139, n. 1–3, pp. 26–36, 2010.
53. J. T. Dobbins III, *Handbook of Medical Imaging.* Volume 1: Physics and psychophysics, SPIE Press, U.S.A., chapter 3, 2000.
54. IEC 62220-1, Medical electrical equipment - Characteristics of digital X-ray imaging devices - Part 1-1: Determination of the detective quantum efficiency - Detectors used in radiographic imaging, 2015.
55. K, Medjoubi, T. Bucaille, S. Hustache, J.-F. Bérar, N. Boudet, J.-C. Clemens, P. Delpierre, B. Dinkespiler, "Detective quantum efficiency, modulation transfer function and energy resolution comparison between CdTe and silicon sensors bump-bonded to XPAD3S", *J. Synchr. Rad.*, vol. 17, pp. 486–495, 2010.
56. J. Marchal, "Discriminator threshold dependence of the noise power spectrum in single-X-ray-photon counting silicon strip detectors", *J. Instrum.*, vol. 5, p. P11002, 2010.
57. F. C. Brunner, J. C. Clemens, C. Hemmer, C. Morel, "Imaging performance of the hybrid pixel detectors XPAD3-S", *Phys. Med. Biol.*, vol. 54, pp. 1773–1789, 2009.
58. K. S. Kalluri, M. Mahd, S. J. Glick, "Investigation of energy weighting using an energy discriminating photon counting detector for breast CT", *Med. Phys.*, vol. 40, n. 8, 2013.
59. R. Bellazzini, A. Brez, G. Spandre, M. Minuti, M. Pinchera, P. Delogu, P.L. de Ruvo, A. Vincenzi, "PIXIE III: A very large area photon-counting CMOS pixel ASIC for sharp X-ray spectral imaging", *JINST*, vol. 10, p. C01032, 2015.
60. E. Kraft, F. Glasser, S. Kappler, D. Niederloehner, P. Villard, "Experimental evaluation of the pile-up trigger method in a revised quantum-counting CT detector", *Proc. of SPIE*, vol. 8313, p. 83134A, 2012.
61. D. Lee, K. Park, K. T. Lim, G. Cho, "Energy-correction photon counting pixel for photon energy extraction under pulse pile-up", *NIM A*, vol. 856, pp. 36–46, 2017.
62. G M. Gustavsson, F. U. Amin, A. Bjorklid, A. Ehliar, C. Xu, C. Svensson, "A high-rate energy-resolving photon-counting ASIC for spectral computed tomography", *IEEE Transactions on Nuclear Science*, vol. 59, n. 1, pp. 30–39, 2012.
63. C. Ullberg, M. Urech, N. Weber, A. Engman, A. Redz, F. Henckel, "Measurements of a dual-energy fast photon counting CdTe detector with integrated charge sharing correction", *Proc. of SPIE*, vol. 8668, p. 86680P, 2013.
64. R. Ballabriga, G. Blaj, M. Campbell, M. Fiederle, D. Greiffenberg, E.H.M. Heijne, X. Llopart, R. Plackett, S. Procz, L. Tlustos, D. Turecek, W. Wong, "Characterization of the Medipix3 pixel readout chip", *JINST*, vol. 6, p. C01052, 2011.
65. A. Krzyżanowska, G. W. Deptuch, P. Maj, P. Gryboś, R. Szczygieł, "Characterization of the photon counting CHASE Jr., chip built in a 40-nm CMOS process with a charge sharing correction algorithm using a collimated X-ray beam", *IEEE Transactions on Nuclear Science*, vol. 64, n. 9, pp. 2561–2568, 2017.
66. R. Ballabriga, M. Campbell, E. H. M. Heijne, X. Llopart, L. Tlustos, "The Medipix3 prototype, a pixel readout chip working in single photon counting mode with improved spectrometric performance", *IEEE Transactions on Nuclear Science*, vol. 54, n. 5, pp. 1824–1829, 2007.
67. J. Hoff, G. W. Deptuch, F. Fahim, P. Gryboś, P. Maj, D. P. Siddons, R. Szczygiel, M. Trimpl, T. Zimmerman, "An on-chip charge cluster reconstruction technique in the miniVIPIC pixel readout chip for X-ray counting and timing", IEEE Nuclear Science Symposium and Medical Imaging Conference (NSS/MIC), Seattle, WA, pp. 1–11, 2014.
68. M. Campbell, J. Alozy, R. Ballabriga, E. Frojdh, E. Heijne, X. Llopart, T. Poikela, L. Tlustos, P. Valerio, W. Wong, "Towards a new generation of pixel detector readout chips", *JINST*, vol. 11, p. C01007, 2016.

12 Photon Counting Detectors Viewed as Nonlinear, Shift-Variant Systems

Thomas Koenig
Ziehm Imaging GmbH, Nuremberg, Germany
Mayo Clinic Graduate School of Biomedical Sciences,
Rochester, Minnesota, United States

CONTENTS

12.1 INTRODUCTION

12.1.1 Photon Counting

Photon counting x-ray detectors have been a subject of intense study in both academic and industrial research for many years [1–18]. As opposed to conventional, energy integrating detectors, they are capable of resolving individual photon interactions, instead of only summing up the total energy released within a pixel during exposure. By doing so, they are also able to quantify the energy released during such an interaction, and so the abilities to count photons and to measure their energies are connected.

Most photon counting detectors obtain their spectroscopic capabilities by quantifying a voltage that is the output of some combination of a charge sensitive amplifier and a pulse shaper [19]. If this voltage output is above the reference voltage applied to a comparator, an associated counter is incremented, and ultimately read out. The reference voltage can then be calibrated to represent photon energies and so acts as an energy threshold that enforces counting only those photon events with an energy above it. Moreover, electronic noise that adversely affects energy integrating detectors at low x-ray exposures manifests as the occurrence of low-energy events in photon counting detectors. Setting an energy threshold above a detector's noise floor suppresses this dark-current and makes the resultant frames remain unexposed in the absence of radiation. This enables photon counting detectors to work at very low x-ray fluxes [20] and even be sensitive to environmental radiation. In fact, this is what gives such a detector its ability to count photons in the first place.

When asking other researchers about the main benefits of these detectors, though, the most common answer I have been given in the past is not that these detectors count photons. Instead, it appears that their capability to record spectral information is what stimulates most of the interest that has driven the field. Not only does this aim at augmenting detection concepts that so far have produced x-ray images that are mostly grayscale. Especially in medical imaging, and in particular computed tomography (CT), it also promises to improve on approaches that target material decomposition and contrast agent quantification [4, 21–25], such as multisource CT, fast tube voltage switching or multilayer detectors [26]. While replacing such concepts by a single detector that provides energy information is an attractive goal that has also stimulated my own research for many years, it represents a line of thinking that prevents asking a different, but very important question: How well does a photon counting detector count photons? Often, this question remains unasked, and so the main purpose of this chapter is to enable readers to both understand and answer this question when working with photon counters. While I will revisit the most important of their aspects in this chapter, I will assume some basic familiarity with the technology that has already been explained throughout the previous chapters of this book. Also, none of the data presented below was novel scientific research at the time of my writing. Instead, I want to use my previous research to shed light on counting detectors from a different angle and provide a view that, in my opinion, has not been made sufficiently explicit in the past.

12.1.2 Nonlinearity Resulting from Shift-Variance

Often, photon counting detectors are implicitly considered devices offering spectral information as an additional feature to regular, energy integrating detectors. A counting detector is then viewed as a device offering multiple energy bins, and its energy resolution is modeled as a convolution integral applied to the incoming x-ray spectrum. In other words, measuring a photon's energy E is assumed to be subject to a certain probability distribution, making it appear having an energy E', and so forth.

Obtaining a good energy resolution is by itself a challenging problem. The reason for this can be found in the detection principle of a counting detector, which I will now briefly sketch. A pixelated application specific integrated circuit (ASIC), containing all the necessary pulse shaping, discrimination and counting structures, is bump-bonded to an opaque sensor. Typical sensor materials include silicon (Si) [27], cadmium telluride (CdTe) [28], cadmium zinc telluride (CZT) [29], as well as gallium arsenide (GaAs) [30]. During detector operation, a high voltage is applied to such a sensor, typically some hundreds of volts per millimeter. This is done in a manner such that in the absence of radiation, ideally no current will flow. While Si-sensors require rectifying characteristics to act in the desired fashion due to a rather small band gap, both CdTe, CZT as well as GaAs offer band gaps large enough to be operated as semi-insulators.

Once a photon interacts with the sensor by complete or partial absorption, it generates a cascade of electron-hole pairs that immediately start drifting to opposite sides of the sensor under the electric field applied. This process generates free charge that can be measured and that is proportional to the energy released during photon interaction. The drifting charge then constitutes an induced charge at the entrance of the charge-sensitive amplifier that is present within each of the ASIC's pixels, and the quantification of this charge occurs as outlined above. Yet, there is no way to force this charge to end up at a single pixel only. In fact, many events will occur close to pixel boundaries such that the generated currents will flow through a multitude of pixels, as illustrated in Figure 12.1.

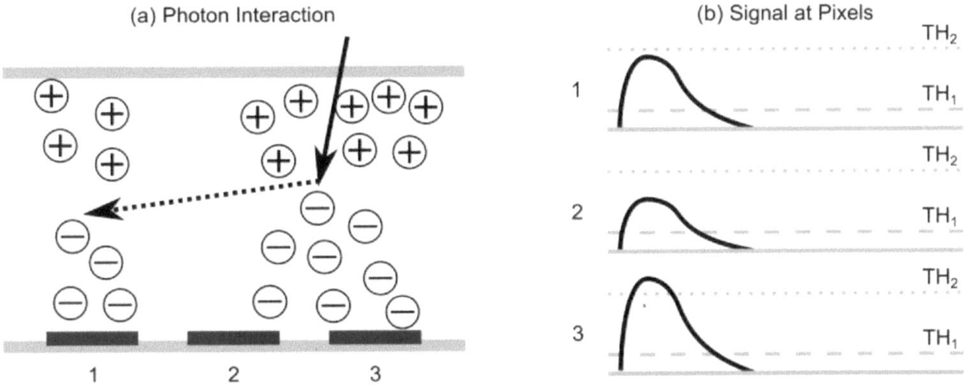

FIGURE 12.1 (a) An incident photon (solid line) generates a photo-electron, which causes a cascade of secondary electrons and the emission of a characteristic secondary photon (dotted line, also called fluorescence). In this example, the resulting total free charge generated by this event is spread across three pixels. (b) A voltage threshold leads to a binary decision as to whether a counter pertaining to a particular threshold and pixel is incremented. For the low threshold TH_1, three events are recorded, while for the high threshold TH_2, only one event is counted by the third pixel. Thresholds even higher would lead to ignoring this particular interaction completely, making it appear as if it never occurred.

It is easy to see that each of these individual pixels will then be deceived into reporting events of lower energies, biasing the measured energy spectrum. The strength of this bias is usually quantified in terms of a detector's energy response function (ERF), which describes its response to a well-defined, monoenergetic photon energy (and which is therefore a function of it). Figure 12.2 shows that the charge sharing (and fluorescence) bias revealed by an ERF

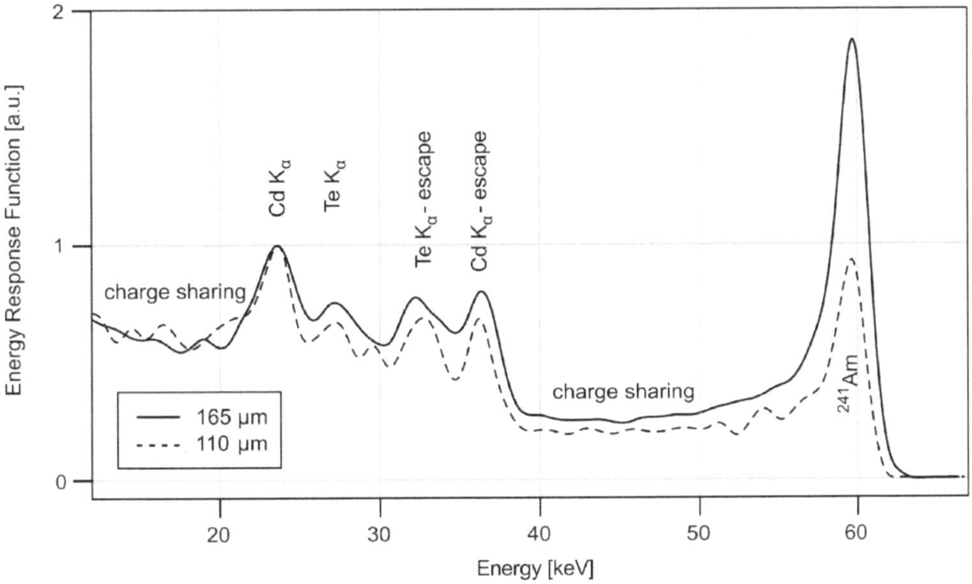

FIGURE 12.2 Energy response functions for 60 keV monoenergetic photons impinging on 1 mm thick CdTe sensors bonded to two Medipix2MXR detectors with pixel pitches of 110 and 165 μm [9]. In addition to the 60 keV peak, the sensor's K_α lines are also visible. Connected to this is the occurrence of those discrete energies that represent the remaining photo-electrons, called escape peaks. Both curves were normalized to one at the Cd-fluorescence.

strongly depends on the pixel pitch. As the very essence of this chapter, I will now explain why this ERF does *not* represent the kernel of a convolution integral, and discuss the consequences arising from this fact.

12.1.3 Photon Counting versus Energy Integrating Detectors

The key to understanding photon counting detectors is knowing that their response is intrinsically position sensitive and thus no longer shift-invariant. Although the charge induced at the pixelated anode is conserved in good approximation, the amount of this charge is not what is reported by a photon counting detector upon readout. This is due to the binary decision-making that occurs for each and every interaction separately, and that we have encountered in Figure 12.1.

This decision-making introduces nonlinearity and can have a substantial impact on the detector's efficiency and noise properties. Depending on a photon's energy, its site of interaction relative to the pixel matrix and the energy thresholds applied, it may be counted once, multiple times, or not at all. This behavior constitutes shift-variance. While a varying count per incoming photon contributes an additional source of noise [31], a photon not being counted at all behaves as if it penetrated the detector without interaction. Both effects mimic reduced absorption efficiency by increasing image noise. In a certain sense, this corresponds to a convolution kernel that loses normalization to a total sum of one, depending on the site of interaction.

In contrast, energy integrating detectors perform digitization upon readout only. Also, light that may have spread to neighboring pixels reduces the intensity measured by the pixel pertaining to the original site. Consequently, the total energy released is conserved to much larger a degree within energy integrating detectors, which allows modeling them assuming a linear, shift-invariant behavior.

This strategy fails for photon counting detectors. Due to their detection principle, their inherent difference to energy integrating devices is that there is no such thing as "half a count". Instead, counting detectors require more sophisticated modeling strategies [32], the most successful of which are probably those based on cascaded systems analysis [33, 34]. Discussing them goes beyond the scope of this chapter, and so I will move on to presenting concepts to restore shift-invariance. Along with this, I will discuss those consequences of shift-variance that go beyond spectroscopic resolution: threshold dependent point spread functions (PSFs) as well as detective quantum efficiencies (DQEs).

12.2 RESTORING SHIFT-INVARIANCE

Claiming back shift-invariance is something that needs to be addressed during detector design. There exist two major and very different types of approaches that can be used to reach this goal: increasing the pixel size, or allowing pixels to communicate with each other.

12.2.1 Large Pixels

12.2.1.1 Energy Response versus Spatial Resolution

From the above considerations it becomes immediately clear that the pixel size, or pitch, is a fundamental quantity that defines the degree of shift-variance. The smaller the pixel is, the more likely it is for a charge cloud or a secondary photon to escape to its neighbors. Thus, increasing the pixel size may appear as a valuable option to more and more suppress these unwanted effects. Indeed, Figure 12.2 demonstrates a notable dependence of a detector's spectroscopic performance on the pixel pitch.

In order to assess whether a benefit can be expected from larger pixels, it is crucial to understand that increasing the pixel area must occur in hardware prior to signal height analysis. Simply binning detector pixels after readout, on the contrary, will not restore any uncounted photons or incorrectly measured photon energies. Put differently, there exists no linear, shift-invariant filter that could be applied and that would correctly mimic larger pixels.

As a natural drawback of this approach, the size of the resulting image matrix decreases. This may or may not come as a loss of spatial resolution, depending on other system parameters such as the extent of the x-ray source employed. In some cases, designing larger pixels may be the best way to go. Of course, this will be counterproductive if obtaining a high spatial resolution is the main design goal for a specific detector.

12.2.1.2 Energy Response versus Count Rate Linearity

Other than image resolution, there is one more severe disadvantage of large pixels, which is connected to the processing speed of single events within an ASIC and which does not have a direct analogy in energy integrating detectors. Indeed, for a photon counting detector to count individual events, it is important for these events to be separated in time to avoid their fusion. This applies to the analog signal processing prior to signal height analysis as well as the digital part of the detector that feeds and increments its counters. Usually, it is the analog fusion of events that is the limiting part here.

This effect of analog event fusion is called pulse pile-up and is illustrated in Figure 12.3. It represents another source of nonlinearity that is due to finite signal processing times [35, 36]. Pile-up is the limiting factor of the input x-ray flux that can be reasonably handled by a photon counting detector, as above a certain point the ASIC's output count rate will no longer be proportional to the input rate. The onset of this effect is proportional to a pixel's area: the larger the area, the lower the number of photons per unit area and time that can be processed correctly. Measurements demonstrating this effect will be presented further below.

Noteworthy, the amount to which a detector suffers from pile-up also depends on the energy threshold that pertains to a given counter. As can be inferred from Figure 12.3, a higher energy threshold makes it more likely for the fusion product of two signals to intermediately drop below the threshold and to correctly trigger the counting of separate events. A finely tuned threshold can then be used to push detector linearity up to very high levels. However, this strategy cannot restore energy resolution lost to pile-up as it delivers linearity only for one particular threshold setting. Also, this fine tuning needs to be tailored to a certain photon energy. In particular for wide x-ray spectra as those produced by an x-ray tube, this is no longer viable because different photon energies are absorbed differently within an object. Consequently, the spectrum that reaches the detector depends on object composition, and it is no longer possible to perform this fine-tuning without prior knowledge even if energy resolution is not of interest.

Hence, choosing large pixels restores shift-invariance to some degree. However, this bears significant drawbacks, most importantly a loss of spatial resolution and a reduction of the maximum input count rate at which a detector can be operated in a reasonable manner. Therefore, in order to

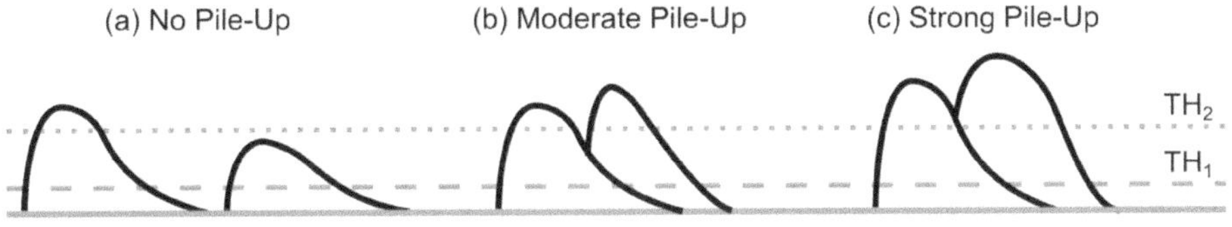

FIGURE 12.3 Schematic of the origin of pulse pile-up, and its dependence on the energy threshold setting. (a) Two pulses processed by a pixel are well separated in time, and so no pile-up occurs. (b) Two pulses partially overlap. At this particular setting of the energy thresholds TH_1 and TH_2, the second threshold is able to separate the two pulses, while the first threshold counts a single event only. (c) The two pulses overlap to a degree that causes both thresholds to report a single event.

achieve both shift-invariance, high count rates as well as a high spatial resolution, it is necessary to make substantial changes to a detector ASIC that go beyond adjusting the pixel pitch. These will be discussed next.

12.2.2 Inter-Pixel Communication

12.2.2.1 Working Principle

The previous sections identified the sharing of charge between neighboring pixels as the source to degrading a photon counting detector's performance. Most prominently, this charge sharing is due to the generation of a charge cloud close to a pixel boundary. However, the emission of secondary x-rays can also contribute a large part, in particular by incoherently scattered x-rays within sensors of low atomic number such as Si, or characteristic x-rays emitted predominantly by sensors of higher atomic numbers such as CdTe. The general concept to recombine these shared charges is therefore to establish a communication among a neighborhood of pixels that allows them to determine the correct total charge and the particular pixel that is most likely to be closest to the initial site of interaction [3, 37]. Doing this carefully allows establishing a neighborhood that dynamically forms around this very site. It is therefore possible to obtain a high spatial resolution without jeopardizing energy resolution. Moreover, it promises to restore shift-invariance to a good degree by yielding detector responses that are much less position sensitive.

While different names exist to label such concepts, the most well-known is that of *charge summing*, a technology that has been brought forward by the Medipix3 collaboration. This collaboration, a member of which I have been for some years myself, has produced chip designs that have significantly influenced the scientific discussion in the field of photon counting and spectral imaging. Most notably, the design of the Medipix3 ASIC [3] as well as its successor, the Medipix3RX [10], can be considered milestones in the development and understanding of restoring shift-invariance in photon counting detectors. The Medipix collaborations are centered at CERN, the European Organization for Nuclear Research, and their work generally features a strong academic component. This is why in particular the Medipix3RX represents one of the best studied implementations of inter-pixel communication, and most of my considerations below are based on the literature published about this particular chip [14, 38–40].

A scheme of a single pixel contained in this chip is given in Figure 12.4. The charge sensitive amplifier can be found to the very left. At its entrance, the charges induced by the charge cloud traveling through the sensor are formed. The use of the feedback capacitance C_F converts this input charge to an output voltage. If charge summing is switched off, this voltage will be fed into two discriminators that trigger their associated counters in the way explained before. The chip indeed allows operation in this so-called single pixel mode (SPM), which enables an easy assessment of the benefits of charge summing.

Activating charge summing mode (CSM) brings two features into play. The first one is indeed represented by the summing of the charges that arrive from a pixel's neighbors. The second one is connected to the actual hit allocation. It is performed by the arbitration logic and hence represents a feature contained within the chip's digital part. This logic determines the pixel that will be assigned an individual hit and ensures that a hit is counted only once. In short, a pixel will be assigned a hit if it has the highest charge deposition compared with its neighbors. However, the event will only be counted if the associated discriminator detects a summed charge above the associated threshold.

A number of examples of how this charge summing and hit allocation acts is depicted in Figure 12.5. Panels a & b correspond to the behavior of individual pixels. In this case, whether a particular pixel increments a counter depends on where a charge cloud travels relative to the pixel matrix (and of course the level of the pixel's energy threshold). As discussed before, this behavior is the very origin of shift-variance in a photon counting detector.

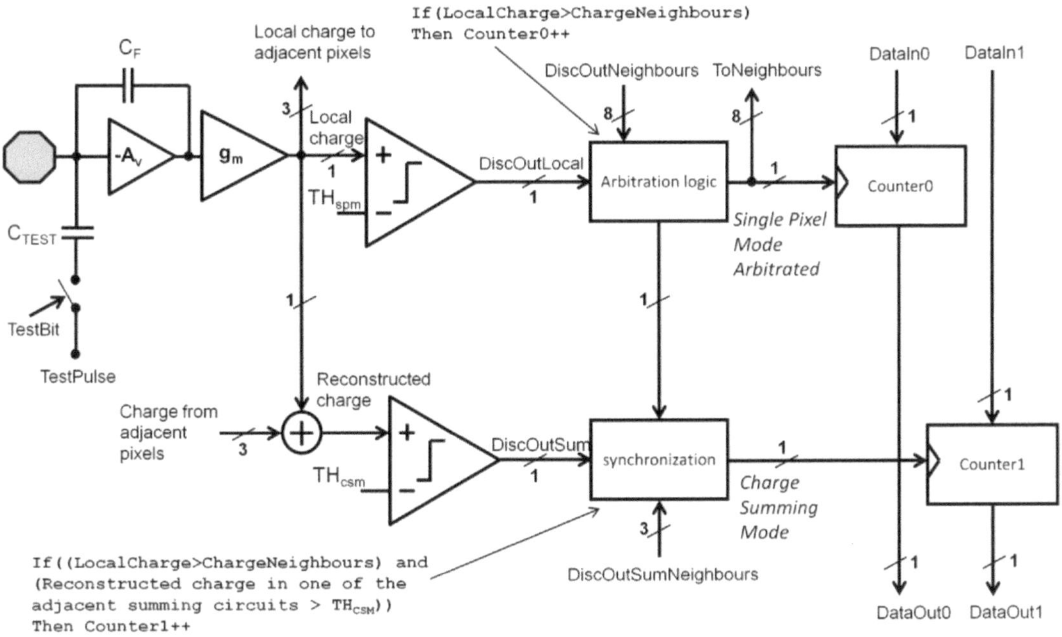

FIGURE 12.4 Schematic of a pixel cell used in the Medipxi3RX and implementing charge summing functionality. Figure courtesy of Rafael Ballabriga, CERN [3].

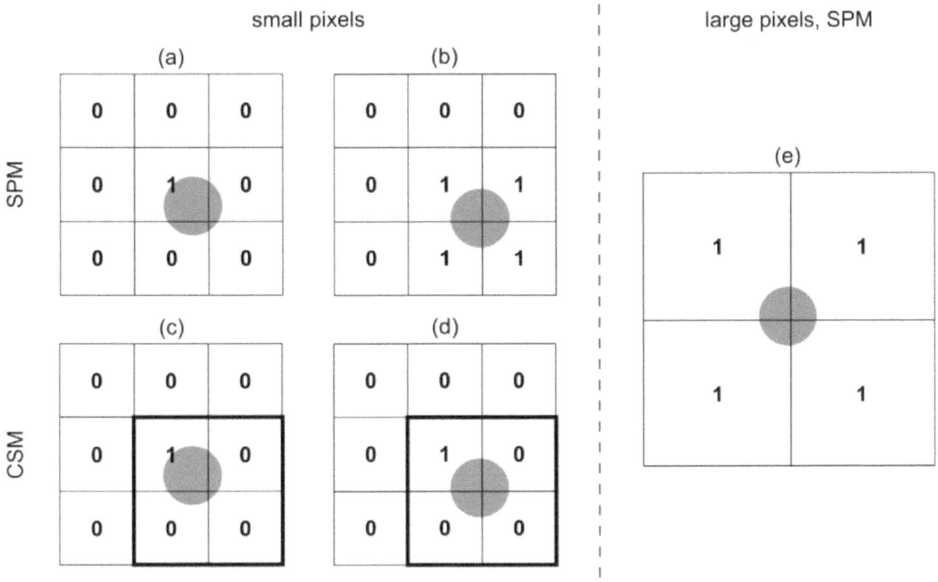

FIGURE 12.5 Examples of hit allocations in single pixel mode (SPM, a & b) and charge summing mode (CSM, c & d). Thin lines represent pixel boundaries, thick lines correspond to the collection areas in CSM which form adaptively around the charge cloud (gray circles), inhibiting border hits. To the right, an array of large pixels operated in SPM is shown, which does not prevent border hits. The numbers indicate counter increments, assuming suitably low energy thresholds.

In contrast to this, panels c & d illustrate hit allocation when inter-pixel communication is active within the Medipix3RX. It establishes a charge collection area that adaptively forms around the charge cloud. If this charge cloud is not too large, it will be impossible for it to hit the adaptive collection area at its boundaries. Charge summing therefore does not simply yield the ERF of individual pixels that have four times the area, as shown in panel (e). Instead, its ERF can be expected to be superior due to the absence of border hits, which still occur for the larger pixel. This is what carries the potential to restore shift-invariance.

12.2.2.2 Energy Response

The measurements depicted in Figure 12.6 demonstrate that this strategy is indeed very successful at achieving much better a performance also in practice. In addition, it also gives a good impression of how detrimental charge sharing can be if it is not accounted for. While the ERF pertaining to the CSM measurement is not perfectly Gaussian (the fluorescence and escape peaks remain to some extent), the advantage of inter-pixel communication is obvious. However, comparing Figures 12.2 and 12.6, we find that the energy resolution within the peaks has become worse by using charge summing, owing to the increased electronic noise that arises with establishing inter-pixel communication. However, exchanging the long tail that is caused by charge sharing against some moderate deterioration in peak width is certainly a trade worth making, as I will corroborate further below.

12.2.2.3 Effects on Dead Time

The additional complexity introduced by replicating and distributing charge among pixels brings along drawbacks that, at first, appear similar to larger pixels when count rates are considered. Indeed, collecting and comparing charge from multiple pixels leads to an increased (analog) dead

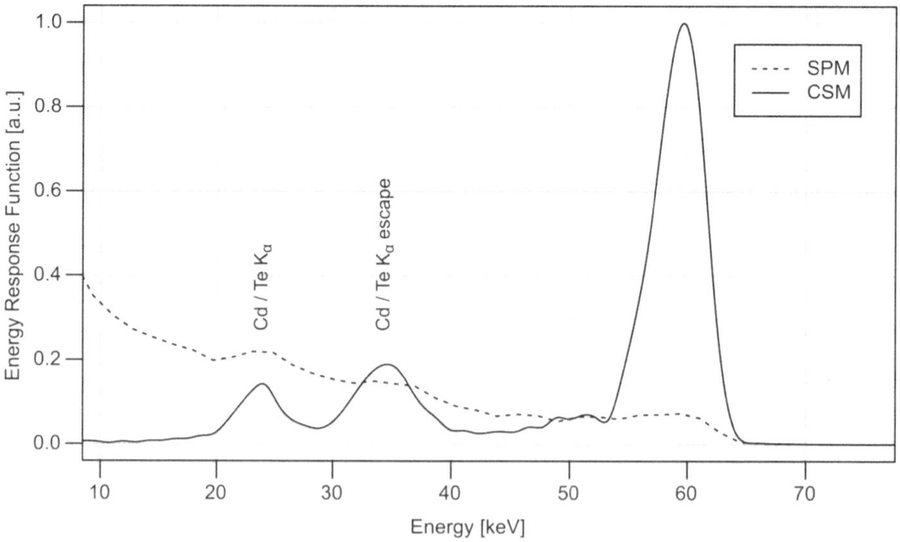

FIGURE 12.6 Energy response functions for 60 keV monochromatic photons, recorded with a Medipix3RX detector bump bonded to a 2 mm thick CdTe sensor at a pixel pitch of 110 μm [38]. The curves pertain to measurements in charge summing mode (CSM) and in single pixel mode (SPM). Even in CSM, some characteristic x-rays from the sensor escape the collection volume and are fused to a single peak here at around 25 keV. When comparing these measurements to Figure 12.2, be aware that this detector exhibited a sensor of twice the thickness, resulting in substantially more charge sharing.

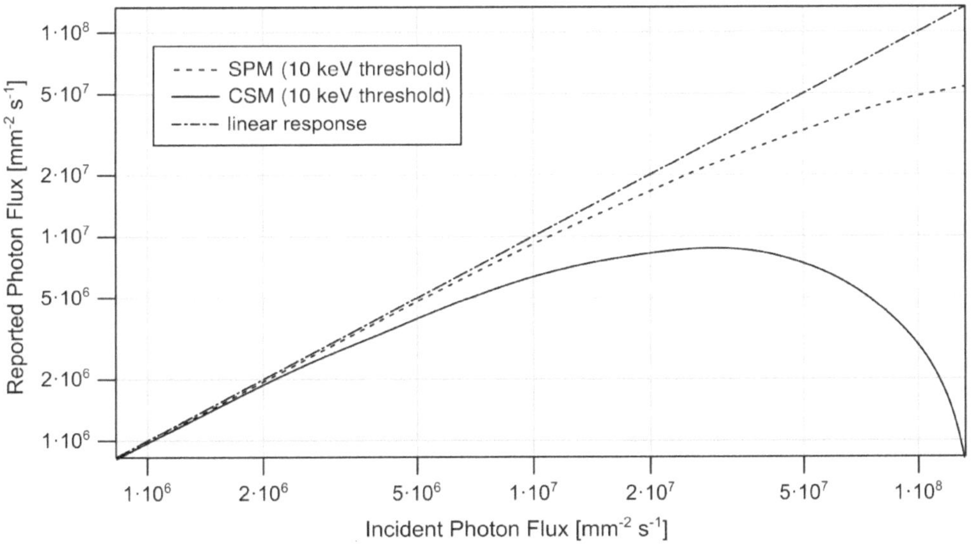

FIGURE 12.7 Count rate linearity measured with 25 keV monochromatic photons and the same detector as in Figure 12.6 [38].

time. Figure 12.7 shows that the Medipix3RX ASIC enters the pile-up regime substantially earlier when charge summing is activated. Measurements conducted at the ANKA synchrotron at the Karlsruhe Institute of Technology by my colleagues and myself [38] determined a factor of a little more than four regarding the differences in this critical flux. This finding was indeed notable, as charge summing incorporates information from neighborhoods of nine pixels. In fact, we found that the spectral resolution provided by charge summing is closer to a ninefold increase in pixel area, which led us to concluding that charge summing offers a net benefit regarding the trade-off between energy resolution and count rate. Therefore, pixels offering charge summing can likely be made smaller than those who do not, while exhibiting similar spectral resolution. In other words, at a comparable energy resolution a detector that employs charge summing is likely to be able to tolerate higher x-ray fluxes than one that was built using larger pixels.

12.2.2.4 Detective Quantum Efficiency

We can therefore conclude that charge summing is a very powerful concept to restore shift-invariance, and so I will now turn back to the question I raised at the beginning of this chapter: How well does a photon counting detector count photons? After all, achieving a high dose efficiency is of utmost concern particularly in the medical field, and spectral resolution is second to that in most cases. So, in order to answer this important question, it is best to adhere to a quantity that can also be determined for other types of detectors and that has been established for many decades: the DQE. Most generally, it is defined in Fourier space as the ratio of the output to the input signal-to-noise ratio (SNR), at a given spatial frequency ν:

$$\mathrm{DQE}(\nu) = \frac{\mathrm{SNR}_{\mathrm{out}}^2}{\mathrm{SNR}_{\mathrm{in}}^2}(\nu)\,. \quad (12.1)$$

Being a quantity critical to compare system performance, a lot of care needs to be taken to measure the DQE precisely. Luckily, an easy way exists to determine it for photon counting detectors at a spatial frequency of $\nu = 0$ [31]. Briefly, a detector is operated at exposure times short enough to identify individual hits within the resulting frames. A clustering algorithm is then employed to quantify the probability distribution of the number of counts produced by a single hit. The first- and second-order moments of these so-called hit multiplicities m then directly give the DQE(0) as:

$$\mathrm{DQE}(0) = \frac{\langle m \rangle^2}{\langle m^2 \rangle} \epsilon , \tag{12.2}$$

where ϵ denotes the sensor's absorption efficiency. Being connected to these multiplicities, the zero-frequency DQE is a direct indicator of shift-invariance, reaching a value of one in the case of a perfect detector that always responds to an incoming photon by a single count only.

Hence, we can use the DQE(0) to finally study how well photon counting detectors count photons, the result of which is given in Figure 12.8a. It shows two curves, the upper one corresponding to a measurement using CSM, and the lower one giving the regular behavior pertaining to independent pixels. The underlying experiment was carried out using monochromatic photons with an energy of 88 keV, varying a single energy threshold, recording thousands of frames and performing the cluster analysis as described. Studying the figure, it becomes obvious that independent pixels quickly lose their counting efficiency when the threshold is raised. This loss of efficiency starts from a pixel's borders, as this is where charges are shared and events are split into a multitude of low-energy events that eventually drop below a threshold. As the threshold increases, this insensitive region grows toward a pixel's center, reducing its active area. Consequently, more and more photons remain uncounted, and radiation dose is wasted.

This observation is especially important for spectral applications, where energy thresholds are also placed at higher levels, which is a prerequisite for material decomposition. In fact, Figure 12.8a tells us that leaving pixels to act independently during detector design will eventually provide us with material-specific images that contain more noise.

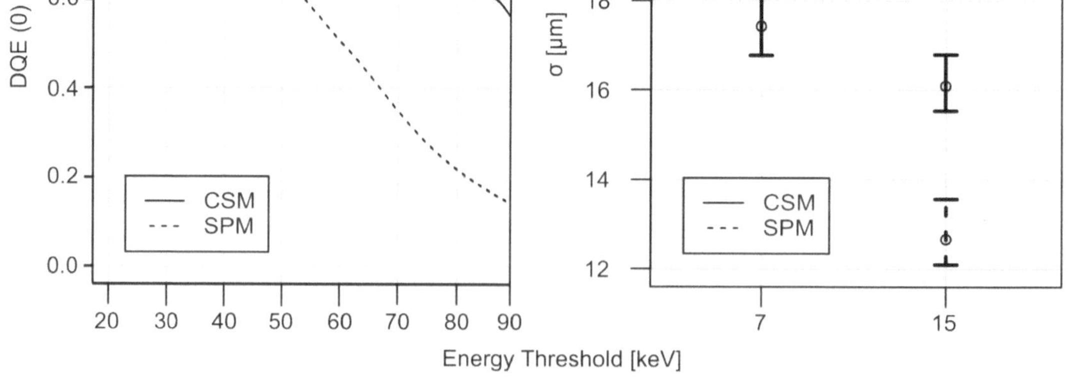

FIGURE 12.8 (a) DQEs obtained for a spatial frequency of zero as a function of the energy threshold and a photon energy of 88 keV [39]. Note that the curves do not reach zero at the photon energy due to a finite energy resolution. (b) Width of a spatially averaged point spread function, measured for photons of 25 keV energy [41]. SPM: single pixel mode; CSM: charge summing mode. All measurements were performed with the same detector as those shown in Figures 12.6 and 12.7.

Activating charge summing provides us with a different behavior and enables maintaining a comparably high DQE throughout most of the threshold range. Strikingly, the DQE is even observed to improve when the threshold crosses 25 keV. How can this be? The explanation is that these threshold settings exceed the energies of those characteristic photons that are emitted by the CdTe sensor and that travel beyond the volume formed by charge summing. Suppressing the counting of these photons, which experience an exponential absorption, indeed removes noise from an x-ray image by reducing the average number of the pixels responding to a single interaction, as well as their variance. Since in these cases a detector may still recover the charges stemming from the initial site (if the threshold is not too high), the original interaction is not lost and we are left with a cleaner image. This is reflected by the DQE measurement.

12.2.2.5 Spatial Resolution

Beyond increasing image noise, both charge sharing as well as long-ranged secondary photons constitute yet another, mostly unwanted effect that degrades image quality, blurring, and so they contribute to a detector's PSF. Based on our previous considerations, we can now infer that operating pixels independently of each other will rapidly cut-off this PSF at its tails when a threshold is raised. Indeed, this effect has been proven experimentally [42], and we can find additional confirmation in Figure 12.8b. The same figure also demonstrates that charge summing is much less prone to showing this effect, as it is able to capture many events originating from charge sharing and sensor fluorescence. Indeed, the threshold dependence of a photon counting detector's modulation transfer function (MTF) varies much less with the energy threshold when charge summing is enabled.

The PSF is a concept known from shift-invariant, linear system's theory and, by definition, represents the kernel of a convolution integral. So how could we measure it at all to arrive at the results shown in Figure 12.8b, knowing that detectors without charge summing are not shift-invariant? The truth is, we just did and applied the usual methods known from shift-invariant systems to arrive at an effective, spatially averaged PSF. The fact that we do see a threshold dependence simply reflects the shortcomings of linear system's theory when trying to describe counting detectors, and therefore demonstrates a lack of shift-invariance. However, the threshold dependence of the PSF is no artifact. It does correspond to a physical increase of image sharpness, and one may argue whether it represents a desired effect or not. Clearly, sharper images are a good thing, but then the associated loss in DQE still needs to be considered. Since the DQE is a function of the MTF for frequencies larger than zero, there may well exist a scenario in which an improved MTF counteracts a loss of apparent absorption efficiency due to charge sharing. However, it is reasonable to believe that such cases represent a minority in medical imaging, given the rapid drop of the DQE witnessed in Figure 12.8a. Still, there exist experiments beyond medical imaging that do profit from an adjustable PSF. As an example, this effect was exploited to explain one of the many origins of the visibility contrast encountered in x-ray grating interferometry [41].

12.3 EFFECTS ON IMAGE QUALITY

We have now developed a sound understanding of the consequences of losing shift-invariance, and so it is time to turn to inspecting actual images. We will do so using the important example of spectrally resolved CT scans of a phantom containing solutions of iodine and gadolinium. Exhibiting K-edges at 33 and 50 keV, these contrast agents represent a well-accepted standard to study the spectral imaging properties of a photon counting detector.

12.3.1 Energy Resolved CT Images

A CT scan of a phantom containing iodine and gadolinium is shown in Figure 12.9. It was acquired using a Medipix3RX equipped with a 2-mm CdTe sensor and operated in both SPM (top row) as well as CSM (bottom row). The tube voltage was set to 120 kV to provide a broad spectrum of x-ray energies.

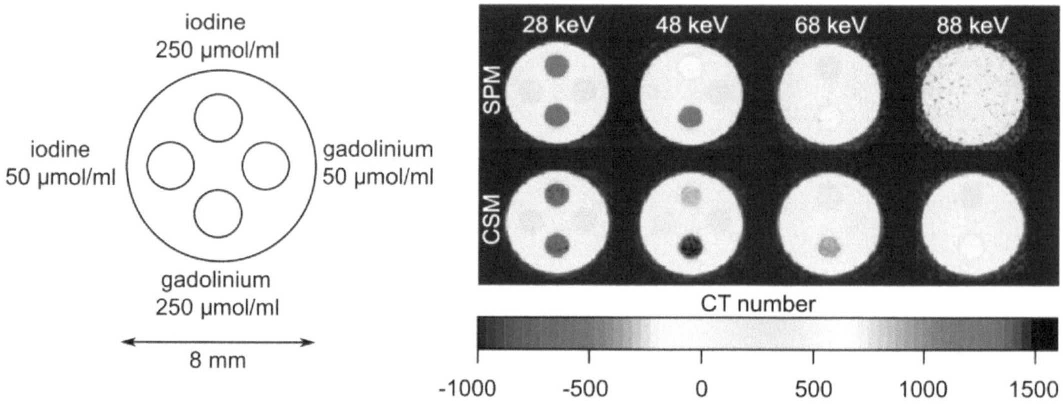

FIGURE 12.9 Left: Phantom made from PMMA, containing iodine and gadolinium contrast agents at two concentrations. Right: Slices extracted from two spectral CT scans of this phantom [39], using energy thresholds ranging from 28 keV to 88 keV. No further binning into energy windows was performed, that is, there was no upper bound on photon energies in each of the four channels. SPM: single pixel mode; CSM: charge summing mode.

The probably most striking difference between the two modes of operation is represented by the noise visible for the energy threshold of 88 keV. Here, the reduced DQE in SPM, as observed in Figure 12.8a, leads to a substantial noise increase, compared to the CSM scan.

The next feature that differentiates the two scans is the visibility of the gadolinium K-edge. It manifests itself in the CSM measurement (bottom capillary) when raising the threshold from 28 keV to 48 keV, but not in the SPM scan. Last but not least, the contrast of the capillaries with regard to the PMMA background is strongly increased when activating CSM, owing to the better spectroscopic resolution that is a defining characteristic of this mode.

To summarize, both noise and contrast are improved when shift-invariance is restored by employing charge summing. The first effect is due to an improved DQE, the second one because of a much better spectral resolution. In combination, both lead to a twofold improvement in contrast-to-noise ratio [39] (CNR). The CNR is known to be proportional to the square of the radiation dose. Consequently, charge summing allows us to lower x-ray exposure by a factor of four to arrive at the same image quality as we obtained in SPM. This reduction of radiation dose is substantial.

Ultimately, we are now ready to find out how this translates to the accuracy of material decomposition, the probably most exciting application of multi-energy CT.

12.3.2 Material Decomposition

In Figure 12.10 we find material-specific images that were extracted from the spectral CT-scans shown in Figure 12.9. Material decomposition was performed in the CT domain using a linear model, that is, the material-specific images are linear combinations of the multi-energy images. The model was trained using a least squares regression to recover the ground truth [39].

Inspecting Figure 12.10, it is not hard to again find a difference in noise when comparing SPM with CSM, the former showing a comparably strong noise component that is visible for each of the three materials. In particular, the difference in density between the PMMA phantom material (1.18 g/cm^3) and the water contained within the contrast agent solutions (1 g/cm^3) is barely visible here. Charge summing, on the contrary, resolves this density contrast much better. It also reveals the existence of the lower of the two gadolinium concentrations, whose existence is mostly concealed within the SPM scan.

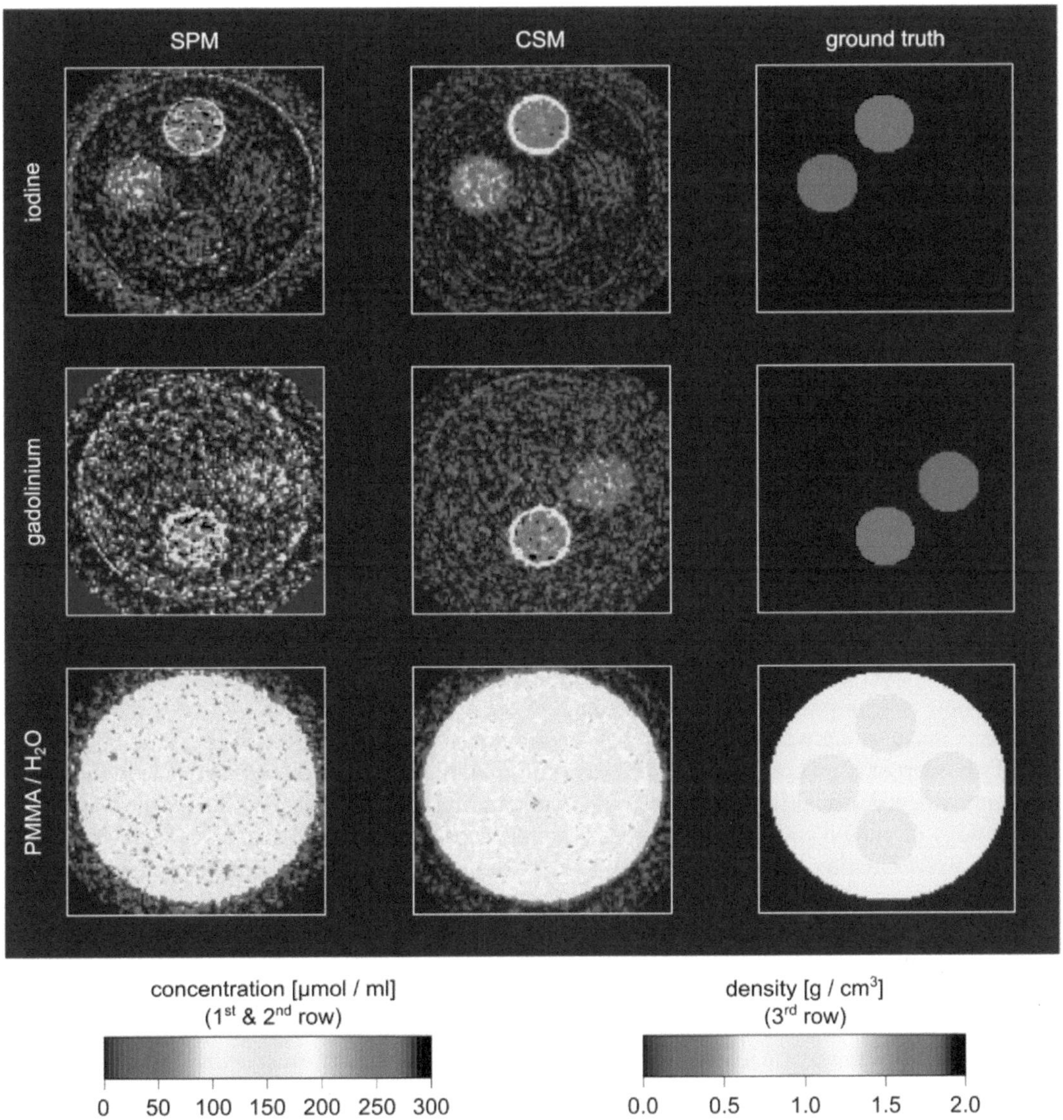

FIGURE 12.10 Material-specific images extracted from the two spectral CT scans shown in Figure 12.9 [39]. SPM: single pixel mode; CSM: charge summing mode.

The attentive reader who closely examines these material-specific CT slices will also identify another important difference between the two modes of operation: The SPM measurement is notably sharper than its CSM counterpart, which is best visible when comparing the two iodine images. It is tempting to blame the threshold dependent PSF as the origin of this behavior, and certainly this effect contributes to some extent. However, charge summing introduces yet another source of blurring to a photon counter: If the energy of a secondary photon is larger than the energy deposited at the original site of interaction, a hit will be assigned to where the secondary photon was reabsorbed. This can be directly concluded from the working principle of charge summing, which ensures to assign a hit to the pixel receiving most of the charge. While this effect does not increase image noise, it represents a source of blurring especially for characteristic x-rays, which are emitted isotropically within the CdTe sensor under study, and with a yield of more than 80%. Hence, the only way to efficiently suppress this blurring is to use photon energies that are at least twice the energy of the largest fluorescence energy occurring.

12.4 SUMMARY & OUTLOOK

Linearity and shift-invariance are properties that are convenient to assume when describing signal and image processing systems. They allow to construct models in a time- or position-invariant fashion and so can help limit both analytic as well as computational complexity. Even though these assumptions are almost never perfectly fulfilled, many systems can still be treated as if they were. Conventional, energy integrating detectors are examples of such behavior if one carefully handles the subtraction of dark-current and the saturation of scintillators at high x-ray fluxes. Most importantly, their response to radiation exhibits, in good approximation, translational invariance in the detector plane. Even though photodiodes usually do not cover a pixel completely, it does not really matter where a photon interacts with the scintillator within this plane.

As I have explained in this chapter, photon counting detectors behave differently. First of all, they are highly nonlinear due to a binary decision-making that each and every pulse recorded within a pixel is subject to. The decision to make here is whether to increment a counter or not. There is only yes or no, but nothing in-between. Unlike the digitization in energy integrating detectors, which is performed upon readout after exposure, this represents a source of error that applies to every single event. In a certain sense, this represents a rounding error of a number between zero and one, and that sometimes becomes zero, and sometimes one. As we have seen, this results in a quantization error that can have a large impact on image quality.

I have demonstrated how this quantization error, caused by nonlinearity, introduces shift-variance. Charge sharing, the reabsorption of characteristic x-rays as well as incoherent scattering all lead to a varying number of pixels responding to an initial photon interaction. A detector's DQE relates to the average and, in particular, to the variance of this number. This variance is directly connected to image noise, along with lost events that remain undetected because they occurred too close to a pixel's border, or if an energy threshold was set too high. Energy thresholds are indeed the core to the binary decision-making that enables photon counting, but they are also the reason for why the technology of photon counting offers spectroscopic capabilities. Representing a sought-for feature, energy discrimination suffers even more from shift-variance because it requires spreading energy thresholds across a large part of the x-ray spectrum under consideration. The loss of counts due to shift-variance can be extreme in these applications because high energy thresholds make pixels become more and more insensitive to the incoming radiation, by shrinking a pixel's active area more and more toward its center. The resulting split events are only recorded by the lower energy thresholds (if at all), and severely distort a detector's ability to discriminate photons by their energy.

Indeed, it was the desire to obtain an improved spectroscopic performance, not to improve DQE, that stimulated researchers around the world to propose and successfully implement a strategy to restore shift-invariance: inter-pixel communication. If designed with care, a clever combination of analog and digital features allows to establish an adaptive neighborhood that centers around each individual hit. If a charge cloud's size is smaller than this charge collection area, it is no longer possible for it to be split into multiple low-energy events. No matter whether a photon hits a pixel at its borders or at its center, it is correctly counted, and its energy is correctly measured.

Deviations from this ideal behavior arise by inevitable effects such as the emission and potential reabsorption of characteristic x-rays within the sensor, along with incoherently scattered photons. These do not have a finite range, and so some of them are able to travel beyond what is covered by a collection area. How many these are depends on the sensor material and the extent of the adaptively forming collection area. The pixel size therefore remains a crucial design element that goes beyond spatial resolution.

Inter-pixel communication also has drawbacks. First of all, it requires a thorough design to be implemented successfully. Next, the necessary changes to the analog electronics contained within a pixel are both substantial and technologically challenging. This also raises the costs to manufacture such ASICs on an industrial scale with a high yield. Last but not least, there are also disadvantages during operation, one of which is the increase in noise, usually reported as the equivalent noise charge (ENC). While the negative effects of the resulting peak broadening are easily outweighed by the almost complete suppression of a charge sharing tail, an increased ENC also affects the minimum threshold that can be set during operation without flooding the counters with noise. As an example, an ENC increase of around a factor of two was reported for the Medipix3RX when activating charge summing [10].

Another effect that can arise from inter-pixel communication is the allocation of an event to the wrong pixel that can occur in the case of a secondary photon carrying away more than half of the primary photon's energy. This represents a compelling example of how a lack of shift-invariance trades low noise for high sharpness.

X-ray detectors are tools used in x-ray imaging. As such, photon counting detectors must not only be compared to and benchmarked against each other. Instead, all competing technologies must be considered in a fair and unbiased comparison to assess whether photon counting brings a true benefit. Energy integrating detectors, in fact, comprise a wide range of technologies and commercial designs. While those flat panel detectors that employ thin film transistors on amorphous silicon have been the hallmark of modern cone beam x-ray imaging, this technology is now being replaced by one relying on CMOS electronics more and more. CMOS technology is also the basis of photon counting detectors and enables integrating complex and low-noise signal amplification electronics into each individual pixel. Consequently, the x-ray images produced by CMOS-based energy integrating detectors are known to show very little readout noise or dark current. Unlike photon counting detectors, energy integrating detection concepts based on CMOS technology do not suffer from the multiple counting of events, or their complete loss. In addition, they are a lot cheaper to fabricate in comparison to photon counting detectors (at the time of writing). It will therefore be very interesting to see which concept will prevail, and it may well be that different applications will require different kinds of detectors even in the distant future. Either way, there will be an abundance of questions to study and comparisons to make, and the science of x-ray detection is very likely to remain an exciting field for many years to come.

REFERENCES

1. M. Campbell et al. "Readout for a 64 × 64 pixel matrix with 15-bit single photon counting". In: *IEEE Trans. Nucl. Sci.* 45 (3) (1998), p. 751.
2. X. Llopart et al. "Medipix2: A 64-k pixel readout chip with 55-μm square elements working in single photon counting mode". In: *IEEE Trans. Nucl. Sci.* 49 (5) (2002), p. 2279.
3. R. Ballabriga et al. "The Medipix3 prototype, a pixel readout chip working in single photon counting mode with improved spectrometric performance". In: *Nuclear Science Symposium Conference Record, 2006. IEEE.* 6 (2007), p. 3557.
4. J. Schlomka et al. "Experimental feasibility of multi-energy photon-counting K-edge imaging in pre-clinical computed tomography". In: *Phys. Med. Biol.* 53 (15) (2008), p. 4031.
5. T. G. Schmidt. "Optimal "image-based" weighting for energy-resolved CT". In: *Med. Phys.* 36 (7) (2009), p. 3018.
6. B. Henrich et al. "PILATUS: A single photon counting pixel detector for x-ray applications". In: *Nuclear Instruments and Methods in Physics Research Section A: Accelerators, Spectrometers, Detectors and Associated Equipment.* 607 (1) (2009), p. 247.
7. M. F. Walsh et al. "First CT using Medipix3 and the MARS-CT-3 spectral scanner". In: *J. Inst.* 6 (01) (2011), p. C01095.
8. S. Kappler et al. "First results from a hybrid prototype CT scanner for exploring benefits of quantum-counting in clinical CT". In: *Medical Imaging 2012: Physics of Medical Imaging.* 8313. International Society for Optics and Photonics, 2012, p. 83130X.
9. T. Koenig et al. "Imaging properties of small-pixel spectroscopic x-ray detectors based on cadmium telluride sensors". In: *Phys. Med. Biol.* 57 (21) (2012), p. 6743.
10. R. Ballabriga et al. "The Medipix3RX: a high resolution, zero dead-time pixel detector readout chip allowing spectroscopic imaging". In: *J. Inst.* 8 (02) (2013), p. C02016.
11. K. Taguchi and J. S. Iwanczyk. "Vision 20/20: Single photon counting x-ray detectors in medical imaging". In: *Med. Phys.* 40 (10) (2013), p. 100901.

12. H. Chen et al. "A photon-counting silicon-strip detector for digital mammography with an ultrafast 0.18 μm CMOS ASIC". In: *Nuclear Instruments and Methods in Physics Research Section A: Accelerators, Spectrometers, Detectors and Associated Equipment.* 749 (2014), p. 1.
13. M. Persson et al. "Energy-resolved CT imaging with a photon-counting silicon-strip detector". In: *Phys. Med. Biol.* 59 (22) (2014), p. 6709.
14. E. Hamann et al. "Performance of a medipix3rx spectroscopic pixel detector with a high resistivity gallium arsenide sensor". In: *IEEE Trans. Med. Imag.* 34 (3) (2015), p. 707.
15. S. Faby et al. "Performance of today's dual energy CT and future multi energy CT in virtual non-contrast imaging and in iodine quantification: A simulation study". In: *Med. Phys.* 42 (7) (2015), p. 4349.
16. K. C. Zimmerman and T. G. Schmidt. "Experimental comparison of empirical material decomposition methods for spectral CT". In: *Phys. Med. Biol.* 60 (8) (2015), p. 3175.
17. Z. Yu et al. "Evaluation of conventional imaging performance in a research whole-body CT system with a photon-counting detector array". In: *Phys. Med. Biol.* 61 (4) (2016), p. 1572.
18. M. Bochenek et al. "IBEX: Versatile readout ASIC with spectral imaging capability and high count rate capability". In: *IEEE Trans. Nucl. Sci.* 65 (6) (2018), p. 1285.
19. R. Ballabriga et al. "Review of hybrid pixel detector readout ASICs for spectroscopic x-ray imaging". In: *J. Inst.* 11 (01) (2016), p. P01007.
20. P. Vagovič et al. "X-ray Bragg magnifier microscope as a linear shift invariant imaging system: Image formation and phase retrieval". In: *Opt. Express.* 22 (18) (2014), p. 21508.
21. M. Firsching et al. "Contrast agent recognition in small animal CT using the Medipix2 detector". *In: Nucl. Instr. and Meth. A.* 607 (1) (2009), p. 179.
22. C. O. Schirra et al. "Spectral CT: A technology primer for contrast agent development". In: *Contrast Media Mol Imaging.* 9 (1) (2014), p. 62.
23. T. Koenig et al. "Pooling optimal combinations of energy thresholds in spectroscopic CT". In: *Proc. SPIE, Medical Imaging: Physics of Medical Imaging.* 9033 (2014), pp. 90331A–90331A.
24. M. Touch et al. "A neural network-based method for spectral distortion correction in photon counting x-ray CT". In: *Phys. Med. Biol.* 61 (16) (2016), p. 6132.
25. S. Leng et al. "Spectral performance of a whole-body research photon counting detector CT: Quantitative accuracy in derived image sets". In: *Phys Med Biol.* 62 (17) (2017), p. 7216.
26. C. H. McCollough et al. "Dual- and multi-energy CT: Principles, technical approaches, and clinical applications". In: *Radiology.* 276 (3) (2015), p. 637.
27. M. Zuber et al. "Characterization of a 2x3 timepix assembly with a 500 um thick silicon sensor". In: *J. Inst.* 9 (05) (2014), p. C05037.
28. P. M. Shikhaliev, S. G. Fritz, and J. W. Chapman. "Photon counting multienergy x-ray imaging: Effect of the characteristic x rays on detector performance". In: *Med. Phys.* 36 (2009), p. 5107.
29. H. Ding, J. L. Ducote, and S. Molloi. "Breast composition measurement with a cadmium-zinc-telluride based spectral computed tomography system". In: *Med. Phys.* 39 (3) (2012), p. 1289.
30. E. Hamann et al. "Investigation of GaAs:Cr timepix assemblies under high flux irradiation". In: *J. Inst.* 10 (01) (2015), p. C01047.
31. T. Michel et al. "A fundamental method to determine the signal-to-noise ratio (SNR) and detective quantum efficiency (DQE) for a photon counting pixel detector". In: *Nucl. Instr. and Meth. A.* 568 (2) (2006), p. 799.
32. S. Faby et al. "An efficient computational approach to model statistical correlations in photon counting x-ray detectors". In: *Med. Phys.* 43 (7) (2016), p. 3945.
33. J. Tanguay et al. "Detective quantum efficiency of photon-counting x-ray detectors". In: *Med Phys.* 42 (1) (2015), p. 491.
34. X. Ji et al. "Impact of anti-charge sharing on the zero-frequency detective quantum efficiency of CdTe-based photon counting detector system: Cascaded systems analysis and experimental validation". In: *Phys Med Biol.* 63 (9) (2018), p. 095003.
35. K. Taguchi et al. "An analytical model of the effects of pulse pileup on the energy spectrum recorded by energy resolved photon counting x-ray detectors". In: *Med. Phys.* 37 (8) (2010), p. 3957.
36. K. Rink et al. "Investigating the feasibility of photon-counting K-edge imaging at high x-ray fluxes using nonlinearity corrections". In: *Med. Phys.* 40 (10) (2013), p. 101908.
37. C. Ullberg et al. "Measurements of a dual-energy fast photon counting CdTe detector with integrated charge sharing correction". In: *Proc. SPIE.* 8668 (2013), pp. 86680P–86680P.
38. T. Koenig et al. "Charge summing in spectroscopic x-ray detectors with high-Z sensors". In: *IEEE Trans. Nucl. Sci.* 60 (6) (2013), p. 4713.

39. T. Koenig et al. "How spectroscopic x-ray imaging benefits from inter-pixel communication". In: *Phys. Med. Biol.* 59 (20) (2014), p. 6195.
40. E. Frojdh et al. "Count rate linearity and spectral response of the Medipix3RX chip coupled to a 300 μm silicon sensor under high UX conditions". In: *J. Inst.* 9 (04) (2014), p. C04028.
41. T. Koenig et al. "On the origin and nature of the grating interferometric dark-field contrast obtained with low-brilliance x-ray sources". In: *Phys. Med. Biol.* 61 (9) (2016), p. 3427.
42. L. Tlustos et al. "Imaging properties of the Medipix2 system exploiting single and dual energy thresholds". In: *IEEE Trans. Nucl. Sci.* 53 (1-2) (2006), p. 367.

13 Signal Generation in Semiconductor Detectors for Photon-Counting CT

Xiaochun Lai, Liang Cai, Kevin Zimmerman, and Richard Thompson
Canon Medical Research Inc. Vernon Hills, Illinois, USA

CONTENTS

13.1 INTRODUCTION

As an emerging spectral computed tomography (CT) technique, photon-counting CT has great potential of changing clinical CT applications and has been of great research and development interest both within academia and industry. A typical photon-counting CT employs photon-counting detectors (PCDs) based on semiconductors, like cadmium zinc telluride (CZT), cadmium telluride (CdTe), or silicon (Si). PCDs record individual photons' interaction position and deposited energy, enabling a CT scanner to reveal patient's mass attenuation under different x-ray energies. This technique has potentials to reduce imaging noise and radiation dose, improve image resolution, achieve better material decomposition accuracy, enable multiple contrast imaging, and other new clinical applications [1].

The detector response of a PCD – *that is*, the recorded energy as a function of incident energy – is critical for detector design, performance evaluation, as well as performing material decomposition. The PCD response involves a complicated signal generation process, which includes various physics effects, such as x-ray interaction, fluorescence escape and re-abortion, charge sharing caused by charge transportation, etc. In this chapter, we will review the signal generation process in a typical PCD.

13.2 X-RAY INTERACTION WITHIN A SEMICONDUCTOR

Photon energies of a clinical CT range from 20 keV to 160 keV. Photoelectric interaction, Compton scattering, and Rayleigh scattering occur when a photon in this energy range interacts with the sensor. Compton scattering and photoelectric interaction play dominant roles, while Rayleigh scattering mainly dominates in the every low energy range (<10 keV). For example, when 122 keV photons interact with CdTe, 82.4% of the interactions are the photoelectric absorption, 10.7% Compton scattering, 6.9% Rayleigh scattering.

In the photoelectric interaction, a photon will be absorbed by a bonded electron in an atom. The inner shell electrons have a larger absorption cross section compared to that of the outer shell electrons. If the photon energy (E_γ) is higher than the electron binding energy (E_0), the electron will escape from the atom binding shell, and become a free electron with a kinetic energy of E_e given by:

$$E_e = E_\gamma - E_0. \tag{13.1}$$

The free and energetic electron will interact with the sensor, CdTe or CZT, through scattering, ionization, and Bremsstrahlung radiation. It could travel some distance away from the initial interaction position. The maximum travel distance can be described by Kanaya-Okayama (KO) radius [2]:

$$R_{KO} = 2.76 \times 10^{-7} \frac{A}{\rho Z^{\frac{8}{9}}} E_e^{\frac{5}{3}}, \tag{13.2}$$

where R_{KO} has a unit of μm, and A, Z, and ρ are effective mass number, atomic number, and density with a unit of g/cm^3, respectively. For a 120-keV gamma-ray, the free electron has a kinetic energy around 95 keV, and R_{KO} is around 34 μm.

After the photon-electron leaves the atom's binding shell, a vacancy is created, and the atom becomes excited. The de-excitation occurs through Auger electron ejection or x-ray fluorescence (k-shell fluorescence is around 27–31 keV for Te, 23–26 keV for Cd). As shown in Table 13.1, the Auger electron ejection counts for 25% of de-excitation events in CdTe, and the Auger electron travels a few microns. X-ray fluorescence events count the other 75%. The characteristic x-ray can possibly trigger a sequence of events. It could travel 100 μm away from the initial interaction position, x-ray fluorescence of a Te atom could be absorbed by a Cd atom through the photoelectric effect, and a second x-ray fluorescence could be generated through the de-excitation process of the Cd atom. This phenomenon will distribute the initial photon deposited energy in a much larger area compared to the travel range of the initial electron. As shown in Figure 13.1, the radius covering 95% deposited energy can be as large as 180 μm. This will play a significant role in the detector response, including the energy resolution and the detection efficiency, which will be covered in the later sections.

In Compton scattering, an incident photon is scattered by an electron with an angle, θ, along the original incident direction and part of the photon energy will be transferred to the electron. If the

TABLE 13.1
De-excitation Events for Photoelectric Interaction in CZT [3]

Fluorescence Number	Ratio (%)
0 (Auger)	25
1	45
2	25
>3	5
Fluorescence only	75
All events	100

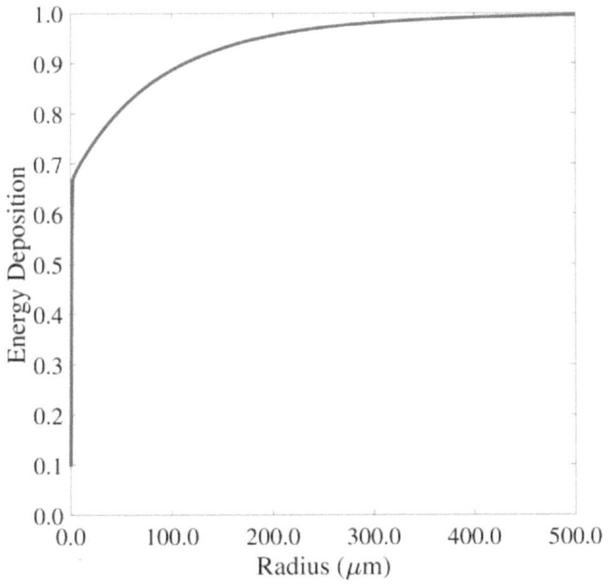

FIGURE 13.1 Energy deposition distribution when one million 60 keV x-rays interact with a CZT crystal. The x-axis is the distance away from the initial interaction position. The y-axis is percentage of energy deposited within the corresponding radius.

electron can be assumed to be free and at rest when the Doppler effect is not taken into account, the remaining energy of the scattered photon is described by [4],

$$E'_\gamma = \frac{E_\gamma}{1 + \frac{E_\gamma}{m_0 c^2}(1 - \cos\theta)}, \tag{13.3}$$

where $m_0 c^2 = 511$ keV is rest mass energy of an electron. For example, depending on the scattered angle, θ, the scattered photon energy for the 122 keV incident photon ranges from 122 keV to 82.6 keV, and the corresponding recoiled electron has an energy from 0 keV to 39.4 keV. Since the number of inner shell electrons is significantly less than that of outer shell electrons, Compton scattering mainly happens in the outer shell electrons and the characteristic x-ray escape effect can be ignored compared the photoelectric interaction.

13.2.1 Initial Charge Cloud Generated by Photon Interactions

Compton scattering and the photoelectric interaction will transfer either part or all of the photon energy to the interacted electron. The electron loses its energy through scattering, ionization of atoms, and Bremsstrahlung radiation. Consequently, the interaction generates phonons (lattice vibration) or electron-hole pairs in CdTe or CZT. The process of the electron-hole pair (N_{eh}) generation could be modeled as a Poisson process. Since the number of electron-hole pairs is on the order of 10,000, the process could be approximated by a Gaussian distribution:

$$P(N_{eh}) = \frac{1}{\sqrt{2\pi F \bar{N}_{eh}}} \exp\left[-\frac{(N_{eh} - \bar{N}_{eh})^2}{2F\bar{N}_{eh}}\right], \tag{13.4}$$

where the variance of the distribution, $F\bar{N}_{eh}$, illustrates the sub-Poisson behaviors of the process. For CdTe or CZT, the Fano factor F is around 0.12 [5]. The mean, $\bar{N}_{eh}$ is equal to E_e / ζ, where ζ is the

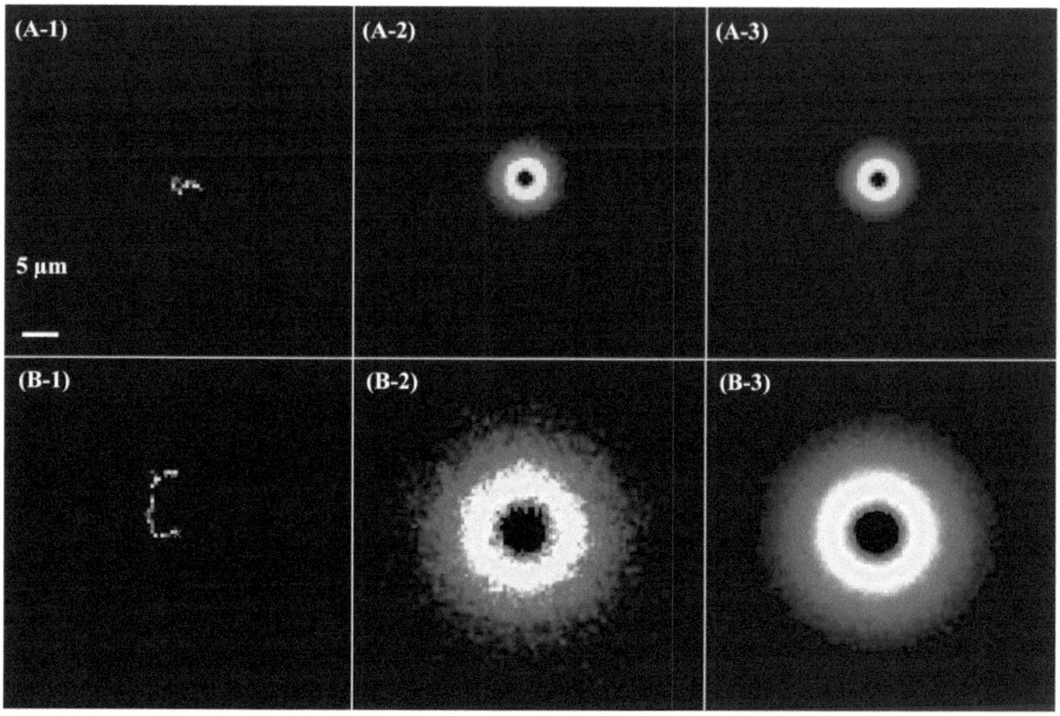

FIGURE 13.2 (A-1) charge distribution for a single 31 keV electron; (A-2) charge distribution for 10,000 electrons with energy of 31 keV; (A-3) charge distribution for 100,000 electrons with energy of 31 keV; except the photon energy, (B-1), (B-2), and (B-3) are similar to that of (A-1), (A-2), and (A-3), respectively. The photon has energy of 91 keV.

energy needed for generating an electron-hole pair. For CZT, it is 4.64 eV. E_e is the photon energy, here we assume the detector absorb all the photon energy. For a 122-keV photon, there are around 26,300 electron-pairs produced by the photoelectric effect.

The initial charge cloud (electrons and holes) spatial distribution can be assumed to be the same as the electron energy deposition profile. For a single electron interaction, it is quite random, as shown in Figure 13.2. But when we evaluate the detector response, the average behavior of hundreds or even thousands of events will be considered. Figure 13.2A and Figure 13.2B also show the charge distribution profile over 10 k and 100 k events with energy at 31 keV and 91 keV. The maximum distance that an electron can penetrate can be calculated by the KO radius in Eq. 13.2. However, it is significantly overestimated by charge cloud size. Figure 13.3 shows the radius covering 95% of the initial charge, which roughly equals to $0.42R_{KO}$.

13.3 CHARGE TRANSPORTATION

The detector is biased to collect the charges generated by x-ray interaction. The charges will drift along the electric field, *that is*, electrons drifting to the anodes and holes moving toward the cathode. The drift velocity of electrons and holes is proportional to the electric field strength, $\boldsymbol{E}_a$,

$$\boldsymbol{V}_{e/h} = \mu_{e/h}\boldsymbol{E}_a, \tag{13.5}$$

where $\mu_{e/h}$ is the electron/hole mobility. For CZT, the mobility is typically about $1000\ \text{cm}^2/\text{Vs}$ for electrons and $80\ \text{cm}^2/\text{Vs}$ for holes. If a 900-V bias voltage is applied to a 2-mm CZT

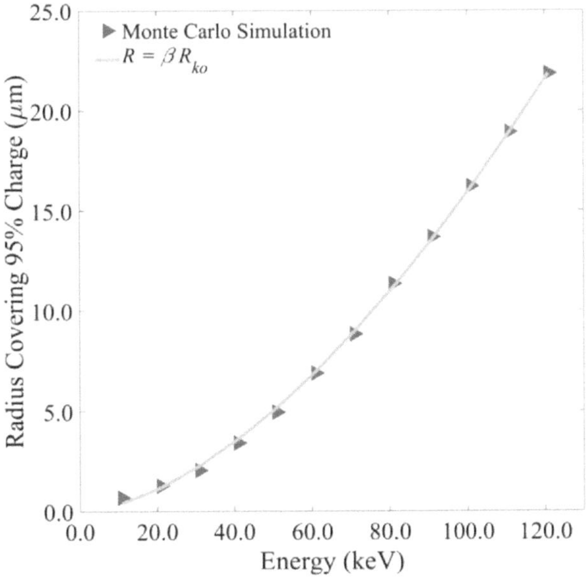

FIGURE 13.3 Radius covering 95% of charge, the solid triangle is derived from charge cloud generated by 10,000 electrons and solid curve shows βR_{KO}, where β equals to 0.42 and R_{KO} is the KO radius (Eq. 13.2).

crystal, it will generate an electric field with a strength of 450 V/mm. It takes around 44 ns for electrons to travel from the cathode to the anode pixel. The holes move around ten times slower than electrons.

When drifting along the electric field, random thermal motions of electrons (holes) will expand the charge cloud size. If we assume the initial charge cloud has a Gaussian distribution, the charge cloud will evolve as a Gaussian distribution with a standard deviation given by,

$$\sigma_T = \sqrt{2Dt + \sigma_0^2}, \tag{13.6}$$

where σ_0 is the initial size, and D is the diffusion coefficient, which is calculated by the *Einstein relation*,

$$D = \mu_{eh}\frac{KT}{e}, \tag{13.7}$$

where D is proportional to the electron/hole mobility, $\mu_{e/h}$, the Boltzmann constant (K), and the absolute temperature, T, in Kelvin; and e is the charge of an electron. At room temperature (25°C), $\frac{KT}{e}$ equals to 2.57 mV.

During charge transportation, crystal defects could trap the charge and prevent them from being collected by the electrodes. The duration of an electron and hole from its generation to being trapped is defined as the lifetime, $\tau_{e/h}$. For a hole in the CZT, the typical value is around 1 μs, and for the electrons, the value is around 3 μs. Since the electron lifetime is significantly larger than its drift time, electron trapping can be ignored. However, the hole drift time has a similar order of its lifetime, and it prevents the holes from being fully collected by the cathode. Consequently, it will degrade the detector energy resolving performance.

In the above, we discussed that the charge cloud distribution is affected by the applied electric field, the thermal diffusion, and charge trapping. The charge cloud size also is affected by self repulsion between electrons/holes. All of these factors are coupled together. For this case, there is no

TABLE 13.2
Materials Properties of CZT [6]

Electron Mobility (μ_e)	Electron Lifetime (τ_e)	Hole Mobility (μ_h)	Hole Lifetime (τ_h)	Permittivity (ϵ)
1000 cm²/Vs	3 μs	80 cm²/Vs	1 μs	9.4×10^{-13} F / cm

simple solution, like Eq. 13.6, anymore. To accurately model these effects, we have to solve charge transportation partial differential equations. For the electron cloud, we have,

$$\frac{\mathrm{d}}{\mathrm{d}t} q_{em}(\boldsymbol{r},t) = D_e \nabla^2 q_{em}(\boldsymbol{r},t) - \mu_e \nabla \cdot (q_{em}(\boldsymbol{r},t)\boldsymbol{E}_e) - \frac{q_{em}(\boldsymbol{r},t)}{\tau_e}, \tag{13.8}$$

$$\frac{\mathrm{d}}{\mathrm{d}t} q_{es}(\boldsymbol{r},t) = \frac{q_{em}(\boldsymbol{r},t)}{\tau_e}, \tag{13.9}$$

where the electron cloud ($q_e(\boldsymbol{r},t)$) includes a moving part ($q_{em}(\boldsymbol{r},t)$) and a trapped part ($q_{es}(\boldsymbol{r},t)$). The moving part will be affected by three terms. The first one is diffusion, *that is,* $D_e \nabla^2 q_{em}(\boldsymbol{r},t)$. The second term is a convectional term, *that is,* $\mu_e \nabla \cdot (q_{em}(\boldsymbol{r},t)\boldsymbol{E}_e)$. It models the charge convection caused by the electric field ($\boldsymbol{E}_e$). The last term is the trapping term, *that is,* $\frac{q_{em}(\boldsymbol{r},t)}{\tau_e}$. Typical material properties of CZT are shown in Table 13.2.

The term, $\boldsymbol{E}_e$, in Eq. 13.8 includes the applied electric field ($\boldsymbol{E}_a$) generated by the high-voltage bias and the electric field generated by the electron cloud itself, which models the charge repulsion effect. Here we did not take into account interaction between holes and electrons, because electrons and holes will be separated in a 0.1 ns time scale and after that the interaction between holes and electrons will be reduced rapidly by the inverse of the distance squared. $\boldsymbol{E}_e = \nabla \phi(\mathbf{r},t)$, which is given by

$$\begin{aligned} \nabla^2 \phi(\mathbf{r},t) &= \frac{1}{\epsilon} q_e(\mathbf{r},t), && \text{if } \mathbf{r} \in V, \\ \phi(\mathbf{r},t) &= f(\mathbf{r}), && \text{if } \mathbf{r} \in \partial V, \end{aligned} \tag{13.10}$$

where ϵ is permittivity of CZT. The boundary condition consists of the high voltage (HV) bias applied between the cathode and anodes.

For the hole cloud, we have,

$$\frac{\mathrm{d}}{\mathrm{d}t} q_{hm}(\boldsymbol{r},t) = D_h \nabla^2 q_{hm}(\boldsymbol{r},t) - \mu_h \nabla \cdot (q_{hm}(\boldsymbol{r},t)\boldsymbol{E}_h) - \frac{q_{hm}(\boldsymbol{r},t)}{\tau_h}, \tag{13.11}$$

$$\frac{\mathrm{d}}{\mathrm{d}t} q_{hs}(\boldsymbol{r},t) = \frac{q_{hm}(\boldsymbol{r},t)}{\tau_h}, \tag{13.12}$$

where the notations of Eqs. 13.11 and 13.12 are the same as Eqs. 13.8 and 13.9, except the subscript "*e*" is for the electron cloud and "*h*" for the hole cloud.

Figure 13.4A shows a 2D profile as the charge cloud drifts toward the anode, and corresponding radius (R_{95}) covering 95% of the charge cloud is shown in Figure 13.4B. The initial size of the charge cloud has a radius around 6.5 μm. The thermal diffusion and charge repulsion expand the radius to around 45.0 μm when the cloud reaches the anode side. The overall size ($2R_{95}$, *i.e.*, 90 μm) is comparable to a small anode pitch, like 250 μm. Figure 13.4B also shows that the model, without considering the repulsion effect, significantly underestimates the charge cloud size by around 20%. When the charge repulsion is not taken into account, only thermal diffusion will expand the charge cloud size, the solution of PDE in Eq. 13.8 is the same as the widely used empirical formula in Eq. 13.6. The empirical formula significantly underestimates the charge cloud size change over time by around 20%.

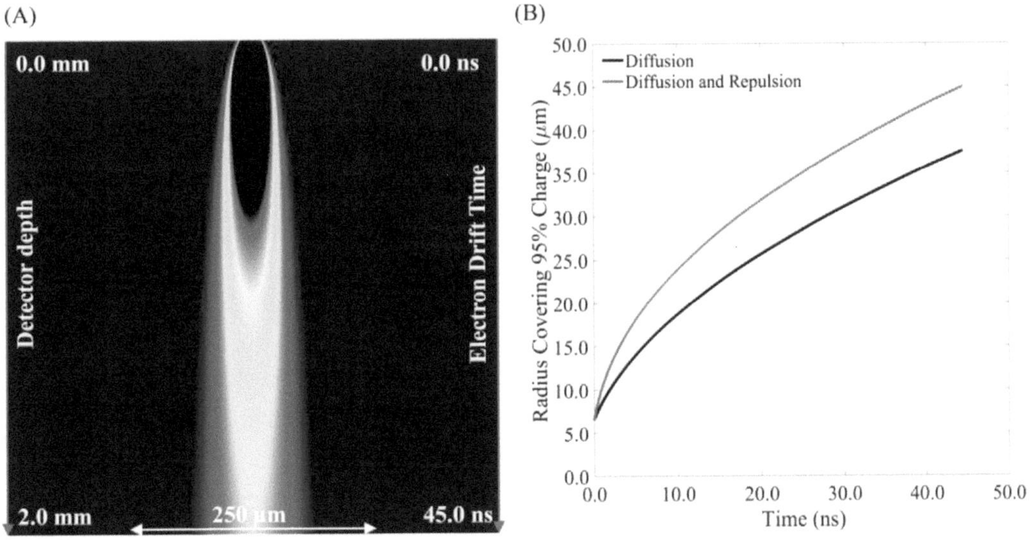

FIGURE 13.4 Illustration of electron cloud distribution change over time when the cloud drifts toward the cathode. (A) is the 2D profile; (B) shows radius covering 95% of the charge cloud. The solid red curve considers both repulsion and diffusion effect, while the solid black curve only incorporates the thermal diffusion effect.

Figure 13.5 shows the charge cloud size evolution for 30 keV, 60 keV, and 120 keV events. The corresponding initial sizes of these charge clouds have a radius around 2.1 μm, 6.5 μm, and 21.0 μm, respectively. The thermal diffusion and charge repulsion expand the radius to 41.8 μm, 45.0 μm, and 51.3 μm as the cloud reaches the anode side. As expected, the cloud size differences are reduced over time.

13.4 SHOCKLEY RAMO THEOREM

As the charge cloud ($q(\boldsymbol{r},t)$) evolves over time and space, it will generate a time-varying electric potential, and induce charges on the electrodes. It is challenging to directly solve the Maxwell equations to get the electric potential because of coupling between the magnetic field and the electric field in these equations. Since the charge density change is sufficiently slow and the quasistatic assumption is satisfied [7], the electric potential could be solved using electrostatics given by,

$$\begin{aligned} \nabla^2\phi(\mathbf{r},t) &= \frac{1}{\epsilon}q(\mathbf{r},t), && \text{if } \mathbf{r}\in V, \\ \phi(\mathbf{r},t) &= f(\mathbf{r}), && \text{if } \mathbf{r}\in \partial V, \end{aligned} \tag{13.13}$$

where ϵ is the dielectric constant of the semiconductor. With the boundary condition, we can solve the equation and get the charge induced in the detector electrodes. There are several approaches that could be used to get the induced charge, like the Green function method [8]. The Shockley-Ramo theorem [9, 10] is also commonly used, and it states that charge Q on an electrode induced by a moving point charge q is given by,

$$Q = -q\psi(\mathbf{r}), \tag{13.14}$$

where $\psi(\mathbf{r})$ are called the weighting potential. Dr. Z. He has published a review paper regarding the Shockley-Ramo theorem, where he proved the theorem through energy conservation [11].

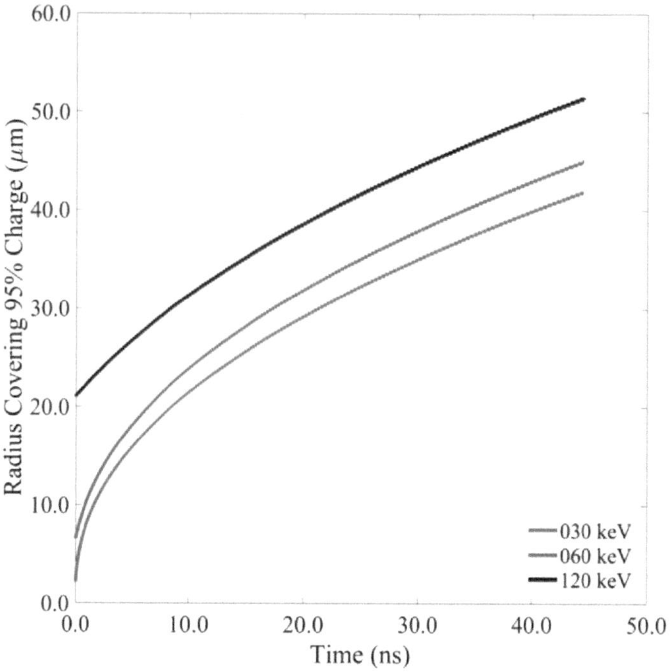

FIGURE 13.5 Charge cloud size with various deposited energy. The simulated electron clouds are generated by energy deposition at the cathode from 30 keV, 60 keV, and 120 keV x-rays, respectively. The corresponding initial sizes have radius of 2.1 μm, 6.5 μm, and 21.0 μm, respectively.

In the following section, we will revisit a proof of Shockley-Ramo theorem [9, 10] to help us better understand weighting potential and expand its application from a point charge to a spatially distributed charge cloud.

Based on the superposition principle, we can decompose the potential in Eq. 13.13, $\phi(\mathbf{r},t)=\phi_0(\mathbf{r},t)+\phi_1(\mathbf{r})$, and $\phi_0(\mathbf{r},t)$ and $\phi_1(\mathbf{r},t)$ satisfy the PDEs given by,

$$\begin{aligned} \nabla^2\phi_0(\mathbf{r},t) &= \frac{1}{\epsilon}q(\mathbf{r},t), \quad \text{if } \mathbf{r}\in V, \\ \phi_0(\mathbf{r},t) &= 0, \quad \text{if } \mathbf{r}\in \partial V, \end{aligned} \tag{13.15}$$

$$\begin{aligned} \nabla^2\phi_1(\mathbf{r}) &= 0, \quad \text{if } \mathbf{r}\in V, \\ \phi_1(t) &= f(\mathbf{r}), \quad \text{if } \mathbf{r}\in \partial V, \end{aligned} \tag{13.16}$$

The term, $\phi_0(\mathbf{r},t)$ is induced by the time varied charge cloud with the ground boundary condition. The term, $\phi_1(\mathbf{r})$ is the static potential generated by the boundary potential of $f(\mathbf{r})$. And the induced charge on the electrodes (anodes or cathode) decomposes to two parts,

$$Q(t)=Q_0(t)+Q_1, \tag{13.17}$$

where $Q_0(t)$ is the electrode charge induced by the time varied field $\phi_0(\mathbf{r},t)$ and Q_1 is the charge on the electrodes induced by the static potential $\phi_1(\mathbf{r})$. Since we are interested in the charge induced by $q(\mathbf{r},t)$, we will focus on the time varied part, $\phi_0(\mathbf{r},t)$, and the corresponding induced charge, $Q_0(t)$. Assuming we are interested in the charge on one specific electrode, $\boldsymbol{i}$, the charge, $Q_0^i(t)$, could be calculated by,

$$Q_0^i(t) = \oint_{\partial V^i} \epsilon \nabla \phi_0(\mathbf{r},t)\,\mathbf{ds}. \tag{13.18}$$

To calculate the charge, we play a math trick as Ramo did in his paper [10] and induce another potential, called the weighting potential, $\psi(\mathbf{r})$,

$$\begin{aligned} \nabla^2\psi(\mathbf{r}) &= 0, \quad \text{if } \mathbf{r} \in V, \\ \psi(\mathbf{r}) &= 1, \quad \text{if } \mathbf{r} \in \partial V^i, \text{ other boundaries equals zero,} \end{aligned} \tag{13.19}$$

where $\psi(\mathbf{r})$ is equal to one volt in the electrode of interest and zero elsewhere.

According to Gauss's theorem, we have

$$\oint_{\partial V} [\phi_0(\mathbf{r},t)\nabla\psi(\mathbf{r}) - \psi(\mathbf{r})\nabla\phi_0(\mathbf{r},t)]\mathbf{ds} = \iiint_V \nabla\cdot[\phi_0(\mathbf{r},t)\nabla\psi(\mathbf{r}) - \psi(\mathbf{r})\nabla\phi_0(\mathbf{r},t)]\,d^3\mathbf{r}. \tag{13.20}$$

Applying the boundary conditions in Eqs. 13.15 and 13.19 into the left-hand side of Eq. 13.20,

$$\oint_{\partial V^i} \nabla\phi_0(\mathbf{r})\,\mathbf{ds} = \frac{Q_0^i(t)}{\epsilon}, \tag{13.21}$$

where equal relation is based on Eq. 13.18.

The right-hand side of Eq. 13.20 can be simplified by using PDEs in Eqs. 13.15 and 13.19

$$\iiint_V \phi_0(\mathbf{r},t)\nabla^2\psi(\mathbf{r}) - \iiint_V \psi(\mathbf{r})\nabla^2\phi_0(\mathbf{r},t) = -\iiint_V \frac{1}{\epsilon}\psi q(\mathbf{r},t)\mathbf{dr}. \tag{13.22}$$

We can get the induced charge on the $\boldsymbol{i}^{th}$ electrode based on Eqs. 13.20, 13.21, and 13.22:

$$Q_0^i(t) = -\iiint_V q(\mathbf{r},t)\psi(\mathbf{r})\mathrm{d}^3\mathbf{r}, \tag{13.23}$$

where the charge induced on the electrode depends on the spatial integration of the product of the charge distribution and the weighting potential.

Based on Eq. 13.19, we can calculate the weighting potential of the electrodes. It is worthy to point out that the weighting potential does NOT physically exist and it is just a virtual potential used to calculate the induced charge at specific electrodes, and it is NOT the potential generated by the bias voltage that we apply to the electrode to collect the charges. Figure 13.6 shows the weighted potential for the different size of anodes in a 2-mm detector, including the parallel plane (an infinitely large anode pixel), and the anodes with pitch sizes of 250 μm and 500 μm. Figure 13.6 shows the corresponding line profiles in the pitch center. The weighting potential strongly depends on the anode size (Figure 13.7). The weighting potential for the parallel plane slowly increase linearly from zero at the cathode to one at the anode. In comparison, the weighting potentials for a small pixel

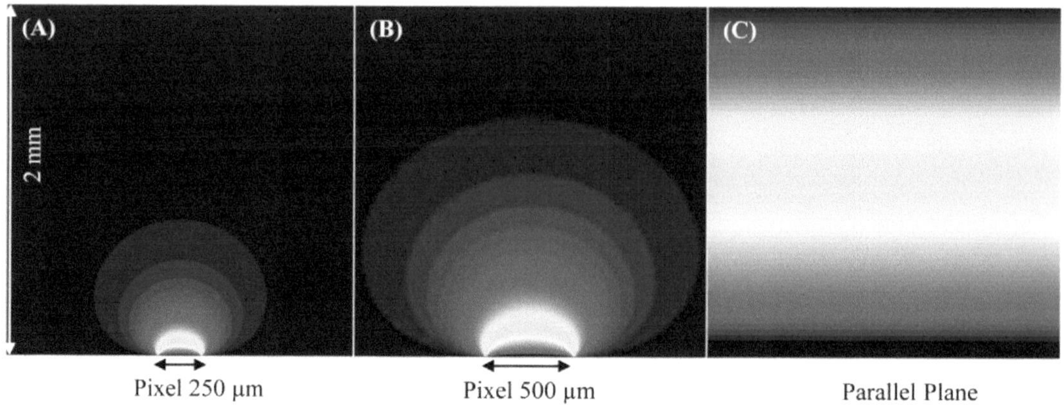

FIGURE 13.6 Weighting potentials for different electrode sizes. (A), (B), and (C) show weighting potential profiles for anode pixel 250 μm, 500 μm, and parallel plane, respectively.

detector has value around zero among most regions and sharply increases to one when the position approaches the anode. Due to weighting potential difference, the induced charge is also strongly dependent on the anode size.

Figure 13.8 shows charge induction on the anodes with varied pitch sizes. The induced charge at the anode has a fast component in the first 22 ns, mainly caused by the electron rapidly drifting toward the anode. It also has a slow component, which ends at 280 ns and is caused by the holes slowly moving toward the cathode. The total portion of the fast component contribution increases as anode size decreases. The fast component contributes 99% of the total induced

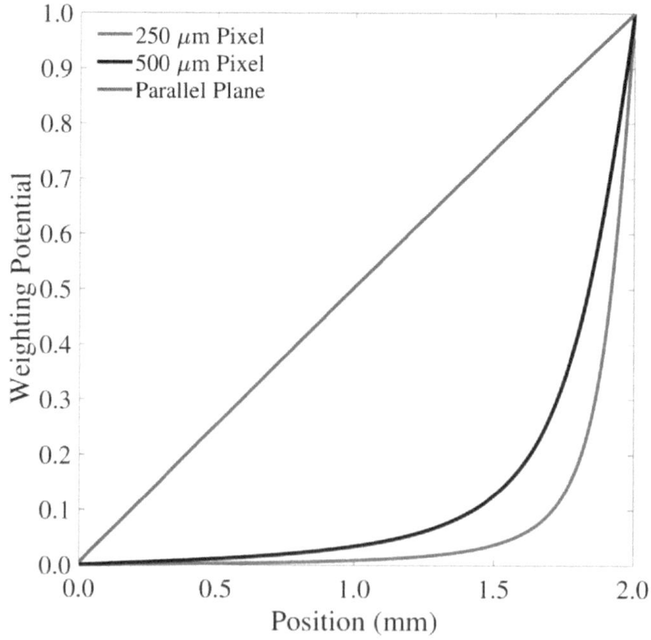

FIGURE 13.7 Weighting potential line profiles at the center of the pixel, with the position starting from the cathode and ending at the anode.

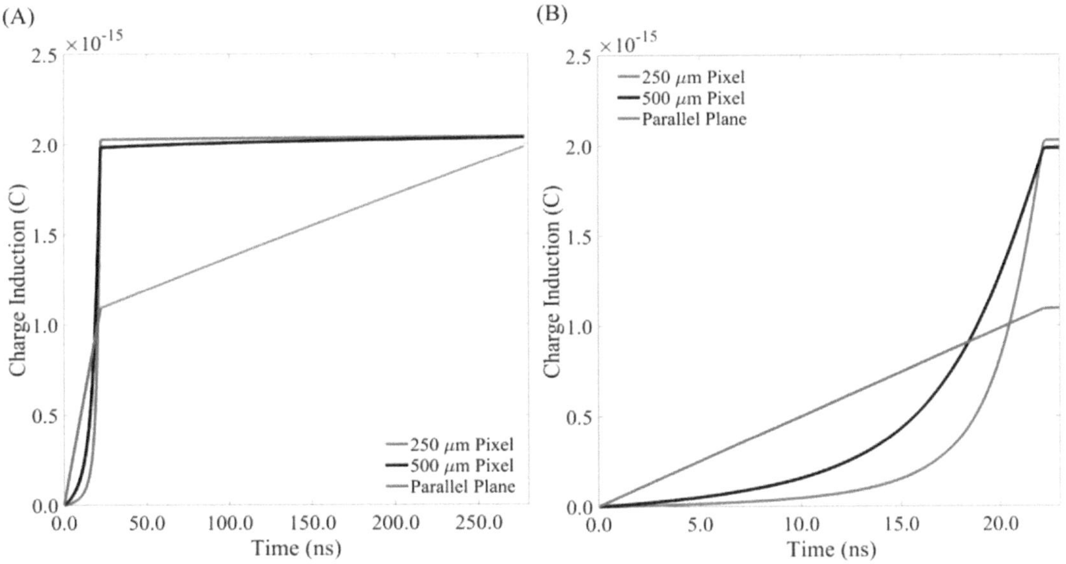

FIGURE 13.8 Charge induction on anodes with varied sizes. (A) shows the induction charge on anode pixel 250 μm, 500 μm, and parallel plane, respectively. 60 keV energy is absorbed at the center of the anode in the lateral direction and 1 mm away from the pixel center in the depth direction, 900 V bias is applied to a 2-mm CZT; (B) shows the first 20 ns profile of induction charge.

charge in the 250 μm anode, 97% in the 500 μm, and 55% in the parallel plane. The total induced charge varies with the anode size. The total induced charge is equal to 98.7% of the charge generated by energy deposition in the 250 μm anode, 98.3% in 500 μm anode, and 96.0% in the parallel plane. The lost part is caused by charge trapping, mainly from hole trapping. Smaller pixel is less impacted by trapping effect, because the charge induced by the electrons contributes to the most part of total induced charge. In Figure 13.8B, for the 250 μm anode, it takes roughly 8 ns for the induced charge increasing from 10% of the total induced charge to 98%, while it takes around 16 ns for the 500 μm anode. The pulse duration determines the minimum dead-time of the anode readout electronics and it applies a critical role in the pile up, which we will discuss in the next section.

13.5 DETECTOR RESPONSE

In the previous few sections, we went through details of physics processes and signal generation that affect detector response. In an ideal case (Figure 13.9A), all the charges generated by a x-ray interaction are collected by a single pixel and the total induced charges are exactly the same as that generated by a x-ray interaction. However, because of charge sharing (Figure 13.9B) or fluorescence x-ray escaping (Figure 13.9C), the charge could be partially collected by multiples pixels and the induced charges on individual pixel are less than that generated by the x-ray interaction. Charge sharing and fluorescence x-ray effect will distort the detector response. As shown in Figure 13.10, besides the primary peak at 60 keV, the recorded spectrum has many events less than 60 keV. The smaller pixel has much more severe distortion. The charge-repulsion effect is also shown in the figure. The readout electronics can implement various correction techniques to sum up charges induced on neighboring pixels to resolve the distortion effects [12, 13]. But such correction schemes may sacrifice the counting capability

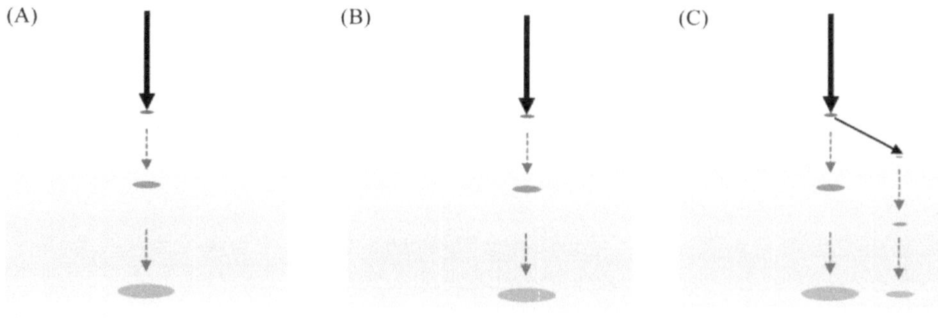

FIGURE 13.9 Illustration of physics processes affecting the detector response. (A), charge is fully collected in one pixel. (B), charge is partially collected by two separated pixels, caused thermal diffusion and charge repulsion. (C), charge is partially collected by two separated pixels, caused by fluorescence x-ray escaping. Here we do not consider hole and electrons trapping effect, since Figure 13.8 shows a minor factor in a small anode detector.

of the detector, which is a critical parameter for photon-counting CT application, and also may increase power consumption.

PCDs are widely used in nuclear molecular imaging [14–18]. However, it is just recently available for clinical CT. This is due to CT applications requiring much higher flux than molecular imaging. With up to several hundred million photon interactions happening per second per square millimeter, it is highly possible that two photons interact with the same pixel in a short time interval. Part or full charge induction process could overlap with each other (Figure 13.11). This phenomenon is called pile up. This effect will distort the recorded photon energy. And if two events happen too close, the post-processing electronics could treat these two events as one. Two solutions could be used to reduce pile-up effect from the detector design perspective. One is

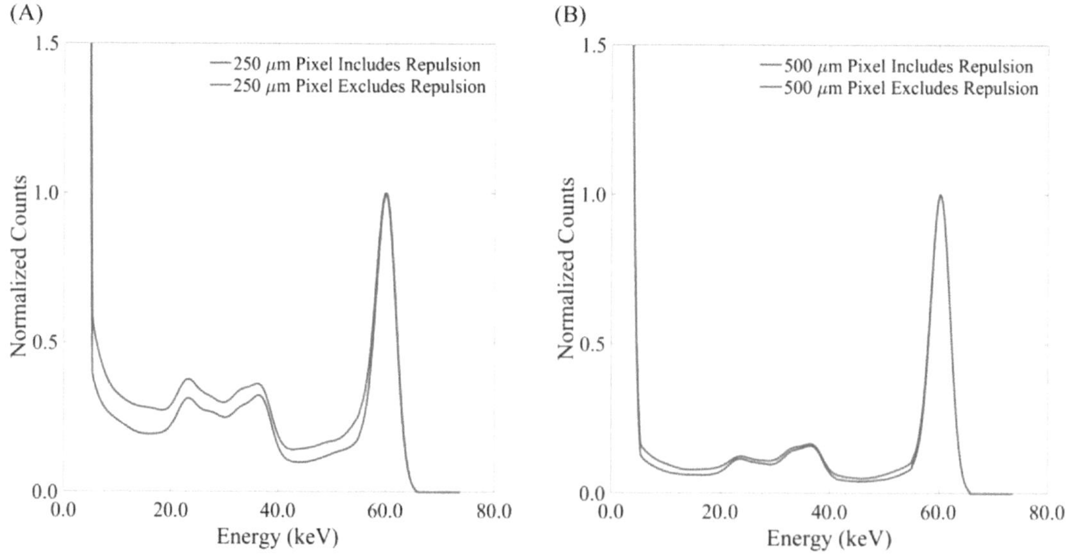

FIGURE 13.10 Detector response with varied anode sizes, when 60 keV photons interact with the crystal. The spectra are post-smoothed by a Gaussian filter with a 5-keV full width at half maximum (FWHM).

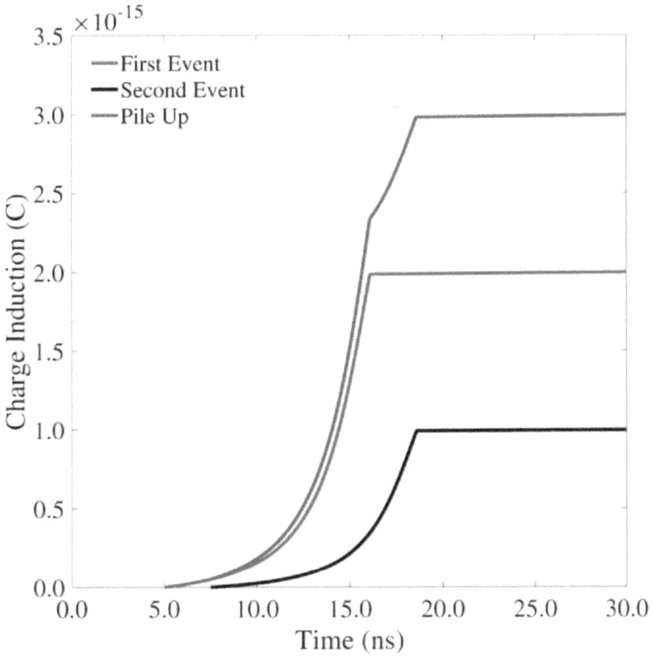

FIGURE 13.11 Illustration of pile up. The first photon interacts with crystal at 5 ns and the second event happens at 7.5 ns later. The induced charge is simulated for a 500-μm anode pitch. A 900-V bias is applied to a 2-mm CZT.

increasing the bias voltage to have a shorter charge drift time for each event. Recent CZT detector designs allow the detector to have a much higher bias voltage without significantly increasing leakage current. The other is reducing the anode pitch size. This has two benefits. One is that the number of events in each readout channel is reduced as pixel area getting smaller. The other is that the small pixel has a shorter induced charge pulse, as in Figure 13.8, which allows us to use a shorter post-processing time (called dead time) for a single pulse. On the other hand, the small pixel will have more severe spectrum distortion as we discussed previously. Figure 13.12 shows simulated x-ray spectra under different flux levels. In the low flux, 500 μm pixel has less spectrum distortion caused by charge sharing and fluorescence escaping and re-abortion. However, in the high flux, the severe pile-up effect distorts the spectrum, while the 250 μm anode pitch has less pile-up impact.

13.6 SUMMARY

In this chapter, we discussed the signal generation process of semiconductor detectors for photon-counting CT. We evaluated the x-ray interaction and fluorescence x-ray escaping and re-abortion through Monte-Carlo simulation and studied the initial charge cloud size dependence on the primary electron kinetic energy. The charge transportation was modeled through partial different equations, which included thermal diffusion, charge self repulsion, and charge trapping. Finally, we derived induced charges on the detector electrodes through the Shockley-Ramo theorem. By taking all these effects into account, we evaluated detector responses under different anode pitch configurations. A detector with a larger pitch has better capability of resolving photon energy information in low flux, because of less fluorescence escaping and re-abortion and charge sharing. However, in the high-flux scenario, detectors with a larger pixel pitch have more severe pile-up effect.

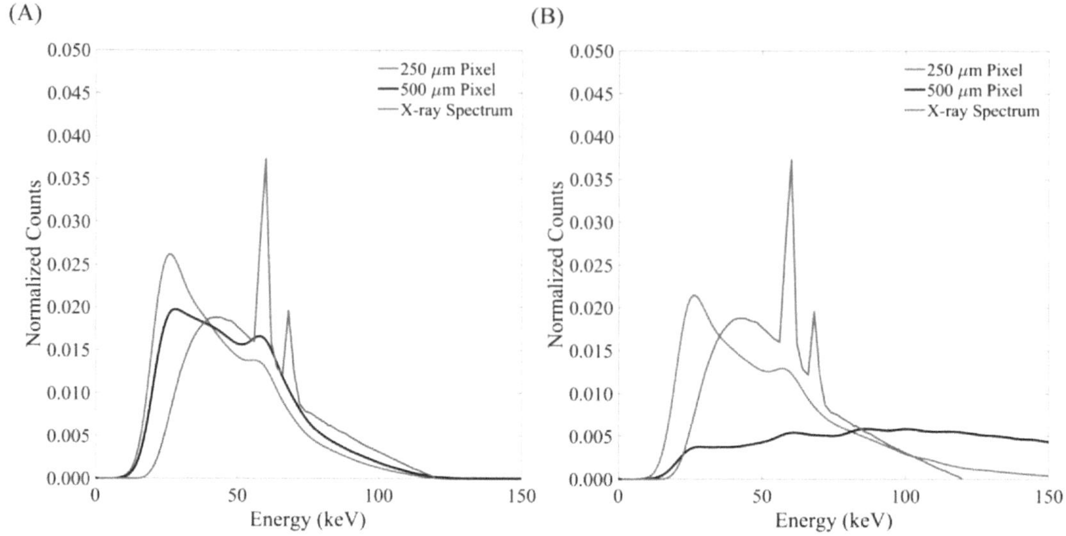

FIGURE 13.12 Detector response under different x-ray flux levels. (A), the detector response when a x-ray flux is 1 Mcps/mm^2. (B), the detector response when a x-ray flux is 200 Mcps/mm^2. Both spectra are post-smoothed by a Gaussian filter with a 5-keV FWHM.

REFERENCES

1. M. J. Willemink, M. Persson, A. Pourmorteza, N. J. Pelc, and D. Fleischmann, "Photon-counting CT: Technical principles and clinical prospects," *Radiology*, vol. 289, no. 2, pp. 293–312, 2018.
2. K. A. Kanaya and S. Okayama, "Penetration and energy-loss theory of electrons in solid targets," *Journal of Physics D: Applied Physics*, vol. 5, no. 1, p. 43, 1972.
3. E. G. d-Aillon, J. Tabary, A. Glière, and L. Verger, "Charge sharing on monolithic CdZnTe gamma-ray detectors: A simulation study," *Nuclear Instruments and Methods in Physics Research Section A: Accelerators, Spectrometers, Detectors and Associated Equipment*, vol. 563, no. 1, pp. 124–127, 2006.
4. R. D. Evans, "The Atomic nucleus krieger," *New York*, 1982.
5. S. Kraft, M. Bavdaz, B. Castelletto, A. Peacock, F. Scholze, G. Ulm, M.-A. Gagliardi, S. Nenonen, T. Tuomi, M. Juvonen et al., "The X-ray response of CdZnTe detectors to be used as future spectroscopic detectors for X-ray astronomy," *Nuclear Instruments and Methods in Physics Research Section A: Accelerators, Spectrometers, Detectors and Associated Equipment*, vol. 418, no. 2, pp. 337–347, 1998.
6. "Semiconductor detector material properties," http://www.umich.edu/~ners580/ners-bioe_ 481/lectures/pdfs/SemiConductor-material_ prop.pdf, accessed: 2019-01-24.
7. J. Larsson, "Electromagnetics from a quasistatic perspective," *American Journal of Physics,* vol. 75, no. 3, pp. 230–239, 2007.
8. J. Eskin, H. H. Barrett, and H. Barber, "Signals induced in semiconductor gamma-ray imaging detectors," *Journal of Applied Physics,* vol. 85, no. 2, pp. 647–659, 1999.
9. W. Shockley, "Currents to conductors induced by a moving point charge," *Journal of Applied Physics,* vol. 9, no. 10, pp. 635–636, 1938.
10. S. Ramo, "Currents induced by electron motion," *Proceedings of the IRE,* vol. 27, no. 9, pp. 584–585, Sept 1939.
11. Z. He, "Review of the Shockley–Ramo theorem and its application in semiconductor gamma-ray detectors," *Nuclear Instruments and Methods in Physics Research Section A: Accelerators, Spectrometers, Detectors and Associated Equipment,* vol. 463, no. 1, pp. 250–267, 2001.
12. R. Ballabriga, M. Campbell, E. Heijne, X. Llopart, L. Tlustos, and W. Wong, "Medipix3: A 64 k pixel detector readout chip working in single photon counting mode with improved spectrometric performance," *Nuclear Instruments and Methods in Physics Research Section A: Accelerators, Spectrometers, Detectors and Associated Equipment,* vol. 633, pp. S15–S18, 2011.

13. C. Ullberg, M. Urech, N. Weber, A. Engman, A. Redz, and F. Henckel, "Measurements of a dual-energy fast photon counting CdTe detector with integrated charge sharing correction," in *Medical Imaging 2013: Physics of Medical Imaging*, vol. 8668, p. 86680P, 2013. International Society for Optics and Photonics, https://doi.org/10.1117/12.2007892.
14. L. Cai, X. Lai, Z. Shen, C. Chen, and L. Meng, "MRC-SPECT: A sub-500 μm resolution MR-compatible SPECT system for simultaneous dual-modality study of small animals," *Nuclear Instruments and Methods in Physics Research Section A: Accelerators, Spectrometers, Detectors and Associated Equipment,* vol. 734, pp. 147–151, 2014.
15. X. Lai and L.J Meng, "Simulation study of the second-generation MR-compatible SPECT system based on the inverted compound-eye gamma camera design," *Physics in Medicine & Biology,* vol. 63, no. 4, p. 045008, 2018.
16. "NM/CT 870 CZT," https://www.gehealthcare.com/en/products/molecular-imaging/nuclear-medicine/nm-ct-870-czt, accessed: 2019-01-24.
17. A. Groll, K. Kim, H. Bhatia, J. Zhang, J. Wang, Z. Shen, L. Cai, J. Dutta, Q. Li, and L. Meng, "Hybrid pixel-waveform (HPWF) enabled CdTe detectors for small animal gamma-ray imaging applications," *IEEE Transactions on Radiation and Plasma Medical Sciences,* vol. 1, no. 1, pp. 3–14, 2017.
18. S. Abbaszadeh and C. S. Levin, "New-generation small animal positron emission tomography system for molecular imaging," *Journal of Medical Imaging*, vol. 4, no. 1, p. 011008, 2017.

14 Application Specific Integrated Circuits (ASICs) for Spectral Photon Counting

Chris Siu,[1] *Conny Hansson,*[2] *and Krzysztof Iniewski*[2]
[1]BCIT, Burnaby, British Columbia, Canada
[2]Redlen Technologies, Saanichton, British Columbia, Canada

CONTENTS

14.1 INTRODUCTION

Traditional X-ray imaging uses one value of μ integrated over all photon energies [Alvarez 1976], while spectral X-ray imagining uses independent photon information on a per energy bin basis [Taguchi 2013]. Multi-energy or spectral X-ray imaging requires use of advanced semiconductor detectors. Semiconductor pixelated detectors, by definition, need to have a high level of segmented multi-channel readout. Several decades ago the only way to achieve this was via massive fan-out schemes to route signals to discrete low-density electronics.

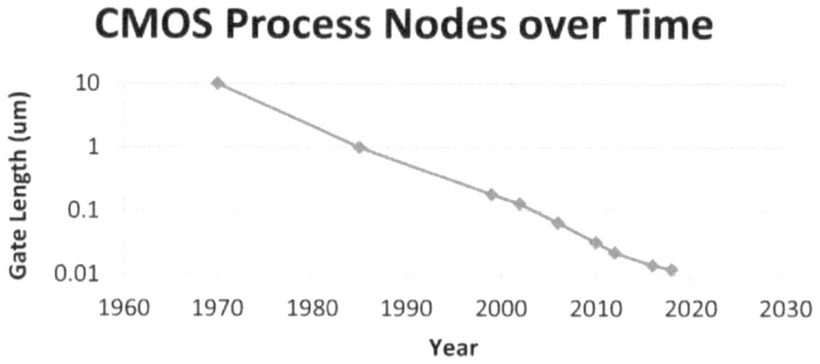

FIGURE 14.1 CMOS process nodes over time.

However, at the present time, complementary metal oxide semiconductor (CMOS) technology can create very dense low power electronics with many channels which can be bonded directly or indirectly (through common carrier PCB) to the detector, allowing for much more compact solutions.

There are different requirements for the CMOS technology used for the analog front-end signal processing, as opposed to that for the digital signal processing. For the analog part of the electronics there is a requirement for a robust technology that has low electronic noise and high dynamic range that typically requires large power supply voltages. Digital signal processing in turn requires very high speed and high density that is more compatible with the more modern low voltage supply, deep submicron processes. The purpose of this chapter is to present a review of available photon counting (PC) application specific integrated circuits (ASICs) that are or can be used in spectral computed tomography (CT).

An interesting perspective on the technology used in ASIC manufacture is provided in Figure 14.1. Here leading-edge ASIC development nodes are plotted against time. While 10 um CMOS process was used back in 1970, it took 10 years to take it down to 1 um. The 0.18 um process was introduced in 1999 and 0.13 um in 2002. That was the time when many photon-counting ASIC were developed, resulting in MEDIPIX ASICs (the Medipix2 collaboration was created in 1999 to develop Medipix2, while Medipix3 was developed in 2004) and many other devices developed in that decade. Relentless progress of Moore's law has enabled state-of-the-art ASICs to be designed in 7 nm process node today. However, extremely high cost of the circuit design and mask manufacture of these ASICs is only justifiable in the highest volume applications, such as cell phones or data servers. With time we expect spectral CT photon-counting ASICs to be designed in very advanced manufacturing nodes at 65 nm/45 nm, but it is unlikely that they will end up being designed in 14/7 nm processes soon as the number of CT scanners would always be orders of magnitude smaller than say cell phones or data servers. The graph in Figure 14.1 is approximately a straight line (in a log-linear scale); however, it needs to be cautioned that the CMOS manufacturing progress may not continue indefinitely due to physical and financial limitations. Most experts predict saturation of progress at 5 nm node although we must note that historically many predictions at much higher levels failed to materialize.

The expected slowdown in Moore's law progress is forcing chipmakers to look for alternate ways to boost ASIC performance. One of the new approaches being proposed relies on connecting large numbers of smaller chips, called chiplets, using silicon interposer technology as schematically shown in Figure 14.2. Instead of carving new ASICs from silicon as single chips, semiconductor companies will assemble them from multiple smaller pieces of silicon. Whether that approach becomes adopted by the semiconductor industry, and whether X-ray

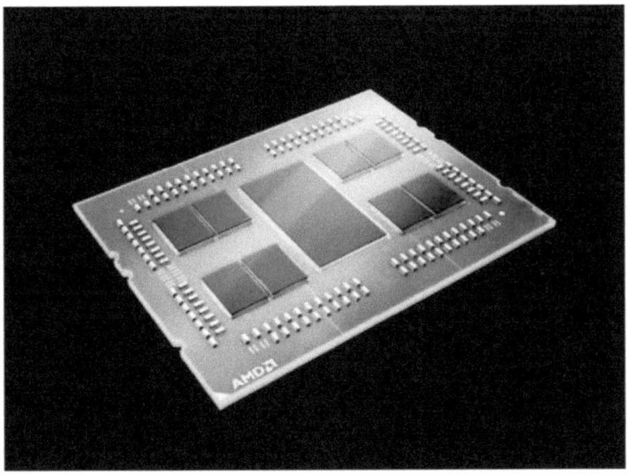

FIGURE 14.2 AMD's Epyc server processor combines nine chiplets. Source: www.amd.com.

photon devices will be assembled that way remains to be seen, but it could possibly serve an alternative approach to existing Moore's law.

14.1.1 Direct Conversion

Direct conversion radiation detectors offer new capabilities for X-ray imaging over currently used indirect conversion detectors. These capabilities include the ability to differentiate the energy of the incoming photons, variable energy weighting, noise reduction to the quantum statistical limit, as well as increased spatial resolution. These advantages in turn enable new applications such as material/tissue decomposition for CT, as discussed in this book and in the literature [Altman 2015; Boussel 2015; McCollough 2015; Persson 2014]. In direct conversion detectors, as opposed to indirect detection detectors, the absorbed X-ray imaging photons generate individually detectable and measurable electric current pulses without the production and detection of optical photons as an intermediary step. Since the signals are immediately available at the output of the detectors, they can be sensed with ASIC electronics, which can significantly reduce sources of noise and expensive infrastructure overhead. Detectors built with this technique are referred to as hybrid pixel detectors, and spectral photon counting (SPC) is a use case for a detector that can do both PC and energy discrimination.

SPC detectors are made of scintillator/semiconductors sensors and associated electronics. The sensor material is usually a solid-state semiconductor, such as silicon (Si), Germanium (Ge), Gallium Arsenide (GaAs), Cadmium Telluride (CdTe), or Cadmium–Zinc Telluride (CdZnTe/CZT). The advantages of silicon include high charge-collection efficiency, ready availability of high quality, high-purity silicon crystals, and established methods for test and assembly driven by the $400 billion annual revenue semiconductor industry. The main challenge is the relatively low photo-electric cross section, which limits the detection efficiency and leads to a large fraction of Compton scatter in the detector. Although low detection efficiency can to some degree be addressed by edge-on geometries, degradation due to Compton scatter remains. High Purity Germanium detectors (HPGe) offer superior detector spectral performance, due to the low pair creation energy of the material, but therefore require operation at liquid nitrogen temperature. It is therefore not practical in several applications that for various reasons are resource limited, including food inspection, space, and portable detection systems.

Several research groups and commercial companies have been investigating CdTe and CZT as sensor materials for PC applications. The higher atomic number of these materials result in higher

TABLE 14.1
Basic Properties of Selected Semiconductor Materials Used for Radiation Detection

Material	Ge	Si	CZT	TlBr	HgI_2
Average Z	32	14	49	80	80
Density (g/cm³)	5.32	2.33	5.78	7.56	6.4
Resistivity (Ω-cm)	50	1e5	1e10	1e12	1e12

absorption and less detector scattering, but, on the other hand, the higher K-edge fluorescent yield and energies lead to degraded spectral response and cross-talk between detector elements that needs to be controlled. Also, manufacturing of large size crystals of these materials used to present practical challenges, and these crystals suffered from lattice defects and impurities that lead to charge trapping. Charge trapping, in turn, limits the charge-collection efficiency for individual events and may cause both short-term and long-term polarization effects that prevent proper operation of those sensors.

Recent advances in CdZnTe (CZT) growth and device fabrication have enabled to dramatically improve hole transport properties and reduce polarization effects [Iniewski 2014; Iniewski 2015; Iniewski 2016; Iniewski 2017; Pennicard 2017; Prekas 2014; Strassburg 2011; Szeles 2008]. As a result, high flux operation of CZT sensors at rates more than 250 Mcps/mm^2 is now possible and has enabled multiple medical imaging original equipment manufacturers (OEMs) to start building prototype spectral CT scanners [Altman 2015; Boussel 2015; Kappler 2012; McCollough 2015; Persson 2014; Redlen 2016]. CZT sensors are also finding new commercial applications in non-destructive testing (CT) and baggage scanning. For that reason, the focus of this chapter is on CZT sensors; however, our major findings are applicable to other direct conversion technologies as well, including GaAs and CdTe. Other emerging materials like Thallium Bromide (TlBr) and Mercury Iodide (HgI_2) are being explored scientifically but their use in commercial application is several years away at best. A summary of basic properties of selected semiconductor materials is shown in Table 14.1.

14.1.2 ASIC Readout Integrated Circuits

One of the major advantages of PC detectors is electronics noise rejection. A well-designed detector has an ASIC electronics threshold high enough to reject noise pulses while still counting useful signals. Therefore, quantum-limited operation of the PC detector can be achieved, as image noise is determined mostly by statistical variations of X-ray photon flux. On the contrary, traditional energy-integrating detectors suffer from electronics noise that is mixed with useful photon signals and separating it from statistical noise is not possible.

Electronic noise rejection is important because its magnitude for currently used digital X-ray detectors is not negligible, and a high SNR is essential for X-ray imaging systems. An example of the CZT readout system is shown schematically in Figure 14.3. After converting the CZT-generated charge to voltage via the charge-sensitive amplifier (CSA), and subsequently shaping the signal, given enough gain in the system, the signal would be ready for digitization. Figure 14.3 shows a typical block diagram of the ASIC electronics used for CZT sensors; other semiconductor sensors use very similar architectures. This configuration is primarily used for systems with a low number of bins (up to 6–8), while other high-spectroscopy systems for CZT use other implementations. Typically, the signal is compared with a user-selected threshold voltage (or multiple threshold voltages for multi-energy systems) to produce a 1-bit trigger signal

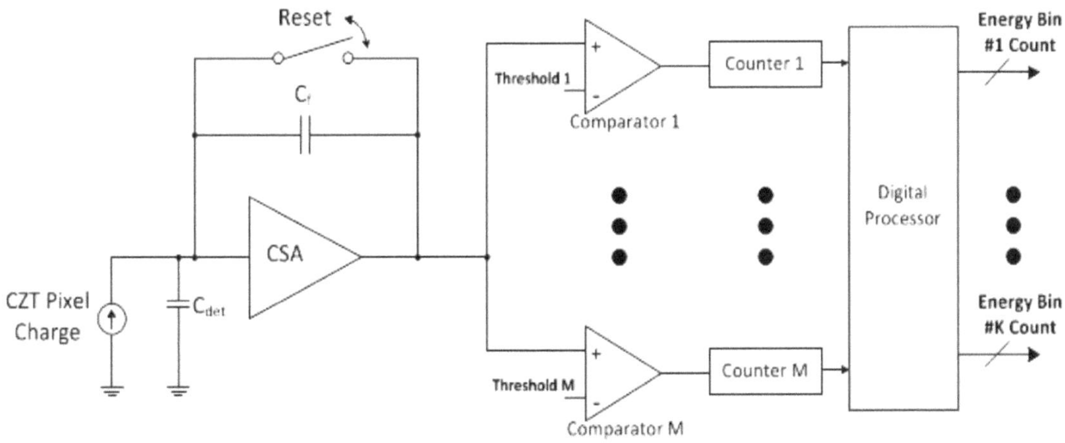

FIGURE 14.3 Schematic representation of the signal processing in the readout system with M multiple thresholds.

indicating the detection of the pulse. In parallel, the value of the shaped signal is sent to the analog to digital converter (ADC) converter with n-bit accuracy. The conversion resolution is typically between 8 and 16 bits depending on the system accuracy, noise levels, and degree of signal precision achieved. By using more signal comparators, the ASIC can easily be designed to accommodate multiple threshold voltages. The corresponding digital counters can be readout simultaneously effectively creating multi-energy PC system.

14.1.3 Pixelated Detector Design

Radiation detectors absorb and convert radiation into electric signals. In all cases discussed here the radiation energy must be high enough to cause ionization in the sensing material. The resulting charges are electron-hole pairs. The amount of charge, Q, generated by an ionizing event is proportional to energy deposited in the detector. Almost all imaging applications require either discriminating or measuring Q and, in some cases, its time of arrival (ToA).

The detector has at least two electrodes, but frequently has a larger number, especially on its anode side (e.g., pixelated-, strip-, co-planar, or Frish grid-detectors). For imaging applications pixelated detectors are typically being used. An electric field is generated in the detector, most often by applying a voltage between the pixelated (or segmented) electrodes on one side, and a common electrode on the opposite side. Under this electric field, the negative ionized charge of electrons, Q_n, moves toward one or more anodes, inducing a charge flow in each. The positive ionized charge of holes, Q_p, moves toward the cathode (at the origin of creation $Q_p=-Q_n$, but due to carrier trapping there will be differences in charge collection of electrons and holes). In most compound semiconductor sensors such as GaAs, CdTe, or CdZnTe holes move much slower than electrons and that property has major impact on operating detector at high-flux rates as discussed later in this chapter.

Depending upon the type of detector and the application, the charge can be readout event by event (as typically done in spectroscopy) or it can be integrated from several events in the given channel and readout later (as typically done in PC). Reading out the signals from radiation sensors requires highly specialized electronics, usually referred to as ASIC "front-end" electronics. Design of these electronics circuits usually entails stringent requirements in terms of the signal-to-noise ratio, dynamic range, linearity, and stability as discussed later in section 13.3.2.

There are two critical parameters that determine precision of the PC pixelated detectors: pixel pitch and sensor thickness. The pixel pitch affects the energy resolution (ER) of the spectrum due to well-known small-pixel effect. When pixels are smaller, the system is less dependent on the signal from holes which are susceptible to slow drift and trapping. As a result, the smaller the pixel pitch, the better the ER. However, smaller pixel pitch leads to increased charge-sharing which, if left uncorrected, leads to loss of detector efficiency and ER. In practical CT, PC systems the pixel pitch between 0.25 mm and 1 mm is typically used. In the follow-up discussion we will assume that charge-sharing has been either corrected for or pixel pitch is large enough for this effect to be negligible. Detailed discussion of charge-sharing effects is provided elsewhere in this book.

The sensor thickness affects detector quantum efficiency (QE). For typical X-ray tube voltages used in human body CT of 140 keV the required minimum CZT thickness is typically 2 mm which is easy to manufacture. CdTe and GaAs sensor must currently limit their thickness due to polarization effects; typically, 1.6 mm in CdTe case and 1 mm for GaAs, which reduces their QE significantly below values achieved by CZT sensors. The origin of this effect can be traced back to high densities of impurities and defects that in turn lead to severe charge-carrier trapping. Under high-flux conditions, the trapped charge builds up inside the detector affecting its stability, and in extreme condition leads to complete collapse of electric field and device operation. It is quite possible that with further improvement in material science polarization problems in CdTe and GaAs will be solved eventually as industry is investing significant efforts in solving these problems, but currently the leading sensor materials for PC detectors is CZT. From the ASIC perspective, which is the topic of this chapter, the type of the sensor material does not matter as long as the ASIC is ready to readout the negative charge of electrons. However, some ASICs have been designed for readout of positive charge (holes); therefore, they are not usable with CdTe/CZT and will be treated separately for that reason in our ASIC comparison.

14.1.4 Detector Energy Resolution (ER)

Detector ER expresses ability of the detector to resolve spectral features, the lower the value the better. In a typical CZT-based system ER varies from 2 keV to 10 keV depending on the pixel size, sensor thickness, material transport properties, and ASIC electronics being used. Full discussion of these factors is presented in the detector section of this book.

In general X-ray readout ASICs can be divided into two broad classes: spectroscopic and PC devices, as shown in Figures 14.4 and 14.5. Spectroscopic devices offer better ER (usually under 3 keV) but low-count rate, too low for spectral CT applications. The PC ASICs offer worse ER values (typically 4–10 keV) but can operate at rates of hundreds of millions of counts per second per mm^2. The detailed review of the state-of-the-art PC ASICs is given later in this and follow-up chapters.

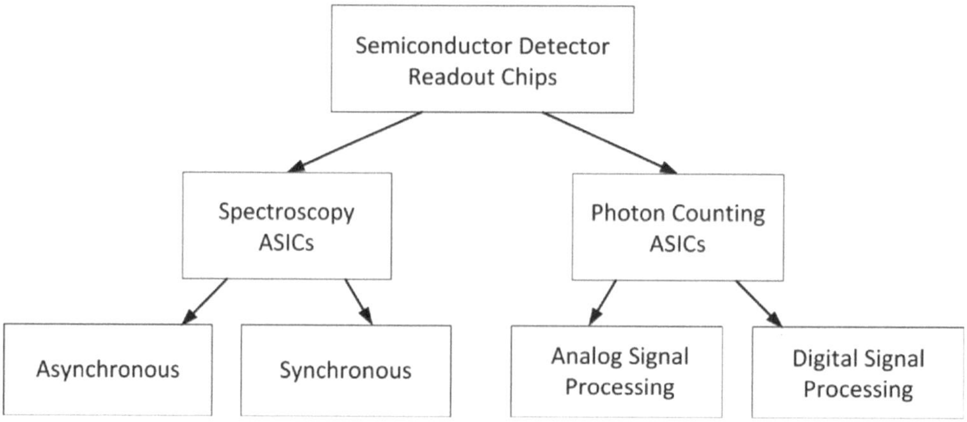

FIGURE 14.4 Classification of the readout ASICs based on modes of signal processing.

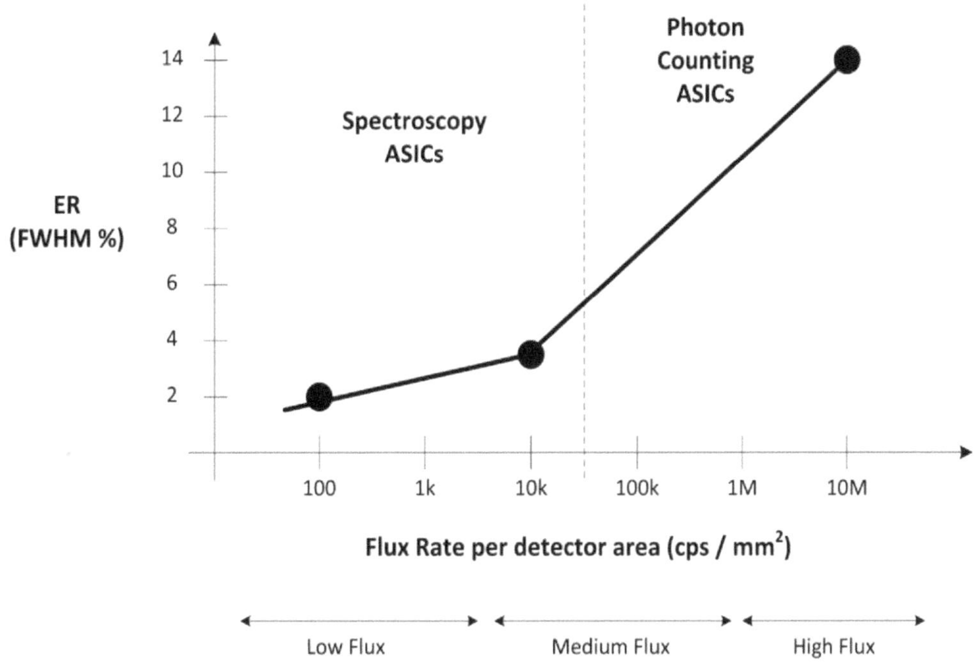

FIGURE 14.5 Classification of the readout ASICs into spectroscopic and PC devices based on the incoming flux rate. The dots represent average circuit performance at the particular flux rate and it is not tied to specific ASICs.

14.2 ASIC DESIGN

14.2.1 Analog Front End

CZT detectors typically operate in a single photon detection mode where an electric charge generated by one photon needs to be collected by the readout electronics. As the amount of generated charge is small (about 2 fC for a 50-keV photon) a very sensitive analog circuitry is required to amplify that charge. In spectroscopic applications the amount of charge, which directly corresponds to the photon energy, needs to be precisely determined. In PC applications only binary decisions are required but the count rate might be very high creating its related challenges. The purpose of this section is to explain some of the design considerations that are important when building semiconductor readout electronics system.

Analog signal processing can be divided into the following steps:

- Amplification – The input charge signal is amplified and converted to a voltage signal using a charge amplifier. A main characteristic of the amplification stage is equivalent noise charge (ENC) which is required to be as low as possible in order not to degrade intrinsic detector ER. Another important consideration for the charge sensitive amplifier (CSA) operation is a dark current compensation mechanism. A solution that accommodates continuous compensation for dark currents up to several nAs levels while maintaining low ENC is desired. Gain and resulting maximum input charge are important considerations here.
- Signal shaping/filtering – The time response of the system is tailored to optimize the measurement of signal magnitude or time and the rate of signal detection. The output of the signal chain is a pulse whose pulse height is proportional to the original signal charge, that is, the energy deposited in the detector. The pulse shaper transforms a narrow detector current pulse to broader pulse (to reduce electronic noise), and with a gradually rounded maximum at the peaking time to facilitate measurement of the amplitude. The pulse shaper (after the CSA), strictly speaking, transforms a "step-like" pulse at the CSA output into a "shaped" signal tailored to the specifications of

the system. A solution that provides effective signal shaping while maximizing the channel count rate needs to be applied. The importance of the frequency response of the shaper is of primary importance here as this circuit is strongly designed to ensure the noise is cut out.

- Pulse detection – The input pulse, broadened by the shaping process, needs to be detected against a set-up threshold value. The threshold level is a critical parameter that determines whether the event is recognized as a true event or false reading caused by noise. As a result, the threshold value is typically adjustable both globally and at the pixel level. The peak detection value determines energy level information. A solution that prevents temperature drift of the peak detector (PD) needs to be used.
- Channel multiplexing/counting – In case of ASIC spectroscopy all parallel channels of the channel readout ASIC need to have their signals multiplexed at the output before being sent out to an external ADC. The key requirement to channel multiplexing and signal shaping is a maximum channel count rate determined by the given application. In case of PC devices, all channels need to be associated to counters, for all energy bins used by the CT scanner.

14.2.2 Charge Sensitive Amplifier (CSA)

In both cases of spectroscopy and PC, the low-noise amplification is required to reduce the noise contribution from the processing electronics (such as the shaper, PD, and ADC) to negligible amount; good design practice dictates maximizing this amplification while avoiding overload of subsequent stages. Also, in both cases, low-noise amplification would provide either a charge-to-voltage conversion (e.g., source follower, charge amplifier), or a direct charge-to-charge (or current-to-current) amplification (e.g., charge amplifier with compensation, current amplifier). Depending upon this choice, the shaper would be designed to accept a voltage or a current, respectively, as its input signal.

In a properly designed low-noise amplifier, the noise is dominated by processes in the input transistor. If CMOS technology is employed in the design, the input transistor is referred as the "input MOSFET", although the design techniques can easily be extended to other types of transistors, such as the JFET, the bipolar transistor, or the hetero-junction transistor. The design phase, also known as "input MOSFET optimization", consists of sizing the input MOSFET for maximum resolution, and has been studied extensively in the literature. The optimization process involves many parameters: technology parameters, amplifier transfer function, size of the transistor, noise parameters, operating region of the input transistor (weak-moderate-strong inversion). The amplifier which is responsible for charge to voltage conversion is typically referred to as CSA.

14.2.3 Equivalent Noise Charge (ENC)

A key metric of the CSA is the ENC. The ENC expresses an amount of noise that appears at the ASIC chip input in the absence of useful input signal and is a key chip parameter that affects the ER of the readout system. Following the standard approach, the total ENC can be divided into three independent components: the white thermal noise associated with the input transistor of the CSA (ENC_{th}), the flicker noise associated with the input transistor of the CSA ($ENC_{1/f}$), and the noise associated with the detector dark leakage current (ENC_{dark}). Noise arising in other components connected to the ASIC input node such as the bias resistor is generally made negligible in a properly designed system. For a first-order shaper the ENC components can be approximately expressed as:

$$ENC_{th}^2 = (8/3)kT/(T_{peak} * g_m) * C_{tot}^2 \tag{14.1}$$

$$ENC_{1/f}^2 = K_f/2 * WL * C_{tot}^2/C_{inp}^2 \tag{14.2}$$

$$ENC_{dark}^2 = 2q * I_{dark} * T_{peak} \tag{14.3}$$

$$\text{ENC} = (ENC_{th}^2 + ENC_{1/f}^2 + ENC_{dark}^2)^{1/2} \tag{14.4}$$

where g_m is the transconductance of the CSA input transistor, T_{peak} is the shaper peaking time, K_f is the CSA input transistor flicker noise constant, W and L are input transistor width and length, and I_{leak} is the detector leakage current. C_{tot} is the sum of the detector capacitance C_{det}, the gate-source and gate-drain capacitances of the input transistor C_{inp}, and any other feedback or parasitic capacitance at the CSA input originating from the chip package, ESD diodes and PCB traces. Clearly, particular values are strongly dependent on the chosen technology for the ASIC design and packaging as well as on the chosen connectivity scheme between CZT detector and the chip.

It can be easily shown that the optimum peaking time is given by the condition where ENC_{th} is equal to ENC_{leak} leading to the following expression:

$$T_{opt}^2 = 4\ kT\ C_{tot}^2 / (3 g_m q I_{leak}) \tag{14.5}$$

The optimum shaping time derived from (Eq. 14.5) is typically a fraction of a microsecond, sometimes a few microseconds, and frequently implemented in spectroscopic ASICs. This optimum value however is way too large for PC applications as it would lead to severe pile-up as described later in this chapter. The spectral CT ASIC needs to have the shaping time of the order of several ns to be able to cope with very large count rates existent in CT scanners. We will compare the available shaping times when discussing various ASIC design implementations.

ENC is typically measured in the lab by measuring the output noise and referring it back to the input knowing the overall gain of the system. It is also possible to measure channel performance using the oscilloscope. By acquiring the channel shaper output signal on the oscilloscope at 1 MHz sampling frequency (for example 5 msec observed time on 5000 points), the fast fourier transform (FFT) can be applied to the acquired data and the resulting spectrum calculated for each frequency. The result of these calculations is ENC value expressed in number of electrons, typically in the hundreds of electrons range depending what electronics is used, the count rate, and the loading capacitance at the CZT input.

Based on the equations for these noise components, several conclusions can be drawn regarding the optimization (i.e., minimization) of the ENC for a given design:

- The input transistor width W has opposing effects on ENC. Increasing W increases total input capacitance, which in turn increases ENC. However, increasing W also reduces device thermal noise and flicker noise and, therefore, there is an optimal width W which results in a minimum ENC.
- Increasing the input transistor bias current I_D results in an increase in g_m transconductance and a corresponding decrease in ENC (via reduction in device thermal noise). Increased power consumption is the trade-off here.
- The input transistor should use the minimum available gate length for the given process to reduce the total capacitance and increase transconductance.
- Other significant relationships which are dependent on the process that is used to implement the ASIC circuitry are generally outside the designers' control (once the process to implement the ASIC has been chosen) include: increasing the detector capacitance increases ENC, increasing the flicker noise increases ENC, increasing the detector leakage current increases ENC [Geronimo, 2014; Michalowska 2011]

14.2.4 Signal Shaping

The low-noise CSA amplifier is typically followed by a high-pass or band-pass filter, frequently referred to as shaper, most often responding to an event with a pulse of defined shape and finite duration (width) that depends on the time constants and number of poles in the transfer function. The shaper's purpose is twofold: first, it limits the bandwidth to maximize the signal-to-noise ratio; second, it restricts the pulse width in view of processing the next event. Extensive calculations have been made in the literature to optimize the shape, which depends on the spectral densities of the noise and system constraints (e.g., available power and count rate).

Optimal shapers are difficult to realize, but they can be approximated, with results within a few percent from the optimal, either with analog- or digital-processors, the latter requiring analog-to-digital conversion of the charge amplifier signal (anti-aliasing filter may be needed). In the analog domain, the shaper can be realized using time-variant solutions that limit the pulse width by a switch-controlled return to baseline, or via time-invariant solutions that restrict the pulse width using a suitable configuration of poles. The latter solution is discussed here as it minimizes digital activity in the front-end channels.

In a front-end channel, the time-invariant shaper responds to an event with an analog pulse, the peak amplitude of which is proportional to the event charge, Q. The pulse width, or its time to return to baseline after the peak, depends on the bandwidth (i.e., the time constants) and the configuration of poles. The most popular unipolar time-invariant shapers are realized either using several coincident real poles or with a specific combination of real and complex-conjugate poles. The number of poles, n, defines the order of the shaper. Designers sometimes prefer to adopt bipolar shapers, attained by applying a differentiation to the unipolar shapers (the order of the shaper now is n-1). Bipolar shapers can be advantageous for high-rate applications, but at expenses of a worse signal-to-noise ratio.

The next important stage in the detector system is pulse-shaping amplifiers, which improve S/N of the amplifiers, restores baseline, and serves as a filter. In typical spectral CT readout systems, the shaping time varies from several ns to fraction of μs. The shaping time is defined as the time-equivalent of the standard deviation of the Gaussian output pulse. In the laboratory, it is measured as the full width of the pulse at half of its maximum value (FWHM). FWHM value is greater than the shaping time by a factor of 2.35.

The DC component of the shaper from which the signal pulse departs is referred to as the output baseline. Since most extractors process the pulses' absolute amplitude, which reflects the superposition of the baseline and the signal, it is important to properly reference and stabilize the output baseline. Non-stabilized baselines may fluctuate for several reasons, like changes in temperature, pixel leakage current, power supply, low-frequency noise, and the instantaneous rate of the events. Non-referenced baselines also can severely limit the dynamic and/or the linearity of the front-end electronics, as in high-gain shapers where the output baseline could settle close to one of the two rails, depending on the offsets in the first stages. In multiple front-end channels sharing the same discrimination levels, the dispersion in the output baselines can limit the efficiency of some channels.

14.2.5 Peak Detection

PD is one of the critical blocks in the spectroscopic signal detection system as accurate photon energy is determined by the detected peak amplitude. Standard PDs may be sampled or asynchronous solutions. Sampled PDs are more precise but suffer from high-circuit complexity and dissipate high power. Asynchronous PDs have simpler structure but suffer from lower output precision [Dlugosz 2007].

In PC system readouts an accurate photon energy is not needed. It is sufficient to determine whether the photon energy is between two selected values, so the detected event can be classified into particular energy bin. This is easily accomplished by comparing a shaped signal against a set of threshold voltage references. An example of the 128-channel signal processing ASIC is shown in Figure 14.6. A typical PC ASIC implementation contains hundreds of channels frequently implemented with multiple energy bins. Example of typical implementations are shown later in this chapter.

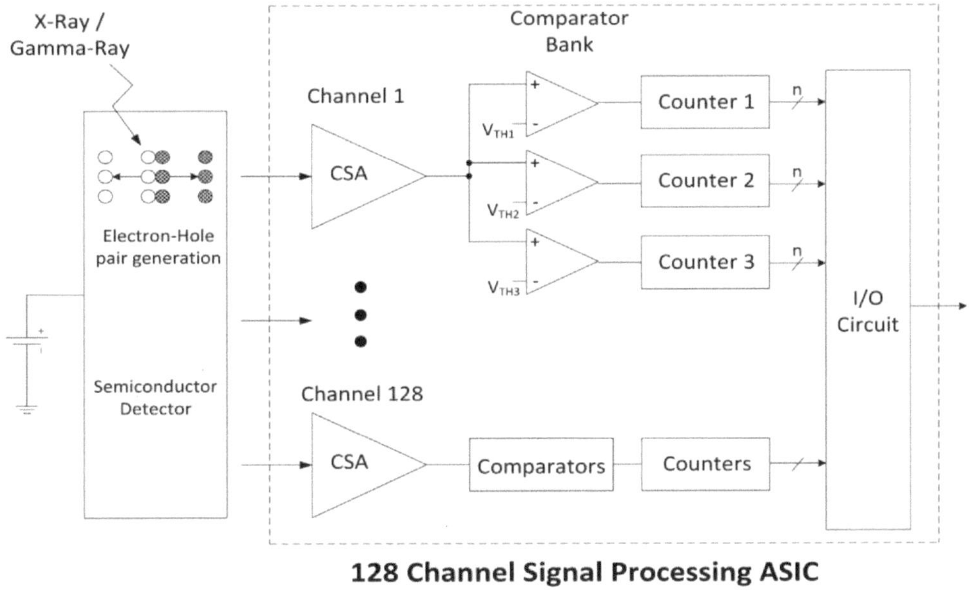

FIGURE 14.6 Block diagram of 128-channel PC ASIC.

14.3 ASIC OPERATIONAL ISSUES

14.3.1 THRESHOLD EQUALIZATION

Before calibration of a pixelated detector, the ASIC chip has to be equalized in order to minimize the threshold dispersion between pixels. This requirement results from the fact that the threshold that the pixel sees is applied globally but the off-set level of the pixel can be slightly different due to process variations affecting the baseline of the preamplifier resulting from transistor mismatch in CMOS processes. The equalization is typically performed with a threshold adjustment digital to analog converter (DAC) in each pixel. The resolution of the adjustment DAC is usually in the range of 3–6 bits depending on particular ASIC implementation. The standard way to calculate the adjustment setting for each pixel this is by scanning the threshold and finding the edge of the noise, then aligning the noise edges. These adjustments correct for the off-set level of the pixel but gain variations can still deteriorate the ER at a given energy. To correct for the gain mismatch either test pulses or monochromatic X-ray radiation must be used for the equalization. Equalizing at the energy of interest instead of the zero level might be also preferred.

14.3.2 ENERGY CALIBRATION

Depending on the ASIC architecture, there are two types of energy calibration that needs to be done: calibration of the threshold and calibration of the time over threshold (ToT) response (if applicable). For PC chips as Medipix3 the only calibration required is the one of the thresholds while in ToT ASICs such as Timepix-3 chips the ToT response must be calibrated as well. Virtually all spectroscopic ASICs need to undergo energy calibration procedures.

To calibrate the threshold, we need monochromatic photons or at least radiation with a pronounced peak. These can be obtained from radioactive sources, by X-ray fluorescence or from synchrotron radiation. In practice one typically utilizes Am-241 and Co-57 point sources although other techniques based on the sharp edges of the K-edge filter have been utilized as well. To find the corresponding energy for a certain threshold the threshold is scanned over the range of the peak obtaining an integrated spectrum. The data is then either directly fitted with an error or sigmoid function or first differentiated and then fitted with a Gaussian function. From this fit the peak position and ER can be extracted. Repeating the procedure for multiple peaks the result can then be fitted with a linear function and the relation between threshold setting in DAC steps or mV and deposited energy in the detector found.

14.3.3 Charge-Sharing Corrections

For imaging applications, the semiconductor sensor must be pixelated to localize the incoming photons. The pixel size is a topic of design tradeoffs: a large pixel creates a low-resolution image; whereas a small pixel suffers from effects such as charge-sharing as described below and elsewhere in this book.

Once generated inside the sensor material, due to the absorption of an X-ray photon, the free charge carriers (electrons and holes) drift toward the electrodes under the influence of an applied electric field. The drift is accompanied by diffusion, which causes the charge cloud to spread out before reaching the electrodes. If the charge cloud is close to the edge of the pixel, it will be shared by adjacent pixel(s); this phenomenon is known as charge-sharing. Charge-sharing leads to distortion in the energy spectrum, most notably in the form of a low-energy tail.

To explain the techniques used for charge-sharing correction, it is helpful to review charge-sharing using the diagrams in Figure 14.7. Suppose that a pixelated detector is divided into nine pixels, as shown in (7a). If an X-ray photon strikes pixel 5 near the center as in (7b), then most of the charge will be localized to that pixel, and very little charge-sharing will occur. However, if the photon lands near the pixel boundaries as in (7c), then the charge will be shared amongst pixels 1, 2, 4, and 5, and assuming the thresholds of the pixels are set low enough to detect the charge, low-energy events will be detected in these pixels, creating the low-energy tail in the spectrum.

To retain the energy information of the incoming photons, the system must recognize that a single photon event has spread its charge into a cluster of pixels, determine where the photon has most likely landed (usually selected as the pixel with the largest charge deposition), and assign all surrounding charge to that single pixel. This process is schematically illustrated in Figure 14.8.

A typical approach to this problem is to sum the charge in the detector as implemented in Medipix3, where the analog charge is summed in a 2×2 cluster before being compared to the threshold. This method of correction can solve both true charge-sharing and the effects of fluorescence photons. The advantage of this approach (compared to signal processing after quantization) is that it can handle much higher interaction rates and also that even charge below the threshold is summed as long as one pixel is triggered. However, since this correction has to be implemented in the ASIC architecture this complicates the chip design and is less flexible. There is also a practical limit to over how many pixels the summation can be done. The importance of charge summing when using CZT detectors with small pixels is clearly visible in cases where the energy spectrum of 110 μm pixels bump bonded to Medipix3 are compared in both single pixel and in charge summing modes [Ballabriga 2016].

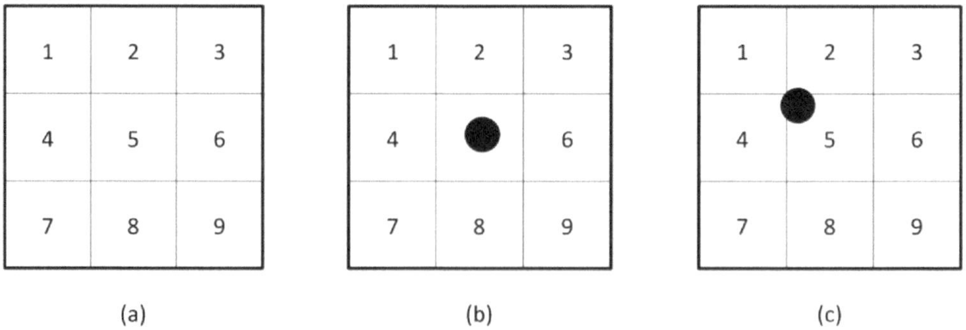

FIGURE 14.7 Schematic illustration of the pixelated sensor (a), with charge generated in the center (b), and at the boundary between the pixels (c).

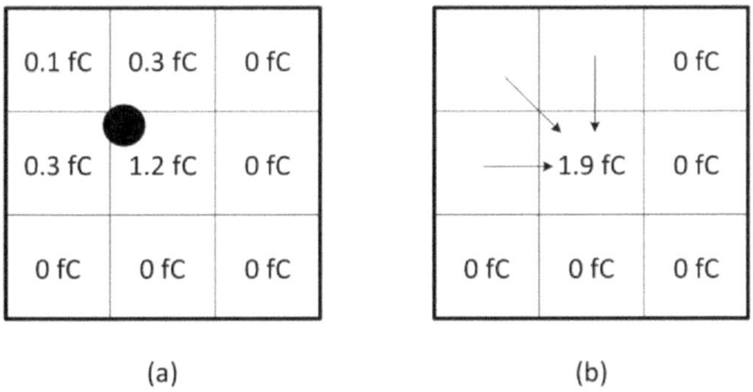

FIGURE 14.8 Charge-sharing between the pixels (a) and charge-summation to the dominant pixel (b). The diagonal contribution (0.1 fC in this example) is frequently ignored.

For an ideal semiconductor sensor, where inter-pixel gap surface charge recombination is negligible, it is possible to correct for the charge-sharing as explained above. The correction principle relies on the fact if two events are detected simultaneously it is very likely that they originated from one event. However, it is also possible that events were created as a result of Compton effect or they truly represent two independent events. Practical implementation of this correction depends on system requirements, details of charge event electronics design, and count rate used. In some cases increased deadtime, system activity, and noise levels can negate benefits of reconstructing some of the charge-shared events.

In practical sensor the surface recombination processes might not be negligible. In that case the charge summation process will not be complete as portion of the charge will be lost in the inter-pixel gaps as illustrated in Figure 14.9. It has been reported that in typical sensors charge-loss of 10–15% might be experienced and proper ways of recalibrating that loss might have to be developed.

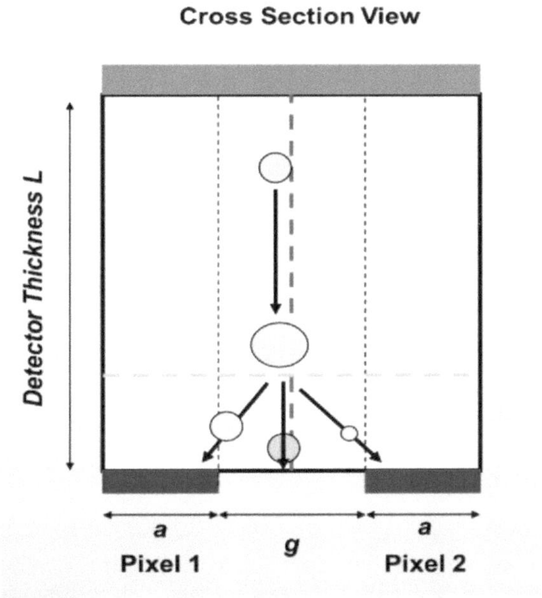

FIGURE 14.9 Schematic illustration of the charge-loss effect.

14.3.4 Pile-Up Effects

In any real detector system, to accurately differentiate between two events, a minimum time separating these events are needed. This minimum separation time is referred to as the deadtime, τ, of the system. The exact behavior of a detector system when one or multiple events occur within the deadtime set by a previous event is dictated by the architecture of that system and can depend on the physical processes in the sensor, or delays in the pulse processing chain or readout electronics. Two closely related phenomena are usually considered during these conditions: pile-up and count loss.

Pile-up usually refers to when the pulse being induced on the readout electronics from one event temporally interacts with the pulse from another event. This is illustrated in Figure 14.10, where the top graph shows the current pulses generated by photons interacting with the sensor (i.e., the events), and the bottom graph shows the corresponding voltage pulses observed for these events at the output of the shaper. For the first three events, no temporal overlap occurs and each pulse, both existence (i.e., counting) and pulse height (i.e., energy determination), is easily distinguishable from the others. However, for pulse four and five, the two events temporally interact, and the net effect is a super positioning of the pulse heights and the final determined pulse height will be a convolution of the two, resulting in an error in energy determination. For non-energy discriminating detectors, this in itself would not be an issue, only the potential count loss would. However, for an energy discriminating detector, such as the once used for spectral PC computed tomography (PCCT), this would lead to a distorted measured spectral response. The pile-up effect shown in Figure 14.10 is a traditional analogue electronic illustration of this effect, where the time constant of the shaper often sets the limitation for pile-up onset (pile-up resolution time) and dictates the maximum count rates allowable before spectral distortion occurs. However, if, for example, a peak hold circuit following on from the shaper is used to hold the peak value for readout, and a second event would occur before the peak hold value had been readout, the highest peak height pulse would eventually be readout. This can lead to both a loss in count and a distorted spectral response, as described above, without the pulses necessarily being temporally overlapping.

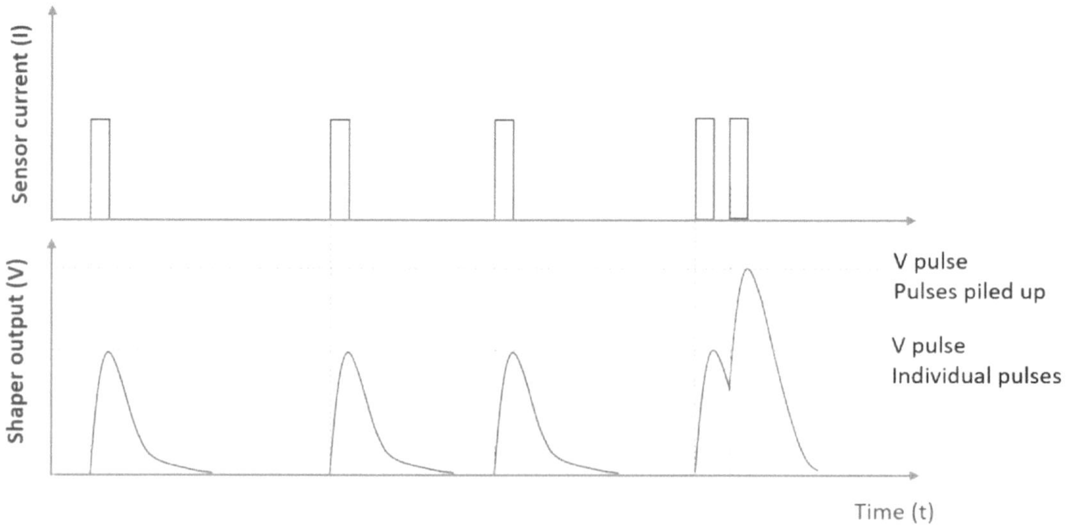

FIGURE 14.10 The effect of two pulses arriving close to each other (i.e., pile-up), and the resulting effect on the measured pulse height. For the final two pulses illustrated, two potential effects come into play: 1. Two pulses are counted as one (count loss), and 2. The final pulse height detected is incorrectly determined to be higher than it should be for any one pulse (i.e., error in determined photon energy).

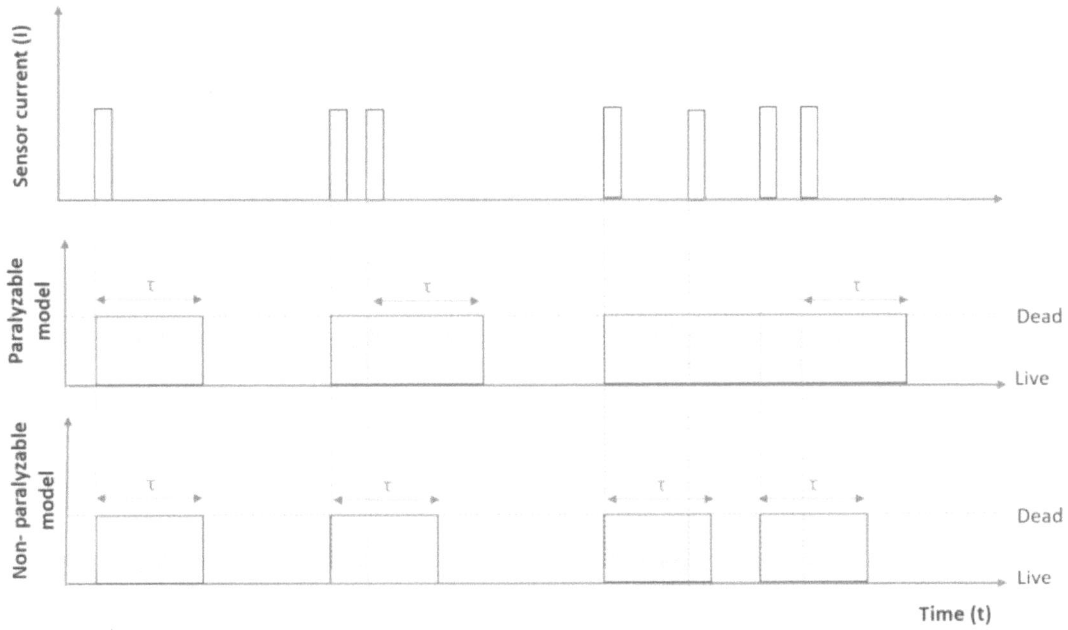

FIGURE 14.11 The response from a paralyzable (middle graph) and non-paralyzable (bottom graph) detector to the same incoming event sequence (top graph). As can be seen, for low-count rates the (pulse one) both systems accurately determine the count. For higher count rates (pulse 2 to 7) the effect of increasing periods of non-responsive behavior for the paralyzable model starts to play a significant role. The total counts measured for the illustrated time is 4 out of 7 for the non-paralyzable detector, and 3 out of 7 for the paralyzable detector.

When discussing deadtime count loss in detector systems, two idealized behaviors are usually referenced – those dictated by the paralyzing and non-paralyzing deadtime models. These models relate the three primary metrics of deadtime, true count, *T*, and measured count, *M*, to each other; the difference between the true count and measured count being the count loss. The main difference between the non-paralyzable and the paralyzable model is in how the detector system reacts when a second event occurs within the deadtime of the first event. The response of systems adhering to both these models to the same incoming count rate scenario is illustrated in Figure 14.11.

In the case of a non-paralyzable system, a first event would occur, and for the timespan of the deadtime, the system could not differentiate any other event, making the system nonresponsive (also referred to as dead). If a second event would happen within the timespan of the deadtime of this first event, that second event would not be counted (count loss), and the system would remain dead until the end of the deadtime as set by the first event. This behavior can be seen for pulse 2 and 3 in the third graph in Figure 14.11. For a paralyzing system, the two events would also be counted as one (count loss); however, the system would remain nonresponsive until the timespan of one deadtime had elapsed from the time when the second event was registered. This behavior can be seen for pulse 2 and 3 in the second graph in Figure 14.11.

The behavior of these two systems can be further contrasted and is illustrated in the response seen to pulse 4 to 7 in Figure 14.11. Once a high-enough event rate occurs the paralyzing system would consistently have events happening within the deadtime of the previous event, and the system would never come out of a nonresponsive mode, that is, the nonresponsive period would be indefinite, resulting in a measured count of 1. This phenomenon is in effect what gives the names to the paralyzing and non-paralyzing models. The non-paralyzing model on the other hand would lose the counts occurring during the deadtime of the first event but would then become responsive. As such, the measured count under these conditions for a non-paralyzable system would be given by the time measured divided by the length of the deadtime. A more detailed description of the response to various event rates for the two models is given in the following section. It should however be noted, as mentioned earlier in the text, that the non-paralyzable and paralyzable models are idealized behaviors, and any real detector system would have a response that would fall somewhere between these two extremes as dictated by the response of the detector system architecture.

As described previously, both the paralyzable and non-paralyzable model sets out to connect the deadtime, τ, the true count, T, and measured count, M, for a detector system. For a non-paralyzing system, the amount of time the system is nonresponsive is a set value, as illustrated in Figure 14.2, and the total amount of nonresponsive time in any measured interval is set by the measured number of counts and the deadtime, that is, $M \times \tau$. As such, the rate of loss is given by $T \times M \times \tau$. Considering that the rate of loss also can be written as T-M, this gives $T\text{-}M = T \times M \times \tau$, and when solving for n gives us the following description for the non-paralyzable model [Knoll 2000]:

$$T = \frac{M}{1-(M \times \tau)} \tag{14.6}$$

For the paralyzing model, as can be seen in Figure 14.11, the nonresponsive period is not always a set value. However, it can be shown that the distribution of intervals between random events occurring at an average rate is given by [Knoll 2000]:

$$P(\Delta t)\, d\Delta t = T \times e^{T \times \Delta t}\, d\Delta t \tag{14.7}$$

were the left-hand term is the probability observing an interval within $d\Delta t$ of Δt. Since any two events occurring within a deadtime of each other in a paralyzable system would end up with a non-responsive period exceeding τ, integrating the above expression from τ to ∞, and multiplying for the true rate, T, gives us the following description for the paralyzable model:

$$M = T \times e^{-T \times \tau} \tag{14.8}$$

The variation in true count versus the measured count for an ideal detector (T=M), a detector following the non-paralyzing model, and a detector following the paralyzing model can be seen in Figure 14.12.

For very low rates the three models line up. As the rates increases, however, the probability of two events occurring within a short time span of each other increases, and the non-paralyzing

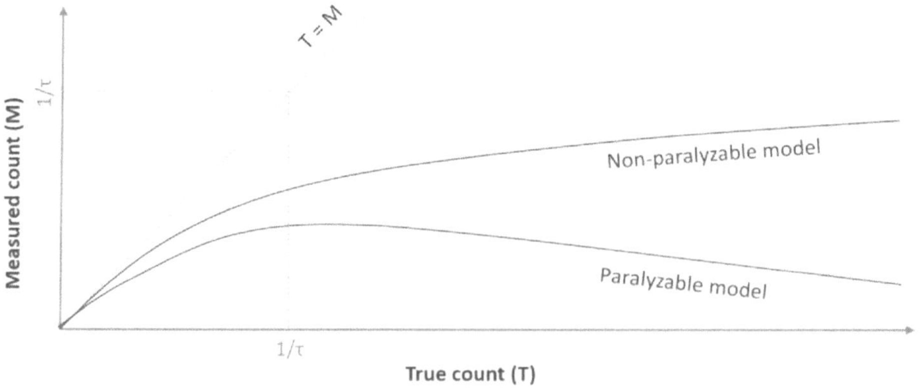

FIGURE 14.12 Illustration of the variation between true count and measured count for the paralyzable and non-paralyzable model. It should be noted that when operating a detector system following the paralyzable model in count rates exceeding $1/\tau$, an ambiguity in the corresponding true count to and measured count occurs.

or paralyzing nature of the system starts taking affect and influencing the measured counts. For the paralyzing model, operating at rates exceeding the peak measured count (i.e., $1/\tau$) introduces an ambiguity in trying to determine the true count, since any one measured count could correspond to two values of true count, which can be hard to differentiate. Additionally, operating under conditions where the count loss exceeds 30–40% is often advised against [Knoll 2000], since small measured count variations correspond to a large variation in true count. As such, any error in the measurement will result in a large error in the accuracy of the estimated true count.

14.4 ASIC IMPLEMENTATION EXAMPLES

In this section, we describe several ASICs used for PCCT that have been reported in the literature. The list is obviously not complete as there are over 100 ASICs worldwide, some existing as low-channel test chips and some have properties that would make them not suitable for applications in CT, such as a low-count rate handling capability. In addition, some commercially used ASICs are not reported here due to lack of complete information about their performance. An excellent review of a broad scope PC ASICs has been provided in [Awadalla 2015; Ballabriga 2016; Iwanczyk 2015]. In this section we will limit the discussion to the selected ASICs that are already used or can be potentially used in spectral CT scanners.

14.4.1 Timepix/Medipix Family from CERN

The Medipix3 collaboration is centered at CERN, the European Organization for Nuclear Research, and its work generally features a strong academic component. As a result Medipix3RX ASIC represents the first implementation of PC, and inter-pixel communication. Literature published about this chip is very extensive [Awadalla 2015; Ballabriga 2016; Iwanczyk 2015].

Timepix1 is a pixel detector ASIC developed in the framework of the Medipix2 collaboration. The pixel matrix consists of 256 × 256 pixels with a pitch of 55 μm, which gives a sensitive area of about 14 × 14 mm. The original Timepix ASIC was designed in a 0.25-μm CMOS process and contained about 500 transistors per pixel. The chip has one threshold and can be operated in PC, ToT or ToA modes. The principles of the different operating modes are described in detail in the literature.

In the PC mode the counter is incremented once for each pulse that is over the threshold. In ToT mode the counter is incremented as long as the pulse is over the threshold. Lastly, in ToA mode the pixel starts to counts when the signal crosses the threshold and keeps counting until the shutter is closed. Timepix was followed by Timepix3 designed in 0.13 um with better performance and a more extensive feature set. Timepix3 is a data driven chip which means the hit information is sent to the readout system as a 48-bit data packet containing simultaneously time and energy information. The time bin is 1.56 ns. Timepix4 will be designed to be versatile for dealing with high fluxes and for particle time stamping with time bin of 200 ps.

While Timepix is a general purpose chip the Medipix is aimed specifically at X-ray imaging [Ballabriga 2016]. In this chapter we will focus on Medipix3RX variant of the chip. It can be configured with up to eight thresholds per pixel and features analog charge summing over dynamically allocated 2 × 2 pixel clusters (i.e., an area of 220 × 220 um). The finer pixel pitch of the ASIC is 55 μm. Silicon die can be bump bonded in this mode called, fine pitch mode, the chip can then be run with either two thresholds per pixel in single pixel mode or with two thresholds per pixel in charge summing mode. Optionally the chip can be bump bonded with a 110 μm pitch then combining counters and thresholds from four pixels. Then operation is possible in single pixel mode with eight thresholds per pixel or in charge summing mode having eight thresholds and summing charge of a 220 × 220 μm^2 area but keeping a spatial resolution of 100 μm. In such a mode the ASIC is being used in the MARS CZT scanner discussed earlier.

Being a very versatile and configurable chip there is also a possibility to utilize the two counters per pixel and run in continuous read/write mode where one counter counts while the other one is being readout. This eliminates the readout dead-time but come a cost losing one threshold since both counters need to be used for the same threshold. Finally, the charge summing mode is a very important feature to combat contrast degradation by charge-sharing in semiconductors detectors with small pixels and its utility has been described previously in this chapter and elsewhere in this book [Butler 2018].

14.4.2 ChromAIX Family from Philips

Two proprietary multi-energy resolving ASICs called ChromAIX1 [Steadman 2011] and two have been designed to support spectral CT applications. In order to enable K-edge imaging, at least three spectrally distinct measurements are necessary; for a PC detector the simplest choice is to have at least the same number of different energy windows. With increasing number of energy windows the spectrum of incident X-ray photons is sampled more accurately, thus improving the separation capabilities.

The ChromAIX1 ASIC accommodates a sufficient number of discriminators to enable K-edge imaging applications [Steadman 2011]. Post-processing allows separating the photoelectric effect, Compton effect, and one or possibly two contrast agents with their corresponding quantification. The ASIC is a pixelated integrated circuit that has been devised for direct flip-chip connection to a direct converting crystal like CZT. The design target in terms of observed count rate performance is 10 Mcps/pixel, which corresponds to approximately 27.2 MHz/pixel periodic pulses, assuming a paralyzable deadtime model.

Although the pixel area in CT is typically about 1 mm^2, both the ASIC and direct converter features a significantly smaller pixel, or sub-pixel. In this way significantly higher rates can be achieved at an equivalent CT pixel size, while further improving the spectral response of the detector via exploiting the so-called small-pixel effect. The sub-pixel should not be made too small, since charge-sharing effects then start to deteriorate the spectral performance. Very small pixels would need counter-measures as implemented in Medipix3 described previously, the effectiveness of which at higher rates remains doubtful due to charge-sharing effects.

The ChromAIX ASIC consists of a CSA and a pulse shaper stage, as any other PC device. The CSA integrates the fast transient current pulses generated by the direct converter, providing a voltage step-like function with a long exponential decay time. The Shaper stage represents a band-pass filter that transforms the aforementioned step-like function into voltage pulses of a defined height. The height of such pulses is directly proportional to the charge of the incoming X-ray photon. A number of discriminator stages are then used to compare a predefined value (i.e., energy threshold) with the height of the produced pulse. When the amplitude of the pulse exceeds the threshold of any given discriminator, the associated counter will increment its value by one count.

In order to achieve 10 Mcps observed Poisson rates, which would typically correspond to incoming rates exceeding 27 Mcps, a very high bandwidth is required. The two-stage approach using a CSA and a Shaper allows achieving such high rates while relaxing the specification of its components. The design specification in terms of noise is 400e-, which corresponds to approximately 4.7 keV FWHM. Simulations of the analogue front-end have been carried out to evaluate the noise performance of the channel. According to these simulations the complete analogue front-end electronic noise, that is, of CSA, shaper and discriminator input stage together, amounts to approximately 2.51 mVRMS, which in terms of ER corresponds to approximately 4.0 keV FWHM for a given input equivalent capacitance.

The ChromAIX1 consisted of a 4×16 pixel array at 300 um pitch. The ChromAIX2 was meant to consolidate the performance of its predecessor and to allow integration on a CT gantry for evaluation [Steadman 2017]. The pixel pitch has been increased from the 300 um featured in ChromAIX1 to 500 um. The larger pixels ensure a better energy response as it is less affected by charge-sharing.

The chip provides a fast shaper of 10 ns peaking time and nominal 23.5 ns deadtime at equivalent 25 keV threshold. The 23.5 ns deadtime ensures 10 Mcps/pixel output count rate (OCR). Each pixel is equipped with five independent energy thresholds and the corresponding counters with a bit-depth of 16 bits. Other changes from version 1 to 2 include larger channel support (from 4×16 to 22×32), higher observable count rate (from 13.5 Mcps/ch to 15.5 Mcps/ch) and lower ENC (from 350e- down to 260e-). The ChromAIX2 is used in the Philip's CZT scanner described previously in the book that has been installed at University of Lyon and other medical facilities. Due to its practical importance and superior performance we are devoting an entire follow-up chapter for its coverage.

14.4.3 PILATUS3 and IBEX from Dectris

The PILATUS3 ASIC [Loeliger 2012], designed in 0.25 μm CMOS, has been deployed in system supporting a pixel size of 172 um × 172 um. Photon rates up to 10 M photons per second per pixel are achieved, via the use of count correction to mitigate the pile-up effect. PILATUS3 uses DECTRIS's *Instant Retrigger Architecture*, which re-evaluates the pulse shaper output after a programmable amount of time. The delay for re-evaluation is nominally set to be slightly higher than the pulse width of a single photon; hence, this strategy works well for monochromatic sources. If the output is still above threshold this delay, it is assumed that pile-up has occurred, and the counting circuit is retriggered. This technique prevents the count rate from freezing due to multiple photon arrivals.

The improvement due to the Instant Retriggering Architecture is shown in Figure 14.13. The red curve shows the ASIC count when retriggering is disabled and the count rate paralyzes as the input photon flux is increased. With the retriggering enabled in the green curve, the count rate versus input flux relationship remains linear for much longer, until the processing capability of the ASIC is exceeded. Note that Figure 14.13 results follow very closely mathematical modeling of Figure 14.12.

A block diagram of the circuitry per pixel is shown in Figure 14.14. The output of the CSA and pulse shaper is fed into a comparator. A global threshold is set for all comparators such that, if the photon is detected by the pixel, the comparator will increment a 20-bit counter dedicated to that pixel. There is also a 6-bit local threshold adjustment for each threshold, such that the variations across different pixels may be accounted for in a calibration procedure.

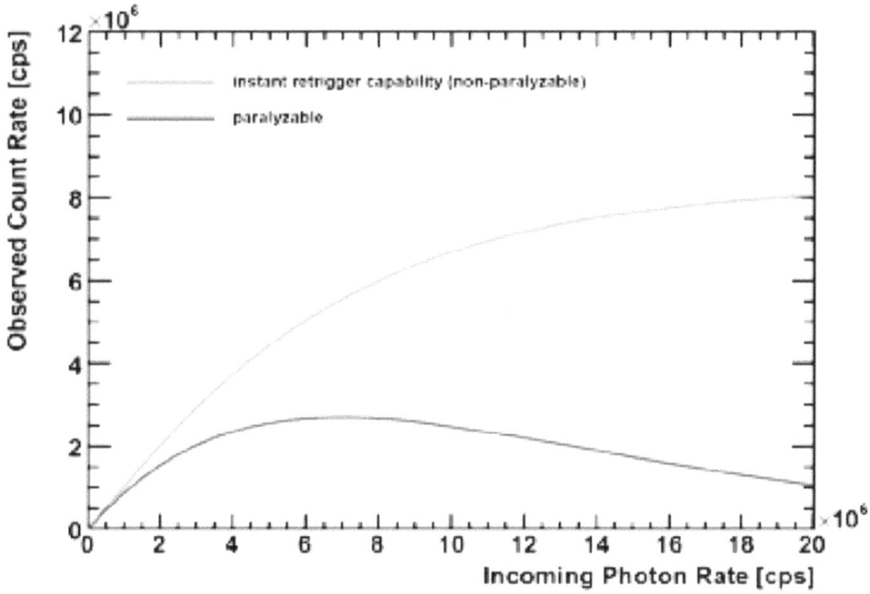

FIGURE 14.13 PILATUS3 output count rate vs. input flux rate.

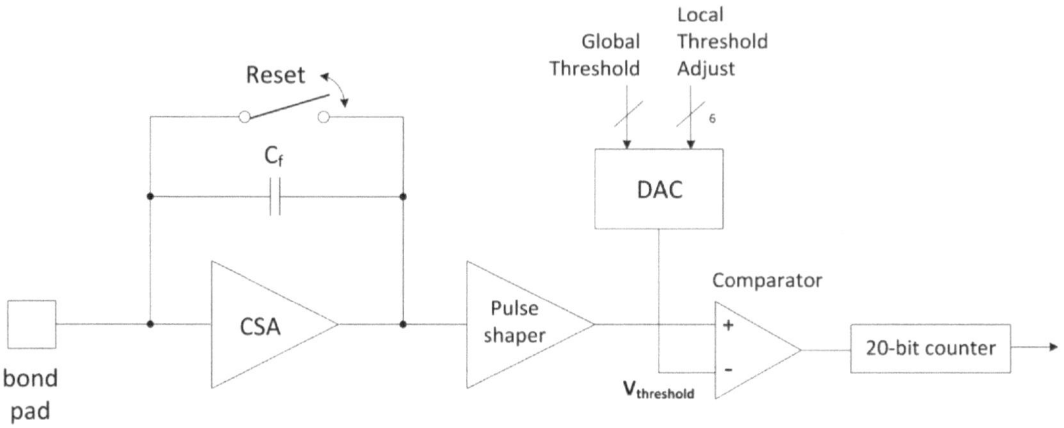

FIGURE 14.14 PILATUS3 pixel circuitry: block diagram.

A more recent product from DECTRIS is the IBEX ASIC [Bohenek 2018], which is designed in 0.11 μm CMOS, and supports a pixel size of 75 μm × 75 μm. IBEX also uses DECTRIS's *Instant Retrigger Architecture* to support a high-count rate. As such, it has a count rate similar to PILATUS3, up to 10 M photons per second per pixel.

With the smaller pixel size, IBEX can support higher resolution images and is less susceptible to pile-up. There are also other features that IBEX offer compared to PILATUS3:

- Dual threshold per pixel
- Pixel merging
- Adjustable gain for wide energy range

For each pixel, IBEX has two independent comparators after the CSA. These comparators have separate energy thresholds, allowing polychromatic X-ray sources to be used. This is in addition to a 6-bit local threshold trim, which is present in the PILATUS3 circuitry (Figure 14.15).

IBEX also has the capability to merge a 2 × 2 grid of pixels together, effectively changing the pixel size to 150 μm × 150 μm and supporting four energy thresholds. Furthermore, since the amount of charge generated by a detector is proportional to the X-ray energy, a fixed gain in the CSA will set a certain dynamic range. In order to expand the dynamic range, IBEX implements an adjustable gain in the CSA and measures X-ray up to 140 keV. One way to change the gain in a CSA is to use different feedback capacitor values as shown in Figure 14.16.

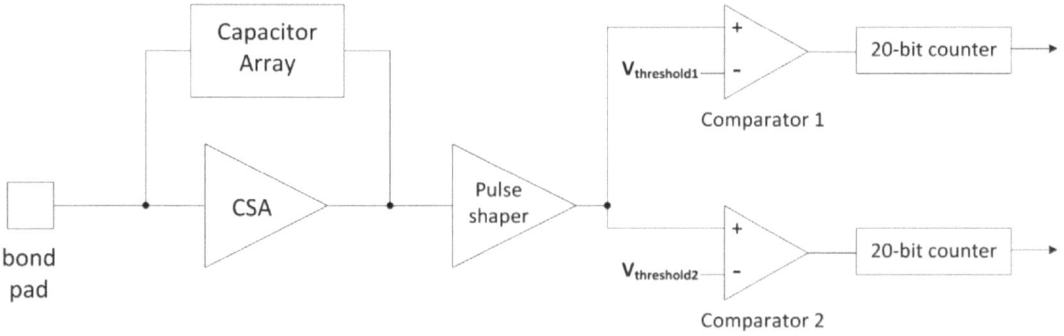

FIGURE 14.15 IBEX pixel circuitry: block diagram.

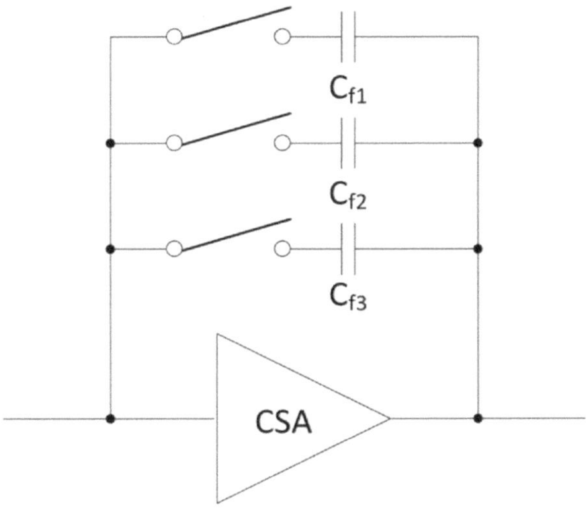

FIGURE 14.16 IBEX adjustable gain CSA.

14.4.4 KTH/Prismatic ASIC

As mentioned in introductory section, several different sensor materials have been considered for use in PCCT detectors, with CdZnTe and CdTe being the most prevalent choice. However, several ASICs have been developed with Si as the targeted sensor material, one of which is the KTH/Prismatic ASIC. For ease of access, the relative positive and negative characteristics of these three material systems for use as sensor materials have been re-iterated in Table 14.2. It should also be noted that for Si, unlike CdZnTe and CdTe, the charge signal induced on the detector front end is due to hole transport and not electron transport.

As seen in Table 14.2, the main drawback of using Silicon as the sensor material is the low absorption coefficient of this material. To overcome this drawback the KTH/Prismatic detector utilize a silicon strip detector configuration, with an edge on illumination geometry, as can be seen in Figure 14.17.

The detector module itself consist of five ASICs, as seen on the right side of Figure 14.17, wire bonded to the Si sensor, seen on the left side of Figure 14.17. The sensor consists of 16 segments of strip contacts (going from top to bottom), each segment having 50 strips (going from left to right). The length of the sensor is 30 mm allowing for the poor absorption coefficient to be compensated for, and the strip lengths are gradually increasing with subsequent segment to ensure similar count rates for each channel. The width of the sensor is 20 mm and the thickness 0.5 mm. As the strip

TABLE 14.2
Strength and Weaknesses of the CdTe, CdZnTe, and Si Material System for Use as Sensor Materials

Positive for Silicon	Negative for Silicon	Positive for CZT/CdTe	Negative for CZT/CdTe
Mature, cheap technology	Low absorption	High absorption	Comparatively immature, expensive technology
High charge carrier mobility	High probability of Compton scattering	Low probability of Compton scattering	Lower mobility
Minimal effect of K-edge fluorescence escape			Significant effect of K-edge fluorescence escape, polarization effects (CdTe)

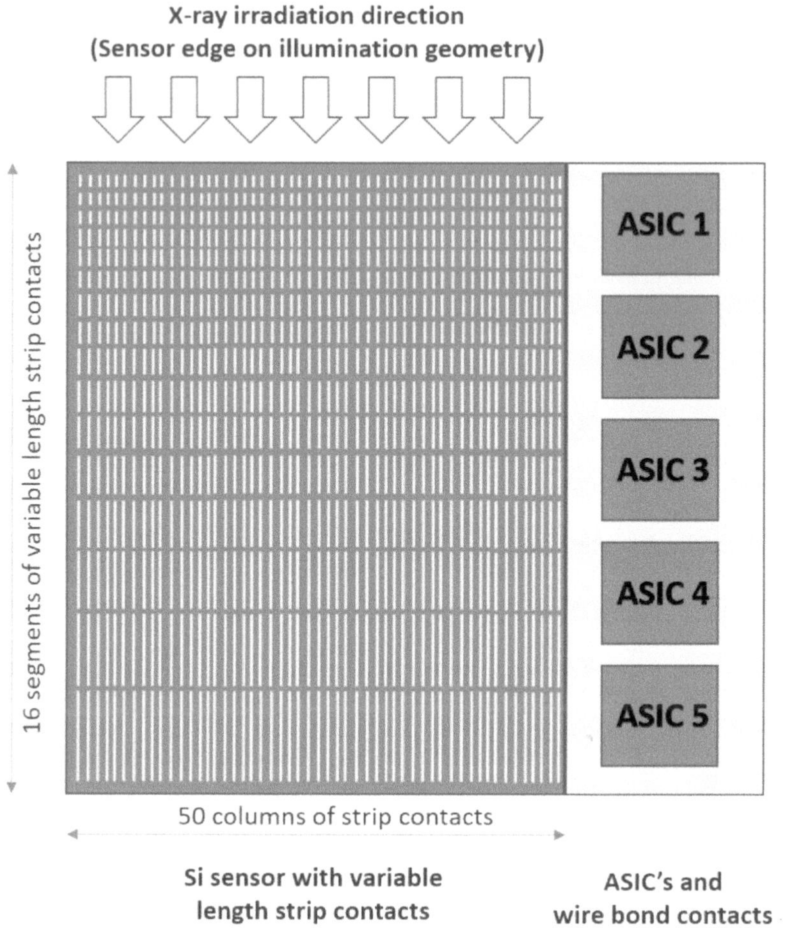

FIGURE 14.17 Diagram of the KTH/Prismatic Silicon strip detector module. The detector consists of five ASICs (right), wire bonded to the Si sensor (left). The sensor is divided into 16 segments (top to bottom) of strip contacts with increasing strip length. The detector is operated in edge on illumination configuration to overcome the poor detection efficiency of Si.

pitch is 0.4 mm, the resulting pixel pitch size is therefore 0.4 mm × 0.5 mm, with a varied voxel volume as dictated by the strip length.

The KTH/Prismatic ASIC has been developed in 180 nm CMOS technology, on a 5-mm × 6.6 mm die area, and consist of 160 analogue channels and a digital count/readout section, and the chip can be clocked using either a 100-MHz or a 200-MHz clocking signal [Liu 2016]. Each analogue channel consists of a CSA, a Semi-gaussian Shaping Amplifier with a pole-zero cancelation circuit, and an additional Gm-C filtering stage, as can be seen in Figure 14.18. It should be noted that the shaping time for the shaping amplifier is variable with the option to set it to 10 ns, 20 ns, 40 ns, and 60 ns available. To minimize the effect of the long shaping time of the Shaper, a novel filter reset scheme was implemented where, once a pulse has been detected, the filter output is reset after a set time period. This time period is set so that the output of the filter is reset to zero shortly after having reached it maximum peak height and the magnitude of this period is altered according to the chosen shaping time. Using this reset scheme a 17-Mcps/channel count rate capability has been measured using test pulses [Liu 2016], while measuring an approximate 30% loss of counts when exposing the detector to fluxes of 485 Mphotons/s/mm^2 (average non-paralyzable deadtime estimated to be 20.2+/-5.2 ns) [Gustavsson 2012].

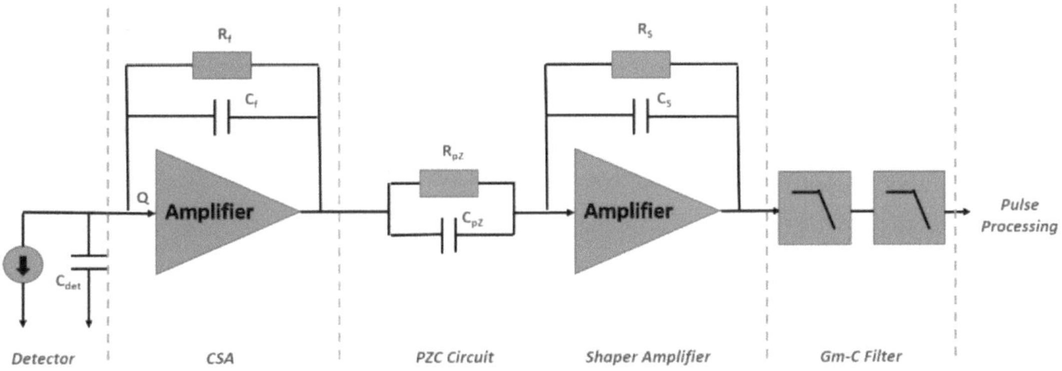

FIGURE 14.18 Illustration of analogue channel designed for the KTH/Prismatic detector. Each channel has a CSA, Shaper with Pole-zero cancelation, and Gm-C filter associated with it.

Following the analogue chain, a pulse amplitude detection procedure has been implemented using eight comparators that are clocked by the main clocking frequency (100 MHz or 200 MHz) and connected directly to the filter output. Once the input signal exceeds a comparator level, it turns on and sets a digital register, effectively creating a digital PD. The peak height of any pulse is determined by finding the highest comparator register that has been triggered after a set time period. This time period is programmed to be a number of clock cycles following the lowest comparator register having been triggered. Once the highest comparator level has been identified, the counter corresponding to the comparator register with the highest value is incremented.

The ASIC power consumption for this ASIC was measured to be 670 mW when using a 100 MHz clocking frequency, and 800 mW at a 200-MHz clocking frequency. The power per channel was determined to be 5 mW, of which 4.1 mW is drawn by the analogue block [Liu 2016]. The average ENC noise for a channel was measured to be 192 electrons for an open input and 214 electrons with a 3-pF capacitance load on the front end [2016]. An overview of the ASIC parameters can be seen in Table 14.3.

TABLE 14.3
Overview of Various Performance Parameters for the KTH/Prismatic ASIC

Process	180 nm CMOS
Die area	5 mm × 6.6 mm
Number of channels	160
Pitch	400 um[1]
Pixel area	500 um × 400 um[2]
Count rate per channel	17 Mcps@100 Mhz[3]
Total power	800 mW@200 MHz; 670 mW@100 MHz
Power per channel	5 mW/channel (4.1 mW from the analogue block)
Number of bins per channel	8
ENC	192e-@0 pF; 214e-@3 pF

[1] Set by the strip pitch.
[2] Set by the strip pitch × *Si* sensor thickness.
[3] Measured with test pulses.

14.5 ASIC PERFORMANCE COMPARISON

Several high-flux readout ASICs have been proposed, designed, and fabricated for high-count CZT based systems, CERN group provided a very comprehensive ASIC summary [Ballabriga 2016]. As discussed in this and follow-up chapters various ASICs deal with the following common key design issues in a different way. The following is the list of key parameters to be considered:

- Power dissipation (per channel and per mm^2)
- OCR
- ENC and related ER
- Number of energy bins
- Pixel pitch that determines charge-sharing and pile-up effects
- Sensor anode rise time that determines ballistic deficit
- Frequency response of baseline restoration
- Leakage current compensation required to compensate for sensor dark current
- 3-D or 4-D tiling depending on use of Thru Silicon Via (TSVs) or interposer technology

In the following chapters, various comparison of performance characteristics from the perspective of addressing those key design issues are provided. To establish fair comparison between various ASICs one can establish Figure of Merit (*FOM*) formulas that reflect the final application in spectral CT. It needs to be pointed out that some of the above design considerations depend largely on the sensor design and not the ASIC design or implementation technology. For example, key detector characteristics are closely tied to the selected sensor pixel pitch.

The first design trade-off is common to all electronics: power versus speed. It is usually possible to improve the speed of circuit operation by increasing the dissipated power and PC is not an exception to that simple rule. There are limits of course, probably the most visible in the microprocessor design space: microprocessor speed has been increasing over the years with each process generation until they reach 3–4 GHz speed barrier. It has taken significant effort by Intel and others to finally reach 5 GHz operating speed on selected models.

A simple FOM for CT ASICs can be created for the comparison as follows:

$$FOM = OCR/P_{diss} \tag{14.9}$$

where OCR is the count rate per unit area, and P_{DISS} is the power dissipation per unit area. This *FOM* metric attempts to capture the conversion efficiency in terms of power consumption. Precise calculation of this *FOM* has been difficult. ASIC power dissipation consists of the static power dissipation, which is present regardless of the X-ray activity, and dynamic power, which is typically proportional to the flux rate. For example, KTH ASIC dissipates 800 mW@200 MHz, but only 670 mW@100 MHz clock frequency. Static power dissipation typically dominates the total power consumption and consists of 50–90% of the total power dissipation but exact percentage is largely dependent on the chip architecture. Unfortunately, not all references quote static and dynamic power components separately so precise FOM1 calculations are difficult.

Similar challenges exist with OCR values. In paralyzable ASICs, the OCR-ICR curve has a maximum point so the assessment of the maximum count rate is difficult. For non-paralyzable (NP) ASICs the selection of the maximum OCR is more difficult as theoretically OCR continues to increase even for large ICR values. In practice even for NM ASICs, there is some limitations on the maximum obtainable OCR. In addition, the measurement of OCR is very dependent on the measurement conditions (energy spectrum, threshold, etc.) so precise comparisons are again difficult.

The ER of the sensor-ASIC sub-system is an important parameter that determines number of photon energy bins that can be used in various imaging applications and minimum detectable energy. Neither ER nor number of energy bins is captured by FOM definition in (Eq. 14.9). In addition, we have found that more critical parameters are those responsible for maximum count rate due to pile-up and charge-shared events that determine system efficiency. Important design trade-offs are discussed in detail in the following three chapters of this book.

With deep-submicron CMOS technology, it becomes cost-effective to integrate digital functionality onto the ASIC. Typically, for each pixel, the ASIC processes the charge information into N energy bins, with counters for each bin. In essence, a rough energy spectrum is created for each pixel on-chip, and this data is then transmitted over a high-speed low voltage differential signaling (LVDS) interface at the readout time. Consequently, it is becoming easier to implement more energy bins, from 6 to 8 typically, to enable multi-contrast K-edge imaging for example.

Critical parameters for high-flux CT scanner operation include *OCR*, minimum detectable energy (E_{min}), and spectrum ER. The maximum count rate is directly related to electron rise time at the anode and can be limited by sensor polarization effect or ASIC shaping time. ER is dependent on the pixel pitch through small pixel effect, input capacitance loading due to contributions from pixel, interposer and input CSA capacitances, sensor dark current as well as high voltage bias (*HV*) and the amount of charge-sharing. Finally, the minimum detectable energy depends on ER, but usually for most of hybrid pixel detectors available, this minimum detectable energy is usually much smaller than the energy at which there are fluorescence photons emitted.

To provide more insights on how different ASIC deal with the above trade-offs further work on various FOM measures needs to be done. Such comparisons need to be used carefully as other factors like process node, die size, packaging, price, yield, chip reliability (radiation hardness), and availability might equally matter. Nevertheless we believe that this section allowed the reader to get some taste of the spectral ASIC performance space that might be useful for individual explorations.

14.6 CONCLUSION

Traditional CT systems use energy integrating scintillator detectors to measure the X-ray attenuation of the imaged object. These systems do a superb job of detecting human bodies abnormalities and are employed in most hospital emergency departments in the world. However, their clinical applications are limited due to their inability to differentiate the energy of the incoming X-ray photons.

Color or spectral CT enables detecting small tissue abnormalities that might result in major illnesses like cancer. Early detection requires the capacity to perform spatially resolved material identification at high throughput. Achieving the necessary tissue discrimination capabilities relies on the development of cost-effective multi-pixel, energy-sensitive based systems.

Semiconductor direct-conversion sensor-based CT spectral imaging is bringing new clinical information to the diagnosis and characterization of many diseases. Spectral functionality brings additional contrast to the image that makes subtle disease more conspicuous and brings chemical composition to the diagnosis to better characterize disease. This makes CT more cost effective, by reducing the need for downstream tests, especially in cancer, vascular disease, and kidney stones diagnosis.

First generation spectral CT scanners are currently being tested using phantom as well as in first clinical trials as discussed in detail in this book. Further improvements in ASIC design are expected to further scanner performance. Future ASICs will have to deal with increased channel rates in excess of 500 Mcps/mm^2, provide good spectroscopic performance with ENC of 500e- or better, dissipate low enough power, ideally lower than 0.1 mW per channel and provide four-side buttability for flexibility in designing large scanner field of view (FoV).

One limiting factor that the future ASICs will have to deal with is charge-sharing, which as explained above creates a characteristic low-energy tail and leads to a reduced contrast and distorted spectral information. The distortion in the energy spectrum is more pronounced at fine pixel pitch. To counteract this problem there are two possibilities, either to use larger pixels with reduced spatial resolution or to implement charge summing on a photon by photon basis. As charge-sharing correction, as implemented in Medipix3 or similar devices, is intrinsically slow other, faster schemes might have to be developed.

More advanced CMOS processes, 65 nm or below, might have to be used for chip implementations, to fully benefit from Moore's law relentless chip evolution. Modern ASICs used currently in cell phones utilize already 14 nm CMOS processes with 7 nm generation knocking at the door. Spectral CT market size might not be able to afford 7/14 nm chip implementations, but it can likely do better than the 0.13 um process employed in state-of-the-art PC ASIC space. There are however many advantages and drawbacks/challenges in going downscale toward 65 nm and 45 nm processes! Only future will tell how advanced spectral CT chip become.

14.7 ACKNOWLEDGMENT

The authors would like to acknowledge Dr. Rafael Ballabriga, CERN for his insightful comments and suggestions to improve the manuscript.

REFERENCES

[Altman 2015] A. Altman, Quantified characteristics of lesions and diseases using photon counting spectral CT without contrast injection: Are there enough opportunities and sensitivity? *1st Spectral Photon Counting CT Workshop*, Lyon, France, September 2015.

[Alvarez 1976] R. E. Alvarez, A. Macovski, Energy-selective reconstructions in x-ray computerised tomography, *Physics in Medicine & Biology* 21, 733 (1976).

[Awadalla 2015] S. Awadalla (Ed.), Solid-state radiation detectors: Technology and applications, in *Devices, Circuits, and Systems*, CRC Press, 2015, Boca Raton, FL.

[Ballabriga 2016] R. Ballabriga, J. Alozy, M. Campbell, E. Frojdh, E. Heijne, T. Koenig, X. Llopart, J. Marchal, D. Pennicard, T. Poikela, L. Tlustos, P. Valerio, W. Wong and M. Zuber, Review of hybrid pixel detector readout ASICs for spectroscopic x-ray imaging, *Journal of Instrumentation*, 2016 JINST 11 P01007, doi:10.1088/1748-0221/11/01/P01007.

[Bohenek 2018] M. Bochenek, S. Bottinelli, Ch. Broennimann, P. Livi and T. Loeliger, IBEX: Versatile readout ASIC with spectral imaging capability and high count rate capability, *IEEE Transactions on Nuclear Science* 65(6), 1285–1291 (June 2018).

[Boussel 2015] L. Boussel, D. Barness, Pre-clinical application with in vivo photon counting technology: Preliminary results, *1st Spectral Photon Counting CT Workshop*, Lyon, France, September 2015.

[Butler 2018] A. Butler, Mars Collaboration, First living human images from a MARS photon-counting 8-energy CT, *IEEE NSS-MICS*, October 2018, Sydney, Australia.

[Dlugosz 2007] R. Dlugosz, K. Iniewski, High-precision analogue peak detector for x-ray imaging applications, *Electronics Letters* 43(8), (April 2007).

[Geronimo 2014] G. De Geronimo, P. O'Connor, *MOSFET optimization in deep submicron technology for charge amplifiers*, IEEE Symposium Conference Record Nuclear Science, 2004, 10.1109/NSSMIC.2004.1462062.

[Gustavsson 2012] M. Gustavsson, F. Ul Amin, A. Bjorklid, A. Ehliar, C. Xu and C. Svensson, A high-rate energy-resolving photon-counting ASIC for spectral computed tomography, *IEEE Transactions on Nuclear Science* 1(59), 30–39 (2012).

[Iniewski 2014] K. Iniewski, CZT detector technology for medical imaging, *Journal of Instrumentation* 9(11), C1100 (November 2014), DOI: 10.1088/1748-0221/9/11/C11001.

[Iniewski 2015] K. Iniewski, CZT growth, characterization, fabrication and electronics for operation at > 100 Mcps/mm^2, *3rd Workshop on Medical Applications of Spectroscopic X-ray Detectors*, CERN, Geneva, April 2015.

[Iniewski 2016] K. Iniewski, CZT sensors for computed tomography: From crystal growth to image quality, *Journal of Instrumentation* 11, (December 2016).

[Iniewski 2017] K. Iniewski et al, 4-side buttable CZT detector modules for spectral CT, *4th Workshop on Medical Applications of Spectroscopic*, CERN, Geneva, May 2017.

[Iwanczyk 2015] J. Iwanczyk (Ed.), Radiation detectors for medical imaging, in *Devices, Circuits, and Systems*, CRC Press, 2015, Boca Raton, FL.

[Kappler 2012] S. Kappler, T. Hannemann, E. Kraft, B. Kreisler, D. Niederloehner, K. Stierstorfer and T. Flohr, First results from a hybrid prototype CT scanner for exploring benefits of quantum-counting in clinical CT, *Proc. SPIE* 8313, (2012).

[Knoll 2000] G. Knoll, *Radiation Detection and Measurement*, John Wiley and Sons, 2000.

[Liu 2016] X. Liu, F. Groenberg, M. Sjolin, S. Karlsson and M. Danielsson, Count rate performance of a silicon-strip detector for photon-counting spectral CT, *Nuclear Instruments and Methods in Physics Research A* 827, 102–106 (2016).

[Loeliger 2012] T. Loeliger, C. Brönnimann, T. Donath and M. Schneebeli, *The new PILATUS3 ASIC with instant retrigger capability*, 2012 IEEE Nuclear Science Symposium and Medical Imaging Conference Record (NSS/MIC), *10.1109/NSSMIC.2012.6551180.*

[McCollough 2015] C. McCollough, S. Leng, L. Yu, J. Fletcher, Dual- and multi-energy CT: Principles, technical approaches, and clinical applications, *Radiology* 276(3), 637–653 (2015).

[Michalowska 2011] A. Michalowska, O. Gevin, O. Limousin and X. Coppolani, *Multi-dimensional optimization of charge preamplifier in 0.18 μm CMOS technology for low power CdTe spectro-imaging system*, 2011 IEEE Nuclear Science Symposium Conference, Valencia, 2011, 10.1109/NSSMIC.2011.6153985.

[Persson 2014] M. Persson, Ben Hubber, S. Karlsson, X. Liu, H. Chen, C. Cu, M. Yveborg, H. Bornefalk and M. Danielsson, Energy-resolved CT imaging with a photon-counting silicon-strip detector, *Physics in Medicine and Biology* 59, 6709–6727 (2014).

[Pennicard 2017] D. Pennicard, B. Pirard, O. Tolbanov and K. Iniewski, Semiconductor materials for x-ray detectors, *MRS Bulletin* 42(06), 445–450 (June 2017), DOI: 10.1557/mrs.2017.95.

[Prekas 2014] G. Prekas, The effect of crystal quality on the behaviour of semi-insulating CdZnTe detectors for x-ray spectroscopic and high flux applications, *IEEE NSS-RTSD-MICS*, October 2014, Seattle.

[Redlen 2016] http://redlen.ca/hitachi-and-redlen-technologies-announce-agreement-on-joint-development-for-next-generation-medical-photon-counting-ct-system/, Vancouver, Canada, March 2016.

[Szeles 2008] C. Szeles, S. Soldner, S. Vydrin, J. Graves and D. Bale, CdZnTe semiconductor detectors for spectroscopic x-ray imaging, *IEEE Transactions on Nuclear Science* 55(1), 572–582 (March 2008).

[Strassburg 2011] M. Strassburg, C. Schroeter and P. Hackenschmied, CdTe/CZT under high flux irradiation, *Journal of Instrumentation* 6, (January 2011).

[Steadman 2011] R. Steadman, C. Herrmann, O. Mülhens and D. Maeding, ChromAIX: Fast photon-counting ASIC for spectral computed tomography, *Nuclear Instruments and Methods in Physics Research Section A Accelerators Spectrometers Detectors and Associated Equipment* 648, (August 2011), DOI: 10.1016/j.nima.2010.11.149.

[Steadman 2017] R. Steadman, C. Herrmann and A. Livne, ChromAIX2: A large area, high count-rate energy-resolving photon counting ASIC for a spectral CT prototype, *Nuclear Instruments and Methods in Physics Research Section A Accelerators Spectrometers Detectors and Associated Equipment* 862, (May 2017), DOI: 10.1016/j.nima.2017.05.010.

[Taguchi 2013] K. Taguchi, J. Iwanczyk, Vision 20/20: Single photon counting x-ray detectors in medical imaging, *Medical Physics* 40(10), 100901 (2013).

15 ChromAIX
Energy-Resolving Photon Counting Electronics for High-Flux Spectral CT

Roger Steadman[1], Christoph Herrmann[1], and Amir Livne[2]
[1]Philips Research Europe, High Tech Campus, Eindhoven, Netherlands
[2]Philips Healthcare, Haifa, Israel

CONTENTS

15.1 INTRODUCTION

While in recent years the focus in clinical computed tomography (CT) has been to reduce the X-ray dose by image reconstruction methods, technology (especially in the area of X-ray conversion materials) has in the mean-time matured such that single photon-counting detectors seem possible, which allow for significantly improved exploitation of spectral information when compared to known dual-energy CT approaches.

The advent of energy-discriminating photon-counting detectors will result in a further significant increase of sensitivity (X-ray and contrast agent dose reduction) and higher specificity (improved quantification, e.g., due to elimination of beam hardening [1, 2]), while requiring lower dose than current state-of-the-art CT [3].

Exploiting energy information of the impinging photons of the polychromatic emission of the X-ray tube allows distinguishing the two main physical causes of energy-dependent attenuation (Photoelectric effect and Compton effect). This energy dependency is not resolved in conventional CT detectors, causing so-called beam-hardening artefacts. Correction algorithms in place are limited and the remaining artefacts can potentially lead to misdiagnosis [1]. Energy-resolving detectors will eliminate beam-hardening artefacts.

Currently a number of dual-energy methods based on conventional indirect conversion detectors are available (dual source [4], tube kVp switching [5], and dual layer stacking [6]) that can provide two spectrally distinct measurements, allowing Photoelectric and Compton effects to be distinguished. There is however more information to be obtained, further contributing to higher diagnostic specificity. The capability of simultaneously providing a number of spectrally distinct measurements not only allows distinguishing between photoelectric and Compton interactions, but also discriminating contrast agents that exhibit a K-edge discontinuity in the absorption spectrum, referred to as K-edge imaging [7, 8]. By acquiring more than two spectral measurements, advanced material decomposition based on K-edge imaging can be achieved. That is, a contrast agent exhibiting a K-edge discontinuity in the CT-relevant energy range can be clearly separated from other materials present in the body (e.g., separation of a Gadolinium contrast agent and calcification). The diagnostic value resides not only in providing contrast-agent only images, but also in the capacity to resolve the local mass density of the contrast agent, thus allowing additional quantification [8].

This requires the introduction of direct-conversion sensors and energy-resolving photon-counting readout electronics both fast enough to separate individual X-ray photons, referred henceforth to as photon-counting Spectral CT. Such detectors are based on direct converting sensors (e.g., CdTe or CdZnTe) and high-rate photon counting electronics.

15.2 ENERGY-RESOLVING PHOTON COUNTING ELECTRONICS

Photon counting electronics are front-end readout channels capable of determining the amount of impinging photons per unit time and per pixel. Figure 15.1 shows a simple block diagram of a typical energy-resolving readout channel consisting of a charge sensitive amplifier (CSA), a Shaper, and a number of energy discriminators. Most photon-counting application specific integrated circuits (ASICs) are based on such a topologies or variations thereof. The CSA integrates the total charge carried by the current pulse generated inside the direct converter material (Si, CdTe, CZT, etc.). It generates a step-like response to an impinging photon, which is then subsequently filtered by the Shaper stage. This stage reduces the high-frequency noise of the first stage [9] and produces a voltage pulse, the height of which is proportional to the charge of the sensor current pulse, and therefore to the energy of the X-ray photon. As Figure 15.1 depicts, most photon-counting ASICs integrate the CSA, Shaper, and energy discriminators within the pixel, often including the threshold analog to digital converter (ADC) also within a pixel.

Single-stage designs have also been demonstrated to work [10]. An advantage of a two-stage amplifier with a CSA is the possibility to provide, via a fast voltage buffer, the CSA output voltage to the outside world for measuring the charge collection time inside the sensor with a fast oscilloscope.

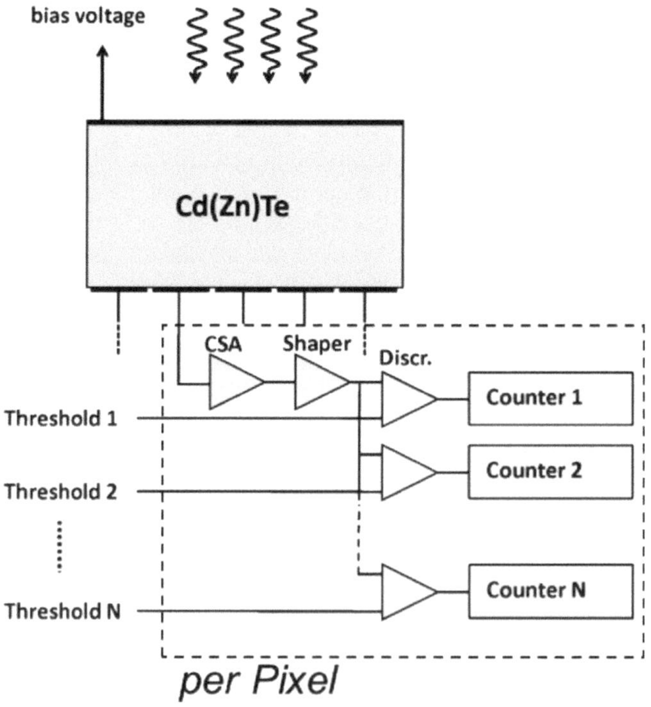

FIGURE 15.1 Typical energy-resolving photon-counting readout channel.

The amplitude of the Shaper voltage pulse can then be compared against a plurality of energy discriminators in order to coarsely classify each event as to its energy. For each event that triggers a discriminator, a corresponding counter is increased to accumulate the number of photons per unit time and energy range, which exceed the discriminator's energy threshold. The energy discrimination may be single-sided (i.e., all energy counters below the photon energy are increased) or double-sided (i.e., only the counter associated to an energy range (or bin) is incremented in correspondence to the registered energy of the impinging photon).

Photon counting electronics are mostly defined by their rate capability and their energy resolution. The capability to distinguish impinging photons, which are deposited within a short time interval defines the rate capability of the ASIC. Photon counting is generally described as "noiseless." That is, if an energy threshold is sufficiently above the electronic noise of the analogue front-end, the number of registered counts only depends on the number of impinging photons undisturbed by electronic noise, while the number of these photons is still governed by Poisson statistics. Electronic noise however still manifests itself by contributing to the energy resolution, that is, the accuracy by which the energy of a known photon can be determined. For a monochromatic source, the energy resolution is determined by the width of the visible photo-peak in a measured spectrum. The wider the photo-peak is, the worse is the energy resolution.

Multiple examples of photon counting electronics can be found in the literature. State-of-the-art examples are the Medipx3 [11], Pilatus3 [12], Ibex [13], XPAD3[14].

Another characteristic of photon-counting detectors is the problem of the low-energy tail: due to charge sharing or K-fluorescence cross-talk between neighboring pixels, many of the recorded events appear with a smaller energy than that of the absorbed X-ray photon. Hence, either the pixel must be chosen large enough or some charge summing logic is needed to correct for this. Circuitry for charge summing, however, limits the achievable count rate support [15].

To pave the way toward human Spectral CT, Philips has developed proprietary photon-counting readout ASIC called ChromAIX (*krəumæks*, Chrome, Greek: color, AIX: ASIC for imaging with X-ray).

To show the experimental feasibility of such electronics, a test ASIC (ChromAIX1, referred to ChromAIX in literature) was reported in [16, 17]. ChromAIX1 achieved observable count rates (OCRs) exceeding 13.5 Mcps/pixel, corresponding to an impinging rate (input count rate, ICR) of 37 Mcps/pixel. The OCR closely followed the expectations from a Paralyzable model [18]. It incorporated four independent energy thresholds and input referred rms-noise lower than 350 e^-. ChromAIX1 consisted of a 4 × 16 pixel array at an isotropic pitch of 300 μm.

ChromAIX2 [19], as described here in more details, is meant to consolidate the performance of its predecessor and to allow integration on a CT gantry for evaluation. To this end a prototype scanner using ChromAIX2 has been developed and installed in a clinical environment. Exemplary results are shown in [20–27].

The ChromAIX2 already exhibits a large area coverage to facilitate evaluating the Spectral CT image quality, and is 3-side-buttable to support a CT scanner of about 2 cm isocenter coverage. Larger pixels (500 μm) were chosen to improve spectral performance (improved low-energy tail) at the cost of the count rate support Table 15.1 presents a juxtaposition of key parameters.

15.3 CHROMAIX2 PIXEL DESIGN

The ChromAIX2 ASIC features 22 × 32 pixels at an isotropic pitch of 500 μm. The ASIC is 3-side tile-able, allowing to arrange many ASICs side by side in a row of two along the gantry rotation axis. Such an arrangement therefore may yield up to 64 slices at a 500-μm pitch. Along one of its sides, the ASIC features the I/O and power connections.

The pixel pitch has been increased from the 300 μm featured in ChromAIX1 to 500 μm. The larger pixels ensure a better energy response as it is less affected by charge sharing.

TABLE 15.1
Key Parameters of the ChromAIX ASIC Family

	ChromAIX1	**ChromAIX2**
Pitch	300 × 300 μm² pixels	500 × 500 μm² pixels
OCR_{max}	13.5 Mcps/pixel → 150 Mcps/mm²	15.5 Mcps/pixel → 62 Mcps/mm²
Deadtime	τ = 27 ns	τ = 23.8 ns
Pile-up characteristic	Paralyzable	Paralyzable
Pixels	4 × 16 pixels	22 × 32 pixels
Buttability	2 side buttable	3 side buttable
Dimensions	5.5 × 7.7 mm²	11 × 19 mm²
Thresholds	4	5
Threshold resolution	0.5 keV/LSB	0.5 keV/LSB
Noise	ENC 350 e⁻	ENC 260 e⁻
Leakge compensation	Static 20 nA	Static/Dynamic 200/(60/600) nA
Dynamic leakage bandwitdh	n/a	10 kHz

The analogue front-end consists of a two-stage amplifier topology. Figure 15.2 shows a simplified block diagram of the pixel electronics. The first stage is a CSA followed by a pole-zero cancellation network. The second stage is a fast Shaper with a less than 10 ns peaking time and nominally 23.5 ns deadtime at an equivalent 25 keV threshold. A deadtime of 23.5 ns offers sufficient margin to ensure achieving OCRs significantly higher than the specified 10 Mcps/pixel. Figure 15.3 shows the simulated waveform at the output of the Shaper stage.

Each pixel is equipped with five independent energy thresholds and the corresponding counters with a bit-depth of 16 bits. In order to enable K-edge imaging applications, the number of spectrally distinct measurements must equal or exceed the number of desired energy decomposed images. To obtain separate photoelectric, Compton and K-edge images, a minimum of three thresholds are required [7]. Furthermore, dual-contrast applications [26, 27] require that the readout channel

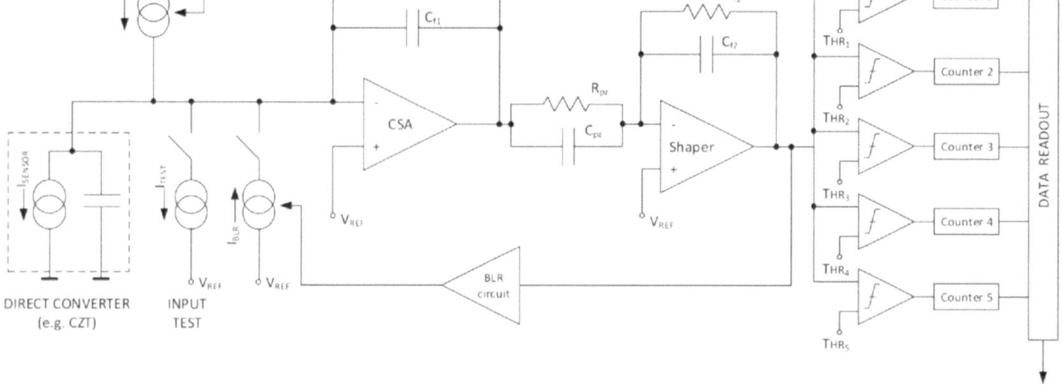

FIGURE 15.2 Simplified block diagram of the ChromAIX2 front-end circuit (Reprinted from [19], with permission from Elsevier).

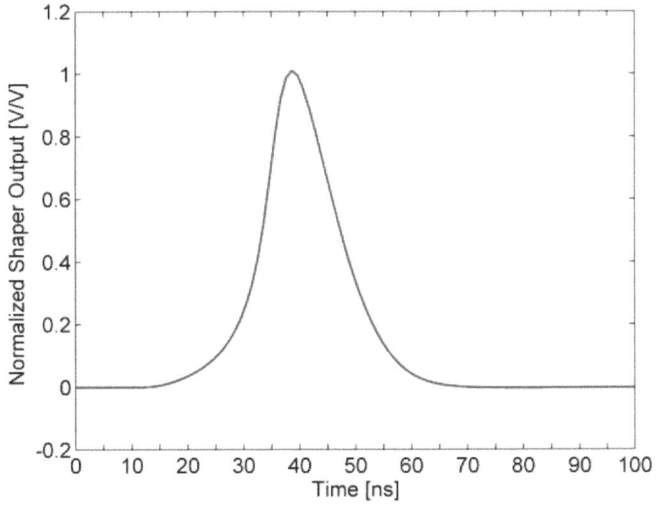

FIGURE 15.3 Normalized Shaper output waveform from simulations in response to a Cd (Zn)Te current transient equivalent to 100 keV (Reprinted from [19], with permission from Elsevier).

is equipped with at least four energy thresholds. The choice of five energy thresholds therefore addresses these needs with some additional flexibility, for example allowing the use of the 5th threshold as a measure of pile-up [28]. The thresholds are implemented as single-sided bins, that is, each of them counts all photons above the equivalent threshold energy. Energy windowing is obtained by subtraction of the single-sided bins later in the image chain when required. The thresholds each consist of a 9-bit digital to analog converter (DAC) covering a range exceeding 160 keV and with a resolution of 0.5 keV/lsb.

In contrast to the ChromAIX1 device, a baseline restoration circuit (BLR) has been included in the front-end for dynamic leakage current compensation (see specification in Table 15.1). The BLR senses the baseline at the Shaper output and compensates any deviation from the reference potential by injecting a current at the input node. Although the ASIC is temperature compensated, a BLR circuit has been introduced to stabilize the baseline in response to changes of the sensor's leakage current. The BLR circuit can be completely switched off if unnecessary and it has been equipped with two current compensation ranges. The low-current range can compensate leakage currents and drifts of up to 60 nA. A high-current mode that can deal with up to 600 nA is also available to accommodate a plurality of sensors and material qualities. The BLR has been designed to effectively cancel out any drifting current with a bandwidth of up to 10 kHz.

The ChromAIX2 is also equipped with a pixel-specific static leakage current compensation circuit. It consists of a current source controlled by a 9-bit DAC. The 9-bit DAC is controlled via the pixel registers and it can compensate up to 200 nA of leakage current. The CSA output is monitored with a reference comparator allowing to determine the crossing of the baseline for increasing compensation currents. To this end, an adequate 9-bit value can be found that compensates the CSA output in absence of X-ray radiation with an accuracy of approximately 0.4 nA. Since each pixel has its own 9-bit DAC, the full array can be compensated for any pixel-dependent leakage current drained by the sensor.

A number of test features have been included on the ASIC allowing to fully assess its performance. For simplicity, Figure 15.2 only shows a current source at the input node. This DC current source is specific to each pixel and controlled by a 9-bit DAC capable of sourcing up to approximately 900 nA. To emulate impinging photon rates, the DC current is strobed by an

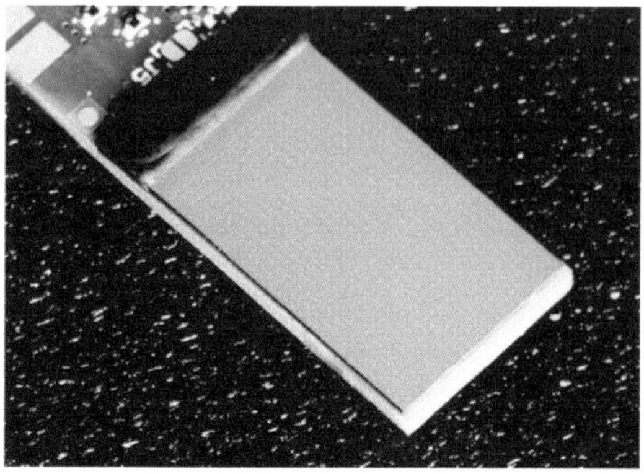

FIGURE 15.4 Photomicrograph of the ChromAIX2 ASIC (Reprinted from [19], with permission from Elsevier).

external high-frequency generator. The frequency and pulse width of the external generator can therefore be used to precisely inject charge pulses and test the performance of the front-end circuits in a well-defined manner. In order to allow testing the leakage current compensation circuits (both static and BLR), the strobe signal can be disabled so that a DC current is injected at the input node.

The ASIC is equipped with a 14-bit ADC converter that allows monitoring a plurality of internal nodes. The ADC can be used as a voltage mode acquisition device or as a current monitoring tool. In the voltage mode, it can be used to measure the programmable Bandgap reference or the internal temperature sensor with a resolution of 0.03°C/lsb. The current-mode option for the ADC can be used to monitor the input node of any one pixel at a time, allowing to gauge the leakage current of the sensor or the current of the internal test pulser. All pixel inputs can therefore be calibrated to offer very similar test conditions, which are necessary to assess the performance of the ASIC in terms of dispersion (e.g., count-rate) across the array. The ADC itself can also be calibrated by injecting precise external currents if required. The ADC output is mapped as an additional pixel in the array and the acquired measurement is therefore available on the projection data. All the aforementioned measureable parameters can in turn also be connected to a plurality of analogue outputs for alternative monitoring options.

The data readout of the ChromAIX2 fulfils the stringent requirements of clinical CT, supporting frame rates higher than 10 kHz and negligible acquisition deadtime, that is, acquisition and readout cycles are concurrent so that effectively no X-ray photon is lost.

The ChromAIX2 has been manufactured in a 0.18 μm process. Figure 15.4 shows a photo of the device mounted onto an evaluation substrate.

15.4 ELECTRICAL CHARACTERIZATION

The internal current pulser circuit has been used to inject well defined charge packets at the input node in order to characterize the inherent count-rate performance of the ChromAIX2. The current is strobed by using an external arbitrary pulse generator which has been programmed to deliver *Poissonian* interarrival times of the pulse injection at subsequently increased frequencies. The results of such a measurement allow assessing if the front-end adheres to the expectation from the Paralyzable model [18]. Figure 15.5 shows the results of injecting fixed amounts of electric charge equivalent to 65 keV photons for a threshold set at 25 keV. In Figure 15.5, the Paralyzable curve delivered by the ASIC can be compared to the Paralyzable theory with a deadtime of 23.8 ns. The variance of the acquired data for 1000 independent acquisitions is also shown, again following

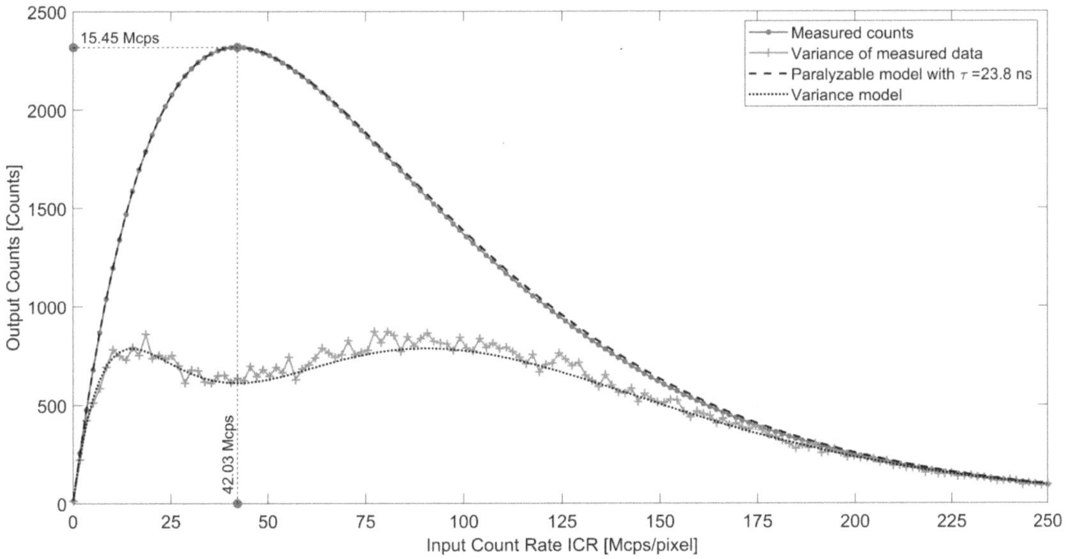

FIGURE 15.5 Observed counts and variance performance of the ChromAIX2 for an exemplary pixel, acquired for 65 keV equivalent input photons at a 25-keV threshold and 150 μs frame time. Count rate points calculated with 150 μs frame time. Paralyzable model for rate and variance shown for comparison (Reprinted from [19], with permission from Elsevier).

very closely the expectation from theory. Equations (Eq. 1 and Eq. 2) show the Paralyzable theory for the mean count-rate and the variance respectively, from [29].

$$E(Y) = \lambda e^{-\lambda\tau} \tag{15.1}$$

$$Var(Y) = \lambda e^{-\lambda\tau}\left[1 - \left(2\lambda\tau - \lambda\tau^2\right)e^{-\lambda\tau}\right], \tag{15.2}$$

where λ is the mean photon rate, τ is the deadtime of the detector, *E(Y)* is the estimate of the mean observed rate and *Var(Y)* is the variance of counts.

For the exemplary pixel shown in Figure 15.5, a maximum OCR of 15.45 Mcps/pixel has been reached, corresponding to an ICR of approximately 42 Mcps/pixel. The ChromAIX2 ASIC can therefore register OCRs beyond 61 Mcps/mm². The full array has been evaluated in calibrated input conditions. The mean maximum OCR for the full array is μ_{rate} = 15.2 Mcps/pixel with σ_{rate} = 0.3 Mcps/pixel, corresponding to a deadtime of τ = 24 ns with σ_τ = 0.5 ns. The deadtime dispersion is consistent with corner simulations. Figure 15.6 shows the distribution of the rate across the array.

The inherent ASIC noise performance is evaluated by analyzing the S-curve resulting from carrying out a threshold scan with a monochromatic input injection. The S-curve is defined by the transition of registered counts when the threshold(s) is subsequently increased until it corresponds to a larger equivalent energy than the impinging photons. In this case, the internal pulser is again used to emulate a monochromatic periodic pulse train, allowing to set up a precise charge at a frequency and thereby easily acquiring good statistics. Figure 15.7 shows an exemplary S-curve obtained by a threshold scan with a 100-keV equivalent input charge at a rate of 5 MHz. The width S-curve is a direct indication of the electronic noise of the channel. For the exemplary pixel shown in Figure 15.7, the noise is 2.73 keV full width at half maximum (FWHM), corresponding to an input referred noise equivalent to 260 e^-, thereby fulfilling the maximum design specification. All pixels in the array exhibit a similar noise performance with a mean noise level of 262 e^- with σ_{noise} = 17 e^-. The results for one channel per pixel and the full array are shown in Figure 15.8.

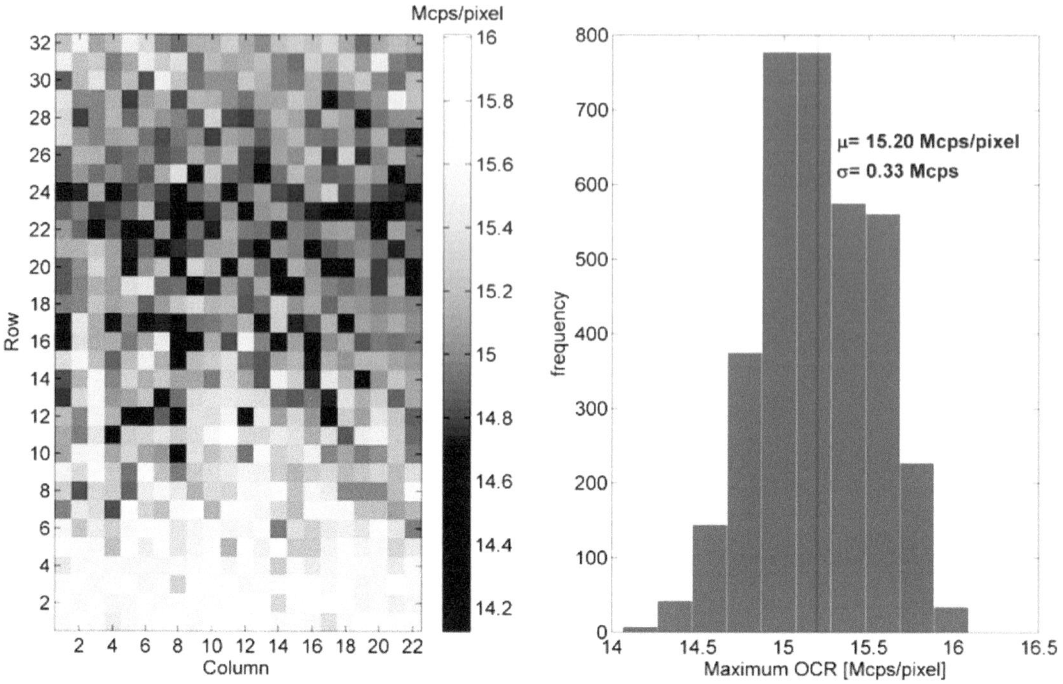

FIGURE 15.6 Rate dispersion across the array. Maximum rate (left) shown for one channel/pixel. Histogram (right) of the maximum rate for the full array, with μ_{rate} = 15.2 Mcps/pixel and σ_{rate} = 0.33 Mcps (Reprinted from [19], with permission from Elsevier).

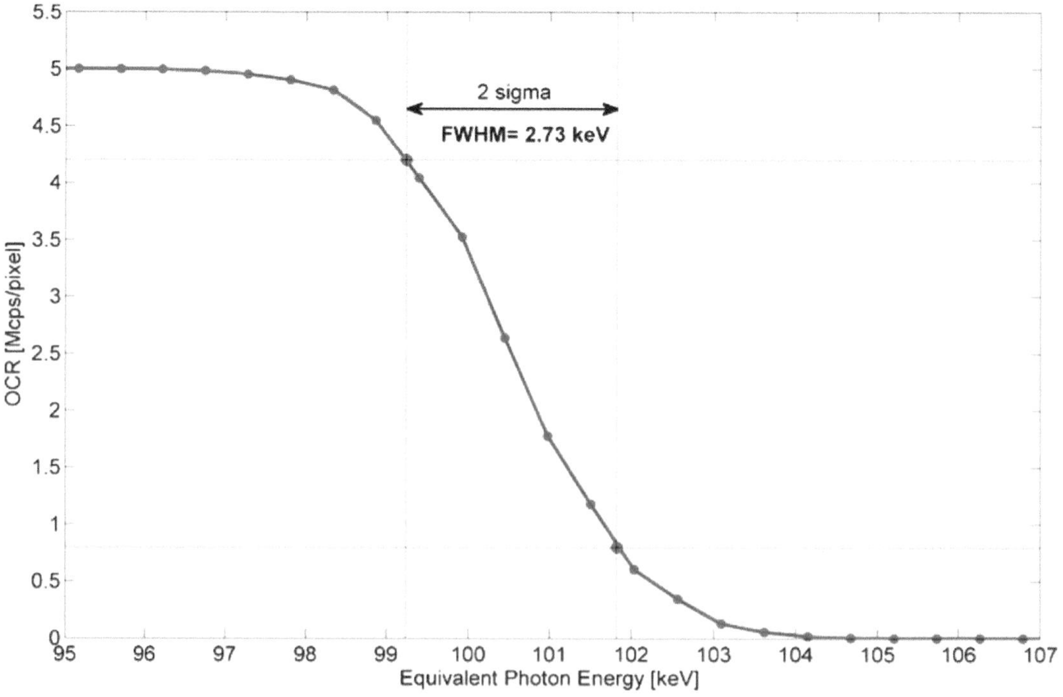

FIGURE 15.7 S-curve of a threshold scan for an exemplary pixel showing FWHM = 2.73 keV, equivalent to 260 e^- ENC (Reprinted from [19], with permission from Elsevier).

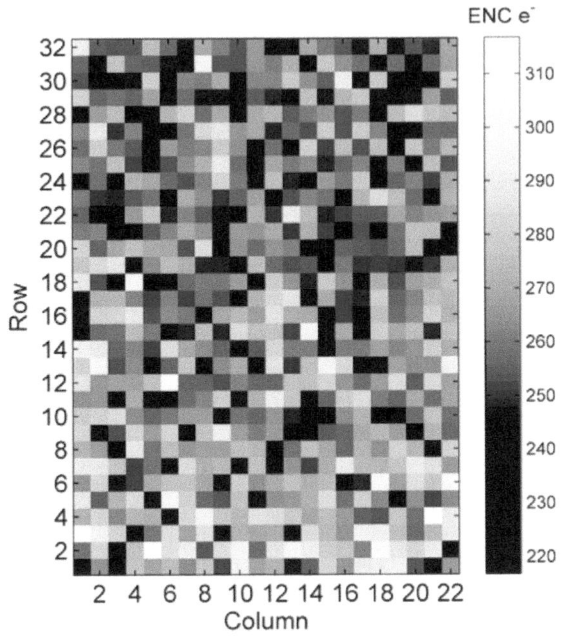

FIGURE 15.8 Noise dispersion in e- for one channel/pixel across the full array, μ_{noise} = 262 e- and σ_{noise} = 17 e- (Reprinted from [19], with permission from Elsevier).

The BLR has also been thoroughly characterized. Figure 15.9 shows the signal attenuation properties of the BLR circuit when a frequency-modulated leakage current is fed into the input node. A biased sine modulation has been used with an amplitude of 40 nA and offset of 20 nA. For increasing frequencies the resulting attenuation at the Shaper output has been characterized. At a sine frequency of 200 Hz, the measured attenuation is approximately -35 dB and as expected follows

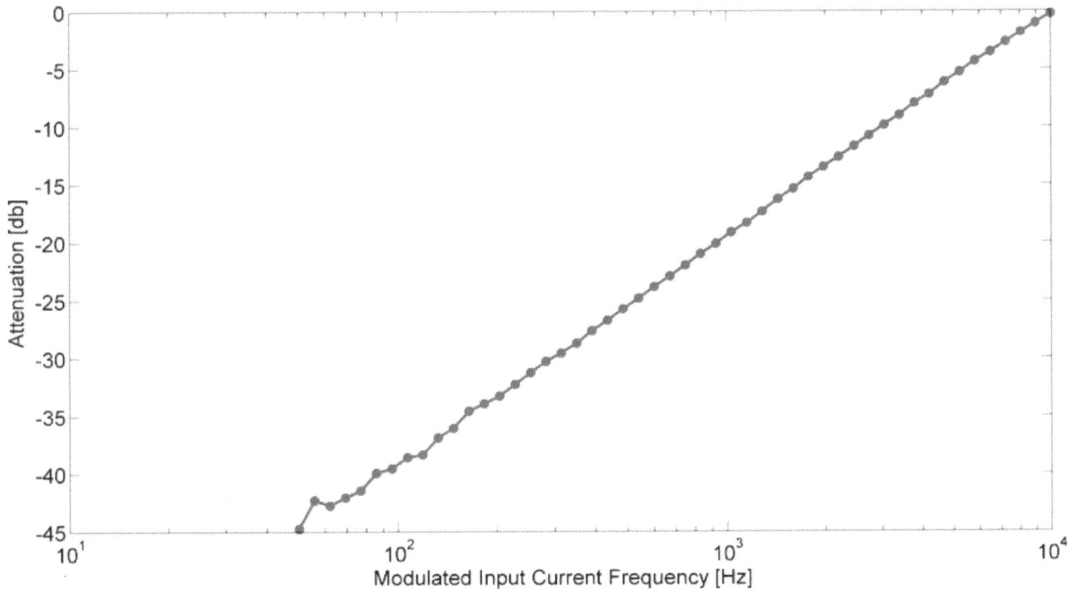

FIGURE 15.9 Attenuation of the BLR as a function of frequency (Reprinted from [19], with permission from Elsevier).

a 20-dB/dec slope. The -3 dB corner frequency is approximately at 9 kHz, slightly lower than the design specification of 10 kHz.

15.5 CHARACTERIZATION WITH X-RAYS

Following the thorough electrical characterization to assess the inherent performance of the ASIC, ~11 × ~16 × 2 mm³ CZT samples with the same native pixel pitch as the ASIC have been flip-chip assembled onto the ChromAIX2. Figure 15.10 shows the result of a (photo-peak normalized) differentiated threshold scan acquired with an 11-GBq ^{241}Am source. The threshold scan is acquired by registering the accumulated counts (single-sided) above a threshold being subsequently increased across the full-energy range. The low-energy events registered in the spectrum are caused by K fluorescence (both Cd and Te, with peaks in the 29–34 keV range) and charge sharing contribution expected from a 500-μm pixel pitch (no collimation used in this experiment). An FWHM of 8% has been achieved.

Spectra have also been acquired with an X-ray tube (Comet MXR-161 3 kW) set to 2 mA and 120 kVp at a distance of 65 cm. Figure 15.11 shows the results obtained with such a tube. The depicted measurement corresponds to averaging all pixels in the array after having been energy calibrated. The characteristic lines of the X-ray tube can be clearly seen.

Count-rate measurements with X-ray have also been carried out with an X-ray Tube (Philips MRC200 0.8 mm focus, tungsten target) at 120 kVp. For each pixel the five thresholds have been set from 30 to 70 keV in 10 keV steps. Rate measurements have been acquired for X-ray tube currents from 3 mA to 30 mA. The source to detector distance (SDD) was set to 30 cm to achieve sufficiently high-impinging rate. A 5-mm Al filter was used. The results can be seen in Figure 15.12. Each trace in Figure 15.12 represents the total number of photons above the corresponding threshold. Rates exceeding 15 Mcps/pixel have been achieved for the highest threshold. For the 30 keV

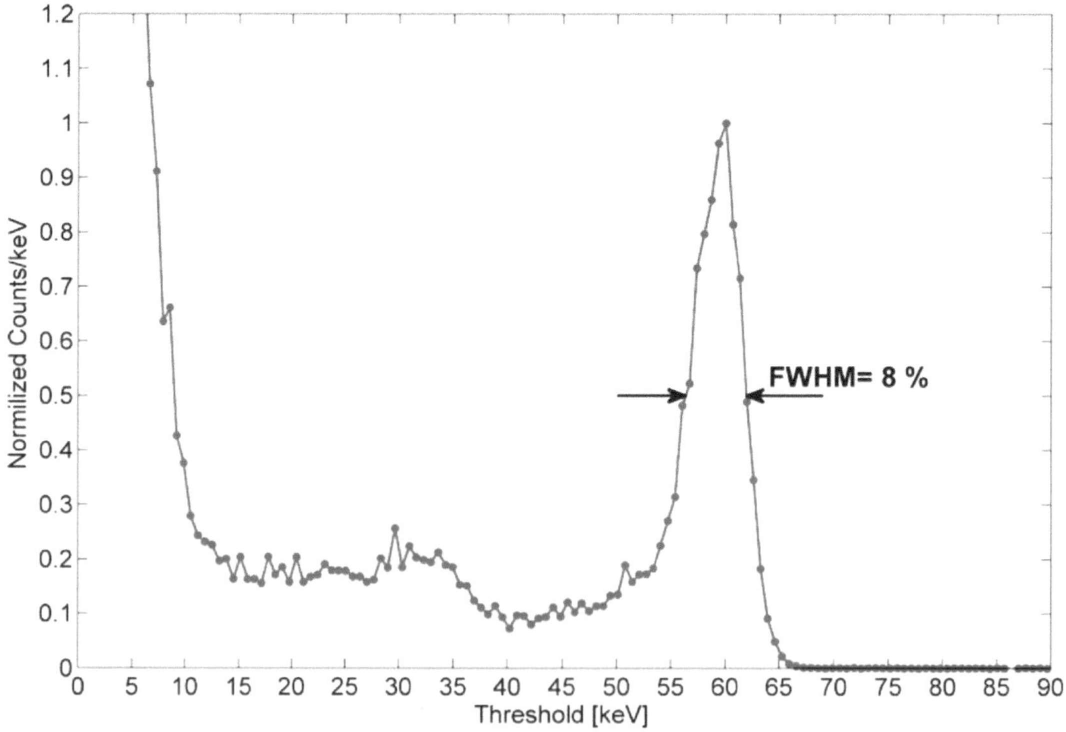

FIGURE 15.10 ^{241}Am spectrum obtained with a CZT sampled flip-chip bonded to the ChromAIX2. FWHM = 8% (Reprinted from [19], with permission from Elsevier).

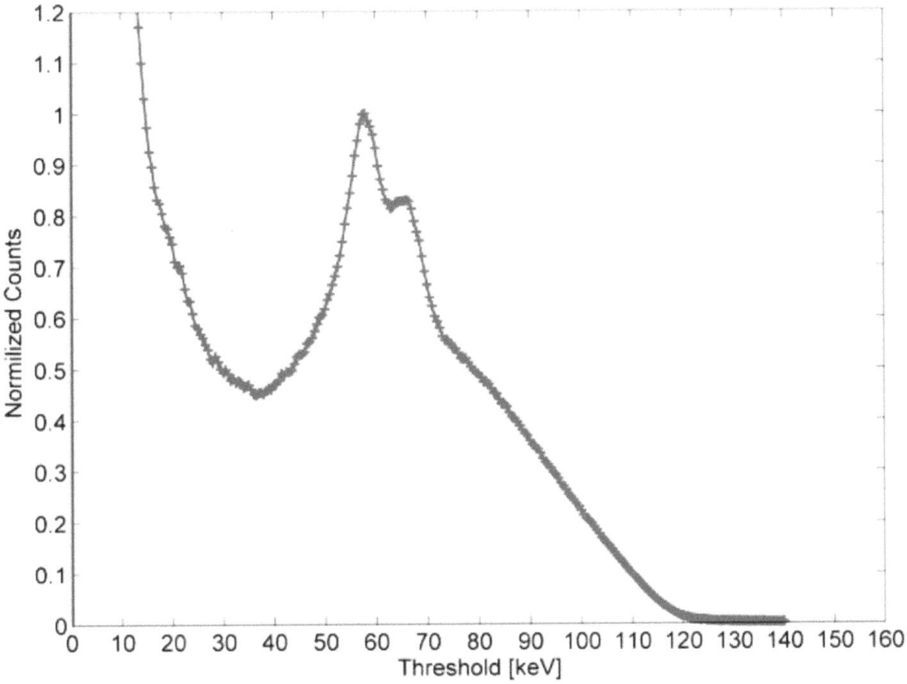

FIGURE 15.11 Tube spectrum obtained from a threshold scan with 120 kVp cathode voltage (Reprinted from [19], with permission from Elsevier).

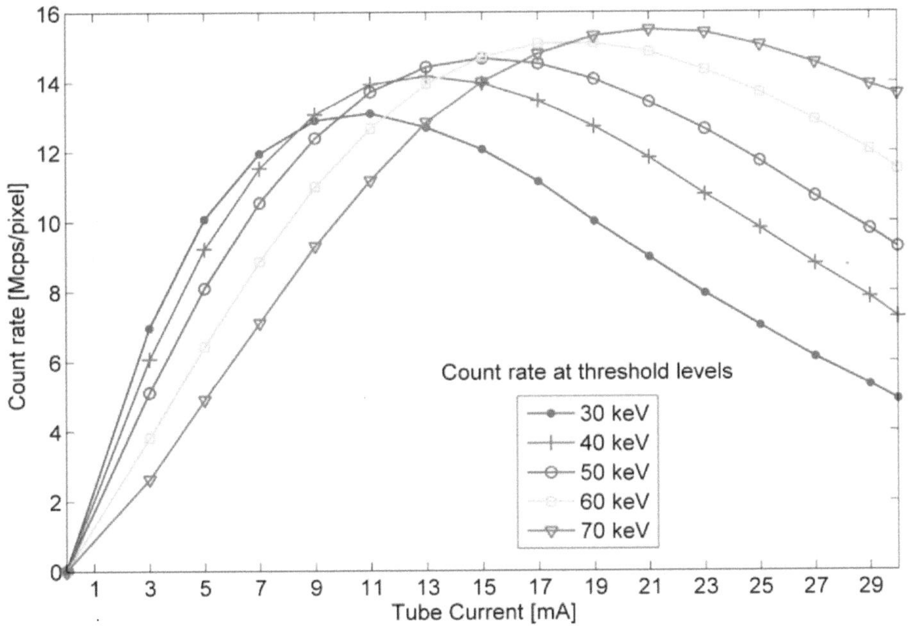

FIGURE 15.12 Rate performance of the CZT and ChromAIX2 with an X-ray tube swept for 1–29 mA. Exemplary pixel with the five-threshold set to 30, 40, 50, 60, and 70 keV (Reprinted from [19], with permission from Elsevier).

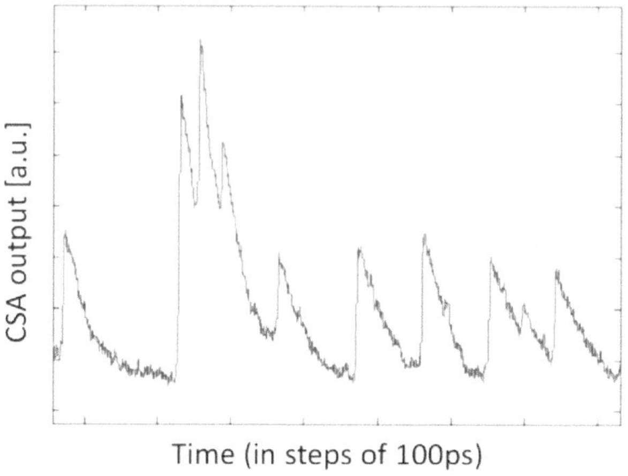

FIGURE 15.13 Pulse train at the CSA output measured with an oscilloscope connected with a fast buffer.

threshold, a rate of approximately 13 Mcps/pixel has been observed. The count-rate obtained with electrical pulses for a 25-keV threshold exceeded 15 Mcps/pixel (see Figure 15.5). There are several factors that contribute to the somewhat reduced count-rate when compared to the electrical characterization. The most relevant difference is the polychromatic nature of the impinging X-rays for the measurement shown in Figure 15.12. As mentioned earlier, for the electrical characterization monochromatic pulses were used. The Paralyzable model does not apply in the case of X-ray measurements and full understanding of the count-rate curve requires an in-depth analysis of the response function of the detector (e.g., [30]) and the pile-up model [31, 32]. The transient response of the CZT sensor can be modeled to an (time-mirrored) exponential-like waveform, as opposed to the rectangular input used for electrical measurements. This difference affects the effective peaking time of the Shaper, contributing to slightly different equivalent deadtimes. One other aspect which contributes to the count-rate curve is the presence of excess counts caused by charge sharing and induction as they account for a higher pile-up regime than it would be expected from the impinging rate.

15.6 SENSOR CHARGE COLLECTION TIME MEASUREMENTS

Using the fast buffer, which can be connected to a subset of pixels, it is possible to monitor the CSA output using a fast oscilloscope, so that CSA output pulse trains can be observed. The time it takes for each of the steps to reach the maximum is an upper bound for the charge collection time inside the sensor. Figure 15.13 shows such an exemplary pulse train from which an estimate of the charge collection time can be extracted. Based on these data, the charge collection time (sometimes also called CZT rise-time) was found to be not higher than 11 … 13 ns for Redlen CZT with 500 μm pitch at an external E-field strength of 450 V/mm.

15.7 CONCLUSION

The ChromAIX2 ASIC has been developed to fulfill the very stringent specifications required to enable energy-resolving Spectral CT. The analogue front-end has been shown to achieve OCRs exceeding 15 Mcps/pixel with electrical excitation at a threshold of 25 keV and an equivalent monochromatic input of 65 keV. The count-rate measurements have been found to follow very closely the expectation from the Paralyzable model for both mean rate and variance of the counts. Measurements with X-ray also show that the combination of the ChromAIX2 and a CZT crystal adhere to the specifications, exceeding 13 Mcps/pixel. The inherent input referred noise of the front-end has been experimentally measured to be 262 e^-. Tests with a ^{241}Am source yielded an FWHM of 8%.

To validate the new applications, clinical benefits and performance of energy-resolving photon-counting CT, the ChromAIX2 ASIC has been integrated onto a Philips CT prototype. Initial results based on this prototype have been published showcasing, among other applications, simultaneous dual-contrast agent experiments with K-edge imaging [26, 27].

REFERENCES

1. So A, Hsieh J, Li JY, Lee TY. Beam hardening correction in CT myocardial perfusion measurement. *Physics in Medicine & Biology*. 2009 Apr 27;54(10):3031.
2. Feuerlein S, Roessl E, Proksa R, Martens G, Klass O, Jeltsch M, Rasche V, Brambs HJ, Hoffmann MH, Schlomka JP. Multienergy photon-counting K-edge imaging: Potential for improved luminal depiction in vascular imaging 1. *Radiology*. 2008 Dec;249(3):1010–1016.
3. Taguchi K, Iwanczyk JS. Vision 20/20: Single photon counting X-ray detectors in medical imaging. *Medical Physics*. 2013 Oct 1;40(10):100901.
4. Johnson TR, Krauss B, Sedlmair M, Grasruck M, Bruder H, Morhard D, Fink C, Weckbach S, Lenhard M, Schmidt B, Flohr T. Material differentiation by dual energy CT: Initial experience. *European Radiology*. 2007 Jun 1;17(6):1510–1517.
5. Xu D, Langan DA, Wu X, Pack JD, Benson TM, Tkaczky JE, Schmitz AM. Dual energy CT via fast kVp switching spectrum estimation. In *SPIE Medical Imaging*. 2009 Feb 26:72583T–72583T. International Society for Optics and Photonics.
6. Carmi R, Naveh G, Altman A. Material separation with dual-layer CT. In *IEEE Nuclear Science Symposium Conference Record*, 2005 Oct 23;4:3. IEEE.
7. Roessl E, Proksa R. K-edge imaging in X-ray computed tomography using multi-bin photon counting detectors. *Physics in Medicine and Biology*. 2007 Jul 17;52(15):4679.
8. Schlomka J, Roessl E, Dorscheid R, Dill S, Martens G, Istel T, Bäumer C, Herrmann C, Steadman R, Zeitler G, Livne A. Experimental feasibility of multi-energy photon-counting K-edge imaging in pre-clinical computed tomography. *Physics in Medicine and Biology*. 2008 Jul 8;53(15):4031.
9. Nygård E, Aspell P, Jarron P, Weilhammer P, Yoshioka K. CMOS low noise amplifier for microstrip read-out design and results. *Nuclear Instruments and Methods in Physics Research Section A: Accelerators, Spectrometers, Detectors and Associated Equipment*. 1991 Mar 15;301(3):506–516.
10. Kraft E, Fischer P, Karagounis M, Koch M, Krueger H, Peric I, Wermes N, Herrmann C, Nascetti A, Overdick M, Ruetten W. Counting and integrating readout for direct conversion X-ray imaging: Concept, realization and first prototype measurements. *IEEE Transactions on Nuclear Science*. 2007 Apr;54(2):383–390.
11. Ballabriga R, Campbell M, Llopart X. ASIC developments for radiation imaging applications: The medipix and timepix family. *Nuclear Instruments and Methods in Physics Research Section A: Accelerators, Spectrometers, Detectors and Associated Equipment*. 2018 Jan 11;878:10–23.
12. Loeliger T, Brönnimann C, Donath T, Schneebeli M, Schnyder R, Trüb P. The new PILATUS3 ASIC with instant retrigger capability. In Nuclear Science Symposium and Medical Imaging Conference (NSS/MIC), 2012 IEEE 2012 Oct 27, pp. 610–615.
13. Bochenek M, Bottinelli S, Broennimann C, Livi P, Loeliger T, Radicci V, Schnyder R, Zambon P. IBEX: Versatile readout ASIC with spectral imaging capability and high count rate capability. *IEEE Transactions on Nuclear Science*. 2018 May 2.
14. Brunner FC, Dupont M, Meessen C, Boursier Y, Ouamara H, Bonissent A, Kronland-Martinet C, Clemens JC, Debarbieux F, Morel C. First K-edge imaging with a micro-CT based on the XPAD3 hybrid pixel detector. *IEEE Transactions on Nuclear Science*. 2013 Feb;60(1):103–108.
15. Koenig T, Hamann E, Procz S, Ballabriga R, Cecilia A, Zuber M, Llopart X, Campbell M, Fauler A, Baumbach T, Fiederle M. Charge summing in spectroscopic X-ray detectors with high-Z sensors. *IEEE Transactions on Nuclear Science*. 2013 Dec;60(6):4713–4718.
16. Steadman R, Herrmann C, Mülhens O, Maeding DG. ChromAIX: Fast photon-counting ASIC for spectral computed tomography. *Nuclear Instruments and Methods in Physics Research Section A: Accelerators, Spectrometers, Detectors and Associated Equipment*. 2011 Aug 21;648:S211–S215.
17. Steadman R, Herrmann C, Mülhens O, Maeding DG, Colley J, Firlit T, Luhta R, Chappo M, Harwood B, Kosty D. ChromAIX: A high-rate energy-resolving photon-counting ASIC for spectral computed tomography. In *Medical Imaging 2010: Physics of Medical Imaging*. 2010 Mar 22;7622:762220. International Society for Optics and Photonics.
18. Knoll GF. *Radiation Detection and Measurement*. John Wiley & Sons; 2010 Aug 16.

19. Steadman R, Herrmann C, Livne A. ChromAIX2: A large area, high count-rate energy-resolving photon counting ASIC for a spectral CT prototype. *Nuclear Instruments and Methods in Physics Research Section A: Accelerators, Spectrometers, Detectors and Associated Equipment.* 2017 Aug 1;862:18–24.
20. Si-Mohamed S, Bar-Ness D, Sigovan M, Cormode DP, Coulon P, Coche E, Vlassenbroek A, Normand G, Boussel L, Douek P. Review of an initial experience with an experimental spectral photon-counting computed tomography system. *Nuclear Instruments and Methods in Physics Research Section A: Accelerators, Spectrometers, Detectors and Associated Equipment.* 2017 Nov 21;873:27–35.
21. Cormode DP, Si-Mohamed S, Bar-Ness D, Sigovan M, Naha PC, Balegamire J, Lavenne F, Coulon P, Roessl E, Bartels M, Rokni M. Multicolor spectral photon-counting computed tomography: In vivo dual contrast imaging with a high count rate scanner. *Scientific Reports.* 2017 Jul 6;7(1):4784.
22. Kim J, Bar-Ness D, Si-Mohamed S, Coulon P, Blevis I, Douek P, Cormode DP. Assessment of candidate elements for development of spectral photon-counting CT specific contrast agents. *Scientific Reports.* 2018 Aug 14;8(1):12119.
23. Si-Mohamed S, Cormode DP, Bar-Ness D, Sigovan M, Naha PC, Langlois JB, Chalabreysse L, Coulon P, Blevis I, Roessl E, Erhard K. Evaluation of spectral photon counting computed tomography K-edge imaging for determination of gold nanoparticle biodistribution in vivo. *Nanoscale.* 2017;9(46):18246–18257.
24. Dangelmaier J, Bar-Ness D, Daerr H, Muenzel D, Si-Mohamed S, Ehn S, Fingerle AA, Kimm MA, Kopp FK, Boussel L, Roessl E. Experimental feasibility of spectral photon-counting computed tomography with two contrast agents for the detection of endoleaks following endovascular aortic repair. *European Radiology.* 2018 Feb 19:1–8.
25. Boussel L, Coulon P, Thran A, Roessl E, Martens G, Sigovan M, Douek P. Photon counting spectral CT component analysis of coronary artery atherosclerotic plaque samples. *The British Journal of Radiology.* 2014 Jul 4;87(1040):20130798.
26. Muenzel D, Bar-Ness D, Roessl E, Blevis I, Bartels M, Fingerle AA, Ruschke S, Coulon P, Daerr H, Kopp FK, Brendel B. Spectral photon-counting CT: Initial experience with dual–contrast agent K-edge colonography. *Radiology.* 2016 Dec 2:160890.
27. Muenzel D, Daerr H, Proksa R, Fingerle AA, Kopp FK, Douek P, Herzen J, Pfeiffer F, Rummeny EJ, Noël PB. Simultaneous dual-contrast multi-phase liver imaging using spectral photon-counting computed tomography: a proof-of-concept study. *European Radiology Experimental.* 2017 Dec 1;1(1):25.
28. Kappler S, Hölzer S, Kraft E, Stierstorfer K, Flohr T. Quantum-counting CT in the regime of count-rate paralysis: Introduction of the pile-up trigger method. In *SPIE Medical Imaging* 2011 Mar 3:79610T–79610T. International Society for Optics and Photonics.
29. Yu DF., Fessler JA. Mean and variance of single photon counting with deadtime. *Physics in Medicine and Biology.* 2000 Jul;45(7):2043.
30. Roessl E, Daerr H, Engel KJ, Thran A, Schirra C, Proksa R. Combined effects of pulse pile-up and energy response in energy-resolved, photon-counting computed tomography. In Nuclear Science Symposium and Medical Imaging Conference (NSS/MIC), 2011 IEEE 2011 Oct 23, pp. 2309–2313.
31. Roessl E, Daerr H, Proksa R. A Fourier approach to pulse pile-up in photon-counting X-ray detectors. *Medical Physics.* 2016 Mar 1;43(3):1295–1298.
32. Roessl E, Bartels M, Daerr H, Proksa R. On the analogy between pulse-pile-up in energy-sensitive, photon-counting detectors and level-crossing of shot noise. In *SPIE Medical Imaging.* 2016 Mar 25:97831H–97831H. International Society for Optics and Photonics.

16 Modeling the Imaging Performance of Photon Counting X-Ray Detectors

Jesse Tanguay[1] *and Ian Cunningham*[2]
[1]Assistant Professor, Department of Physics, Ryerson University, Toronto, Ontario, Canada
[2]Imaging Research Laboratories, Robarts Research Institute, and Department of Medical Biophysics, The University of Western Ontario, London, Ontario, Canada

CONTENTS

16.1 INTRODUCTION

In this chapter, we summarize recent work on mathematical modeling of the performance of photon-counting x-ray imaging detectors. Modeling enables understanding of relationships between the fundamental physics and engineering of x-ray detectors and the quality of the medical images they produce – an important aspect of image science.

State-of-the-art approaches for modeling are the culmination of over 70 years of academic research. Seminal works include those of Albert Rose whose research on the photographic process and the human visual system led to an understanding of relationships between image quality and the quantum nature of light.[1–3] Building on this work, Rodney Shaw and colleagues introduced a Fourier-based description of the performance of quantum-based imaging systems, including medical x-ray systems.[4] They established relationships between the modulation transfer function (MTF), which describes the spatial resolution of an imaging system, the Wiener noise power spectrum (NPS), which describes the power and texture of image noise, and image signal-to-noise ratio (SNR), quantified objectively in terms of the noise-equivalent number of quanta (NEQ). Using the methods of signal detection theory, Robert Wagner later described the relationships between these Fourier-based metrics of system performance and the detectability of objects in medical images.[5,6] The resulting theory provided a framework for objective evaluation and optimization of medical imaging instrumentation and is still used by academic and industry scientists.

Rabbani, Shaw, and Van Metter subsequently developed a mathematical formalism for modeling the influence of fundamental image-forming processes on the NPS of quantum-based imaging systems.[7,8] They provided tools for modeling the effects of stochastic gain and scatter stages on the NPS, enabling descriptions of, for example, the influence of x-ray conversion gain and emission of optical photons in a scintillating x-ray converter. Ian Cunningham and colleagues expanded this work into a set of tools for modeling the signal and noise properties of medical x-ray detectors, including digital x-ray detectors.[9–13] The resulting set of theoretical tools enables cascaded systems analysis (CSA), in which an imaging chain is broken down into serial and parallel cascades of image-forming processes. CSA is used widely by academia and industry in the development of novel x-ray imaging approaches, including contrast-enhanced breast imaging,[14] x-ray breast tomosynthesis,[15] cone-beam CT,[16–19] phase-contrast x-ray imaging,[20] and iterative image reconstruction.[21] CSA was also used extensively in the development of digital x-ray detectors for medical imaging, see for example references 22 and 23.

CSA was developed for energy-integrating x-ray detectors, which record information in a way that is fundamentally different from photon-counting x-ray detectors. The most important distinction is that photon-counting systems use energy thresholds to distinguish x-ray interaction events from electronic noise and to estimate photon energy. Energy thresholding is a nonlinear operation in which an input signal, which may take on values over the domain of real numbers or real integers, is converted to a value of 1 or 0. Until recently, there did not exist mathematical methods for modeling the influence of energy thresholding on the MTF and NPS of photon-counting x-ray detectors.

In this chapter, we summarize recent efforts to model the performance of photon-counting x-ray detectors. The material presented in this chapter utilizes heavily the mathematical and statistical concepts described by Ian Cunningham in the *SPIE Handbook of Medical Imaging*,[24] Harrison Barret and Kyle Myers in Foundations of Image Science,[25] and Athanasious Papoulis in *Probability, Random Variables and Stochastic Processes*.[26] The reader is referred to these texts to supplement the material presented in this chapter.

16.2 PERFORMANCE METRICS FOR LINEAR SHIFT-INVARIANT IMAGING SYSTEMS

Throughout this chapter we assume photon-counting detectors are linear and shift-invariant. Ian Cunningham provides a comprehensive introduction to linear systems theory in Chapter 2 of the *SPIE Handbook of Medical Imaging* Volume 1: Physics and Psychophysics. We provide a brief introduction here.

16.2.1 Image Signal

In general, a linear system is one for which the system output is proportional to the input. In the context of photon-counting detectors, this requirement can only be satisfied when count rates are low enough that pulse pile-up effects can be ignored. Pulse pile-up occurs when two or more photons deposit energy in a single detector element within the resolving time of the x-ray detector and results in a nonlinear relationship between input and output count rates. A shift-invariant system is one in which the response of the system to an impulse is independent of the location of the impulse. If we let $f(\mathbf{r})$ represent the input to a linear shift-invariant (LSI) imaging system, the average output image $[\bar{i}(\mathbf{r})]$ can be expressed as:

$$\bar{i}(\mathbf{r}) = \bar{G}f(\mathbf{r}) * \text{PSF}(\mathbf{r}) \tag{16.1}$$

where the overline bar represents an average value, **r** is a vector representing position in the image, $\bar{G}$ represents the large-area gain, which has units $[i/f]$, $*$ represents the convolution operator, and PSF(**r**) represents the system point spread function (PSF). For two-dimensional (2D) systems, PSF(**r**) has units of inverse area. The PSF represents the average response of a system to a unit impulse located at the origin, quantifies the spatial resolution of an imaging system and is normalized to unity area.

The Fourier-domain representation of Eq. (16.1) is:

$$\bar{I}(\mathbf{u}) = \bar{G}F(\mathbf{u})\text{MTF}(\mathbf{u}) \tag{16.2}$$

where **u** is a vector representing position in the spatial frequency domain, $F(\mathbf{u})$ represents the Fourier transform of $f(\mathbf{r})$, and the MTF is the Fourier transform of the PSF:

$$\text{MTF}(\mathbf{u}) = FT\left[\text{PSF}(\mathbf{r})\right]. \tag{16.3}$$

The MTF is a unitless, Fourier-based metric of the spatial resolution of an imaging system. The MTF is always equal to 1 at 0 spatial frequency. Equation (16.2) shows that the MTF characterizes how particular spatial frequencies are transferred through an imaging system. High spatial frequencies are associated with small objects; low spatial frequencies are associated with large objects. For an ideal imaging system that does not blur the input, the MTF is equal to unity at all spatial frequencies. For ideal digital x-ray imaging detectors, in which the image signal is binned into elements of finite spatial extent, the MTF is equal to the sinc function.

16.2.2 Image Noise

X-ray images are the end result of a series of stochastic processes. At the detection level, the number of x-ray photons incident on an element of a 2D x-ray detector is a Poisson-distributed random variable (RV). This means that if x-ray exposure conditions are held fixed, the number of photons incident on a detector element will vary randomly from one exposure to the next. In addition, the number of photons interacting within an x-ray converter given some fixed number of photons incident on the converter cannot be predicted for any given exposure. Instead, each photon has a probability of interacting with the x-ray converter; whether or not a given photon interacts with an x-ray converter is impossible to predict. The number of secondary quanta (e.g. optical photons in a scintillator, electron-hole (e-h) pairs in a semiconductor) produced by an x-ray interaction also varies randomly from one x-ray interaction to the next. Each of these processes contributes to image noise. Image noise is an important consideration when analyzing the quality of x-ray images, and when determining how medical imaging instrumentation affects image quality.

In the spatial domain, image noise can be quantified in terms of the image autocovariance function, $K(\mathbf{r},\mathbf{r}')$, which describes the covariance between two points in an image:

$$K(\mathbf{r},\mathbf{r}') = E\{\Delta\tilde{i}(\mathbf{r})\Delta\tilde{i}(\mathbf{r}')\} \tag{16.4}$$

where $\Delta\tilde{i}(\mathbf{r})$ represents the random deviation of the image signal $[\tilde{i}(\mathbf{r})]$ from its mean value, and similarly for $\Delta\tilde{i}(\mathbf{r}')$. A system for which the mean signal and variance are independent of location within the image, and for which the autocovariance only depends on the displacement $(\tau = \mathbf{r} - \mathbf{r}')$ between two points in the image is wide sense stationary (WSS). In this case, $K(\tau)$ can be expressed as:

$$K(\tau) = E\{\Delta\tilde{i}(\mathbf{r})\Delta\tilde{i}(\mathbf{r}+\tau)\}. \tag{16.5}$$

The variance of the image signal is obtained by setting $\tau = 0$:

$$\sigma_{\tilde{i}}^2 = K(\tau)\big|_{\tau=0}. \tag{16. 6}$$

The autocovariance characterizes the texture (or correlation) of image noise and the magnitude (or power) of image noise. When WSS conditions are satisfied, Fourier-based approaches can be used to characterize image noise. In the Fourier domain, the power and correlation of image noise are characterized in terms of the image NPS, which is the Fourier transform of the autocovariance function:

$$W(\mathbf{u}) = FT[K(\tau)]. \tag{16.7}$$

For 2D digital x-ray detectors, which only produce signals on a grid of points corresponding to the centers of detector elements, the NPS takes on the following form(27):

$$W_{\text{dig}}(\mathbf{u}) = W_{\text{PS}}(\mathbf{u}) + \sum_{n=1}^{\infty}\sum_{m=1}^{\infty} W_{\text{PS}}(\mathbf{u}+\mathbf{u}_{nm}) \tag{16.8}$$

where $W_{\text{dig}}(\mathbf{u})$ represents the digital NPS, $W_{\text{PS}}(\mathbf{u})$ represents the pre-sampling NPS, which is equal to the NPS of the image signal prior to sampling in discrete detector elements, and $\mathbf{u}_{nm} = (n/\Delta_x, m/\Delta_y)$ where Δ_x and Δ_y represent the sampling intervals in the x and y directions, respectively. The digital NPS is only defined for frequencies up to the Nyquist frequency, which is equal to one-half of the sampling frequency in the x and y directions.

16.2.3 Detective Quantum Efficiency

The preceding sections introduced Fourier-based metrics image signal and noise. The image signal relative to image noise for a 2D digital x-ray detector exposed to a uniform fluence of x-ray photons is characterized in terms of the NEQ(4):

$$\text{NEQ}_{\text{dig}}(\bar{q}_0, \mathbf{u}) = \frac{\bar{q}_0^2 \left|\bar{G}\text{MTF}(\mathbf{u})\right|^2}{W_{\text{dig}}(\mathbf{u})} \tag{16.9}$$

where $\bar{q}_0$ [mm^2] represents the fluence of x-ray photons incident on the x-ray detector. The numerator of the NEQ represents the squared image signal and the denominator represents image noise. It is important to note that the MTF in Eq. (16.9) is the presampling MTF, and does not include the effects of signal aliasing, which is nonlinear. In x-ray imaging, the quantum component of the NPS, that is, that due to random fluctuations in image quanta not including electronic or anatomic noise sources, is proportional to the fluence $\bar{q}_0$. Ignoring all other noise sources the NEQ is therefore proportional to $\bar{q}_0$, which is a property of the incident distribution of quanta, not of the imaging system. Normalizing the NEQ by $\bar{q}_0$ yields the detective quantum efficiency (DQE):

$$\mathrm{DQE_{dig}}(\mathbf{u}) = \frac{\mathrm{NEQ_{dig}}(\bar{q}_0, \mathbf{u})}{\bar{q}_0} = \frac{\bar{q}_0 \left|\bar{G}\mathrm{MTF}(\mathbf{u})\right|^2}{W_{\mathrm{dig}}(\mathbf{u})}. \tag{16.10}$$

The DQE is a normalized measure of the dose efficiency of an x-ray imaging detector, taking on values between 0 and 1 at all spatial frequencies up to the Nyquist frequency. The DQE therefore describes how efficiently an x-ray imaging detector transfers both large (i.e. low frequency) objects and fine (i.e. high frequency) details. The DQE is used widely by the medical imaging community to evaluate the performance of x-ray imaging detectors.

16.3 MODELING SIGNAL AND NOISE IN PHOTON-COUNTING X-RAY DETECTORS

Early efforts to model the performance of photon-counting x-ray detectors include those of Michel and colleagues,(28,29) who developed a model of the zero-frequency DQE under the assumption of low count rates such that pulse pile-up effects are negligible. Michel and colleagues related mathematically the zero-frequency DQE to the first and second statistical moments of what they termed the multiplicity, which is the number of detected photons relative to the number of interacting photons. In photon-counting systems, it is possible to record multiple photons per interaction when photon energy is spread over multiple elements. Michel and colleagues showed that the zero-frequency DQE is proportional to the square of the average multiplicity divided by the second moment of the distribution of multiplicities. They showed that the zero-frequency DQE degrades as the multiplicity increases, which was a novel result. Koenig and colleagues used the multiplicity concept to investigate the DQE of cadmium telluride (CdTe) detectors.(30) More recently, Ji and colleagues modeled theoretically the first and second moments of the multiplicity and calculated the zero-frequency DQE of CdTe detectors.(31)

One of the first efforts to model the frequency-dependent signal and noise properties of photon-counting systems was that of Acciavatti and colleagues.(32,33) They considered a photon-counting detector that applies a single energy threshold to distinguish x-ray interaction events from electronic noise under low count-rate conditions. Energy thresholding was accounted for by interpreting the pre-sampling PSF of an energy-integrating detector as the probability per unit area of counting a photon in an otherwise equivalent photon-counting x-ray detector. This interpretation led to the conclusion that the MTF of a photon-counting detector is equal to that of an otherwise equivalent energy-integrating detector, which has been challenged by recent works, including that of Xu and colleagues and the authors of this chapter.(34,35) By modeling energy thresholding as a binomial selection process, Acciavatti and colleagues related the photon-counting NPS to the probability per unit area of counting a photon. While this contribution is seminal, it is not clear whether or not this approach can be used to model properly the effects of reabsorption of characteristic and/or scattered photons, which is important for CdTe and cadmium zinc telluride (CZT) systems, in addition to amorphous selenium (*a*-Se) systems currently under development.(36–39) In energy-integrating systems, the effects of reabsorption on the NPS cannot be modeled accurately by simply considering the average distribution of deposited energy per interaction. Instead, accurate modeling of the NPS requires a parallel cascades approach that accounts for noise correlations introduced by reabsorption.(11) In addition, the role of thresholding is not modeled explicitly using Acciavatti and colleagues' approach. It is not clear how to apply this methodology to systems that use multiple energy thresholds to count photons in multiple energy bins.

We (i.e. Tanguay, Cunningham and colleagues) developed generic theoretical expressions for the large-area gain, MTF and NPS of photon-counting x-ray detectors operating under low-count-rate conditions.[35,40–43] The large-area gain describes the average number of photons detected in an element per unit x-ray fluence and is directly related to the multiplicity introduced by Michel and colleagues. We modeled explicitly the process of energy thresholding, and showed that the large-area gain and MTF can be obtained from knowledge of the probability density function (PDF) of pre-thresholding, pre-sampling detector signals produced following individual x-ray interactions. We also showed that analytic modeling of the NPS requires knowledge of the joint PDF of pre-thresholding, pre-sampling signals generated in two detector elements as a function of the distance between the elements. This is a substantial deviation from modeling of energy-integrating systems, which only requires knowledge of the first- and second-order statistics, that is, mean values and NPS, of pre-sampling signals. We will show in this chapter that the requirement to model the PDF and joint PDF increases greatly mathematical complexity. Nonetheless, our approach was used by Xu and colleagues, who validated theoretical predictions on a silicon-strip slit-scanning mammography system.[34]

Other modeling efforts include those of Taguchi and colleagues, who separately modeled the effects of pulse pile-up and charge sharing, the latter of which occurs when photon energy is spread over multiple detector elements.[44–46] Taguchi and colleagues, in addition to Roessl and colleagues,[47] modeled analytically the effects of pulse pile-up on the spectrum of recorded energies. Their models accounted for the number of photons interacting within the detector resolving time and the shape of voltage pulses produced by individual x-ray interactions, but they did not consider the effects of pile-up on frequency-dependent metrics of signal and noise, that is, the MTF and NPS. Taguchi also modeled the effects of charge sharing on noise correlations between different energy bins of different elements, which were termed spatio-energetic noise correlations. A similar approach was developed by Faby and colleagues.[48] They quantified spatio-energetic noise correlations in the spatial domain, but did not link these noise correlations to the MTF and NPS, which are directly related to the detectability of objects in medical images.

There have therefore been a number of parallel efforts to model different aspects of image signal and noise in photon-counting x-ray detectors. No single approach has emerged for comprehensive modeling of the combined effects of all important image-forming processes, for example, charge sharing and pulse pile-up. Here, we summarize our recent efforts to model the energy response, large-area gain, MTF and NPS of photon-counting x-ray detectors. We start with a brief introduction to Fourier-based metrics of image quality, proceed to describe generic expressions for these metrics in the context of photon-counting systems, and then present a simplified model of the large-area gain, MTF and NPS of CdTe-based photon-counting x-ray detectors. Where possible, we make connections with the works described above.

16.3.1 General Model of Signal Formation in Photon-Counting X-Ray Detectors

All analyses presented in this chapter assume count rates low enough that pulse pile-up can be ignored, which may be a good approximation for state-of-the-art photon-counting detectors in applications for breast imaging, radiography, fluoroscopy, and angiography, but not likely for computed tomography (CT) applications. We also consider the generic case of a photon-counting x-ray detector that counts the number of photons recorded in one or more energy bins. In all cases, we assume WSS conditions are satisfied.

Photon-counting x-ray imaging detectors can be modeled as conventional (energy-integrating) x-ray detectors operating with low noise and fast readout electronics such that there is little chance of more than one photon interacting in any one detector element within the resolving time of the detector. Images are generated by applying one or more thresholds following individual photon interactions. A model of signal transfer through photon-counting x-ray imaging detectors is illustrated in Figure 16.1. Each stage of the model is summarized below.

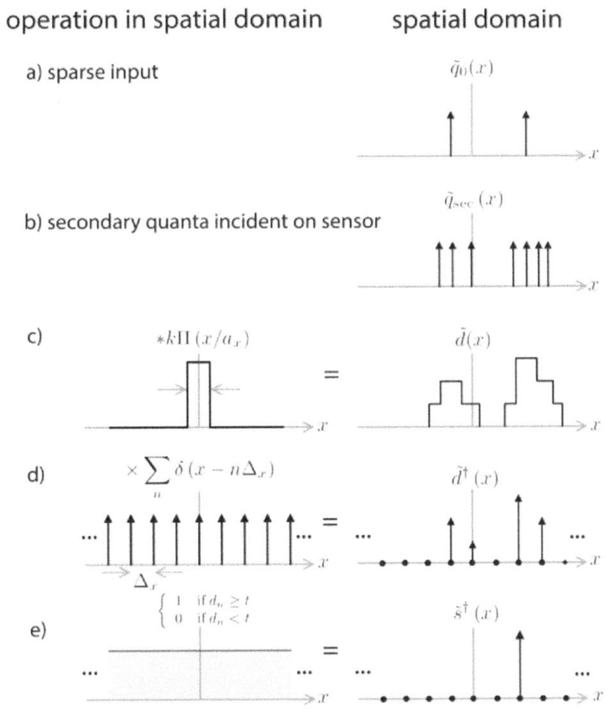

FIGURE 16.1 One-dimensional schematic representation of the process of converting a distribution of incident x-ray quanta ($\tilde{q}_0$) to secondary quanta such as liberated charges in a photoconductor ($\tilde{q}_{sec}$) incident on the sensors, to the detector pre-sampling signal $\tilde{d}$, and then to the thresholded signal $\tilde{d}^{\dagger}$. The superscript † indicates a function consisting of a uniform sequence of delta functions scaled by discrete detector values.

16.3.1.1 Incident X-Ray Quanta, $\tilde{q}_0$

The model starts with a spatio-temporal distribution of x-ray quanta incident on the x-ray converter. Using the methods of point-process theory, the distribution of incident quanta is represented mathematically as a distribution of Dirac delta (δ) functions[25,26]:

$$\tilde{q}_0(\mathbf{r},t) = \sum_{i=1}^{\tilde{N}_0} \delta(\mathbf{r}-\tilde{\mathbf{r}}_i)\delta(t-\tilde{t}_i) \tag{16.11}$$

where $\tilde{N}_0$ is a RV representing the total number of x-ray quanta incident on the x-ray converter during image acquisition, and $\mathbf{r}_i$ and $\tilde{t}_i$ are RVs representing the position and time of the ith photon incidence, respectively. We assume $\{\tilde{\mathbf{r}}_i, i = 1..\tilde{N}_0\}$ is a set of independent and identically distributed RVs, and similarly for $\{t_i, i = 1..\tilde{N}_0\}$. The spatio-temporal distribution $\tilde{q}_0(\mathbf{r},t)$ has units of [mm^{-2}s^{-1}] and its mean value is equal to the incident x-ray fluence rate, $\overline{\dot{q}}_0 = \dot{\overline{N}}_0 / A$ where $\dot{\overline{N}}_0$ [s^{-1}] represents the average total number of photons incident on the x-ray converter per unit time and A represents the detector area.

The first row of Figure 16.1 represents the distribution of photons incident on the converter during a time interval (Δt) of short enough duration that at most one photon is incident on any given detector element. This distribution is represented mathematically as the integral of $\tilde{q}_0(\mathbf{r},t)$ with respect to time:

$$\tilde{q}_{0,j}(\mathbf{r}) = \int_{t_j}^{t_j+\Delta t} \tilde{q}_0(\mathbf{r},t')\,dt' = \sum_{i=1}^{\tilde{N}_0} \tilde{\eta}_{i,j}\delta(\mathbf{r}-\tilde{\mathbf{r}}_i) \tag{16.12}$$

where $\tilde{\eta}_{i,j}$ is a RV that takes on a value of 1 when $t_i \in [t_j, t_j + \Delta t]$ and is 0 otherwise, that is, $\tilde{\eta}_i$ is a Bernoulli RV. The average value of $\tilde{\eta}_{i,j}$ is equal to $\Delta t / T$ where T represents the duration of image acquisition. It is important to note that elements of photon-counting x-ray detectors do not integrate the image signal over a period of time $[t_j, t_j + \Delta t]$ common to all elements. Instead, elements are triggered by energy depositions within the element independent of neighboring elements. The introduction of a common integration period of length Δt in Eq. (16.12) is for mathematical convenience and results in no loss of generality when pulse pile-up can be ignored.

16.3.1.2 Conversion to Secondary Image-Forming Quanta, $\tilde{q}_{sec}$

Figure 16.2 illustrates an x-ray interaction in a semi-conductor-based x-ray converter. Interacting photons produce e-h pairs. An electric field sweeps e-h pairs across the x-ray converter, inducing charge on collecting electrodes, as described by the Shockley-Ramo theorem.(49,50) A detailed description of the Shockley-Ramo theorem is beyond the scope of this chapter; the reader is referred to Ref. 50. The charge induced on collecting electrodes is used to produce a voltage pulse from which interacting photon energy is estimated. The area under the transient current produced following an x-ray interaction is proportional to the total collected charge. We let $\tilde{q}_{\mathrm{sec},j}(\mathbf{r})$ represent the charge distribution induced on collecting electrodes, which can be represented mathematically as a stochastic point processes with an associated mean value $(\overline{q}_{\mathrm{sec},j})$ and NPS, as described in detail by Yao and Cunningham(11) and Barrett and Myers.(25) In this model, we have ignored temporal effects, in which case $\tilde{q}_{\mathrm{sec},j}(\mathbf{r})$ represents the distribution of charges integrated over the duration of charge collection.

16.3.1.3 Collection of Secondary Quanta by Sensor Elements

We let $\tilde{Q}_j(\mathbf{r})$ represent the total number of charges collected in a detector element centered at position $\mathbf{r}$ in the detector plane during time interval Δt. Here, $\tilde{Q}_j(\mathbf{r})$ represents the charges collected in a hypothetical detector element centered at position $\mathbf{r}$ and therefore represents a *pre-sampling, pre-thresholding* signal. This pre-sampling signal is only physically meaningful when evaluated at locations corresponding to the centers of detector elements. Mathematically, $\tilde{Q}_j(\mathbf{r})$ is represented as:

$$\tilde{Q}_j(\mathbf{r}) = \tilde{q}_{\mathrm{sec},j}(\mathbf{r}) * \Pi\left(\frac{\mathbf{r}}{a}\right) \tag{16.13}$$

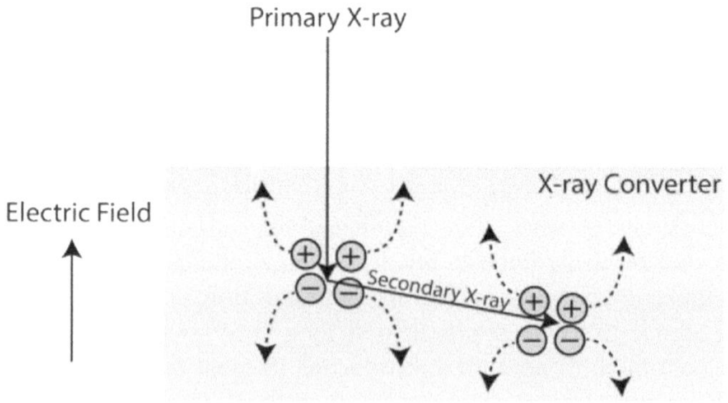

FIGURE 16.2 Schematic illustration of a photoelectric interaction within a semi-conductor-based x-ray converter. The schematic illustrates the case where a primary x-ray photon interacts with a K-shell electron, resulting in the emission of a secondary, characteristic photon that is reabsorbed remotely. Electron-hole pairs are produced at the sites of primary and secondary interactions and then drifted across the x-ray converter by an electric field.

where $a = a_x a_y$ [mm^2] represents the active area of detector elements, $\Pi(\mathbf{r}/a)$ represents a 2D rectangle function of area a, and * represents the convolution operator.

16.3.1.4 Detector Element Signals, $\tilde{d}_j^{\dagger}$

The process of sampling $\tilde{Q}_j(\mathbf{r})$ at locations corresponding to the centers of detector elements is represented mathematically as multiplication with a series of Dirac δ functions. The sampled signal, including the effects of additive electronic noise, is then given by:

$$\tilde{d}_j^{\dagger}(\mathbf{r}) = \left(k\tilde{Q}_j(\mathbf{r}) + \tilde{e}_j(\mathbf{r})\right)\sum_{n=-\infty}^{\infty}\sum_{m=-\infty}^{\infty}\delta(\mathbf{r}-\mathbf{r}_{nm}) \tag{16.14}$$

$$= \sum_{n=1}^{N_x}\sum_{m=1}^{N_y}\tilde{d}_{nm,j}\delta(\mathbf{r}-\mathbf{r}_{nm}) \tag{16.15}$$

where k is a constant of proportionality, N_x and N_y represent the number of detector elements in the x and y directions, respectively, $\mathbf{r}_{nm} = (n\Delta_x, m\Delta_y)$ where Δ_x and Δ_y represent the element-to-element spacing in the x and y directions, respectively, and $\tilde{d}_{nm,j}$ is given by:

$$\tilde{d}_{nm,j} = \tilde{d}_j(\mathbf{r})\Big|_{\mathbf{r}=\mathbf{r}_{nm}} = k\tilde{Q}_j(\mathbf{r})\Big|_{\mathbf{r}=\mathbf{r}_{nm}} + \tilde{e}_{nm,j} \tag{16.16}$$

where $\tilde{d}_j(\mathbf{r})$ is a pre-sampling representation of $\tilde{d}_{nm,j}$, representing the signal from a hypothetical detector element centered at position $\mathbf{r}$, and $\tilde{e}_{nm,j}$ represents the electronic noise contribution to element nm on readout j. The additive electronic noise $\tilde{e}_{nm,j}$ is a zero-mean RV and is typically assumed to be normally distributed.

Since $\tilde{d}_j^{\dagger}(\mathbf{r})$ represents the signal prior to energy thresholding but after sampling, $\tilde{d}_j^{\dagger}(\mathbf{r})$ represents the sampled, pre-thresholding signal. The coefficient in front of each δ function in the summation in Eq. (16.15) is proportional to the total number of charges collected in the element centered at $\mathbf{r}_{nm}$, which is in turn proportional to the total energy deposited in the element at $\mathbf{r}_{nm}$.

16.3.1.5 Thresholded Signals

Photon counting is achieved by applying a threshold to the sampled, pre-thresholding signal $\tilde{d}_j^{\dagger}(\mathbf{r})$. Ideally, x-ray fluence rates are low enough that each detector element collects energy from at most one photon during the detector resolving time. When this condition is satisfied, pulse pile-up is negligible and the thresholded signal from a detector element centered at $\mathbf{r}_{nm}$ is a Bernoulli RV. A Bernoulli RV is the limiting case of binomial RV in which there is only one trial. (See Papoulis(26) for introductory material on binomial and Bernoulli RVs.)

We consider the general case where photons are counted in energy bins with lower and upper thresholds $\{l_i, i = 1..B\}$ and $\{u_i, i = 1..B\}$, respectively, where B represents the number of energy bins. We let $\tilde{s}_{nm,j}^{i}$ represent the thresholded signal from energy bin i in the element centered at $\mathbf{r}_{nm}$:

$$\tilde{s}_{nm,j}^{i} = \begin{cases} 1 & \tilde{d}_{nm,j} \in [l_i, u_i] \\ 0 & \tilde{d}_{nm,j} \notin [l_i, u_i] \end{cases} \tag{16.17}$$

The sampled and binned image signal is then:

$$\tilde{s}_j^{i,\dagger}(\mathbf{r}) = \tilde{s}_j^{i,}(\mathbf{r})\sum_{n=1}^{N_x}\sum_{m=1}^{N_y}\delta(\mathbf{r}-\mathbf{r}_{nm}) = \sum_{n=1}^{N_x}\sum_{m=1}^{N_y}\tilde{s}_{nm,j}^{i}\delta(\mathbf{r}-\mathbf{r}_{nm}) \tag{16.18}$$

where $\tilde{s}_j^i(\mathbf{r})$ is a continuous pre-sampling representation of $\tilde{s}_{nm,j}^i$. Summing over all time intervals of length Δt yields the photon-counting image signal:

$$\tilde{c}_i^\dagger(\mathbf{r}) = \sum_{j=1}^{T/\Delta t} \tilde{s}_j^{i,\dagger}(\mathbf{r}). \tag{16.19}$$

The signal $\tilde{c}_i^\dagger(\mathbf{r})$ represents the binned image signal and is equal to a series of δ functions at locations corresponding to the centers of detector elements. Each δ function is scaled by the total number of photons counted in the ith energy bin of the corresponding detector element.

16.3.2 Average Photon-Counting Image Signal

In this section we present generic expressions for the average photon-counting image signal. We start by considering Eq. (16.19), which includes a sum over all time intervals Δt. In the extreme limit that at most one photon is incident on the x-ray detector during time interval Δt, the sum over all time intervals becomes a sum over the number of incident photons:

$$\tilde{c}_i^\dagger(\mathbf{r}) = \sum_{j=1}^{\tilde{N}_0} \tilde{s}_j^{i,\dagger}(\mathbf{r}) = \tilde{c}_i(\mathbf{r}) \sum_{n=1}^{N_x} \sum_{m=1}^{N_y} \delta(\mathbf{r} - \mathbf{r}_{nm}) \tag{16.20}$$

where $\tilde{c}_i(\mathbf{r}) = \sum_{j=1}^{\tilde{N}_0} \tilde{s}_j^i(\mathbf{r})$. Taking the expectation value of the preceding equation yields the average photon-counting image signal:

$$E\{\tilde{c}_i^\dagger(\mathbf{r})\} = \sum_{n=1}^{N_x} \sum_{m=1}^{N_y} E\{\tilde{c}_{nm,i}\} \delta(\mathbf{r} - \mathbf{r}_{nm}) \tag{16.21}$$

where $E\{\tilde{x}\}$ represents the expected value of $\tilde{x}$. Since $\tilde{c}_{nm,i}$ is equal to a sum of $\tilde{N}_0$ independent Bernoulli RVs, $\tilde{c}_{nm,i}$ is a Binomial RV with expected value given by:

$$E[\tilde{c}_{nm,i}] = \overline{c}_i \tag{16.22}$$

$$= \overline{N}_0 P(\tilde{d}_{nm,j} \in [l_i, u_i]) \tag{16.23}$$

$$= \overline{N}_0 P(\tilde{d}_1 \in [l_i, u_i]) \tag{16.24}$$

where $P(\tilde{d}_{nm,j} \in [l_i, u_i])$ represents the probability that $\tilde{d}_{nm,j} \in [l_i, u_i]$ given one photon incident on the x-ray detector. In writing Eq. (16.24) we have assumed that $P(\tilde{d}_{nm,j} \in [l_i, u_i]) = P(\tilde{d}_1 \in [l_i, u_i])$ is independent of j, n, and m, which is necessary to satisfy the conditions of wide-sense stationarity.

Letting $p_{d_1}(d_1)$ represent the PDF of $\tilde{d}_{nm,j}$ given one photon incident on the x-ray detector, the average number of photons counted in energy bin i of a detector element is represented mathematically as:

$$\overline{c}_i = \overline{N}_0 \int_{l_i}^{u_i} p_{d_1}(d_1) \mathrm{d}d_1. \tag{16.25}$$

This result shows that modeling of the average photon-counting image signal requires knowledge of the PDF of the pre-sampling, pre-thresholding signal. In contrast, modeling of the average energy-integrating image signal only requires knowledge of the average pre-sampling, pre-thresholding image signal. The PDF $p_{d_1}(d_1)$ accounts for the poly-energetic x-ray spectrum, the random location of x-ray incidence in the detector plane, and all processes that distort incident x-ray spectra, including electronic noise, characteristic emission and subsequent reabsorption, and depth-dependent charge collection and charge sharing. We describe a simple theoretical model for $p_{d_1}(d_1)$ in Section 16.4.

16.3.3 Energy-Response Function

The energy-response function, denoted by $R(\varepsilon, E)$, describes the probability of observing deposited photon energy ε given incident photon energy E. When the charge integrated in a detector element is linearly related to deposited photon energy, the energy-response function is related to the PDF of pre-thresholding detector element signals:

$$R(\varepsilon,E)=\frac{1}{\kappa}p_{d_1}(d_1;E)\Big|_{d_1=\varepsilon/\kappa} \tag{16.26}$$

where κ is a constant of proportionality relating deposited photon energy ε to the pre-thresholding detector signal d_1, that is, $\varepsilon = \kappa d_1$, and $p_{d_1}(d_1;E)$ is the PDF of d_1 for incident photon energy E.

16.3.4 Large-Area Gain and Energy-Bin Sensitivity Functions

We define the large-area gain ($\overline{G}_i$) of energy bin i as the average number of counts recorded in energy bin i (per detector element) normalized by the incident fluence rate:

$$\overline{G}_i = \frac{\overline{c}_i}{\overline{q}_0}. \tag{16.27}$$

With this definition, $\overline{G}_i$ has units of mm^2. Combining Eqs. (16.25) and (16.27), $\overline{G}_i$ is expressed mathematically as:

$$\overline{G}_i = A\int_{l_i}^{u_i} p_{d_1}(d_1)\mathrm{d}d_1. \tag{16.28}$$

For poly-energetic x-ray spectra, $\overline{G}_i$ can be written as:

$$\overline{G}_i = \frac{1}{\overline{q}_0}\int_0^{\infty}\overline{q}_0(E)S_i(E)\mathrm{d}E \tag{16.29}$$

where $\overline{q}_0(E)$ [mm^{-2}keV^{-1}] represents the energy-dependent x-ray fluence, $\overline{q}_0 = \int_0^{\infty}\overline{q}_0(E)\mathrm{d}E$, and $S_i(E)$ represents the sensitivity function for the ith energy bin:

$$S_i(E) = A\int_{l_i}^{u_i} p_{d_1}(d_1;E)\mathrm{d}d_1. \tag{16.30}$$

The sensitivity function, $S_i(E)$, represents the number of photons counted in energy bin i given one photon of energy E incident on the x-ray detector. For an ideal photon-counting x-ray detector, $S_i(E)$ is equal to the quantum efficiency for photon energies lying within the lower and upper limits of the energy bin, in which case adjacent energy bins do not overlap each other. In reality, electronic noise, depth-dependent charge collection and charge sharing result in overlapping energy-bin sensitivity functions, as described in Section 16.4.

Multiplicity. In the case of a photon-counting detector operating with a single, open energy bin, the large-area gain can be related to Michel and colleagues multiplicity[28]:

$$\text{multiplicity} = \frac{\bar{G}}{\alpha a} = \frac{A}{\alpha a} \int_{t}^{\infty} p_{d_1}(d_1) \mathrm{d}d_1 \tag{16.31}$$

where t is a threshold used to identify x-ray interaction events from electronic noise and α represents the quantum efficiency, which is equal to the probability that a photon interacts in the x-ray converter. We note that p_{d_1} accounts for the probability that a photon interacts in a given detector element, and therefore includes a factor of a/A which will cancel with the factor of A/a in Eq. (16.31).

16.3.5 Pre-Sampling Modulation Transfer Function

The pre-sampling MTF is equal to the Fourier transform of the pre-sampling PSF, as described in Section 16.2. In the general case of a photon-counting x-ray detector that bins photons into multiple energy bins, it is necessary to define a pre-sampling MTF (and PSF) for each energy bin. We define the pre-sampling PSF of the ith energy bin as the probability of recording a photon in the ith energy bin of a detector element centered at position $\mathbf{r}$ relative to the site of primary x-ray interaction. Here, "primary" distinguishes x-ray photons incident on the converter from those produced following photoelectric or Compton interactions with the x-ray converter.

The pre-sampling MTF of the ith energy bin is generically represented as[35]:

$$\mathrm{MTF}_i(\mathbf{r}) = FT\left[\frac{1}{\bar{G}_i} \int_{l_i}^{u_i} p_{d_1}(d_1;\mathbf{r}) \mathrm{d}d_1\right] \tag{16.32}$$

where $FT[f(\mathbf{r})]$ represents the Fourier transform of $f(\mathbf{r})$ with respect to $\mathbf{r}$, $p_{d_1}(d_1;\mathbf{r})$ represents the PDF of the pre-thresholding, pre-sampling signal generated in an element centered at position $\mathbf{r}$ relative to the site of a primary x-ray interaction and is related to $p_{d_1}(d_1)$ through the following relationship:

$$p_{d_1}(d_1) = \frac{1}{A} \int p_{d_1}(d_1;\mathbf{r}) \mathrm{d}^2\mathbf{r}. \tag{16.33}$$

For an ideal photon-counting x-ray detector, $p_{d_1}(d_1;\mathbf{r})$ is proportional to a 2D rectangle function of area $a = a_x a_y$ centered at $\mathbf{r}$. In practice, characteristic reabsorption, Coulomb repulsion and diffusion broaden the PSF of some energy bins while narrowing the PSF of other energy bins.[35]

Equation (16.32) shows that modeling the photon-counting MTF requires knowledge of the PDF of the signal from a hypothetical detector centered at position $\mathbf{r}$ relative to the site of a primary x-ray interaction, which can be obtained using the analytic methods described in Section 16.4 or by Monte Carlo methods. It is important to note that $p_{d_1}(d_1;\mathbf{r})$ is not equal to the PSF of an otherwise equivalent energy-integrating system, which represents the PDF of detecting a single secondary quantum in a detector element centered at $\mathbf{r}$. In Section 16.4, we will show that the photon-counting MTF is related nonlinearly to the MTF of an otherwise equivalent energy-integrating x-ray detector.

16.3.6 Photon-Counting Autocovariance and Noise Power Spectrum

In energy-integrating systems, the NPS is the Fourier transform of the autocovariance function of the sampled image signal. In photon-counting systems, in which there may be more than one energy bin, there may be noise correlations between different energy bins in different detector elements. In this case, it is necessary to consider the covariance function between the image signals from different energy bins. Following the work of Taguchi *et al.*,[45,46] we refer to such noise correlations as spatio-energetic noise correlations.

The autocovariance between $\tilde{c}_i^\dagger$ and $\tilde{c}_{i'}^\dagger$ is represented mathematically as:

$$K^\dagger_{c_i,c_{i'}}(\tau)=\sum_{n=1}^{N_x}\sum_{m=1}^{N_y}\sum_{n'=1}^{N_x}\sum_{m'=1}^{N_y}K_{c_i,c_{i'}}(\mathbf{r},\mathbf{r}+\tau)\delta(\mathbf{r}-\mathbf{r}_{nm})\delta(\mathbf{r}+\tau-\mathbf{r}_{n'm'}) \tag{16.34}$$

where $K_{c_i,c_{i'}}(\mathbf{r},\mathbf{r}+\tau)$ represents the pre-sampling covariance function for energy bins i and i'. The pre-sampling covariance function is equal to the covariance between energy bins i and i' of elements separated by τ, and can be shown to be given by[40,41]:

$$K_{c_i,c_{i'}}(\tau)=\bar{N}_0E\left\{\tilde{s}^i(\mathbf{r})\tilde{s}^{i'}(\mathbf{r}+\tau)\right\}. \tag{16.35}$$

At this point, we separate our analysis into two cases: $\tau=0$ and $\tau\neq 0$.

In the $\tau=0$ case, $K_{c_i,c_{i'}}(\mathbf{r},\mathbf{r}+\tau)$ is the covariance between $\tilde{c}_i(\mathbf{r})$ and $\tilde{c}_j(\mathbf{r})$, can be shown to be given by:

$$K_{c_i,c_{i'}}(\tau)\Big|_{\tau=0}=\begin{cases}\bar{c}_i,\ i=j\\ 0,\ i\neq j\end{cases}. \tag{16.36}$$

The result for the $i\neq j$ case follows from the fact that a photon cannot be counted in two energy bins of the same detector element. The $i=j$ case shows that the number of detected photons is Poisson-distributed, that is, the variance of the number of detected photons equals the average number of detected photons. This is a general result, independent of the particular sequence of image-forming processes leading to the detection of a photon.

For $\tau\neq 0$, we note that $\tilde{s}^i(\mathbf{r})$ takes on values of either 1 or 0, and similarly for $\tilde{s}^{i'}(\mathbf{r}+\tau)$, in which case the expected value in Eq. (16.35) becomes:

$$E\left\{\tilde{s}^i(\mathbf{r})\tilde{s}^{i'}(\mathbf{r}+\tau)\right\}=P\left(\tilde{d}_1(\mathbf{r})\in[l_i,u_i]\text{ AND }\tilde{d}_1(\mathbf{r}+\tau)\in[l_{i'},u_{i'}]\right) \tag{16.37}$$

where $P(\tilde{d}_1(\mathbf{r})\in[l_i,u_i]\text{ AND }\tilde{d}_1(\mathbf{r}+\tau)\in[l_j,u_j])$ represents the probability that $\tilde{d}_1(\mathbf{r})\in[l_i,u_i]$ and $\tilde{d}_1(\mathbf{r}+\tau)\in[l_{i'},u_{i'}]$ given one photon incident on the x-ray converter. The covariance function between bins i and i' for $\tau\neq 0$ can then be expressed as[40,41]:

$$K_{c_i,c_{i'}}(\tau)=\bar{N}_0\int_{l_i}^{u_i}\int_{l_{i'}}^{u_{i'}}p_{d_1,d_1'}(d_1,d_1';\tau)\mathrm{d}d_1\mathrm{d}d_1',\quad \tau\neq 0 \tag{16.38}$$

where $p_{d_1,d_1'}(d_1,d_1';\tau)$ represents the joint PDF of signals d_1 and d_1', which represent pre-sampling, pre-thresholding signals from elements separated by distance τ given one photon incident on the x-ray converter.

The digital cross NPS of energy bins i and i' is then given by:

$$W_{\mathrm{dig},c_i,c_{i'}}(\mathbf{u})=W_{c_i,c_{i'}}(\mathbf{u})+\sum_{n=1}^{\infty}\sum_{m=1}^{\infty}W_{c_i,c_{i'}}(\mathbf{u}\pm\mathbf{u}_{nm}) \tag{16.39}$$

where $W_{c_i,c_{i'}}(\mathbf{u})$ represents the pre-sampling cross NPS of bins i and i':

$$W_{c_i,c_{i'}}(\mathbf{u}) = \bar{q}_0 \cdot FT\left[A \int_{l_i}^{u_i}\int_{l_{i'}}^{u_{i'}} p_{d_1,d_1'}(d_1,d_1';\tau)\,\mathrm{d}d_1\mathrm{d}d_1' \right]. \tag{16.40}$$

The NPS of energy bin i is obtained by setting $i = i'$ in Eqs. (16.39) and (16.40), which show that the NPS of energy bin i and the cross NPS of energy bins i and i' are determined by the joint PDF $p_{d_1,d_1'}(d_1,d_1';\tau)$. In Section 16.4 we describe a simple model that can be used to calculate $p_{d_1,d_1'}(d_1,d_1';\tau)$.

Spatio-energetic noise correlations. Taguchi and colleagues introduced the concept of spatio-energetic noise correlations,[45,46] characterized in terms of the covariance between energy bins of nearby detector elements. The framework described above accounts for such correlations. We can use Eq. (16.38) to illustrate this explicitly. To this end, we let $C_{n,m,i,i'}$ represent the normalized covariance between energy bins i and i' of two elements separated by n elements in the x direction and m elements in the y direction:

$$C_{n,m,i,i'} = \frac{\bar{N}_0 K_{c_i,c_i'}(\tau)\big|_{\tau=\tau_{nm}}}{\bar{c}_i\bar{c}_j} \tag{16.41}$$

where $\tau_{nm} = (n\Delta_x, m\Delta_y)$, $K_{c_i,c_{i'}}(\tau)$ is given by Eq. (16.38), $\bar{c}_i$ is given by Eq. (16.25) and $W_{c_i,c_{i'}}(\mathbf{u})$ is the pre-sampling cross NPS between energy bins i and i'. The factor of $\bar{N}_0$ is required to produce a metric that is independent of the number of incident photons.

16.4 EXAMPLE X-RAY DETECTION MODEL

In the preceding sections, we introduced generic mathematical expressions for the large-area gain, energy-bin sensitivity functions, MTF and NPS of photon-counting x-ray detectors. Each of these metrics can be calculated from $p_{d_1}(d_1)$, $p_{d_1}(d_1;\mathbf{r})$, or $p_{d_1,d_1'}(d_1,d_1';\tau)$, as shown in Eqs. (16.28), (16.30), (16.32), and (16.40). In this section, we demonstrate how to model these PDFs. We consider an x-ray imaging detector that can be modeled using the serial cascade of imaging forming processes illustrated in Figure 16.3. The model shown in Figure 16.3 is simplistic in the sense that it does not account for emission and subsequent reabsorption of characteristic x-rays emitted following photon interactions. Proper treatment of reabsorption requires a parallel cascades approach,[11,35,42] and is an ongoing area of research. The stages of the model and how the associated PDFs relate to $p_{d_1}(d_1)$ and $p_{d_1,d_1'}(d_1,d_1';\tau)$ are described below. Derivations are performed assuming mono-energetic photons until stage six, after which results are averaged over the spectrum of photon energies.

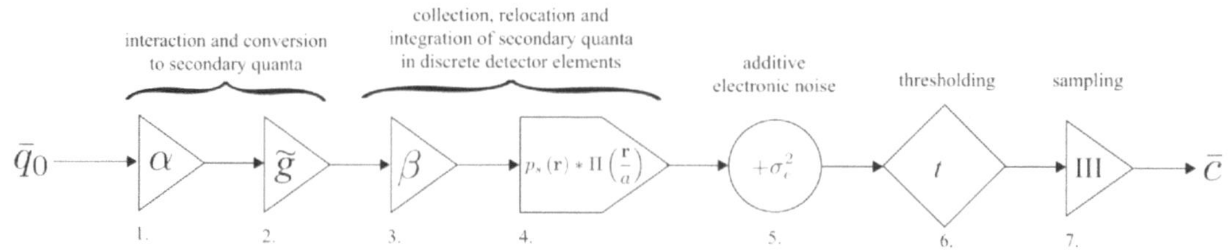

FIGURE 16.3 Schematic illustration of the serial cascade of elementary processes used to model x-ray interaction and detection in a photon-counting x-ray detector.

16.4.1 PDF of Detector Signals, $p_{d_1}(d_1)$

We let n_i represent the total number of image-forming quanta after the ith stage of the model in Figure 16.3. For example, the image-forming quanta after stage one are x-ray photons that have interacted in the x-ray detector. After stage two, the image-forming quanta are e-h pairs. Our goal is to provide an analytic expression for $p_{d_1}(d_1)$ that can be evaluated numerically when given the parameters describing the various stages of the model. As such, in the following, we assume that one photon is incident on the x-ray converter.

16.4.1.1 Stage 1: Quantum Efficiency

The first stage of the cascaded model illustrated in Figure 16.3 represents selection of incident x-ray quanta that interact with the x-ray converter. The probability that a photon interacts in the x-ray converter is equal to the quantum efficiency, which is a function of the energy of incident x-ray photons and the density and atomic number of the x-ray converter. The quantum efficiency is represented mathematically as:

$$\alpha(E) = 1 - e^{-\mu(E)L} \tag{16.42}$$

where E represents the energy of incident photons, $\mu(E)$ represents the energy-dependent linear attenuation coefficient of the x-ray converter and L represents the thickness of the x-ray converter. For compound semi-conductor x-ray converters, the linear attenuation coefficient is given by the mixture rule:

$$\mu(E) = \rho \sum_{i=1}^{N} f_i \left(\frac{\mu}{\rho}\right)_i (E) \tag{16.43}$$

where $(\mu/\rho)_i$ and f_i represent the mass attenuation coefficient and mass fraction of element i, respectively. The linear attenuation coefficient of cadmium telluride is shown in Figure 16.4 for photon energies ranging from 10 keV to 150 keV and selected converter thicknesses.

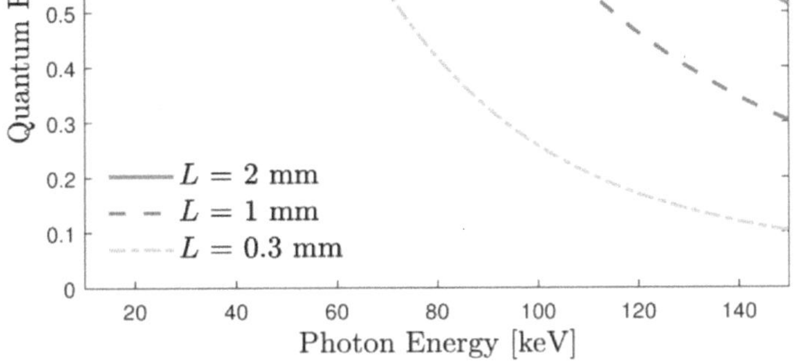

FIGURE 16.4 Quantum efficiency of CdTe x-ray converters for selected thicknesses and photon energies. The quantum efficiency was calculated assuming a mass density of 6 g/cm^3.

After the first stage of the model, the PDF of the number of image-forming quanta takes on a value of α when $n_1 = 1$ and a value of $1-\alpha$ when $n_1 = 0$. Therefore:

$$p_{n1}(n_1) = (1-\alpha)^{1-n_1} + \alpha^{n_1}, \; n_1 \in \{0,1\} \tag{16.44}$$

where we have dropped the dependence on energy for notational convenience. The first term in Eq. (16.44) accounts for the case where incident photons do not interact with x-ray converter. The second term accounts for the case where a photon interacts with the converter. For any successful spectroscopic x-ray imaging detector, the lowest energy threshold will be high enough such that counts are not recorded in elements in which there was no energy deposited. In this case, the first term will go to 0 after stage six of the model in Figure 16.3. It is therefore safe to neglect the first term in Eq. (16.44) in the following analysis.

16.4.1.2 Stage 2: Conversion to Secondary Quanta

The second stage of the model in Figure 16.3 represents conversion of x-ray quanta to e-h pairs, and is therefore a gain stage, in which each interacting x-ray photon produces many e-h pairs. The average conversion gain is approximately given by:

$$\bar{g} = \frac{E}{w} \tag{16.45}$$

where w [keV] represents the average energy required to liberate one e-h pair. The w-values of CdTe and CZT are on the order of 5 eV. For comparison, the w-values of silicon and amorphous selenium, the latter of which is used in clinically available direct conversion x-ray imaging detectors, are ~4 eV and 45 eV, respectively.

Conversion of x-ray quanta to e-h pairs is a stochastic process, and it is therefore necessary to describe not only the mean gain, but also the variance and PDF of the number of e-h pairs liberated following an x-ray interaction. In this model, we assume the number of e-h pairs produced following a single photon interaction is Poisson-distributed with mean value given by Eq. (16.45):

$$p_g(g) = \mathcal{P}(g;\bar{g}) = \frac{e^{-\bar{g}}\bar{g}^g}{g!} \tag{16.46}$$

where $p_g(g)$ represents the probability that g charges are liberated following an x-ray interaction, and $\mathcal{P}(g;\bar{g})$ represents the Poisson distribution with mean value $\bar{g}$ evaluated at g. When the Poisson assumption is satisfied, $\sigma_g/\bar{g} = \sqrt{w/E}$, demonstrating that the photo-peak width relative to the incident photon energy decreases with increasing photon energy.

The PDF of the number of image quanta after the second stage of the model is given by:

$$p_{n2}(n_2) = \sum_{n_1=0}^{n_1} p_{n_1}(n_1)\, p_{n_2}(n_2|n_1) = \alpha\, p_g(n_2) \tag{16.47}$$

where $p_{n_2}(n_2|n_1) = p_g(n_2)$ represents the PDF of n_2 (i.e. the number of liberated e-h pairs) given n_1 x-ray interactions. Note that we have not included the first term in Eq. (16.44) when carrying out the summation in Eq. (16.47) for reasons discussed above. As such, $p_{n_2}(n_2)$ is not properly normalized because it does not integrate to unity. As discussed above, this does not introduce errors in our analysis for energy thresholds above the electronic noise floor. The energy-response function after conversion of x-ray quanta to e-h pairs is illustrated in Figure 16.7 for photon energies relevant for mammography, x-ray angiography, general radiography and CT.

16.4.1.3 Stage 3: Charge Collection

The third stage of the model represents integration of charges by collecting electrodes. This stage only accounts for loss of the total number of charges due to incomplete charge collection; stage four accounts for integration of charges in detector elements. It should be noted that charge collection is somewhat of a misnomer, as the electrodes do not collect the charges liberated from x-ray interactions. Instead, the flow of charges liberated from x-ray interactions induces charge on collecting electrodes.(49,50) In the following, we assume an ideal weighting potential, in which case depth-dependent charge induction on collecting electrodes is ignored. Inclusion of non-ideal weighting potentials is an area of ongoing research.

The total charge induced on all electrodes relative to the charge produced following an x-ray interaction is determined by the electric field in the x-ray converter and the distance charges travel before undergoing a recombination or charge trapping event. The average distance a charge carrier travels before undergoing a recombination or trapping event is typically characterized in terms of the mobility lifetime product, denoted by $\mu\tau$ [cm^{2}V^{-1}], which describes the average distance traveled per unit electric field. The charge induced on electrodes relative to the number of charges produced following an x-ray interaction at depth z can be approximated by the Hecht relationship(51):

$$\beta(z) = \frac{\mu_e\tau_e V}{L^2}\left(1 - e^{-\frac{(L-z)L}{\mu_e\tau_e V}}\right) + \frac{\mu_h\tau_h V}{L^2}\left(1 - e^{-\frac{zL}{\mu_h\tau_h V}}\right) \quad (16.48)$$

where V represents the potential difference across the semiconductor, $\mu_e\tau_e$ and $\mu_h\tau_h$ represent the mobility lifetime products for electrons and holes, respectively, and it has been assumed that electrons drift toward the exit surface of the x-ray converter; when electrons are drifted toward the entrance surface, the positions of $\mu_e\tau_e$ and $\mu_h\tau_h$ are swapped in Eq. (16.48). The Hecht relationship is plotted as a function of interaction depth for selected converter thicknesses in Figure 16.5. The product $\mu\tau E$ [cm] represents the mean free drift length. For CZT operating at electric fields relevant for medical imaging applications (i.e. ~3000 V/cm), the mean free drift lengths of electrons and holes are ~3 cm and 1 cm, respectively.(52–54)

We refer to β as the charge collection efficiency. Charge collection efficiencies less than unity increase the width of the distribution of collected charges relative to the total number of collected

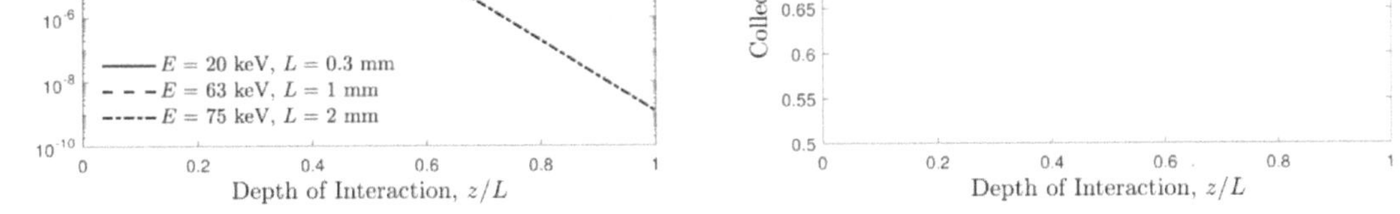

FIGURE 16.5 Left: Probability density function for the depth of interaction for selected photon energies (E) and converter thicknesses (L). Right: Charge collection efficiency as a function of depth of interaction assuming electrons are drifted to the entrance side of the x-ray converter. The charge collection efficiency was calculated assuming electron and hole mobility-lifetime products of 1×10^{-3}cm^{2}V^{-1} and 1×10^{-4}cm^{2}V^{-1}, respectively, and an electric field of 3000 Vcm^{-1}.

charges, which ultimately increases the width of observed photo-peaks, which has two consequences: (1) compromised ability to discern low-energy photons from electronic noise, and; (2) increased overlap between energy-bin sensitivity functions.

Collection of charges by collecting electrodes can be modeled as a binomial collection process where the probability of collecting n_3 charges given n_2 charges liberated at depth $\tilde{z}$ is given by:

$$p_{n3}\left(n_3|\tilde{n}_2,\tilde{z}\right)=\mathcal{B}\left(n_3;\beta(\tilde{z}),\tilde{n}_2\right) \tag{16.49}$$

where $\mathcal{B}(n_2;\beta(z'),\tilde{n}_1)$ represents the binomial distribution with probability of success $\beta(\tilde{z})$ and total number of trials $\tilde{n}_2$. Averaging over $\tilde{n}_2$ yields[(26)]:

$$p_{n3}\left(n_3\right)=\sum_{n_2=0}^{\infty}\mathcal{B}\left(n_3;\beta(\tilde{z}),\tilde{n}_2\right)p_{n2}\left(n_2\right)=\alpha\mathcal{P}\left(n_3;\overline{g}\beta(\tilde{z})\right). \tag{16.50}$$

Equation (16.50) shows that Poisson conversion gain followed by binomial selection yields the same PDF as a single-gain stage with mean gain $\overline{g}\beta(\tilde{z})$. If all processes subsequent to charge collection were depth-independent, we could average over the random depth of interaction at this point in the model. However, below we consider the general case of depth-dependent charge sharing. In this case, averaging over depth z must be performed after charge sharing is incorporated into the model.

The energy-response function after collection of e-h pairs is illustrated in Figure 16.7 for combinations of detector thickness and photon energy relevant for mammography, x-ray angiography, general radiography, and CT. The energy-response functions in Figure 16.7 were calculated using β values averaged over the converter thickness for each combination of photon energy and converter thickness. Figure 16.7 shows that the collection efficiencies in Figure 16.5 result in a modest increase in the width of photo-peaks.

16.4.1.4 Stage 4: Integration of Secondary Quanta in Discrete Detector Elements

Stage four accounts for relocation of secondary quanta from primary interaction sites and subsequent integration of secondary quanta in discrete detector elements. We let $p_\Delta(\Delta)$ represent the probability of detecting a secondary quantum at lateral position Δ relative to the site of a primary interaction. In general, the lateral distance an electron (or hole) travels prior to reaching collecting electrodes is a function of the depth of interaction, the applied electric field, and the converter thickness. Figure 16.6 shows the average distance from the site of primary interactions at which electrons are detected for cadmium telluride. The data presented in Figure 16.6 were extracted from Taguchi and Iwanczyk, which assumes an electric field of 3333 V/cm.[(55)]

The probability that a single secondary quantum is integrated in a square detector element of area $a=a_x a_y$ centered at position $\mathbf{r}$ given a primary interaction at $\tilde{\mathbf{r}}_0$ is given by:

$$P_\Delta\left(\mathbf{r}-\tilde{\mathbf{r}}_0;\tilde{z}\right)=p_\Delta\left(\mathbf{r}-\tilde{\mathbf{r}}_0;\tilde{z}\right)*\Pi\left(\frac{\mathbf{r}-\tilde{\mathbf{r}}_0}{a}\right) \tag{16.51}$$

where * represents the convolution operator. We note here that, when properly normalized to unity and averaged of the depth of interaction, $P_\Delta(\mathbf{r}-\tilde{\mathbf{r}}_0;\tilde{z})$ is equal to the energy-integrating PSF for the model in Figure 16.3.

Similar to charge collection, we model integration of charges in a detector element as a binomial selection process, for which the number of trials is equal to the total collected charge and the probability of success is given by Eq. (16.51). The PDF of the number of quanta integrated in an element centered at position $\mathbf{r}$ given a photon interaction at $\tilde{\mathbf{r}}_0$ is then given by the binomial distribution:

$$p_{n4}\left(n_4|\tilde{n}_3,\tilde{\mathbf{r}}_0,\tilde{z}\right)=\mathcal{B}\left(n_4;P_\Delta\left(\mathbf{r}-\tilde{\mathbf{r}}_0,\tilde{z}\right),\tilde{n}_3\right). \tag{16.52}$$

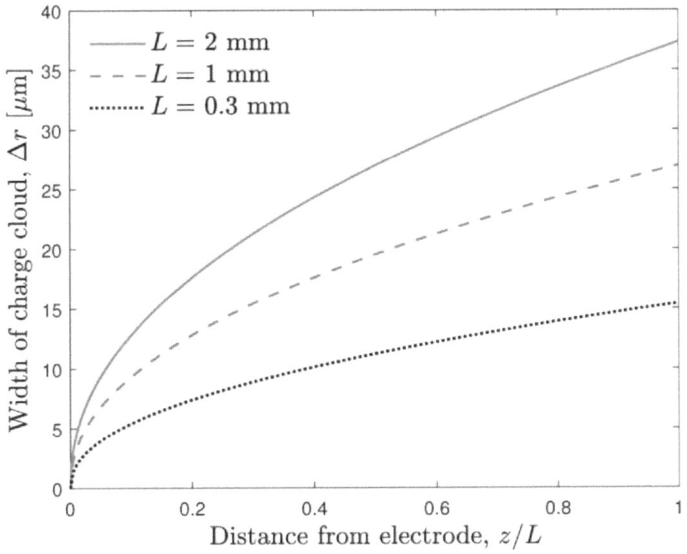

FIGURE 16.6 A plot of the width of charge clouds upon reaching electrodes as a function of distance from electrodes. The charge-cloud width is plotted as a function of normalized distance from electrodes (z/L). Data is extracted from Taguchi *et al.*[55]

Averaging over $\tilde{n}_3$ yields:

$$p_{n4}\left(n_4|\tilde{\mathbf{r}}_0,\tilde{z}\right)=\alpha\mathcal{P}\left(n_4;\mu\left(\mathbf{r}-\tilde{\mathbf{r}}_0,\tilde{z}\right)\right) \tag{16.53}$$

where $\mu(\mathbf{r}-\tilde{\mathbf{r}}_0,\tilde{z})$ represents the average number of photons integrated in an element centered at $\mathbf{r}$ given an interaction at position $\tilde{\mathbf{r}}_0$ and depth $\tilde{z}$:

$$\mu\left(\mathbf{r}-\tilde{\mathbf{r}}_0,\tilde{z}\right)=\overline{g}\beta(\tilde{z})P_\Delta\left(\mathbf{r}-\tilde{\mathbf{r}}_0,\tilde{z}\right). \tag{16.54}$$

Averaging Eq. (16.53) over all possible values of $\tilde{\mathbf{r}}_0$ and $\tilde{z}$ assuming the former is uniformly distributed over the detector area yields:

$$p_4\left(n_4\right)=\frac{\alpha}{A}\int_A\int_0^L\mathcal{P}\left(n_4;\mu(\mathbf{r},z)\right)p_z(z)\mathrm{d}^2\mathbf{r}\mathrm{d}z \tag{16.55}$$

$$=\frac{\alpha}{A}\int_A\left\langle\mathcal{P}\left(n_4;\mu(\mathbf{r},z)\right)\right\rangle_z\mathrm{d}^2\mathbf{r} \tag{16.56}$$

where $p_z(z)$ represents the PDF of the depth of interaction and is equal to an exponential distribution normalized to unity over the thickness of the x-ray detector, as shown in Figure 16.5, and $\left\langle\mathcal{P}\left(n_4;\mu(\mathbf{r},z)\right)\right\rangle_z$ represents the average of $\mathcal{P}\left(n_4;\mu(\mathbf{r},z)\right)$ over all values of z.

The energy-response function after integration of e-h pairs in detector elements is illustrated in Figure 16.7. Figure 16.7 shows that charge sharing produces a low-energy tail extending from the photo-peak down to the electronic noise floor. The low-energy tail is caused by photons that deposit energy in elements neighboring those of primary x-ray interactions. When this occurs, elements neighboring a primary interaction may erroneously record a low-energy photon, resulting in overlap of energy-bin sensitivity functions, as described below. In general, the area under the low-energy tail increases as either the converter thickness increases or the area of elements decreases.

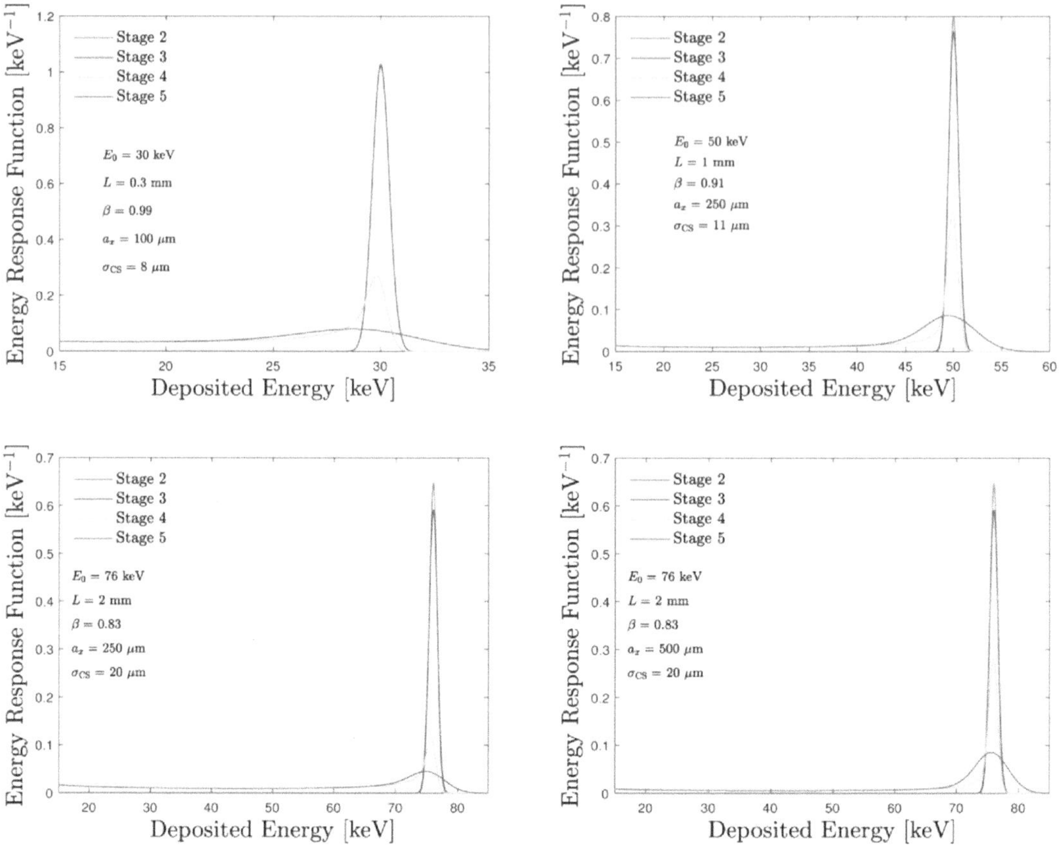

FIGURE 16.7 The energy-response function after each stage of the x-ray detection model illustrated in Figure 16.3. Results for stage five were calculated assuming the electronic noise PDF is a zero-mean normal distribution with a 2.5-keV standard deviation.

16.4.1.5 Stage 5: Electronic Noise

We assume the PDF of the electronic noise contribution is a zero-mean normal distribution with standard deviation σ_e. The PDF of the detector signal given one photon incident on the x-ray converter is then given by:

$$p_{d_1}(d_1) = \alpha\, p_{n_4}(d_1) *_n \mathcal{N}\left(d_1; 0, \sigma_e^2\right) \tag{16.57}$$

$$\approx \frac{\alpha}{A} \int_A \left\langle \mathcal{N}\left(d_1; \mu(\mathbf{r},z), \sigma(\mathbf{r},z)\right)\right\rangle_z \, \mathrm{d}^2\mathbf{r} \tag{16.58}$$

where:

$$\sigma^2(\mathbf{r},z) = \mu(\mathbf{r},z) + \sigma_e^2 \tag{16.59}$$

where $\mathcal{N}(d_1;0,\sigma_e^2)$ represents the zero-mean normal distribution with variance σ_e^2 and $*_n$ represents a convolution with respect to number of quanta. In writing Eq. (16.58) we have set the constant of proportionality (k) in Eq. (16.14) equal to unity, in which case the units of d_1 are number of quanta. In addition, we have assumed $\mathcal{P}(n_4;\mu(\mathbf{r},z)) \approx \mathcal{N}(n_4;\mu(\mathbf{r},z),\sqrt{\mu(\mathbf{r},z)})$, which is a good approximation in regions where $\mu(\mathbf{r},z) \gg 1$. Figure 16.7 shows the influence of electronic noise on the energy-response function for $\sigma_e = 2.5$ keV, which is within the range of electronic noise levels of state-of-the-art photon-counting x-ray imaging detectors.

16.4.1.6 Stage 6: Energy Thresholding

Combining Eqs. (16.25) and (16.58), and integrating over the energy spectrum yields the average number of photons counted in the ith energy bin of a detector element:

$$\bar{c}_i = \int_0^\infty \bar{q}_0(E)\alpha(E) \int_A \int_{\varepsilon_i}^{\varepsilon_{i+1}} \left\langle \mathcal{N}\left(\varepsilon;\mu_E(\mathbf{r},z),\sigma_E(\mathbf{r},z)\right)\right\rangle_z \mathrm{d}\varepsilon \mathrm{d}^2\mathbf{r}\mathrm{d}E \tag{16.60}$$

where we made the change of variables $d_1 = \varepsilon\beta/w$, where ε represents deposited photon energy, ε_i represents the low energy threshold for the ith energy bin, and $\mu_E(\mathbf{r},z)$ and $\sigma_E(\mathbf{r},z)$ are respectively given by:

$$\mu_E(\mathbf{r},z) = EP_\Delta(\mathbf{r}) \tag{16.61}$$

and:

$$\sigma_E^2(\mathbf{r},z) = \frac{Ew}{\beta(z)} P_\Delta(\mathbf{r}) + \frac{\sigma_e^2 w}{\beta(z)} \tag{16.62}$$

where $P_\Delta(\mathbf{r})$ is given by Eq. (16.51).

16.4.2 Large-Area Gain

Combining Eqs. (16.27) and (16.60) yields the photon-counting large-area gain of energy bin i:

$$\bar{G}_i = \frac{1}{\bar{q}_0} \int_0^\infty \bar{q}_0(E)\alpha(E) \int_A \int_t^\infty \left\langle \mathcal{N}\left(\varepsilon;\mu_E(\mathbf{r},z),\sigma_E(\mathbf{r},z)\right)\right\rangle_z \mathrm{d}\varepsilon \mathrm{d}^2\mathbf{r}\mathrm{d}E \tag{16.63}$$

$$= \alpha \left\langle \int_A \int_{\varepsilon_i}^{\varepsilon_{i+1}} \left\langle \mathcal{N}\left(\varepsilon;\mu_E(\mathbf{r},z),\sigma_E(\mathbf{r},z)\right)\right\rangle_z \mathrm{d}\varepsilon \mathrm{d}^2\mathbf{r} \right\rangle_{\bar{q}_0\alpha} \tag{16.64}$$

where $\alpha = \int \alpha(E)\bar{q}_0 \mathrm{d}E / \bar{q}_0$ represents the poly-energetic quantum efficiency and $\langle\rangle_{\bar{q}_0\alpha}$ indicates a weighted average over the spectrum of interacting photon energies $\bar{q}_0(E)\alpha(E)$ [keV^{-1}mm^{-2}]. Equation (16.64) shows that the large-area gain can be represented as a spatio-energetic integral of a normal distribution. The integral with respect to spatial variables represents an average over all possible element locations relative to primary x-ray interactions; the integral over deposited photon energy (ε) accounts for energy thresholding.

Figure 16.8 shows the large-area gain calculated using Eq. (16.64) for a simple photon-counting x-ray detector operating with a single energy threshold to distinguish x-ray interactions from electronic noise. Results are shown for CdTe x-ray converters as a function of the size of detector elements. For angiographic, radiographic, and CT imaging conditions, the large-area gain always exceeds the quantum efficiency due to charge sharing, which results in multiple counting of individual x-ray photons. Charge sharing (combined with energy thresholding) has the opposite effect for mammographic imaging conditions, for which the large-area gain is less than the quantum efficiency. In the case of mammography, charge sharing reduces the large-area gain because the majority of photons have energies less than twice the electronic noise floor. Lowering the electronic noise floor for mammography is expected to increase the large-area gain to a value closer to the quantum efficiency.

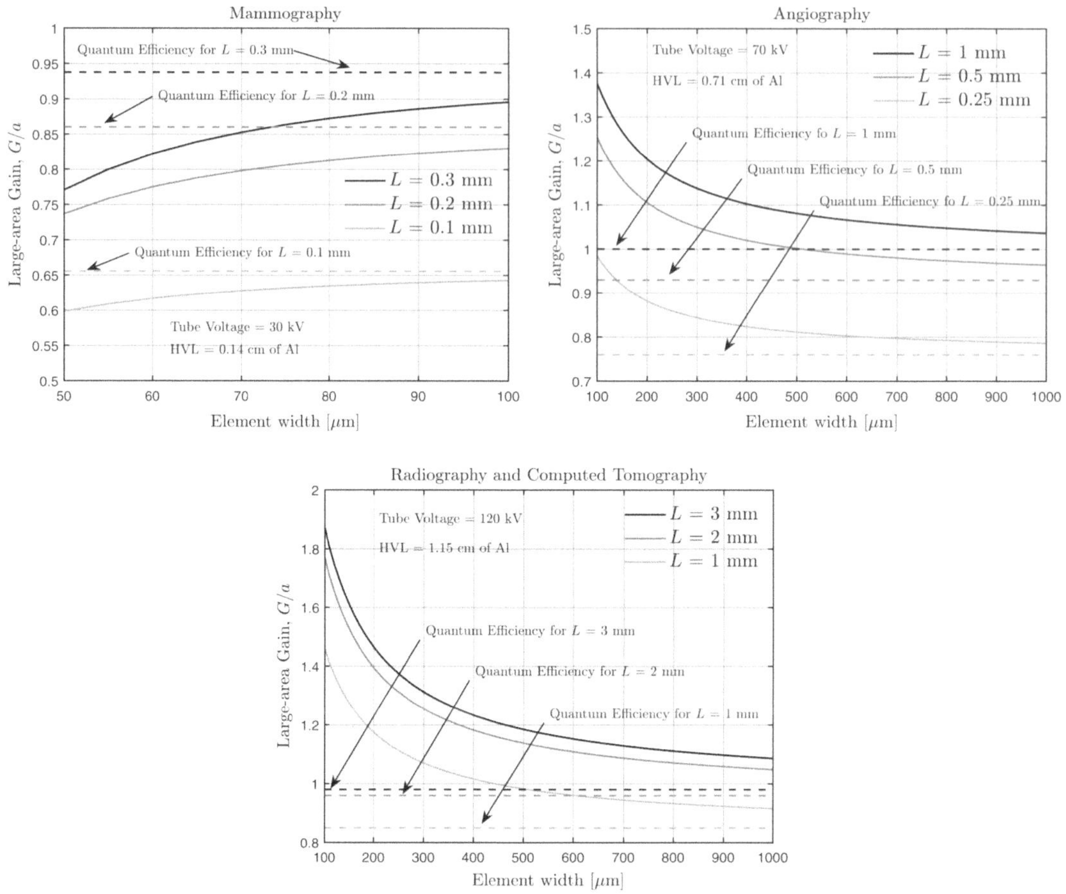

FIGURE 16.8 Large-area gain for mammographic, angiographic, radiographic, and CT imaging conditions. Results are shown for a photon-counting detector operating with a single energy threshold to distinguish x-ray interactions from electronic noise. All calculations were performed for an electronic noise floor of 12.5 keV and an energy threshold equal to the electronic noise floor.

Multiplicity. Combining Eqs. (16.31) and (16.63), the multiplicity for a photon-counting detector operating with a single, open energy bin is given by:

$$\text{multiplicity} = \frac{\bar{G}}{\alpha a} = \left\langle \frac{1}{a} \int_{A} \int_{\varepsilon_t}^{\infty} \left\langle \mathcal{N}\left(\varepsilon; \mu_E(\mathbf{r},z), \sigma_E(\mathbf{r},z)\right)\right\rangle_z \, \mathrm{d}\varepsilon \mathrm{d}^2\mathbf{r} \right\rangle_{\bar{q}_0 \alpha} \tag{16.65}$$

where ε_t represents the energy threshold used to distinguish x-ray interactions from electronic noise. Note that the normal distribution has units of inverse energy, which yields a unitless multiplicity, as required.

16.4.3 Energy-Bin Sensitivity Functions

Combining Eqs. (16.30) and (16.60) yields the energy-bin sensitivity function for the cascaded model illustrated in Figure 16.3:

$$S_i(E) = \alpha(E) \int_{A} \int_{\varepsilon_i}^{\varepsilon_{i+1}} \left\langle \mathcal{N}\left(\varepsilon; \mu_E(\mathbf{r},z), \sigma_E(\mathbf{r},z)\right)\right\rangle_z \, \mathrm{d}\varepsilon \mathrm{d}^2\mathbf{r}. \tag{16.66}$$

Figure 16.9 shows energy-bin sensitivity functions calculated using Eq. (16.66). Also shown are the energy-bin sensitivity functions weighted by the energy spectrum, $q_0(E)$. Calculations are shown for CdTe detectors operating with three energy bins under imaging conditions relevant for contrast-enhanced mammography, angiography, general radiography, and CT. The energy thresholds in Figure 16.9 were not chosen to optimize image quality; they are meant to illustrate

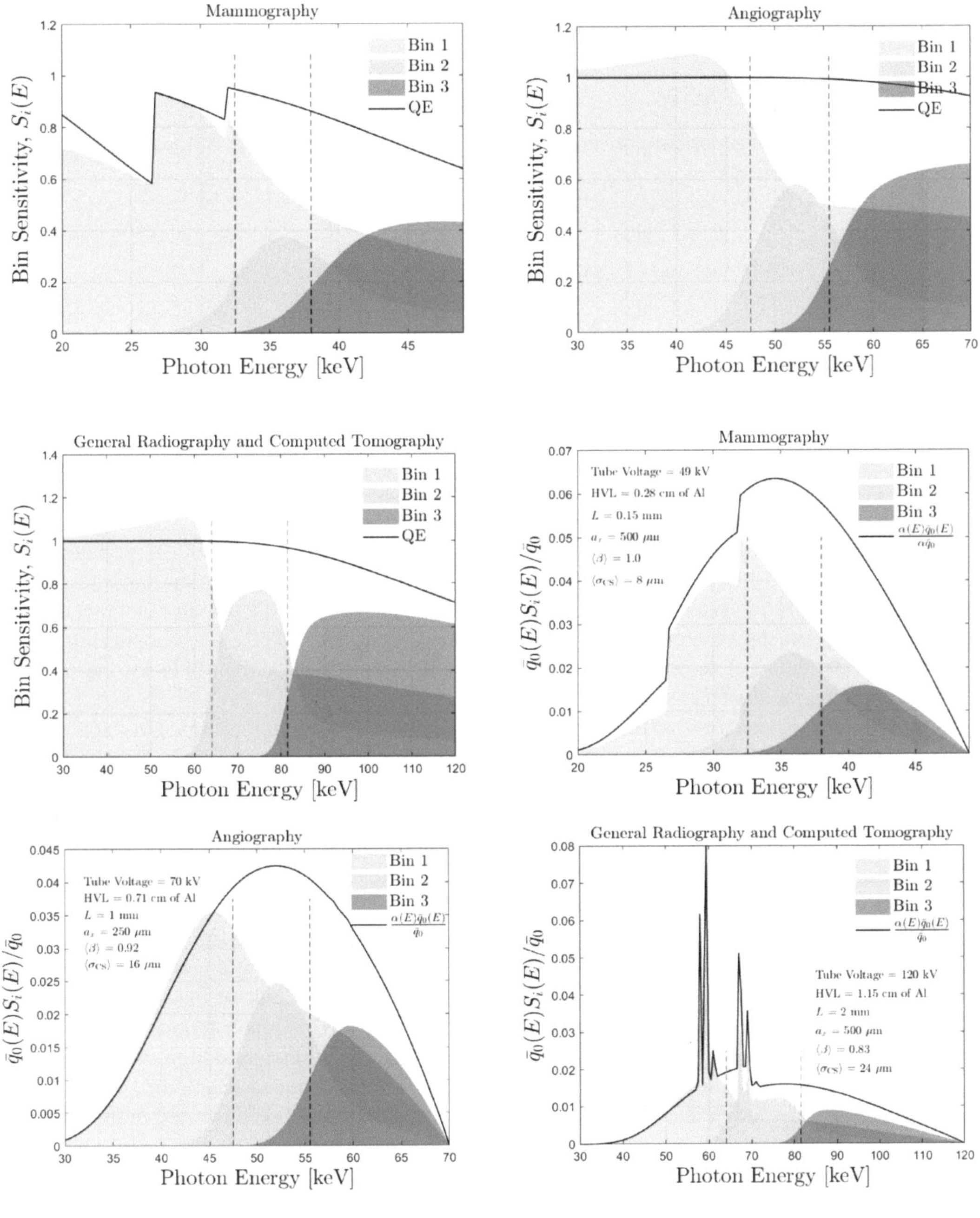

FIGURE 16.9 Energy-bin sensitivity functions for tube voltages, half-value-layers (HVLs), detector thicknesses, and element sizes relevant for contrast-enhanced mammography, angiography, general radiography, and CT. Results are shown for CdTe-based detectors and a 12.5-keV electronic noise floor.

general trends. Figure 16.9 shows that low-energy bins are sensitive to high-energy photons, that is, photons with energies that far exceed the upper threshold of the energy bin. This effect is a result of charge sharing between neighboring detector elements and is most severe for smaller elements, such as those used in mammographic applications. The overlap of bin-sensitivity functions shown in Figure 16.9 is expected to degrade the ability of spectroscopic approaches to produce material-specific images of high quality. A rigorous analysis of the effect of overlapping energy-bin sensitivity functions on image quality is beyond the scope of this chapter, but generally requires a task-based approach accounting for spatial resolution, image noise, and the frequencies of the imaging task.

16.4.4 Pre-Sampling MTFs

Energy-bin MTFs are generically given by Eq. (16.32). Combining Eq. (16.32) with the analysis in the preceding sections yields:

$$\mathrm{MTF}_i(\mathbf{u}) = \bar{G}_i^{-1} FT\left[\alpha \left\langle \int_{\varepsilon_i}^{\varepsilon_{i+1}} \left\langle \mathcal{N}\left(\varepsilon; \mu_E(\mathbf{r},z), \sigma_E(\mathbf{r},z)\right)\right\rangle_z \mathrm{d}\varepsilon \right\rangle_{\bar{q}_0 \alpha} \right] \tag{16.67}$$

where $\bar{G}_i$ is given by Eq. (16.63). The quantity inside the Fourier transform operator in Eq. (16.67) is proportional to the 2D PSF of energy bin i, which is equal to the probability density of recording a photon at position $\mathbf{r}$ relative to the site of a primary interaction. Equation. (16.67) shows that the photon-counting MTF is related nonlinearly to $P_\Delta(\mathbf{r})$ (through Eqs. (16.61) and (16.62)), the latter of which is proportional to the energy-integrating MTF. The nonlinear relationship between the detector PSF and $P_\Delta(\mathbf{r})$ is unique to photon-counting detectors.

The 2D PSF of a CdTe-based photon-counting detector operating with a single open energy bin is shown in Figure 16.10. Results are shown for an angiographic x-ray spectrum as a function of element size. The red squares in Figure 16.10 indicate the boundaries of a detector element centered at the origin. Also shown are the corresponding one-dimensional MTFs. Charge sharing is most severe for the smallest element size (i.e. 100 μm), but has little effect on the MTFs for the combinations of imaging parameters shown in Figure 16.10.

Two-dimensional energy-bin PSFs for selected photon energies for energy bins and detector element sizes relevant for contrast-enhanced mammography, angiography, and CT are shown in Figure 16.11. Figure 16.11 shows that high-energy bins are insensitive to high-energy photons interacting near element boundaries. The opposite is true for lower-energy bins, which, because of charge sharing, are sensitive to high-energy photons interacting near element boundaries. The combination of charge sharing and energy thresholding therefore reduces the sensitive area of detector elements for higher-energy photons and introduces non-stationarity at the sub-pixel level.

Figure 16.12 shows poly-energetic energy bin MTFs calculated using Eq. (16.67) for imaging conditions relevant for contrast-enhanced mammography, angiography, and CT. Also shown is the sinc function, which represents the MTF of an ideal digital x-ray detector in which there are no blurring mechanisms. Figure 16.12 shows that lower energy bins will have reduced spatial resolution relative to high-energy bins. It is interesting to note that the middle- and high-energy bins have MTFs exceeding that of the sinc function. This is a result of the reduced sensitivity of high-energy bins to photons interacting near the boundaries of detector elements, as illustrated in Figure 16.11.

16.4.5 Joint PDF of Detector Signals and Noise Power Spectrum

We showed in Section 16.3.6 that calculating the NPS and cross NPS of energy-bin images produced by photon-counting x-ray detectors requires knowledge of the joint PDF of

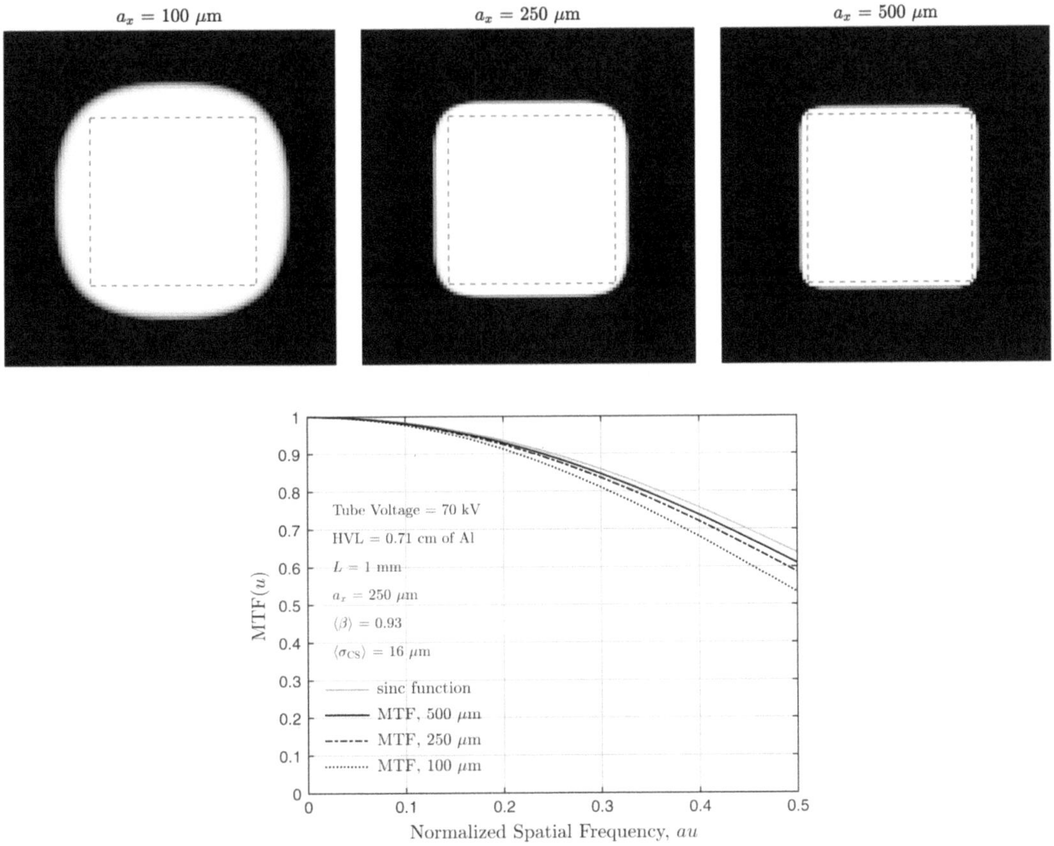

FIGURE 16.10 Two-dimensional PSFs and corresponding one-dimensional MTFs for an RQA5 x-ray spectrum incident on a CdTe photon counting x-ray imaging detector. Results are shown for a simple photon-counting system, in which a single energy threshold is applied to separate photon interaction events from electronic noise. Results are shown for a 12.5-keV electronic noise floor.

pre-sampling, pre-thresholding signals from detector elements separated by a distance $\boldsymbol{\tau}$, that is, $p_{d_1,d_1'}(d_1,d_1;\boldsymbol{\tau})$. In this section we derive a closed-form expression for $p_{d_1,d_1'}(d_1,d_1;\boldsymbol{\tau})$ for the cascaded model illustrated in Figure 16.3 and use the result to calculate the NPS. We drop the dependence on the depth of interaction for notational convenience. Depth-dependent effects can be modeled by averaging the results of this section over the depth of interaction, as was done in the preceding sections.

We first consider the probability that n_4 quanta are detected in an element centered at $\mathbf{r}$ and n_4' quanta are detected in an element centered at $\mathbf{r}+\boldsymbol{\tau}$ given n_3 total quanta collected following an interaction at $\tilde{\mathbf{r}}_0$. When the elements centered at $\mathbf{r}$ and $\mathbf{r}+\boldsymbol{\tau}$ are non-overlapping, the joint PDF of n_4 and n_4' can be modeled as a multinomial distribution with three possible outcomes.[26] In the limit of a large number of collected quanta (i.e. $n_3 \gg 1$), which must be satisfied for viable detector designs, this multinomial distribution can be approximated as the product of two Poisson distributions, yielding the following result:

$$p_{n_4,n_4'}\left(n_4,n_4' \middle| \tilde{\mathbf{r}}_0;\mathbf{r},\boldsymbol{\tau}\right) \approx \alpha \mathcal{P}\left(n_4;\mu\left(\mathbf{r}-\tilde{\mathbf{r}}_0\right)\right)\mathcal{P}\left(n_4';\mu\left(\mathbf{r}+\boldsymbol{\tau}-\tilde{\mathbf{r}}_0\right)\right),\ \boldsymbol{\tau} \notin \left[-\frac{a_x}{2},\frac{a_x}{2}\right]\times\left[-\frac{a_y}{2},\frac{a_y}{2}\right] \quad (16.68)$$

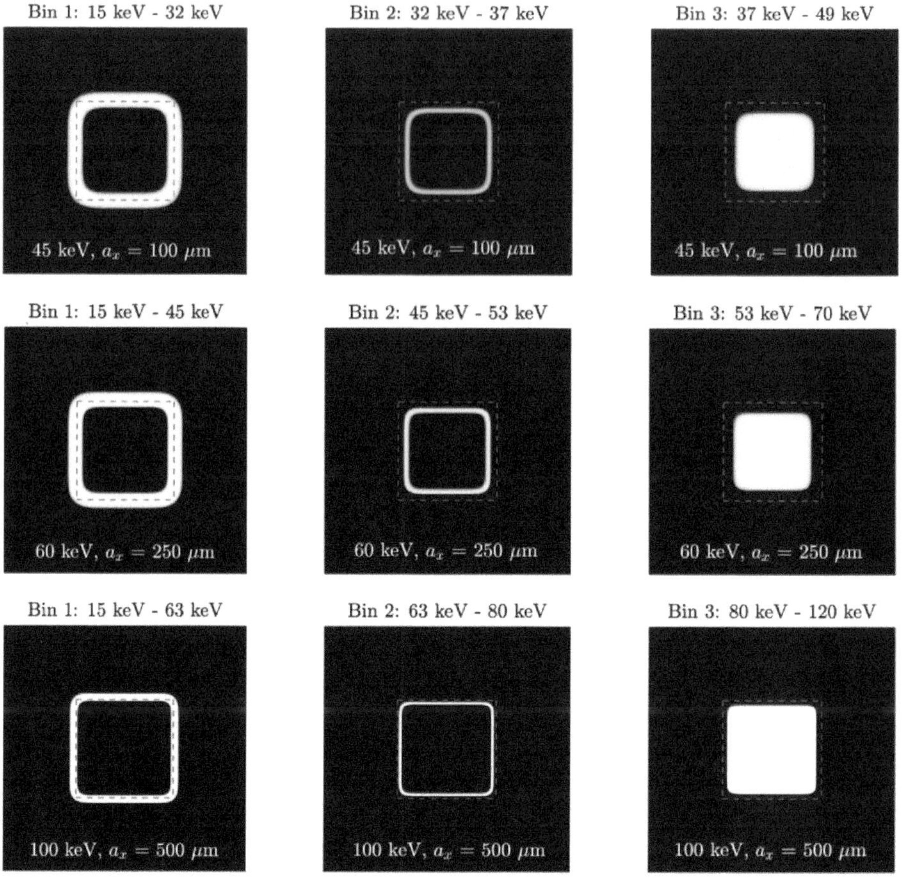

FIGURE 16.11 Two-dimensional energy-bin PSFs for selected photons energies, energy bins, and element sizes. From top to bottom, the combinations of parameters are relevant for contrast-enhanced mammography, angiography, and CT. The red squares indicate the boundaries of detector elements centered at the origin.

where $\mu(\mathbf{r})$ is given by Eq. (16.54) and $\tau \notin \left[-\frac{a_x}{2},\frac{a_x}{2}\right]\times\left[-\frac{a_y}{2},\frac{a_y}{2}\right]$ means that the tip of the vector τ does not lie within a rectangular region defined by the sides of a detector element of width a_x and a_y in the x and y directions, respectively. Averaging over $\tilde{\mathbf{r}}_0$ and accounting for electronic noise yields:

$$p_{d_1,d_1'}\left(d_1,d_1';\tau\right)=\frac{\alpha}{A}\mathcal{N}\left(d_1;\mu(\tau),\sigma(\tau)\right)*\mathcal{N}\left(d_1;\mu(\tau),\sigma(\tau)\right),\ \tau\notin\left[-\frac{a_x}{2},\frac{a_x}{2}\right]\times\left[-\frac{a_y}{2},\frac{a_y}{2}\right] \quad (16.69)$$

where the convolution is with respect to τ. The joint PDF of pre-sampling, pre-thresholding detector signals separated by τ is therefore the self-convolution of a normal distribution with spatially varying mean and standard deviation.

When $\tau = 0$, the detector elements overlap completely, in which case $d_1 = d_1'$ and the joint PDF is given by:

$$p_{d_1,d_1'}\left(d_1,d_1';\tau\right)\Big|_{\tau=0}=\delta\left(d_1-d_1'\right)\frac{\alpha}{A}\int_A\mathcal{N}\left(d_1;\mu(\mathbf{r}),\sigma(\mathbf{r})\right)\mathrm{d}^2\mathbf{r}. \quad (16.70)$$

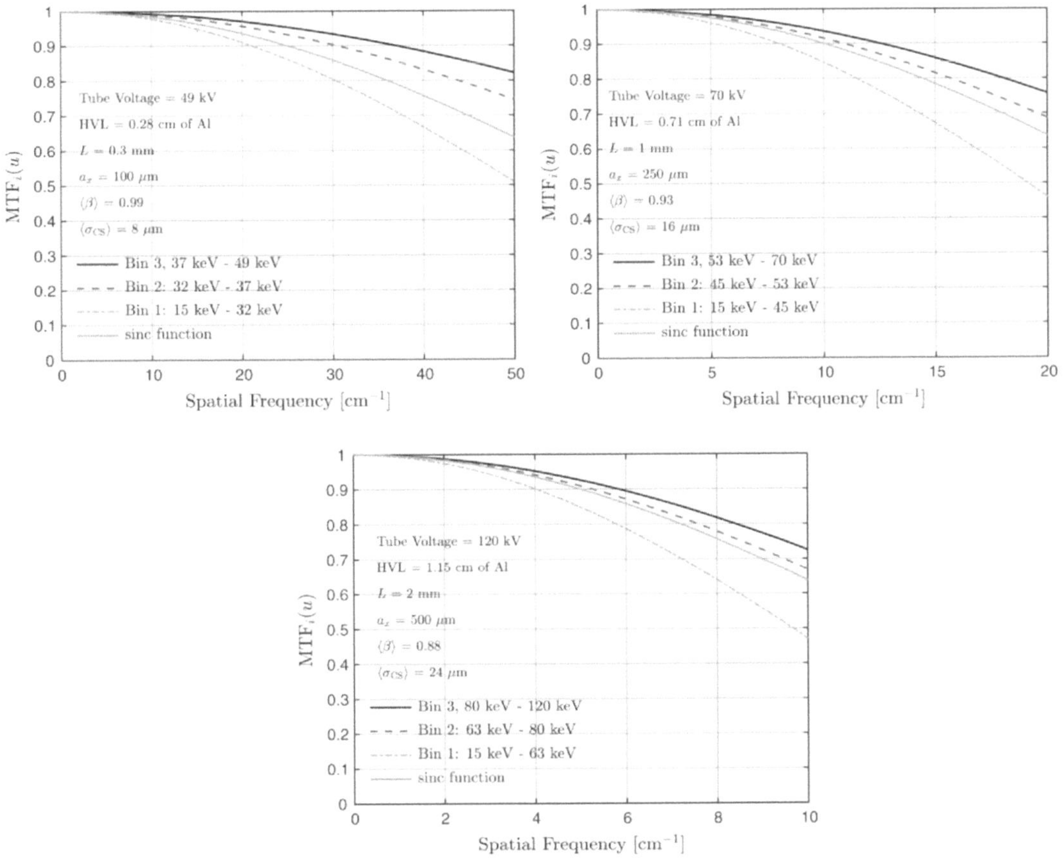

FIGURE 16.12 Energy-bin MTFs for imaging conditions relevant for contrast-enhanced mammography, angiography, and CT from left to right, respectively.

The transition region between $\tau = 0$ and $\tau \notin \left[-\frac{a_x}{2}, \frac{a_x}{2}\right] \times \left[-\frac{a_y}{2}, \frac{a_y}{2}\right]$ corresponds to partially overlapping detector elements and is non-physical. Linear interpolation between complete overlap and no overlap can be used to approximate the joint PDF in the region for which $\tau \in \left[-\frac{a_x}{2}, \frac{a_x}{2}\right] \times \left[-\frac{a_y}{2}, \frac{a_y}{2}\right]$ without introducing errors in the pre-sampling NPS at frequencies lower than $1/a_x$.

Changing from units of quanta to units of energy using $d_1 = \varepsilon\beta / w$ yields:

$$p_{\varepsilon,\varepsilon'}(\varepsilon, \varepsilon'; \tau) = \begin{cases} \delta(\varepsilon - \varepsilon') \dfrac{\alpha}{A} \displaystyle\int_A \mathcal{N}(\varepsilon; \mu_E(\mathbf{r}), \sigma_E(\mathbf{r})) \mathrm{d}^2\mathbf{r}, & \tau = 0 \\ \dfrac{\alpha}{A} \mathcal{N}(\varepsilon; \mu_E(\tau), \sigma_E(\tau)) * \mathcal{N}(\varepsilon'; \mu_E(\tau), \sigma_E(\tau)), & \tau \notin \left[-\dfrac{a_x}{2}, \dfrac{a_x}{2}\right] \times \left[-\dfrac{a_y}{2}, \dfrac{a_y}{2}\right] \end{cases} \tag{16.71}$$

where $p_{\varepsilon,\varepsilon'}(\varepsilon, \varepsilon'; \tau)$ represents the probability density of simultaneously recording energies ε and ε' in detector elements separated by distance τ and $\mu_E(\mathbf{r})$ and $\sigma_E(\mathbf{r})$ are given by

Eqs. (16.61) and (16.62), respectively. The pre-sampling cross NPS between energy bins i and i' is then given by:

$$W_{c_i,c_i'}(\mathbf{u}) = \bar{q}_0 \cdot FT\left[A \int_{\varepsilon_i}^{\varepsilon_{i+1}} \int_{\varepsilon_i'}^{\varepsilon_{i+1}'} p_{\varepsilon,\varepsilon'}(\varepsilon,\varepsilon';\tau) d\varepsilon d\varepsilon' \right]. \tag{16.72}$$

We note here that the relationship between the pre-sampling NPS, the conversion gain, collection efficiency, charge sharing kernel, and the detector aperture function is contained entirely within $p_{\varepsilon,\varepsilon'}(\varepsilon,\varepsilon';\tau)$, which is a piece-wise function that is nonlinear in these variables. In the case of energy-integrating systems, the pre-sampling NPS is linearly related to the square of the Fourier transform of the charge sharing kernel and aperture function. Therefore, compared to CSA of energy-integrating systems, modeling of photon-counting systems does not enable easy, analytical interpretation of relationships between gain and blurring mechanisms and the pre-sampling NPS. This difficulty arises because of energy thresholding, which is nonlinear. Despite the nonlinearity of thresholding, photon-counting detectors operating under low count rates maintain the properties of linearity between input and output and stationarity.

Figure 16.13 shows the normalized pre-sampling and digital NPS of CdTe-based, simple photon-counting x-ray detectors calculated using Eq. (16.72). Also shown is the pre-sampling normalized

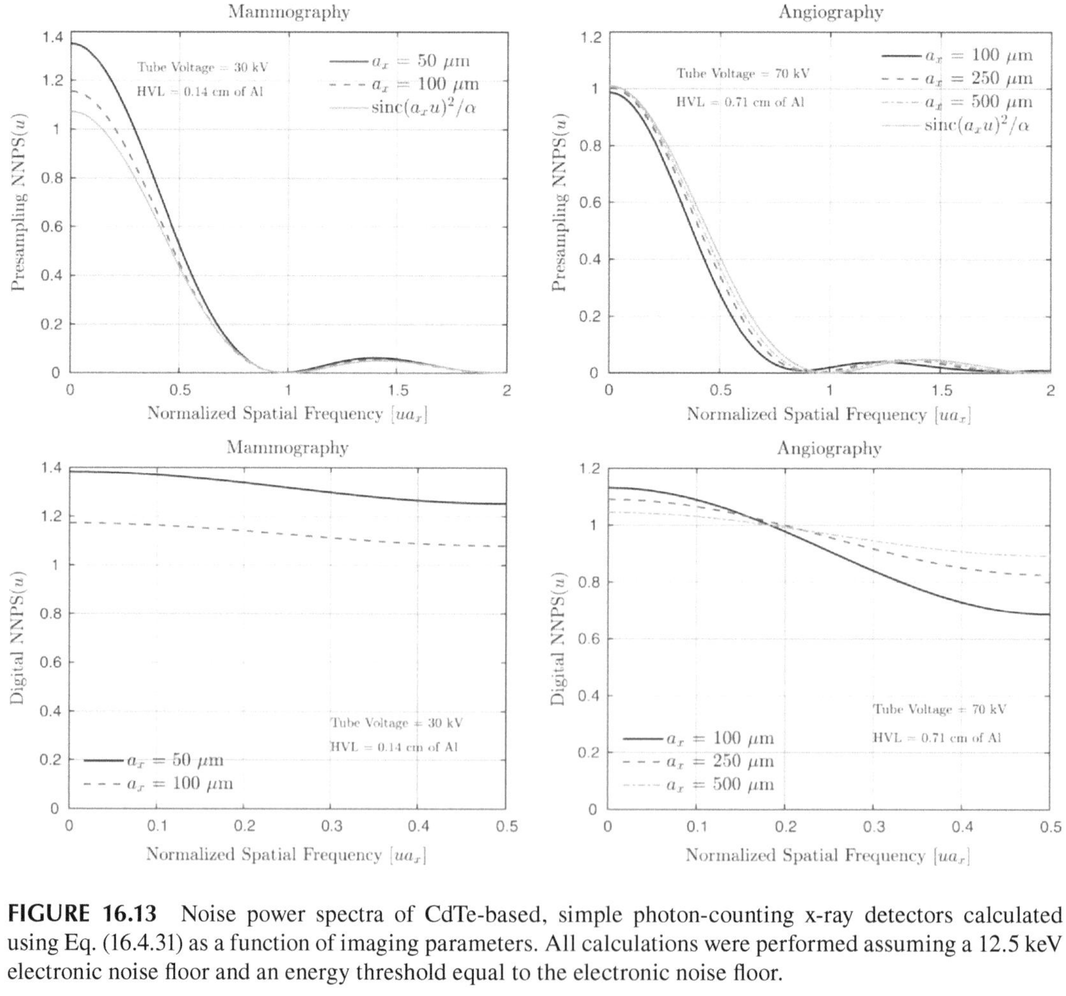

FIGURE 16.13 Noise power spectra of CdTe-based, simple photon-counting x-ray detectors calculated using Eq. (16.4.31) as a function of imaging parameters. All calculations were performed assuming a 12.5 keV electronic noise floor and an energy threshold equal to the electronic noise floor.

noise power spectrum (NNPS) of an ideal digital x-ray detector, for which $\text{NNPS}(u) = \text{sinc}^2(a_x u) / \alpha$. In all cases, the normalized pre-sampling NPS decreases with increasing frequency at a faster rate than the square of the sinc function. This result is due to the slightly reduced MTFs relative to the sinc function. In addition, in the case of mammography and 50 μm detector elements, the normalized pre-sampling NPS is much higher than that of an ideal photon-counting detector. This result is due to the reduced large-area gain relative to the quantum efficiency, which increases image noise relative to the image signal. In the case of angiography, radiography, and CT, the zeros of the pre-sampling noise power spectra do not correspond to those of the sinc function. This mismatch results in noise aliasing at zero spatial frequency. In addition to the zero-frequency value, noise aliasing increases the NNPS at all spatial frequencies, which also occurs in energy-integrating systems.(24)

16.5 SUMMARY AND PROSPECTS

This overview shows that modeling of photon-counting x-ray detectors is a significant challenge. Even the simplified models presented here, which ignore the effects of pulse pile-up, characteristic reabsorption and Compton scattering, require the use of spatio-energetic normal distributions and multivariate normal distributions. As we have shown, this complicating requirement arises from energy thresholding, which is unique to photon-counting systems. We have shown that energy thresholding prevents the application of traditional cascaded systems ideas to photon-counting detectors. As a consequence, a new paradigm requiring modeling of the distribution of all possible pre-thresholding detector signals arising from single photon interactions was developed. This paradigm not only requires modeling of the distribution of pre-thresholding detector signals, but also the joint distribution of pre-thresholding signals from two elements of a photon-counting detector. This is a substantial departure from traditional cascaded systems approaches for modeling of energy-integrating systems.

The models presented here do not enable easy understanding of relationships between the performance of photon-counting detectors and underlying detector parameters. Future work should focus on developing simpler analytic relationships to facilitate such understanding. Until then, it remains to be seen whether or not analytic modeling of photon-counting systems will see as widespread use as cascaded systems modeling of energy-integrating systems. In addition, analytic modeling of photon-counting systems remains limited. A significant limitation is the lack of analytic tools for modeling the effects of reabsorption of characteristic and Compton-scattered x-rays on the photon-counting NPS. In some energy-integrating systems, reabsorption processes are the primary factor leading to a reduction in the DQE at energies immediately above the K-edge energy of the x-ray converter. Accurate modeling of reabsorption requires a parallel cascades approach, and is a focus of ongoing academic research. Future work should also include developing an analytic understanding of combined spatial, temporal, and energetic effects. This would enable theoretical analysis of the influence of charge sharing and pulse pile-up on spectral distortions, spatial resolution and image noise. However, given the expected mathematical complexity, it is possible that such theories may not provide more insight into the underlying physics than a Monte Carlo approach may provide.

Despite these limitations, modeling of photon-counting detectors has come a long way, and there now exist analytic tools that provide insight into frequency-dependent signal and noise properties of photon-counting x-ray imaging detectors. These tools provide a foundation for future theoretical developments and enable task-based modeling of photon-counting x-ray imaging detectors, for example using the methodology developed by Persson and colleagues.(56) Task-based theoretical modeling will enable head-to-head comparisons of different photon-counting technologies in targeted applications, for example, contrast-enhanced breast imaging and vascular imaging, and will enable identifying critical design parameters that must be carefully controlled to maximize imaging quality for a given imaging task. Such approaches are expected to facilitate the design and development of the photon-counting x-ray imaging detectors of the future.

REFERENCES

1. A. Rose, "A unified approach to the performance of photographic film, television pickup tubes, and the human eye," *J. Soc. Motion Pict. Eng.* 47, pp. 273–294, 1946.
2. A. Rose, "The sensitivity performance of the human eye on an absolute scale," *J. Opt. Soc. Am.* 38, pp. 196–208, 1948.
3. A. Rose, "Quantum and noise limitations of the visual process," *J. Opt. Soc. Am.* 43, pp. 715–716, 1953.
4. R. Shaw, "The equivalent quantum efficiency of the photographic process," *J. Photogr. Sci.* 11, pp. 199–204, 1963.
5. R. F. Wagner, "Toward a unified view of radiological imaging systems. Part II: Noisy images," *Med Phys.* 4(4), pp. 279–296, 1977.
6. R. F. Wagner, "Unified snr analysis of medical imaging systems," *Phys. Med. Biol.* 30, pp. 489–519, 1985.
7. M. Rabbani, R. Shaw, and R. V. Metter, "Detective quantum efficiency of imaging systems with amplifying and scattering mechanisms," *J. Opt. Soc. Am. A* 4, pp. 895–901, May 1987.
8. R. V. Metter and M. Rabbani, "An application of multivariate moment-generating functions to the analysis of signal and noise propagation in radiographic screen-film systems," *Med. Phys.* 17(1), pp. 65–71, 1990.
9. I. A. Cunningham, M. S. Westmore, and A. Fenster, "A spatial-frequency dependent quantum accounting diagram and detective quantum efficiency model of signal and noise propagation in cascaded imaging systems," *Med. Phys.* 21, pp. 417–427, Mar 1994.
10. I. A. Cunningham and R. Shaw, "Signal-to-noise optimization of medical imaging systems," *J. Opt. Soc. Am. A* 16, pp. 621–632, 1999.
11. J. Yao and I. A. Cunningham, "Parallel cascades: New ways to describe noise transfer in medical imaging systems," *Med. Phys.* 28, pp. 2020–2038, Oct 2001.
12. S. Yun, J. Tanguay, H. K. Kim, and I. A. Cunningham, "Cascaded-systems analysis and the detective quantum efficiency of single-Z x-ray detectors include photoelectric, coherent and incoherent interactions," *Med. Phys.* 40, pp. 0419161–04191616, 2013.
13. I. A. Cunningham, *Handbook of Medical Imaging*, ch. 2, pp. 79–160. SPIE Press, 2000.
14. Y.-H. Hu, D. A. Scaduto, and W. Zhao, "Optimization of contrast-enhanced breast imaging: Analysis using a cascaded linear system model," *Med. Phys.* 44(1), pp. 43–56, 2017.
15. B. Zhao and W. Zhao, "Three-dimensional linear system analysis for breast tomosynthesis," *Med. Phys.* 35, pp. 5219–5232, Dec 2008.
16. G. J. Gang, D. J. Tward, J. Lee, and J. H. Siewerdsen, "Anatomical background and generalized detectability in tomosynthesis and cone-beam CT," *Med. Phys.* 37, pp. 1948–1965, May 2010.
17. P. Prakash, W. Zbijewski, G. J. Gang, Y. Ding, J. W. Stayman, J. Yorkston, J. A. Carrino, and J. H. Siewerdsen, "Task-based modeling and optimization of a cone-beam CT scanner for musculoskeletal imaging," *Med. Phys.* 38(10), pp. 5612–5629, 2011.
18. G. J. Gang, J. Lee, J. W. Stayman, D. J. Tward, W. Zbijewski, J. L. Prince, and J. H. Siewerdsen, "Analysis of Fourier-domain task-based detectability index in tomosynthesis and cone-beam CT in relation to human observer performance," *Med. Phys.* 38, pp. 1754–1768, Apr 2011.
19. G. J. Gang, W. Zbijewski, J. Webster Stayman, and J. H. Siewerdsen, "Cascaded systems analysis of noise and detectability in dual-energy cone-beam CT," *Med. Phys.* 39, pp. 5145–5156, Aug 2012.
20. E. Fredenberg, M. Danielsson, J. W. Stayman, J. H. Siewerdsen, and M. Aslund, "Ideal-observer detectability in photon-counting differential phase-contrast imaging using a linear-systems approach," *Med. Phys.* 39, pp. 5317–5335, Sep 2012.
21. G. J. Gang, J. W. Stayman, W. Zbijewski, and J. H. Siewerdsen, "Task-based detectability in CT image reconstruction by filtered backprojection and penalized likelihood estimation," *Med. Phys.* 41, p. 081902, Aug 2014.
22. J. H. Siewerdsen, L. E. Antonuk, Y. el Mohri, J. Yorkston, W. Huang, J. M. Boudry, and I. A. Cunningham, "Empirical and theoretical investigation of the noise performance of indirect detection, active matrix flat-panel imagers (AMFPIs) for diagnostic radiology," *Med. Phys.* 24, pp. 71–89, Jan 1997.
23. W. Zhao, G. Ristic, and J. A. Rowlands, "X-ray imaging performance of structured cesium iodide scintillators," *Med. Phys.* 31, pp. 2594–2605, Sep 2004.
24. I. A. Cunningham, *SPIE Handbook of Medical Imaging Vol. 2: Physics and Psychophysics. Chapter 2: Applied Linear Systems Theory.* SPIE, 2000.
25. H. H. Barrett and K. J. Myers, *Foundations of Image Science.* John Wiley &Sons, Hoboken, New Jersey, 2004.

26. A. Papoulis, *Probability, Random Variables, and Stochastic Processes.* McGraw-Hill, Inc., 3rd ed., 1991.
27. I. A. Cunningham, "Applied linear-systems theory," *Handbook of Medical Imaging.* 1, pp. 79–159, 2000.
28. T. Michel, G. Anton, M. Bohnel, J. Durst, M. Firsching, A. Korn, B. Kreisler, A. Loehr, F. Nachtrab, D. Niederlohner, F. Sukowski, and P. T. Talla, "A fundamental method to determine the signal-to-noise ratio (SNR) and detective quantum efficiency (DQE) for a photon counting pixel detector," *Nucl. Instrum. Meth. A.* 568, pp. 799–802, 2006.
29. T. Michel, G. Anton, J. Durst, P. Bartl, M. Bohnel, M. Firsching, B. Kreisler, A. Korn, A. Loehr, F. Nachtrab, D. Niederlohner, F. Sukowski, and P. Takoukam-Talla, "Investigating the DQE of the medipix detector using the multiplicity concept," *IEEE Nuclear Symposium Conference Record.* M06-169, pp. 1955–1959, 2006.
30. T. Koenig, J. Schulze, M. Zuber, K. Rink, J. Butzer, E. Hamann, A. Cecilia, A. Zwerger, A. Fauler, M. Fiederle, and U. Oelfke, "Imaging properties of small-pixel spectroscopic x-ray detectors based on cadmium telluride sensors," *Phys. Med. Biol.* 57, pp. 6743–6759, Nov 2012.
31. X. Ji, R. Zhang, G.-H. Chen, and K. Li, "Impact of anti-charge sharing on the zero-frequency detective quantum efficiency of CdTe-based photon counting detector system: Cascaded systems analysis and experimental validation," *Phys. Med. Biol.* 63, p. 095003, May 2018.
32. R. J. Acciavatti and A. D. A. Maidment, "An analytical model of NPS and DQE comparing photon counting and energy integrating detectors," *Proc. of SPIE.* 7622, p. 76220I, 2010.
33. R. J. Acciavatti and D. A. Maidment, "A comparative analysis of OTF, NPS, and DQE in energy integrating and photon counting digital x-ray detectors," *Med. Phys.* 37, pp. 6480–6495, 2010.
34. J. Xu, W. Zbijewski, G. Gang, J. W. Stayman, K. Taguchi, M. Lundqvist, E. Fredenberg, J. A. Carrino, and J. H. Siewerdsen, "Cascaded systems analysis of photon counting detectors," *Med. Phys.* 41, p. 101907, Oct 2014.
35. J. Tanguay and I. A. Cunningham, "Cascaded systems analysis of charge sharing in cadmium telluride photon-counting x-ray detectors," *Med. Phys.*, 2018.
36. A. Goldan, J. Rowlands, O. Tousignant, and K. Karim, "Unipolar time-differential charge sensing in non-dispersive amorphous solids," *J. Appl. Phys.* 113(22), p. 224502, 2013.
37. J. Stavro, A. H. Goldan, and W. Zhao, "SWAD: Inherent photon counting performance of amorphous selenium multi-well avalanche detector," in *SPIE Medical Imaging*, pp. 97833Q–97833Q. International Society for Optics and Photonics, 2016.
38. J. Stavro, A. H. Goldan, M. Lub, S. Lévelléc, and W. Zhaoa, "SWAD: Transient conductivity and pulse-height spectrum," in *Proc. of SPIE* 10132, pp. 1013208–1, 2017.
39. J. Stavro, A. H. Goldan, and W. Zhao, "Photon counting performance of amorphous selenium and its dependence on detector structure," in *Medical Imaging 2018: Physics of Medical Imaging.* 10573, p. 105735Y, International Society for Optics and Photonics, 2018.
40. J. Tanguay, S. Yun, H. K. Kim, and I. A. Cunningham, "Cascaded systems analyses of photon-counting x-ray detectors," *Proc. of SPIE.* 8668, pp. 0S1–0S14, 2013.
41. J. Tanguay, S. Yun, H. K. Kim, and I. A. Cunningham, "The detective quantum efficiency of photon-counting x-ray detectors using cascaded systems analyses," *Med. Phys.* 40, p. 041913, 2013.
42. J. Tanguay, S. Yun, H. K. Kim, and I. A. Cunningham, "Detective quantum efficiency of photon-counting x-ray detectors," *Med. Phys.* 42, pp. 491–509, Jan 2015.
43. J. Tanguay, J. Stavro, D. McKeown, A. H. Goldan, I. Cunningham, and W. Zhao, "Cascaded systems analysis of photon-counting field-shaping multi-well avalanche detectors (SWADS)," in *Medical Imaging 2018: Physics of Medical Imaging.* 10573, p. 105734V, International Society for Optics and Photonics, 2018.
44. K. Taguchi, E. C. Frey, X. Wang, J. S. Iwanczyk, and W. C. Barber, "An analytical model of the effects of pulse pileup on the energy spectrum recorded by energy resolved photon counting x-ray detectors," *Med. Phys.* 37, pp. 3957–3969, Aug 2010.
45. K. Taguchi, C. Polster, O. Lee, K. Stierstorfer, and S. Kappler, "Spatio-energetic cross talk in photon counting detectors: Detector model and correlated Poisson data generator," *Med. Phys.* 43, p. 6386, Dec 2016.
46. K. Taguchi, K. Stierstorfer, C. Polster, O. Lee, and S. Kappler, "Spatio-energetic cross-talk in photon counting detectors: Numerical detector model (PCTK) and workflow for CT image quality assessment," *Med. Phys.* 45, pp. 1985–1998, May 2018.
47. E. Roessl, H. Daerr, and R. Proksa, "A fourier approach to pulse pile-up in photon-counting x-ray detectors," *Med. Phys.* 43, pp. 1295–1298, Mar 2016.

48. S. Faby, J. Maier, S. Sawall, D. Simons, H.-P. Schlemmer, M. Lell, and M. Kachelrieß, "An efficient computational approach to model statistical correlations in photon counting x-ray detectors," *Med. Phys.* 43, p. 3945, July 2016.
49. S. Ramo, "Currents induced by electron motion," *Proc. IRE.* 27(9), pp. 584–585, 1939.
50. Z. He, "Review of the Shockley–Ramo theorem and its application in semiconductor gamma-ray detectors," *Nuclear Instruments and Methods in Physics Research Section A: Accelerators, Spectrometers, Detectors and Associated Equipment.* 463(1–2), pp. 250–267, 2001.
51. K. Hecht, "Zum mechanismus des lichtelektrischen primarstromes in isolierenden kristallen," *Z. Phys.* 77, pp. 235–245, 1932.
52. A. Ruzin and Y. Nemirovsky, "Methodology for evaluations of mobility-lifetime product by spectroscopy measurements using CdZnTe spectrometers," *J. Appl. Phys.* 82, pp. 4166–4171, 1997.
53. A. Ruzin and Y. Nemirovsky, "Statistical models for charge collection efficiency and variance in semiconductor spectrometers," *J. Appl. Physics* 82(6), pp. 2754–2758, 1997.
54. B. Thomas, M. C. Veale, M. D. Wilson, P. Seller, A. Schneider, and K. Ineiwski, "Characterisation of redlen high-flux cdznte," *J. Instrum.* 12, p. C12045, 2017.
55. K. Taguchi and J. S. Iwanczyk, "Vision 20/20: Single photon counting x-ray detectors in medical imaging," *Med. Phys.* 40, p. 100901, Oct 2013.
56. M. Persson, P. L. Rajbhandary, and N. J. Pelc, "A framework for performance characterization of energy-resolving photon-counting detectors," *Med. Phys.* 45, pp. 4897–4915, Nov 2018.

17 Design Considerations for Photon-Counting Detectors

Connecting Detector Characteristics to System Performance

Scott S. Hsieh
Department of Radiology, Mayo Clinic, Rochester, Minnesota, USA

CONTENTS

17.1 INTRODUCTION

The ultimate goal of any photon-counting detector (PCD) is to improve the ability of the parent x-ray imaging system in accomplishing its imaging task. In the context of diagnostic CT applications, the PCD should provide higher dose efficiency, better detectability, increased spatial resolution, and improved spectral performance compared to conventional, energy-integrating detectors.

It is widely appreciated that the ideal PCD can provide all of these advantages. Conventional detectors suffer from several drawbacks. These detectors implicitly perform energy weighting where photons with higher energy contribute to output signal more than those with lower energy. This nonuniform weighting directly reduces contrast, especially for the detection of iodine, which has greater contrast at lower energies (1). Hence, the ideal detector would weight lower energies more strongly than higher energies, but conventional detectors are the opposite, decreasing dose efficiency (2). Also, energy-integrating detectors have limited fill factor, because light originating in a scintillator pixel must be trapped in that pixel using reflective surfaces. The geometric efficiency of a conventional CT detector can be estimated to be 70% in current systems, although this is implementation-dependent. These reflectors also limit the spatial resolution, because decrease in the pixel pitch would be accompanied by a concomitant increase in reflector density, leading to further decreases in geometric efficiency. PCDs provide an opportunity for improvement in several metrics, but, real PCDs also present non-idealities that degrade performance. This makes the comparison between PCDs and conventional detectors technology-dependent.

Designers of PCDs often assess their detectors using specific metrics such as count rate capability or spectral separation. However, it is their performance in the context of the larger system that ultimately matters. A metric such as spectral separation has value in that it is a surrogate for the systems-level metric of detection of a low-contrast spectral signal.

The purpose of this chapter is to understand the PCD in the broader context of the system, connecting *detector-level* performance metrics with *systems-level* performance metrics to better aid PCD designers in selecting appropriate trade-offs. We will further survey a collection of technologies that can improve the performance of PCDs. We will begin by reviewing common performance metrics used for both detectors and systems. We will then describe PCD parameters that can influence and trade-off between these metrics, and also describe technologies that can improve performance in multiple domains at the cost of greater complexity.

As previously stated, we will focus primarily on the diagnostic CT application. Diagnostic CT imposes particularly demanding flux requirements and uses photons on the order of 50–100 keV. Applications outside of diagnostic CT, and especially those that strive for detection of photons on the order of 10 keV, will naturally lead to very different design choices.

Table 17.1 summarizes the contents of this chapter and links the performance metrics of the CT system with those of the detector and outlines strategies to improve each metric.

17.2 PCD PERFORMANCE METRICS

Several metrics are commonly used or have been proposed to quantify the performance of PCDs. Although the reader may be familiar with many of these, we will provide a brief summary as a reference.

17.2.1 Count Rate Capability

Count-rate capability measures the ability of a PCD to discriminate individual photons that arrive in close temporal proximity. Count rate is the most significant challenge for diagnostic CT (3).

The spectrum and flux of a clinical x-ray tube can be estimated with freely available tools such as Spektr (4) and a typical value for unattenuated beam is 1000 Mcps/mm^2 (million counts per second

TABLE 17.1
Measuring the Performance of a CT System with a Photon-Counting Detector (PCD)

Systems Metric	PCD Metric	Parameters	Technologies
Low-contrast detectability (conventional)	Double counting rate	Pixel size Crystal thickness	Charge summing Anti-coincidence Anti-scatter grid
Low-contrast detectability (spectral)	Spectral separation, energy response function	Pixel size Tube kVp Number of bins	Charge summing K-edge filters Anti-scatter grid Nonlinear reconstruction
Spatial resolution	Pixel pitch	Macropixel binning Pixel size	Advanced source design
Noise at high flux	Count rate, pileup	Pulse-shaping time Pixel size	Dynamic filters Pulse-detection logic
Artifacts	Various	N/A	Calibration Improved substrate material

Note: (Far left) Performance metrics for the CT system. The ultimate goal of a PCD is to improve these metrics. (Middle left) Corresponding metrics of the PCD. Control of these factors can improve the systems performance metrics. (Middle right) Parameters of the detector that could be adjusted to change the balance of PCD performance metrics. In many cases, improving one metric may harm another metric. (Far right) Novel technologies that could enable superior performance, perhaps at the cost of additional complexity.

per square mm) at 1 m away from the focal spot. Count rate can be reported on a per-pixel basis, but in clinical applications the relevant parameter is counts per unit area.

The specific rate that is reported is the characteristic count rate, which is the inverse of the detector dead time. The dead time is the amount of time that the detector is inactive after receiving a photon, and is a semi-theoretical construct for well-defined, idealized paralyzable or nonparalyzable detectors (5). The characteristic count rate for real PCDs, which are neither perfect paralyzable PCDs nor perfect nonparalyzable PCDs, is estimated by fitting the measured reported (or output) count rate to the incident flux (or input count rate) to a curve that is predicted from either an ideal paralyzable or nonparalyzable system.

17.2.2 Energy Response Function

The energy response function (ERF) measures the spectral accuracy of the detector. Although conventions vary, a typical parameterization is that $ERF(E_1,E_2)$ provides the probability that a photon with energy E_2 is measured at an energy E_1. The ERF is conceptually understood to exist prior to binning into discrete energy bins. One way to measure the ERF is to use a radioisotope that emits photons of a known energy, and to sweep the energy threshold to accumulate the integral of the ERF (6). The ERF is usually measured at low flux so that count rate limitations do not impact the accuracy of the measurement.

Figure 17.1 depicts an ERF in the form of a matrix. The ERF is attractive for its simplicity but hides some of the details of the statistics. For example, a photon's energy may be split between multiple pixels, creating multiple counts at the incorrect energy. Double-counting or multi-counting of photons from PCDs negatively impacts noise statistics in the same way as nonuniform weighting for energy integrating detectors. This multiplicity of the events, which affects measurement statistics, is

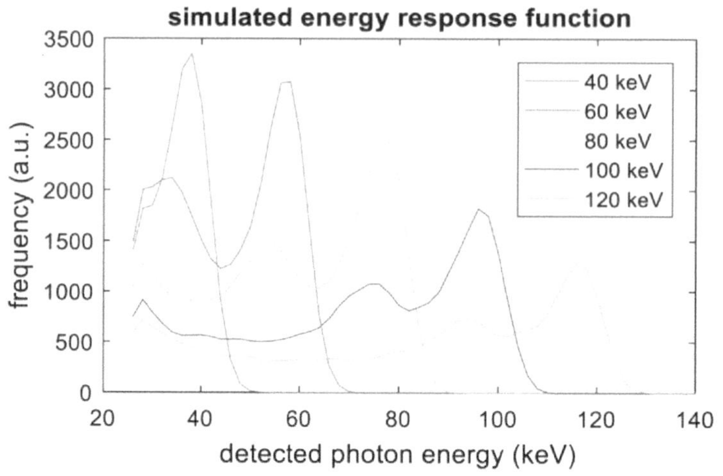

FIGURE 17.1 An example of the energy response function (ERF), showing the relationship between incident monoenergetic photons and the detected response. Five lines are plotted, corresponding to different energies of incident photons. The lines provide a histogram of the detected photon energy. An ideal ERF would be a narrow, tall peak at the correct energy. Real ERFs show degradation from k-escape and charge sharing.

not incorporated into the traditional ERF metric. Simulation studies that neglect possible multiplicity may overestimate the performance of PCD CT systems.

It is possible to extend the ERF to include the correlations and covariance between pixels (7–9). An open-source simulation package, PcTK, has been made available for this task (8). While this extended metric, incorporating correlations, is a fairly complete description of PCD performance except for pileup effects, it is more difficult to measure.

17.2.3 Spectral Separation

Spectral separation is an indicator of performance in spectral tasks. The spectral separation of two energy bins in a PCD is defined as the difference between the mean energies of the photons detected in those bins. This spectral separation must be defined relative to a given incident spectrum. Generally speaking, increasing spectral separation leads to improved imaging performance, but it is possible to construct counterexamples.

17.2.4 Counting Efficiency

To remedy the weakness of ERF at counting multiple events, Ji et al. (10) suggest using the first and second moments of counting statistics. A simplified description for this method is as follows. Given a stable x-ray source, one should measure the mean and the variance of the number of counts detected. With ideal Poisson statistics, the variance should be equal to the mean. If all photons were double-counted, the variance should be twice the mean. In general, the ratio between the variance and the mean of the detected counts gives an indication of the *multiplicity* of the detected events. As with energy-integrating detectors (1), random, unequal weighting of detected photons leads to an effective increase in noise.

The first and second moments can be related to the detective quantum efficiency at zero frequency, DQE(0), if we also have knowledge of the fraction of photons that are not detected. The counting efficiency measure is appropriate for use in *non-spectral tasks* but does not easily relate to performance in *spectral tasks*. Non-spectral tasks are those that can be performed with conventional

CT. Spectral tasks are those that are only possible on spectral CT scanners and include basis material decomposition.

17.3 SYSTEMS PERFORMANCE METRICS

The fundamental task in medical imaging is the detection and classification of pathology. While some pathologies are grossly obvious on any scanner, other pathologies are difficult to detect, either because they are faint (low contrast) or small (high resolution). For these reasons, low-contrast detectability (LCD) has emerged as perhaps the most important performance metric of a CT system. For spectral systems such as PCD-equipped CT scanners, LCD can be understood to be conventional, non-spectral LCD, or an LCD of spectral tasks such as material decomposition or identification of contrast. Besides LCD, system spatial resolution is the second important characteristic.

Another metric of great concern to patients is radiation dose efficiency. In general, radiation dose can always be decreased, but the image quality will suffer. For these reasons, when assessing LCD, it is generally assumed that the radiation dose is fixed. Resolution is typically assessed for high-contrast tasks. The detection efficiency for high-resolution, moderate-contrast tasks is not typically quantified, but PCDs are expected to perform well in this category (11). Clinical examples of small, moderate-contrast imaging targets include urolithiasis (12).

17.3.1 Contrast-to-Noise Ratio (CNR)

The contrast-to-noise ratio (CNR) is a very common measure of detection performance and can be viewed as a surrogate for LCD. Given a target region A containing contrast and a background region B, we define the CNR as:

$$CNR = \frac{|\mu(A) - \mu(B)|}{\sigma(B)}$$

where $\mu(x)$ and $\sigma(x)$ denote the mean and standard deviation of the attenuation of the voxels within the region x, typically measured in Hounsfield Units. The CNR is simple but sometimes misleading. Improvements in spatial resolution will lead to a decrease in CNR even if the visibility of the object remains the same or improves. Smoothing the image with stronger apodization will increase the CNR for larger features. For these reasons, CNR is a potentially misleading metric, when comparing mismatched systems. CNR will also be affected by the use of statistical iterative reconstruction.

17.3.2 Low-Contrast Detectability (LCD): Conventional and Spectral

CNR can be viewed as a simple measure of LCD, but one that is confounded by mismatched resolution or statistical reconstruction. Several improved measures exist (13). The DQE quantifies detectability as a function of frequency, but is derived from linear systems principles and may not apply directly to nonlinear reconstruction, including statistical iterative reconstruction (14). For the detection of a specific task, the DQE can be reduced to a single scalar metric called the detectability index (15). Human observers remain the gold standard, but model observers provide an adequate surrogate in many contexts (16, 17).

While LCD could be measured in either the spectral or conventional (non-spectral or "grayscale") domains, it must be acknowledged that performance in conventional tasks is of overriding importance. After the introduction of dual energy CT in the mid-2000s, there has been a concerted effort to identify applications that would benefit from dual energy techniques. Some of the best use cases have been for kidney stone classification (18) and for the detection of gout (19). Both of these can be considered to be relatively minor applications when viewed as a percentage of total exams. While a wide variety of clinical applications may benefit from spectral overlay (20), it should be understood that dual energy plays a clarifying or adjunct role in most of these applications and often conventional imaging alone is sufficient to make a diagnosis. For these reasons, LCD of non-spectral tasks is an extremely important performance metric.

Conceptually, LCD is easy to understand: for a collection of targets with subtle contrast and given a dose budget, what percentage could be detected by a human observer? Visual inspection of a phantom with inserts of varying contrast is therefore a direct, but very subjective, measure for LCD. Prior knowledge of the insert location will bias most readers, and for these reasons objective measures are preferred. Under linear systems theory, the modulation transfer function (MTF) and noise power spectrum (NPS) can be independently measured and used to predict LCD. Many modern statistical reconstruction algorithms are nonlinear, and measurement of LCD with these algorithms requires model observers.

While LCD of non-spectral targets is of overriding importance, LCD can be also defined for low-contrast spectral targets. The most challenging type of spectral LCD is on objects that have no contrast on grayscale imaging. Most objects that present contrast in a spectral domain will also provide contrast in the conventional or grayscale domain. Some types of reconstruction algorithms can exploit this fact to improve image quality. These forms of advanced reconstruction, such as material decomposition reconstruction, can improve the image quality of spectral images but only provide benefit if there is sufficient contrast in the conventional reconstruction domain.

17.3.3 Spatial Resolution

After LCD, spatial resolution is perhaps the second most important metric for medical imaging modalities. CT is in the curious position in that in-plane resolution has seen minimal improvement over the past three decades (21). Through-plane or z-resolution has seen continuous improvement with the advent of multi-slice CT, but in-plane resolution has remained virtually unchanged. One of the main limitations has been the need for reflective material between scintillating material in energy integrating detectors. These reflective barriers are needed to maintain resolution of conventional detector systems but they also decrease the fill factor of the detector pixel. Further improvement in resolution would lead to further reductions in fill factor and hence lead to unacceptably low-dose efficiency. A very recent system from one vendor seems to have surmounted this barrier (22) and may offer resolution competitive with PCDs with an energy-integrating design.

Virtually all PCDs that have been proposed for inclusion in diagnostic CT systems offer resolution two to four times better than conventional detectors. Conventional detectors have pixel pitch of approximately 1 mm in the detector plane, whereas PCD pixel sizes may range from 0.1 to 0.5 mm. The incremental resolution improvement between 0.5 mm pixels and 0.1 mm pixels is likely to be marginal because the resolution of the CT system will be broadly limited by the x-ray source, unless smaller focal spots are designed. High resolution is indeed an opportunity for PCD systems and may be relevant in a range of clinical tasks (23).

Although high-resolution tasks are often analyzed with very high contrast structures such as a tungsten wire, dose efficiency and detectability at high resolution are also relevant for the classification of the margin of tumors or the detection of small kidney stones (12). Higher detector resolution (11) and higher dose efficiency from improved counting statistics could synergize here to present a significant benefit for these tasks.

17.3.4 Artifacts

Although not the focus of this discussion, another important metric is the level of artifact present in the images. A wide range of imaging artifacts exists in CT (24, 25). It is not possible to create one metric that suitably quantifies all artifacts because each artifact manifests in a different manner. PCDs offer the opportunity to improve beam hardening artifacts because they can perform a material decomposition of the underlying projection data. However, imperfect PCDs may introduce other artifacts like ring artifacts that stem from polarization, pileup, or unstable calibration. The suppression of imaging artifacts is an important real-world consideration that must be solved before PCDs can enter clinical practice.

17.3.5 Electronic Noise

When applied to conventional, non photon-counting CT systems, electronic noise refers to the noise penalty that is imparted in each readout of an energy-integrating detector's noise. Electronic noise is related to the dark current and is sometimes modeled as a Gaussian random variable, although more complex models can be used which are more descriptive (26). A Poisson variable that describes the detected photon flux would possess a variance of N for an expected mean of N, and hence, the signal-to-noise ratio would scale as the square root of N. When the tube current is decreased or the object is very thick, however, the variance of N could be overtaken by the electronic noise floor. The noise floor threshold varies with the design of the readout electronics but is typically in the range of several photons-equivalent. From a systems perspective, electronic noise compounds the noise in the already noisiest measurements and amplifies noise streaks in the reconstructed images.

A large advantage of PCD systems is their rejection of electronic noise. If, however, the lowest level discriminator threshold is set too low and spurious counts appear in a dark scan calibration, this advantage would be lost.

17.3.6 Converting from Detector Metrics to Systems Metrics

Designers of photon-counting systems may be interested in understanding how to relate the figures of merit on the detector system (Table 17.1) with the figures of merit in the final CT scanner. This section provides a brief tutorial of the main steps to assist PCD designers by providing a recipe for the simulation of the entire system.

First, an assumption must be made about the data set and the acquisition protocol. One useful form of data is raw count data from a clinical scanner. Work is presently underway to create an open-source repository for CT raw data (27). A second-best option is to simulate raw count/attenuation data from reconstructed images of a CT scan using forward projection. In either case, the elements in the raw data sinogram can be interpreted to be equivalent absorption lengths of the two basis materials. When k-edge materials are present, such as gadolinium or gold nanoparticles, a three-material decomposition can also be performed. In most cases, the k-edge of iodine is too low to be easily measured. In some cases, assumptions could be used to enrich the basis material decomposition. For example, iodine or bone could be distinguished in the CT scan based on their location, their densities, and thresholding techniques.

At this point, an x-ray tube spectrum can be modeled using publicly available tools (28) and attenuated by the sinogram as well as the material of the bowtie filter (24). The spectrum can then be scaled by the mA of the beam, which may itself vary due to tube current modulation (29). Collectively, this will produce an expected incident count rate and spectrum on the detector for each measurement of the sinogram. Simulations which incorporate charge sharing, pileup, and other non-idealities of interest can now be used. These simulations could include Monte Carlo transport of x-ray photons (30), transport of the electrical charge (31), masking of the pixel by the anti-scatter grid, or a variety of other effects. Depending on the needs of the project, information can be produced using only a simple ERF (32) or by incorporating spatial correlations on top of the ERF (8). The proper choice will depend on the needs of the simulation. As previously mentioned, the PcTK tool has been made publicly available to academic research institutions (8).

The simulated raw data from the PCD must now be translated into basis materials and a reconstruction. Conversion to basis materials is an estimation process with performance bounded by the Cramér-Rao Lower Bound (CRLB). The CRLB could be calculated, or a particular estimator could be used. The difference between the estimated basis materials and the ground truth input is the calculated error. Propagation into the image domain can now be performed using filtered backprojection. This will create an image of a stochastic realization of the noise. Alternatively, unfiltered backprojection of the variance can be used to create a noise map of the variance in the image (33). Assuming deterministic effects can be corrected, it should be appreciated that the main impact of limited count rate, poor ERF, etc. is an increase in the variance in the reconstructed image.

These types of simulations can reveal the protocol-dependent nature of PCD design. For example, count rate is an important criterion for any PCD, and the count rate within CT can reach 1000 Mcps/mm^2. However, 20 cm of tissue will reduce this value to 20 Mcps/mm^2. Although greater flux will be present at the periphery of the object, the bowtie filter will reduce flux in these regions. Furthermore, although the noise performance of the PCD relative to the ideal detector is reduced at high flux, its noise performance may still be increased relative to the ideal detector at low flux. Hence, it may be possible that the maximum noise in the reconstruction remains at the region of highest attenuation and not at the periphery of the patient. The net result is that, unless very high flux is expected in a pediatric population, the count-rate requirements for a PCD could be more modest than one would otherwise expect. The flux requirements depend both on the clinical task and on the acceptable gantry rotation time. Broadly speaking, low contrast targets of interest such as subtle tumors are often found either in the brain (where long rotation times are acceptable) or in the abdomen. At maximum power, modern x-ray sources may reach over 1000 Mcps/mm^2 and may be attenuated to 20 Mcps/mm^2 at the center of a 20 cm patient, as previously described. Assuming that the count-rate capability of the PCD is 100 Mcps/mm^2 and assuming an ideal nonparalyzable detector, an incident flux rate of 20 Mcps/mm^2 implies that 20% of the photons will not be counted.

17.3.7 Photon Counting versus Energy Integrating

A natural question that should be raised at this point is: for the system metrics we have described, how do PCDs compare to conventional, energy-integrating detectors?

Figure 17.2 provides a conceptual illustration comparing these detectors. At low flux, the PCD performs much better due to the elimination of electronic noise. The characteristic flux

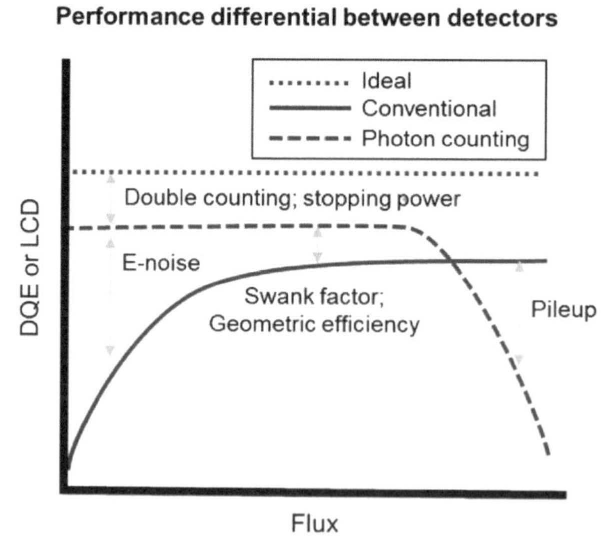

FIGURE 17.2 Performance of PCDs compared to conventional, energy-integrating detectors and the ideal detector for a non-spectral task. This figure assumes fixed dose, so that imaging time is inversely proportional to flux. The ideal detector shows constant DQE or LCD because the total number of photons remains constant.

level at which PCDs become much better than conventional detectors is at the electronic noise floor, which is typically several x-ray photons. On the other hand, at very high flux, pileup effects dominate and PCDs can perform substantially worse. One simple model of image quality requirements is that a radiologist looks for a low contrast lesion (such as a lesion from metastatic cancer) that may appear anywhere in the volume. The dose of the scan will then be increased until the maximum noise level is below an acceptable threshold, so that the radiologist may confidently say that the lesion does not exist anywhere in the scan. Under this model, the relevant metric is the peak or maximum noise, not the average noise. In this case, because PCDs may reduce noise in the center of the image where attenuation and noise are greatest, they increase dose efficiency in most scans.

At moderate flux, the performance of the PCD is less than that of the ideal detector due to multiple counting. As previously described, multiplicity increases noise in reconstructed images (10). Rather than variance being equal to mean counts as one would expect from Poisson statistics, multiple counting causes variance to exceed mean counts. On the other hand, conventional detectors have their own sources of inefficiency. Much of the area of a conventional detector is inactive, because the scintillating layer includes reflectors that reduce the fill factor of the detector. The conventional detector weights photons in proportion to their energy, which is not optimal for the noise statistics of most tasks. In addition, an x-ray photon of a fixed energy can contribute different amounts of electrical signal depending on the location of interaction. These last two effects are sometimes called the Swank factor and add noise to the measurement (1). Energy weighting is especially damaging for iodine contrast imaging at high kVp, where PCDs may see substantial improvements over conventional detectors. Also, PCDs can provide better resolution due to the small pixel size. Experimental measurements on a PCD-equipped system have confirmed these expectations: improved resolution, improved contrast of iodine, and comparable or better noise at matched resolution (34). For the system evaluated, the gap between PCD and conventional at moderate flux was not significant, but the gap could widen in the future. Other systems may show larger gaps between PCD and conventional dual energy (35, 36).

For a material decomposition task, the picture is more complex. A wide range of dual energy implementations are present today, including dual source systems, fast kVp switching, and dual layer detectors, each of which has advantages or disadvantages with regards to spectral separation, temporal separation, and system cost. While an ideal PCD is likely to be better than any of these technologies, real PCDs could perform better than some implementations and worse than other implementations.

17.4 OPTIMIZATION AND TRADE-OFFS

Before describing new technologies that could enable PCDs to achieve superior performance, we will first discuss trade-offs that can be achieved by tuning various design parameters of the PCD. By sacrificing one type of detector-level performance metrics, it may be possible to improve another one and hence achieve a superior design for specific clinical applications.

One of the central challenges for PCD design is charge sharing. Compared to the ideal detector, charge sharing decreases the non-spectral LCD by virtue of double counting. A double-counted photon is weighted twice, whereas other photons are only weighted once. From a statistical perspective, this nonuniform weighting decreases the signal-to-noise ratio. The spectral LCD is degraded even more because high energy photons may be misinterpreted as low energy photons. Because the contrast in a spectral task is determined by the difference between high- and low-energy photons, switching of these signals decreases spectral contrast and hence decreases LCD. A simple explanation is as follows: iodine signal is detected as an increase in low-energy photon attenuation relative to high-energy photon attenuation. However, because high-energy photons are sometimes detected as multiple low-energy events, the difference in low-energy bin and high-energy bin attenuation is reduced, making the detection task more

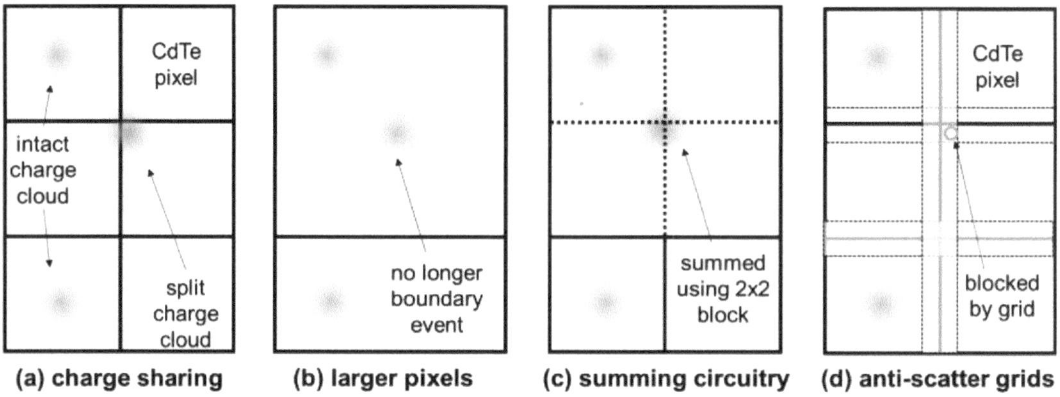

FIGURE 17.3 A comparison of multiple strategies to reduce charge sharing. Detector pixels are shown in black squares. Interaction of photons with the cadmium telluride (CdTe) substrate, producing charge clouds, are shown as spheres. These are drawn as if they are circularly symmetric, but characteristic emission may lead to two effective charge clouds from one photon, spaced tens to hundreds of microns apart. (a) A basic detector without corrections. The orange sphere depicts a charge cloud that is split between multiple pixels. As a result, it is detected multiple times at a reduced energy. (b) Using pixels that are twice the size, fewer boundary events are shown. (c) Charge summing circuitry can add up the energy dynamically found in a 2×2 block. (d) Anti-scatter grids can block photons that would contribute to charge sharing events. However, the geometric efficiency of the detector is reduced.

challenging. Figure 17.3 details a variety of strategies that may be used to reduce or eliminate charge sharing, which will be examined in turn in the following sections.

17.4.1 Pixel Size

Pixel size is perhaps the most important design parameter, and its importance to several system metrics can be seen in Table 17.1. Increasing pixel size decreases charge sharing and improves the ERF, leading to better spectral performance at low flux. However, count-rate capability is inversely proportional to pixel size because, for a fixed level of flux, a smaller pixel receives less flux per pixel. Pixel size therefore controls the balance between count rate and charge sharing. Figure 17.3 shows an example of large pixel size decreasing charge sharing.

Pileup causes rapid and significant deterioration in detector performance. If the incident flux is more than 20% of the characteristic count rate, even the ideal PCD will be outperformed by other approaches (37). On the other hand, current PCDs perform much worse than the ideal PCD regardless. Also, the presence of pileup and increased noise only at the periphery of the scan may be acceptable.

Figure 17.4 shows an example of possible trade-offs that can be achieved by varying the pixel size. The assumed count rate was 15 Mcps per pixel for a 2-mm-thick CdTe pixel and the assumed tube parameters were 140 kVp and 500 mA, and the pulse shape was bipolar. When imaging thick objects, the larger pixel sizes reduce charge sharing effects and provide a modest improvement to variance in the material decomposition. When imaging thin objects at high mA, pileup effects dominate and the smaller pixels perform best. Other assumptions from these simulations and more details are found in Ref. (38). While the tipping point between smaller and larger pixels will vary according to the clinical application and specific scan, there will generally be a competition between pileup and charge sharing that can be adjusted by appropriate choice of pixel size. The choice of the optimal pixel size depends on several factors, including the imaging protocol, the patient size, and the characteristic count rate of the detector.

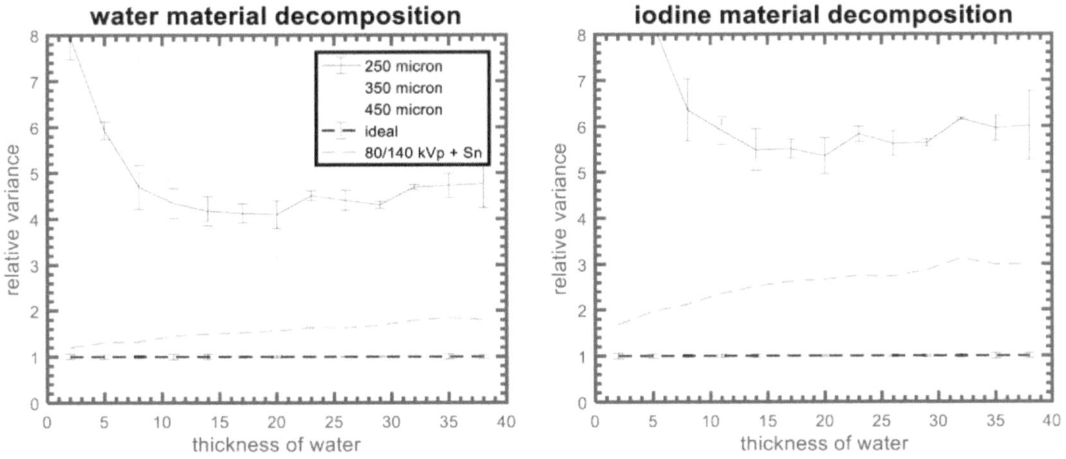

FIGURE 17.4 Relative performance of different pixel sizes for material decomposition tasks. Plots are normalized to the performance of an ideal PCD, so that a relative variance of 1 is ideal performance. These simulated results are sensitive to the incident flux and the assumed characteristic count rate. The characteristic count rate is 15 Mcps per pixel. The flux incident on the detector at 10 and 20 cm of water is about 45 and 7.5 Mcps/mm^2, respectively.

Figure 17.4 also compares the noise in material decomposition of PCDs with an ideal, conventional dual energy implementation (dual kVp with tin filtration). All results have been normalized to an ideal PCD. The ideal PCD outperforms conventional dual energy by a factor of 2, but conventional dual energy outperforms these simulated PCDs by another factor of 2. For PCDs to provide better detectability of spectral objects than conventional dual energy methods, it will be necessary to improve the charge sharing characteristics using technologies such as charge summing.

17.4.2 Electronic Noise

As previously discussed, "electronic noise" in CT commonly refers to the noise penalty that is imparted by the readout electronics of the detector, which amplifies noise streaks in the reconstructed images due to measurements with few photons. Electronic noise can be caused by variance of the dark current.

In this context, PCDs are sometimes described as being free of electronic noise. Given an appropriate choice of threshold for the lowest energy level, their corresponding dark current is zero. But of course, all electronics have noise. The amount of charge that is recorded from a photon is a stochastic process and depends on recombination, depth of interaction, and other factors. PCDs also include dark current that corrupts the energy recorded for any photon. This electronic noise can cause photons near the threshold of an energy bin to be recorded as belonging to the wrong bin.

The strongest effect of electronic noise is in the placement of the lowest level discriminator, or the minimum energy photon that can be reliably distinguished from zero signal. In diagnostic CT, photons that penetrate the human body will generally be above 30 keV. Photons at or below 30 keV that pass through 15 cm of tissue will be attenuated by a factor of approximately 300. Meeting this constraint may require the standard deviation to be less than 7.5 keV (four standard deviations).

Given that this constraint is met, the level of electronic noise appears to have modest impact on spectral performance. Wang et al. contrasted the impact of three different PCD non-idealities: electronic noise, pileup, and spectral accuracy, and found that the least important factor was electronic noise (39). This plot is reproduced in Figure 17.5, and contrast the relative importance of these three

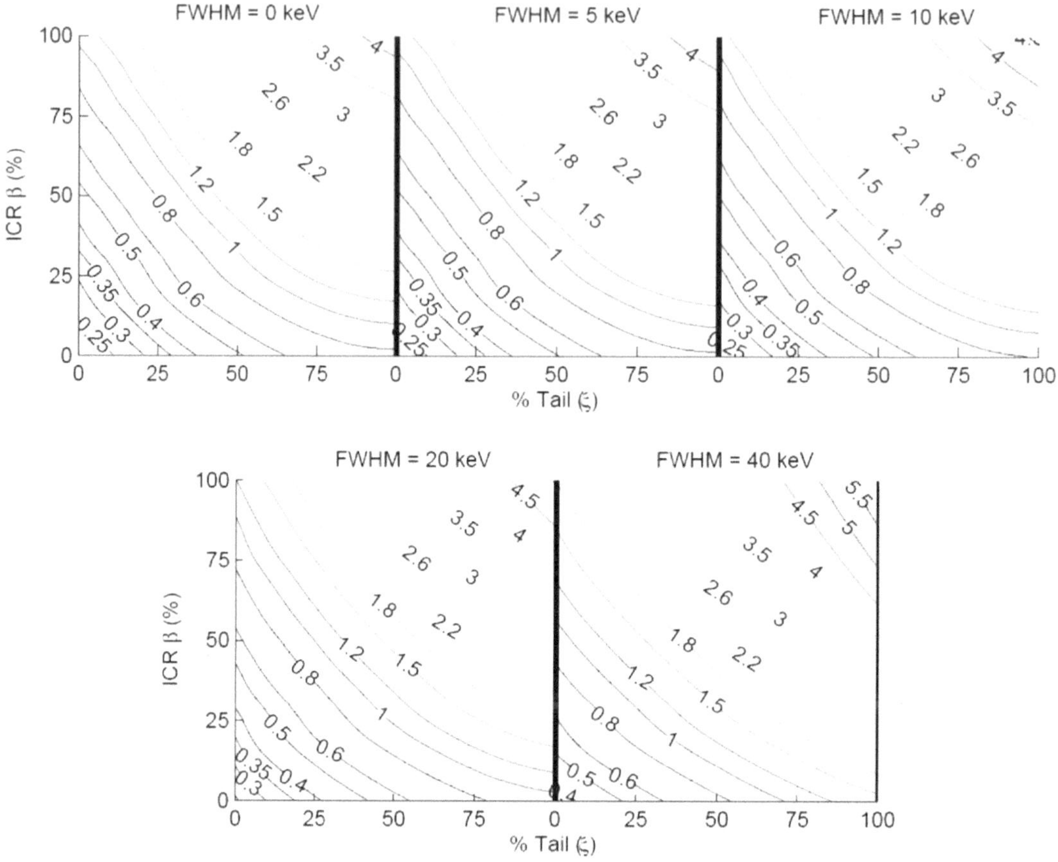

FIGURE 17.5 Effects of three non-idealities on the material decomposition performance of a PCD. Numbers in the plot correspond to an average of the variance of water and iodine materials. The x-axis, ξ, denotes the level of spectral tailing, which is a parameterization of imperfection in the ERF. The y-axis, β, denotes the incident count rate (ICR) as a fraction of the characteristic count rate. Different plots show different levels of electronic noise, as parameterized by full-width half-max (FWHM). The detector uses ten energy bins. Reprinted with permission from "A comparison of dual kV energy integrating and energy discriminating PCDs for dual energy x-ray imaging" by Adam Wang and Norbert Pelc, *SPIE Medical Imaging 2012*, Volume 8313 (39).

factors in material decomposition performance. With some assumptions on the count rate and ERF of the detector, electronic noise of 20 keV FWHM (standard deviation of 8.7 keV for a Gaussian distribution) decreases spectral performance of material decomposition tasks by about 20%.

17.4.3 Pulse-Shaping Time

After pixel size, pulse-shaping time is the next most important parameter at determining count rate and pileup effects. To some extent, pulse shaping can be improved by faster signal processing electronics, and as a general rule faster electronics can lead to increased electronic noise. However, device physics also plays a role. Incident photons frequently interact with the CdTe substrate through the photoelectric effect and produce a K-fluorescence photon that may travel several hundred microns, possibly in the depth direction. The pulse-shaping time should be chosen to group the charges from these events into a single count.

Pulse shaping can also affect the fate of a charge cloud produced near the boundary of a pixel. The induction of signal from these regions may be slower, and a fast pulse-shaping time may fail to integrate the entirety of this charge.

17.4.4 Pixel Thickness

The thickness of the substrate material will directly affect the stopping power of the PCD. For example, a thickness of 1.5 mm CdTe will stop 77% of incident 100 keV photons. On the other hand, 3 mm CdTe will stop 95% of these photons. A thicker substrate is clearly desirable from the perspective of increasing the dose efficiency of the system.

On the other hand, a thicker substrate provides more time for the charge cloud to undergo Coulomb repulsion, diffusion, and trapping. These effects may promote charge sharing, causing one incident photon to be perceived as two detected counts. From the perspective of signal-to-noise ratio, double counting a photon is nearly as harmful as missing the photon entirely. In the context of Figure 17.3, decreasing the pixel thickness would effectively decrease the radii of each charge cloud.

17.4.5 Anti-Scatter Grids

Anti-scatter grids are common in diagnostic CT scanners and consist of attenuating plates (lamellae) placed directly in front of the detector, oriented parallel to the incident radiation. These grids may be centimeters long and spaced 1 mm apart, with characteristic width of 0.1 mm (40). With conventional detectors, these grids can be placed on top of reflector area, so that their penalty to fill factor is neutralized. With PCDs, however, these anti-scatter grids would directly reduce dose efficiency.

The proper utilization of anti-scatter grids with PCDs is not yet established. Reducing the number of lamellae would improve the efficiency of an ideal detector, but for a non-ideal detector that suffers from charge sharing, the inclusion of these grids at the boundaries between pixels could improve performance.

Anti-scatter grids are likely to be included in any diagnostic scanner with an x-ray cone-beam "width" of 4 cm or greater at isocenter. Figure 17.3 shows an example of an anti-scatter grid stopping a photon whose charge would be shared between multiple pixels. For small pixels, including lamellae between every pixel may reduce dose efficiency unless miniaturized lamellae can be manufactured.

17.5 TECHNOLOGIES TO IMPROVE PCD PERFORMANCE

Besides proper selection of detector parameters, a variety of technological advances have been proposed to improve PCD-equipped CT systems. These technologies range from being simple to complex, and may have significant trade-offs that offset their adoption.

17.5.1 Charge Summing

Charge sharing causes large degradations in the ERF. A very powerful method for recovering lost performance is the integration of charge across multiple pixels (41, 42). Charge summing could provide drastic improvements in image quality, but is also complex to implement. In addition, charge summing effectively locks multiple pixels when a photon arrives, so that coincident events that arrive in adjacent pixels may be inappropriately summed. For this reason, the dead time will increase by a factor of 4 or 9 and the pixel size may need to be reduced.

Charge summing is technically complex and many PCDs lack this feature, although some newer designs have included some type of charge summing (10, 43). A variation is anti-coincidence logic,

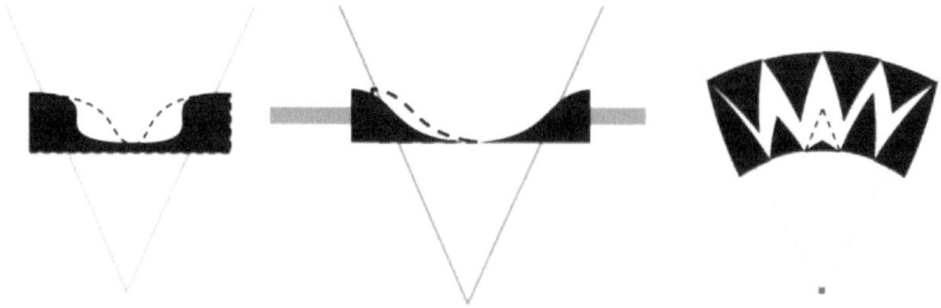

FIGURE 17.6 Three examples of dynamic bowtie filters. The fan beam of the x-ray is shown as a gray triangle, with x-ray source being at the vertex of the triangle. Attenuating material is shown in black, with an alternate dynamic configuration provided in dotted line. (Left) A translating attenuator. When the attenuator translates into or out of the page, the detector changes shape. (Middle) A two-wedge attenuator. The wedges can individually move to accommodate smaller or larger patients. (Right) A piecewise-linear attenuator. Each wedge can individually translate, and the sum of the wedges is a customizable piecewise-linear function with as many control points as there are wedges.

where coincident events are detected after digitization. This can incorporate spectral bin information and hence serve as a digital form of charge sharing correction (44, 45).

17.5.2 Dynamic Bowtie Filters

The "bowtie" filter is a pre-patient attenuating filter that shapes the flux distribution of the beam. The bowtie filter is so named because of its shape, which is thin for rays directed at isocenter but thick for rays directed at the periphery. Conventional bowtie filters are fixed, but dynamic filters could adjust their shape to reduce flux before significant pileup appears on the detector.

Several bowtie filters have been described in the literature (46–50). Figure 17.6 provides three examples. One class of dynamic bowties consists of multiple elements which move to adjust the incident flux on a region-by-region basis. Simpler designs have also been described in the patent literature (51, 52) but may lack the flexibility to deal with pileup because they only present one or two degrees of freedom. A multiple-aperture-device has also been proposed for its rapid switching capabilities but also presents a limited number of degrees of freedom unless more than two devices are used (53). The inclusion of dynamic bowties together with PCDs is expected to decrease peak flux and improve image quality (48, 54).

17.5.3 Pulse Detection Logic

Most PCDs use a bank of comparators to digitize and categorize the incident signal as belonging to predefined energy windows. Once the energy level rises above a threshold voltage, the comparator switches and a counter is incremented. A bank of comparators is simple to implement but may be inefficient at extracting information at high flux. Alternative schemes for detecting pulses may be more efficient at moderate pileup (55). PCDs that perform single-threshold counting alongside charge integration have also been investigated, and this combination of counting-integrating design may be more resistant to pileup because the integrating component is designed to be pileup-immune (56).

17.5.4 Nonlinear Reconstruction Techniques

Statistical iterative reconstruction has become commonplace in diagnostic CT and has the potential to improve detectability, resolution, and dose efficiency. These types of algorithms can be adapted to spectral imaging and may make particular use of the reduced noise in the grayscale imaging

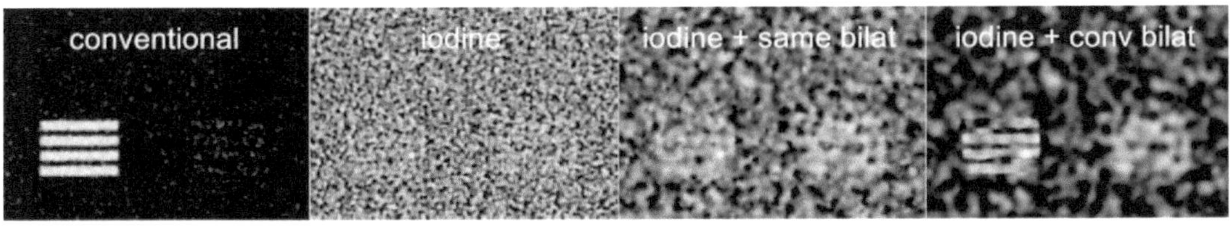

FIGURE 17.7 A simple example of nonlinear reconstruction to improve the performance of spectral images. The object being simulated is two line pair sets with equal iodine but varying water content. A water/iodine decomposition is used. (Far left) Only the left line pairs are easily seen on conventional imaging, because the right line pairs have decreased water content to compensate for increased iodine content. (Center left) In iodine material decomposition, the objects are difficult to see. Note that material decomposition amplifies noise. In a noiseless image, both objects would be visible and equally bright. (Center right) A bilateral filter of the iodine image restores a small amount of image quality. (Far right) A bilateral filter of the iodine image, but guided with the conventional image, restores the left line pair because of contrast in the conventional domain. Its effect on the line pair that is not visible in the conventional domain is greatly reduced.

domain (57). The physical insight underlying these algorithms is that a lesion may be below the limit of detection in a material decomposition reconstruction, but may be visible in a conventional grayscale reconstruction. Hence, apodization or blurring that is guided by the conventional grayscale reconstruction can improve the image quality of material decomposition. Problems may occur if the lesion is not visible with conventional grayscale contrast but presents only spectral contrast. For example, if a calcified plaque has the same CT number as adjacent iodinated blood, the contrast between the two is only spectral. A nonlinear reconstruction that uses the conventional grayscale reconstruction to guide spectral reconstruction would not provide any benefit. However, many real spectral applications, such as the classification of kidney stones or gout, are classification tasks in readily visible and isolated pathology. Nonlinear reconstruction would appear to be perfectly appropriate for these use cases.

Figure 17.7 shows a simple example. The bilateral filter, a simple edge-preserving smoothing technique, is used as a form of nonlinear reconstruction (58). The bilateral filter is a variation of traditional Gaussian smoothing which adapts its smoothing kernel based on both spatial proximity and intensity proximity. Traditional Gaussian smoothing uses only spatial proximity, but by including intensity proximity (similarity of the CT numbers of the two pixels), the bilateral filter avoids smoothing together hard edges. Other, more sophisticated iterative reconstruction packages use optimization of a cost function, which is computationally intensive. While it is impossible to speak broadly of all iterative reconstruction packages, Figure 17.7 illustrates that nonlinear reconstruction methods should be tested carefully. For non-spectral iterative reconstruction, a wide range of tools, including model observers (13) and clinical studies (59), have replaced Fourier metrics such as NPS and MTF. Similar care may be needed to fully characterize spectral nonlinear reconstruction methods.

17.5.5 K-Edge Filters

The x-ray spectrum plays an important role in spectral performance, and in most cases, higher kVp implies a more disparate collection of low- and high-energy photons that can achieve higher spectral separation. K-edge filters can further increase performance by eliminating photons of intermediate energies. In fact, it has been shown that theoretically, dose in intermediate-energy photons is not simply inefficient but actively detrimental to spectral tasks, and that performance would be improved if these photons could be somehow removed on a post-patient basis (60). This is a surprising finding. One approximate explanation is that in spectral imaging, the absorption of low-energy photons suggests photoelectric effect and the absorption of high-energy photons suggests Compton

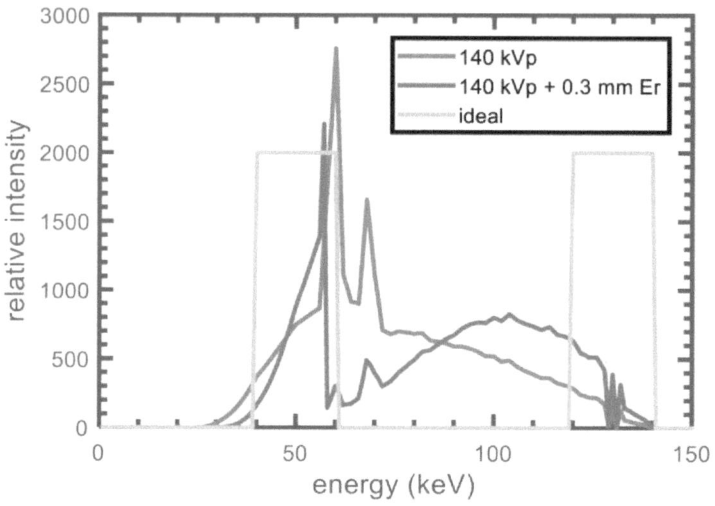

FIGURE 17.8 A 140 kVp spectrum filtered by 20 cm of water, with and without a k-edge filter. The mA for the k-edge filter has been increased by a factor of 4. For a two-bin detector, the ideal spectrum, were it possible, would be two distinct peaks at optimized energies (represented here with finite width of 20 keV), separated by a gap. The gap allows greater spectral separation. The erbium filter brings the spectrum closer to the ideal spectrum.

scattering. Mathematical continuity implies that there must be an intermediate-energy photon whose absorption suggests neither form of contrast. These intermediate-energy photons do not contribute to spectral contrast and their detection in an energy bin harms statistics in the same way that x-ray scatter does. With scatter, even if the average number of scattered photons can be deterministically known and corrected, the noise in Poisson statistics would be amplified. Intermediate-energy photons, which present no spectral information but do contribute statistical noise, appear to function in the same way. In practice, elimination of intermediate-energy photons requires a new energy bin, and dose savings are more readily achieved using a pre-patient K-edge filter (61). K-edge filters can be used with conventional dual energy systems (62), although they are not necessary for dual-source systems because a different filter can be used in each spectrum.

A conceptual illustration of the effect of the k-edge filter on the spectrum is shown in Figure 17.8. A limitation of the k-edge filter is the need for increased tube power.

17.6 DISCUSSION

PCD technology has the potential to improve the image quality and reduce the dose of diagnostic CT systems. In this chapter, we have related the performance metrics of the detector with the performance metrics of the system as a whole. The most important metrics for the end patient are LCD (non-spectral or spectral) and spatial resolution. PCDs have the potential to improve both of these metrics, but this requires appropriate tuning of parameters such as the detector pixel size or pulse-shaping time, and may further benefit from the adoption of new technologies such as charge summing or dynamic bowtie filters.

Currently, the overriding challenge of PCDs for CT applications is the high flux. Systems have recently appeared that have demonstrated capable performance at high flux (34–36, 63). As discussed throughout this chapter, optimizing PCDs for high flux applications is possible if the pixel size is decreased, the pulse-shaping time is decreased, and the thickness of the detector substrate is decreased. Side effects of this optimization may be reduced performance in spectral LCD, increased double-counting of photons, and reduced stopping power. This reduces the performance of the PCD compared to the ideal detector. However, the more practical comparison is to existing, energy-integrating detectors.

Existing PCD designs, optimized for high count rate, may provide comparable or superior non-spectral LCD when compared to conventional detectors (34–36, 63). While their spectral LCD may not be superior to optimized dual energy designs, they can retain their spectral capability without need for activating a specialized protocol. For example, iodine exams of smaller patients, typically performed at lower kVp to maximize contrast-to-noise ratio, may not be suitable for a dual energy protocol that splits dose between 80 kVp and 140 kVp. On the other hand, a PCD-equipped CT system will be able to use the low kVp protocol to maximum benefit and will additionally acquire spectral information that can be used for incidental findings or other post-processing. Finally, PCDs could allow improved resolution in every scan mode.

Further improvements in performance may be possible with charge summing, dynamic bowtie filters, or other technologies discussed in this chapter. Current PCDs may lose photons due to lack of stopping power or double-count photons due to charge sharing. Future PCDs could accurately identify these as single photons, thereby improving non-spectral LCD. Charge summing may enable a dramatic improvement in spectral LCD. While further improvements to the PCD resolution are certainly achievable, the system resolution will be limited by x-ray focal spot characteristics for the foreseeable future.

Attaining maximum performance from PCDs requires efficient estimation of basis material thicknesses from PCD measurements. An efficient estimator for multi-bin detectors is a subject of ongoing research (64, 65), especially in the context of pileup and other non-idealities. Separate, important engineering challenges are present in producing reliable and robust detectors that operate without bias. These and other challenges are addressed elsewhere in this book.

In this chapter, we have focused our attention on CdTe PCDs, but PCDs based on silicon (Si) are also under development (66). Because of the low stopping power of silicon, Si PCDs require larger thicknesses of Si. Photons that interact with Si are much more likely to undergo Compton scattering, leaving behind only a small amount of energy before departing, which in turn, degrades the spectral sensitivity/resolution of PCDs. Very high count rates can easily be achieved with Si because multiple detector layers can be placed in series, with the counting burden distributed between the different layers. The optimization considerations and technologies of Si are substantially different than those of CdTe.

ACKNOWLEDGMENT

The author would like to acknowledge Adam S. Wang, Ph.D. for his input and for valuable discussions.

REFERENCES

1. Swank RK. Absorption and noise in x-ray phosphors. *J Appl Phys.* 1973; 44(9): 4199–4203.
2. Schmidt TG. Optimal "image-based" weighting for energy-resolved CT. *Med Phys.* 2009; 36(7): 3018–3027.
3. Taguchi K, Srivastava S, Kudo H, Barber WC. In: Enabling photon counting clinical x-ray CT. Nuclear Science Symposium Conference Record (NSS/MIC), IEEE; 2009. p. 3581–3585.
4. Punnoose J, Xu J, Sisniega A, Zbijewski W, Siewerdsen J. Technical note: Spektr 3.0 – A computational tool for x-ray spectrum modeling and analysis. *Med Phys.* 2016; 43(8): 4711–4717.
5. Knoll GF. *Radiation Detection and Measurement.* Wiley; 2010.
6. Schlomka J, Roessl E, Dorscheid R, Dill S, Martens G, Istel T, Bäumer C, Herrmann C, Steadman R, Zeitler G. Experimental feasibility of multi-energy photon-counting K-edge imaging in pre-clinical computed tomography. *Phys Med Biol.* 2008; 53(15): 4031.
7. Rajbhandary PL, Hsieh SS, Pelc NJ. In: Effect of spatio-energy correlation in PCD due to charge sharing, scatter and secondary photons. SPIE medical imaging; International Society for Optics and Photonics; 2017.

8. Taguchi K, Stierstorfer K, Polster C, Lee O, Kappler S. Spatio-energetic cross-talk in photon counting detectors: Numerical detector model (pc TK) and workflow for CT image quality assessment. *Med Phys.* 2018; 45(5): 1985–1998.
9. Taguchi K, Polster C, Lee O, Stierstorfer K, Kappler S. Spatio-energetic cross talk in photon counting detectors: Detector model and correlated Poisson data generator. *Med Phys.* 2016; 43(12): 6386–6404.
10. Ji X, Zhang R, Chen G, Li K. Impact of anti-charge sharing on the zero-frequency detective quantum efficiency of CdTe-based photon counting detector system: Cascaded systems analysis and experimental validation. *Phy Med Biol.* 2018; 63(9): 095003.
11. Baek J, Pineda AR, Pelc NJ. To bin or not to bin? The effect of CT system limiting resolution on noise and detectability. *Phys Med Biol.* 2013; 58(5): 1433.
12. Pooler BD, Lubner MG, Kim DH, Ryckman EM, Sivalingam S, Tang J, Nakada SY, Chen GH, Pickhardt PJ. Prospective trial of the detection of urolithiasis on ultralow dose (sub mSv) noncontrast computerized tomography: Direct comparison against routine low dose reference standard. *J Urol.* 2014 Nov; 192(5): 1433–1439. PMCID: PMC4570499.
13. Vaishnav J, Jung W, Popescu L, Zeng R, Myers K. Objective assessment of image quality and dose reduction in CT iterative reconstruction. *Med Phys.* 2014; 41(7): 071904.
14. Richard S, Husarik DB, Yadava G, Murphy SN, Samei E. Towards task-based assessment of CT performance: System and object MTF across different reconstruction algorithms. *Med Phys.* 2012; 39(7Part1): 4115–4122.
15. Gang GJ, Lee J, Stayman JW, Tward DJ, Zbijewski W, Prince JL, Siewerdsen JH. Analysis of Fourier-domain task-based detectability index in tomosynthesis and cone-beam CT in relation to human observer performance. *Med Phys.* 2011; 38(4): 1754–1768.
16. Leng S, Yu L, Zhang Y, Carter R, Toledano AY, McCollough CH. Correlation between model observer and human observer performance in CT imaging when lesion location is uncertain. *Med Phys.* 2013; 40(8).
17. Chen B, Yu L, Leng S, Kofler J, Favazza C, Vrieze T, McCollough C. In: Predicting detection performance with model observers: Fourier domain or spatial domain? SPIE medical imaging; International Society for Optics and Photonics; 2016. p. 978326–978326-8.
18. Primak AN, Fletcher JG, Vrtiska TJ, Dzyubak OP, Lieske JC, Jackson ME, Williams JC, McCollough CH. Noninvasive differentiation of uric acid versus non–uric acid kidney stones using dual-energy CT. *Acad Radiol.* 2007; 14(12): 1441–1447.
19. Choi HK, Al-Arfaj AM, Eftekhari A, Munk PL, Shojania K, Reid G, Nicolaou S. Dual energy computed tomography in tophaceous gout. *Ann Rheum Dis.* 2009 Oct; 68(10): 1609–1612.
20. Johnson T, Fink C, Schönberg SO, Reiser MF. *Dual Energy CT in Clinical Practice.* Springer Science & Business Media; 2011.
21. Kalender WA. X-ray computed tomography. *Phys Med Biol.* 2006; 51(13): R29.
22. Hata A, Yanagawa M, Honda O, Kikuchi N, Miyata T, Tsukagoshi S, Uranishi A, Tomiyama N. Effect of matrix size on the image quality of ultra-high-resolution CT of the lung: Comparison of 512 × 512, 1024× 1024, and 2048× 2048. *Acad Radiol.* 2018.
23. Leng S, Yu Z, Halaweish A, Kappler S, Hahn K, Henning A, Li Z, Lane J, Levin DL, Jorgensen S. Dose-efficient ultrahigh-resolution scan mode using a photon counting detector computed tomography system. *J Med Imaging.* 2016; 3(4): 043504–043504.
24. Hsieh J. *Computed Tomography: Principles, Design, Artifacts, and Recent Advances.* Society of Photo Optical; 2003.
25. Boas FE, Fleischmann D. CT artifacts: Causes and reduction techniques. *Imaging Med.* 2012; 4(2): 229–240.
26. Ma J, Liang Z, Fan Y, Liu Y, Huang J, Chen W, Lu H. Variance analysis of x-ray CT sinograms in the presence of electronic noise background. *Med Phys.* 2012; 39(7Part1): 4051–4065.
27. Chen B, Duan X, Yu Z, Leng S, Yu L, McCollough C. Development and validation of an open data format for CT projection data. *Med Phys.* 2015; 42(12): 6964–6972.
28. Siewerdsen J, Waese A, Moseley D, Richard S, Jaffray D. Spektr: A computational tool for x-ray spectral analysis and imaging system optimization. *Med Phys.* 2004; 31: 3057.
29. Gies M, Kalender WA, Wolf H, Suess C, Madsen MT. Dose reduction in CT by anatomically adapted tube current modulation. I. Simulation studies. *Med Phys.* 1999; 26: 2235.
30. Agostinelli S, Allison J, Amako K, Apostolakis J, Araujo H, Arce P, Asai M, Axen D, Banerjee S, Barrand G. Geant4-a simulation toolkit. *Nucl Instrum Meth A.* 2003; 506(3): 250–303.
31. Faby S, Maier J, Sawall S, Simons D, Schlemmer H, Lell M, Kachelrieß M. An efficient computational approach to model statistical correlations in photon counting x-ray detectors. *Med Phys.* 2016; 43(7): 3945–3960.

32. Faby S, Kuchenbecker S, Sawall S, Simons D, Schlemmer H, Lell M, Kachelrieß M. Performance of today's dual energy CT and future multi energy CT in virtual non-contrast imaging and in iodine quantification: A simulation study. *Med Phys.* 2015; 42(7): 4349–4366.
33. Chesler DA, Riederer SJ, Pelc NJ. Noise due to photon counting statistics in computed x-ray tomography. *J Comput Assist Tomogr.* 1977; 1(1): 64.
34. Yu Z, Leng S, Jorgensen SM, Li Z, Gutjahr R, Chen B, Halaweish AF, Kappler S, Yu L, Ritman EL. Evaluation of conventional imaging performance in a research whole-body CT system with a photon-counting detector array. *Phys Med Biol.* 2016; 61(4): 1572.
35. Blevis I, Daerr H, Rokni M, Hermann C, Istel T, Livne A, Martens G, Peyrin F, Rubin D, Sigovan M, Steadman R, Thran A, Brendel B, Levinson R, Altman A, Zarchin O, Boussel L, Douek P, Roessl E. In: Spectroscopy in computed tomography using pixelated photon counting detectors. Workshop on medical applications of spectroscopic X-ray detectors; Geneva, Switzerland; 2015.
36. Blevis I, Altman A, Berman Y. In: Introduction of philips preclinical photon counting scanner and detector technology development. *IEEE Nuclear Science Symposium and Medical Imaging Conference, San Diego, CA*; 2015.
37. Wang AS, Harrison D, Lobastov V, Tkaczyk JE. Pulse pileup statistics for energy discriminating photon counting x-ray detectors. *Med Phys.* 2011; 38: 4265.
38. Hsieh SS, Rajbhandary PL, Pelc NJ. Spectral resolution and high-flux capability tradeoffs in CdTe detectors for clinical CT. *Med Phys.* 2018; 45(4): 1433–1443.
39. Wang AS, Pelc NJ. In: A comparison of dual kV energy integrating and energy discriminating photon counting detectors for dual energy x-ray imaging. Medical imaging 2012: Physics of medical imaging; International Society for Optics and Photonics; 2012. p. 83130W.
40. Melnyk R, Boudry J, Liu X, Adamak M. In: Anti-scatter grid evaluation for wide-cone CT. SPIE medical imaging; International Society for Optics and Photonics; 2014. p. 90332P–90332P-7.
41. Gimenez E, Ballabriga R, Campbell M, Horswell I, Llopart X, Marchal J, Sawhney K, Tartoni N, Turecek D. Study of charge-sharing in MEDIPIX3 using a micro-focused synchrotron beam. *J Instrum.* 2011; 6(01): C01031.
42. Ballabriga R, Campbell M, Heijne E, Llopart X, Tlustos L. The Medipix3 prototype, a pixel readout chip working in single photon counting mode with improved spectrometric performance. *IEEE Trans Nucl Sci.* 2007; 54(5): 1824–1829.
43. Ullberg C, Urech M, Eriksson C, Stewart A, Weber N. In: Photon counting dual energy x-ray imaging at CT count rates: Measurements and implications of in-pixel charge sharing correction. Medical imaging 2018: Physics of medical imaging; International Society for Optics and Photonics; 2018. p. 1057319.
44. Hsieh SS, Sjolin M. Digital count summing vs analog charge summing for photon counting detectors: A performance simulation study. *Med Phys.* 2018; 45(9): 4085–4093.
45. Lundqvist M, inventor; Mamea Imaging, assignee. Method and arrangement relating to x-ray imaging. Sweden patent US6559453B2. 2003 May 6, 2003.
46. Szczykutowicz TP, Mistretta CA. Design of a digital beam attenuation system for computed tomography: Part I. System design and simulation framework. *Med Phys.* 2013; 40: 021905.
47. Szczykutowicz TP, Mistretta CA. Design of a digital beam attenuation system for computed tomography. Part II. Performance study and initial results. *Med Phys.* 2013; 40: 021906.
48. Hsieh SS, Pelc NJ. A dynamic attenuator improves spectral imaging with energy-discriminating, photon counting detectors. *IEEE Trans Med Imaging* 2015; 34(3): 729–739.
49. Hsieh SS, Pelc NJ. Control algorithms for dynamic attenuators. *Med Phys.* 2014; 41(6): 061907.
50. Liu F, Wang G, Cong W, Hsieh SS, Pelc NJ. Dynamic bowtie for fan-beam CT. *J X-Ray Sci Technol.* 2013; 21(4): 579–590.
51. Arenson JS, Ruimi D, Meirav O, Armstrong RH, inventors; General Electric Company, assignee. X-ray flux management device. United States patent 7330535. 2008 Feb 12.
52. Toth TL, Bernstein T, inventors; General Electric Company, assignee. Method and apparatus of modulating the filtering of radiation during radiographic imaging. United States patent 6836535. 2004 Dec 28.
53. Mathews A, Gang G, Levinson R, Zbijewski W, Kawamoto S, Siewerdsen J, Stayman J. In: Experimental evaluation of dual multiple aperture devices for fluence field modulated x-ray computed tomography. Medical imaging 2017: Physics of medical imaging; International Society for Optics and Photonics; 2017. p. 101322O.
54. Hsieh SS, Pelc NJ. The piecewise-linear dynamic attenuator reduces the impact of count rate loss with photon-counting detectors. *Phys Med Biol.* 2014; 59(11): 2829.
55. Hsieh SS, Pelc NJ. Improving pulse detection in multibin photon-counting detectors. *J Med Imaging.* 2016; 3(2): 023505–023505.

56. Kraft E, Fischer P, Karagounis M, Koch M, Krueger H, Peric I, Wermes N, Herrmann C, Nascetti A, Overdick M. Counting and integrating readout for direct conversion x-ray imaging: Concept, realization and first prototype measurements. *IEEE Trans Nucl Sci.* 2007; 54(2): 383–390.
57. Zhang R, Thibault J, Bouman CA, Sauer KD, Hsieh J. Model-based iterative reconstruction for dual-energy x-ray CT using a joint quadratic likelihood model. *IEEE Trans Med Imaging.* 2014; 33(1): 117–134.
58. Tomasi C, Manduchi R. In: Bilateral filtering for gray and color images. Computer vision, 1998. Sixth International Conference on IEEE; 1998. p. 839–846.
59. Pickhardt PJ, Lubner MG, Kim DH, Tang J, Ruma JA, del Rio AM, Chen GH. Abdominal CT with model-based iterative reconstruction (MBIR): Initial results of a prospective trial comparing ultralow-dose with standard-dose imaging. *AJR Am J Roentgenol.* 2012 Dec; 199(6): 1266–1274. PMCID: PMC3689212.
60. Wang AS, Pelc NJ. Sufficient statistics as a generalization of binning in spectral x-ray imaging. *IEEE Trans Med Imaging.* 2011; 30(1): 84–93.
61. Shikhaliev PM. Photon counting spectral CT: Improved material decomposition with K-edge-filtered x-rays. *Phys Med Biol.* 2012; 57(6): 1595.
62. Yao Y, Wang AS, Pelc NJ. Efficacy of fixed filtration for rapid kVp-switching dual energy x-ray systems. *Med Phys.* 2014; 41(3): 031914.
63. Gutjahr R, Halaweish AF, Yu Z, Leng S, Yu L, Li Z, Jorgensen SM, Ritman EL, Kappler S, McCollough CH. Human imaging with photon counting-based computed tomography at clinical dose levels: Contrast-to-noise ratio and cadaver studies. *Invest Radiol.* 2016 Jul; 51(7): 421–429. PMCID: PMC4899181.
64. Rajbhandary PL, Hsieh SS, Pelc NJ. Segmented targeted least squares estimator for material decomposition in multibin photon-counting detectors. *J Med Imaging.* 2017; 4(2): 023503–023510.
65. Alvarez RE. Estimator for photon counting energy selective x-ray imaging with multibin pulse height analysis. *Med Phys.* 2011; 38(5): 2324–2334.
66. Bornefalk H, Danielsson M. Photon-counting spectral computed tomography using silicon strip detectors: A feasibility study. *Phys Med Biol.* 2010; 55(7): 1999.

18 Photon Counting Detector Simulator
Photon Counting Toolkit (PcTK)

Katsuyuki Taguchi
Radiological Physics Division, The Russell H. Morgan Department of Radiology and Radiological Science, Johns Hopkins University School of Medicine, Baltimore, Maryland, USA

CONTENTS

18.1 INTRODUCTION

Energy sensitive photon counting x-ray detectors (PCDs) and the use of PCDs for x-ray computed tomography (CT) systems have been one of the hottest topics of research in CT community. As discussed in other chapters of this book, PCD-CT is expected to be the future of CT, which not only will improve the currently existing CT imaging applications, but also will enable novel applications such as simultaneous multi-agent imaging that are impossible with the current CT technologies (1). Understandably, many researchers may wish to start new research projects on various topics related to PCD-CT such as detector designs, image reconstruction methods, image analysis algorithms, image quality assessments, and the merit of new clinical applications and protocols.

Unfortunately, not many researchers have an access to PCD-CT scanners and no public PCD-CT data are available at this moment. Therefore, researchers are forced to simulate PCD data in their laboratory, often with unrealistic assumptions, for example, PCDs having an ideal "spectral response" (discussed later) or modeling the spectral response using a symmetric Gaussian distribution. Results and conclusions based on such wrong assumptions would limit the practical and scientific value of the work.

In order to address the issue and help the community, we have developed a PCD cross-talk model (2–4) and made the software available to academic researchers in academic institutions, free of charge. The software is called "Photon Counting Toolkit (PcTK)" (5) and interested readers should visit pctk.jhu.edu for more information. Users can use PcTK to compute the expected recorded spectra or simulate noisy PCD data using a realistic spectral response. In the following sections, we briefly outline how PcTK works and present three use cases of PcTK.

18.2 PcTK

As outlined in other chapters, a spectrum and a photon count recorded by a PCD are different from those that are incident onto the PCD due to two types of interactions. The first type includes charge sharing, K-escape, and fluorescence x-ray emission and its reabsorption (4), which we call "spectral response" in this chapter. They are attributed to interaction physics between incident x-ray photons and detector sensor materials, independent of count rates, occur all the time and everywhere, and thus, cannot be avoided. The second type is pulse pileups that are dependent on the incident count rates and become significant only when the incident count rates are high when the object is thin and the attenuation is small. In other words, pulse pileups could be mitigated by using a low-tube current and the effect is limited to projections that go through a thin part of the object near the skin. The behavior related to the spectral response is mostly dominated by the front-end detection crystals and electrodes, while pulse pileups strongly depend on the counting back-end electronics such as an application specific integrated circuit (ASIC). While both of the factors and their interconnections need to be included in a sophisticated modeling, the PcTK version 3.2 includes only a subset of spectral responses.

PcTK version 3.2 (3) uses the cascaded parallel systems model (Figure 18.1) and computes the probability of a count recorded at energy E_3 given the probability of incident energy E_1, detection, and one of the interaction phenomena. One x-ray photon may simply pass through the PCD with no interaction ((a) in Figure 18.1) or interact with a photoelectric effect with ((c) & (d)) or without (b) fluorescence x-ray emission. PcTK version 3.2 includes neither Compton scattering nor Rayleigh scattering.

One or two electron charge clouds (see Figure 18.2a and 18.2b, respectively) may be generated at the interaction sites, which may be detected by multiple adjacent PCD pixels. When the

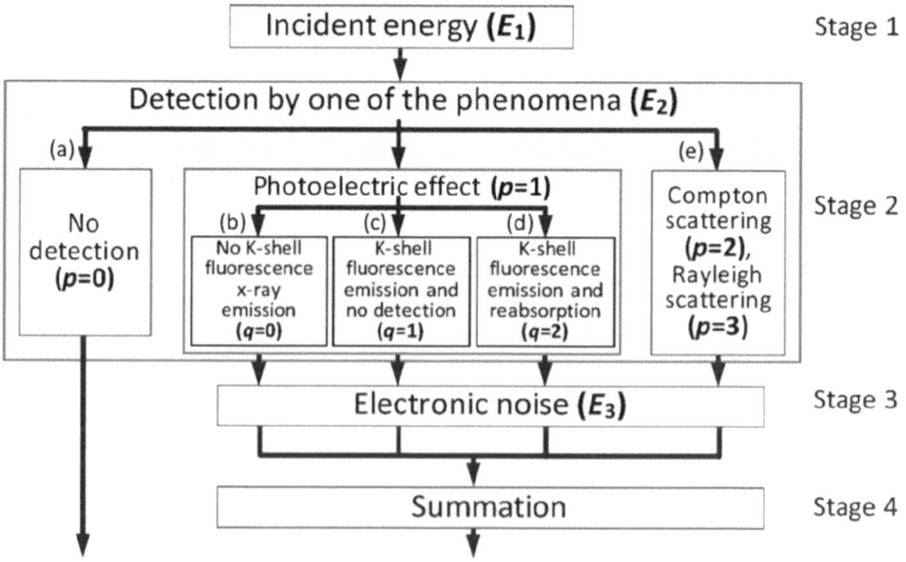

FIGURE 18.1 Cascaded parallel systems modelled through various interaction phenomena, from left, (a) no interaction with PCD ($p = 0$); (b–d) photoelectric effects ($p = 1$) (b) with no K-shell fluorescence x-ray emission ($q = 0$), (c) K-shell fluorescence x-ray emission and its escape from PCD ($q = 1$), and (d) K-shell fluorescence x-ray emission and its reabsorption ($q = 2$); and (e) Compton scattering ($p = 2$) and Rayleigh scattering ($p = 3$). Compton scattering and Rayleigh scattering are *not* included in PcTK version 3.2. The figure is from Ref. (3), where p and q are the primary and secondary interaction types.

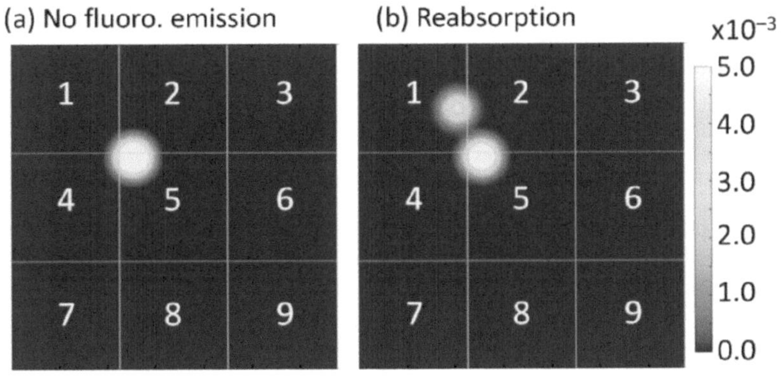

FIGURE 18.2 An example of electron charge distribution over the 3×3 neighboring pixels when (a) a photon with energy 100 keV is incident near the left upper corner of pixel 5 with no fluorescence emission and (b) the primary charge with 76.0 keV is generated at the same location as (a) and the fluorescence x-ray with energy 24.0 keV is absorbed 112 μm away from the primary charge. Note that all of the charge clouds had the same full-width-at-half-maximum size of d_0, although they may appear in different sizes due to windowing. The figures are from Ref. (3).

photon energy is split to more than one pixel, the recorded energy at each pixel is lower than the original energy and one photon produces more than one count. This is called double-counting or *n*-tuple-counting. As a result, PCD data are spatially and energetically correlated. PcTK models the recorded x-ray spectrum with such correlation.

Users provide PcTK several parameters for their PCDs such as the pixel size, the pixel depth, the reference size of electron charges, and the electronic noise. Then PcTK computes the conditional probabilities of energy and count(s) recorded at neighboring 3×3 PCD pixels (see Figure 18.2) when x-rays are incident onto somewhere within the central PCD pixel (pixel 5 in Figure 18.2) and outputs a normalized covariance matrix for 1-keV-width energy windows (Figure 18.3a) or a given energy windows if a user choses so (Figure 18.3b).

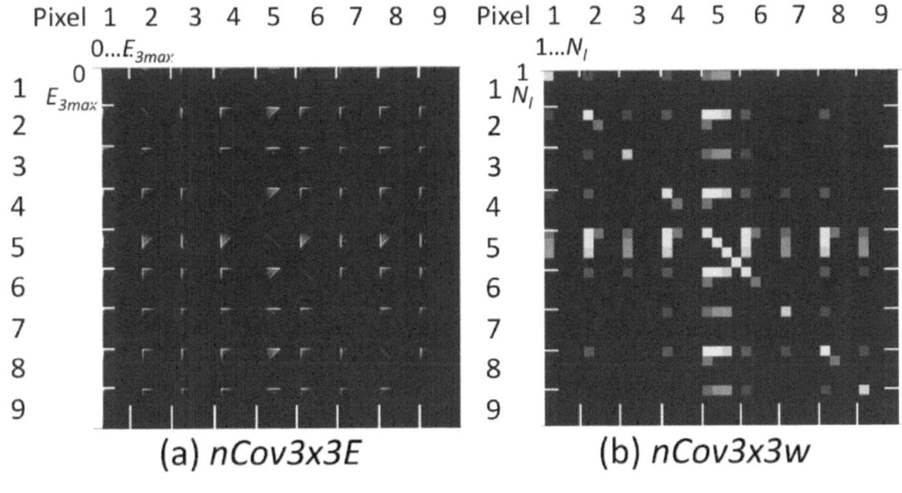

FIGURE 18.3 Normalized covariance matrices for (a) 1-keV-width energy windows *nCov3* × *3E* for $E_1 = 90$ keV and (b) N_l (= 4) energy windows *nCov3* × *3w* for $E_1 = 90$ keV with energy thresholds at 20, 50, 65, and 80 keV. The window scale was (a) (0, 10^{-3}) and (b) (0.0, 0.2). The figures are from Ref. (3).

18.3 USE CASES

In this section, we present three use cases of PcTK. Script files to perform some of the use cases are included in the PcTK package (5).

18.3.1 Use Case 1 (PCD Design)

Use case 1 is to study the effect of various PCD design parameters on distorted recorded spectra (3). Spectra recorded by each of 3 × 3 PCD pixels can be computed from the normalized covariance matrix (Figure 18.3a).

Figure 18.4 shows spectra recorded at the central pixel 5 (Figure 18.4b), edge pixels (Figure 18.4c), or corner/diagonal pixels (Figure 18.4d) when the central pixel receives x-rays. It can be seen that the central pixel received counts at higher energies, while peripheral pixels recorded counts at lower energies. It would be challenging to perform this type of physical experiments due to the presence of penumbra; thus, simulation is valuable for the study. Figure 18.4a shows the spectrum as a sum of nine pixels, which is equivalent to the spectrum that will be recorded with flood field irradiation with no anti-scatter grids (see Subsection 18.3.2).

Figure 18.5 presents the recorded spectra with incident monochromatic x-rays at different energies with flat field irradiation with no anti-scatter grids. The energy-dependent responses can shed light on the contributions of photopeaks, K-escape peaks, fluorescence peaks, continuum, and the noise floor and a better detector design may be found especially if a range of target incident energies can be identified.

Figure 18.6 shows the recorded spectra while changing one of the following three PCD parameters: the pixel size (Figure 18.6a), the reference size of electron charges (Figure 18.6b), and the electronic noise (Figure 18.6c).

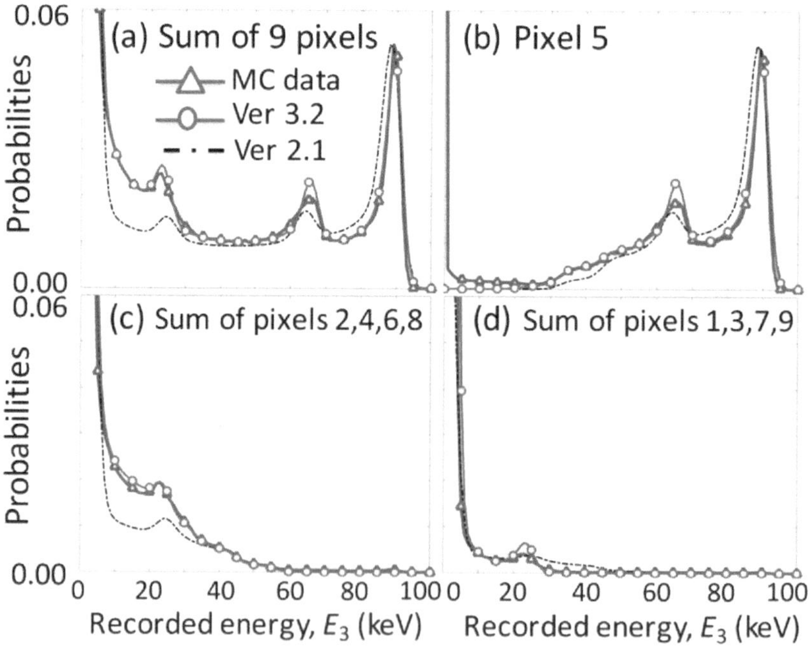

FIGURE 18.4 Comparison of Monte Carlo simulated data, PcTK version 3.2, and PcTK version 2.1 with incident energy $E_1 = 90$ keV, with single pixel irradiation: (a) a sum of all of 3 × 3 pixels; (b) pixel 5; (c) a sum of pixels 2, 4, 6, and 8 (that share an edge with pixel 5); and (d) a sum of pixels 1, 3, 7, and 9 (that share a corner with pixel 5). The agreement between the Monte Carlo simulation and PcTK version 3.2 was excellent. The figures are from Ref. (3).

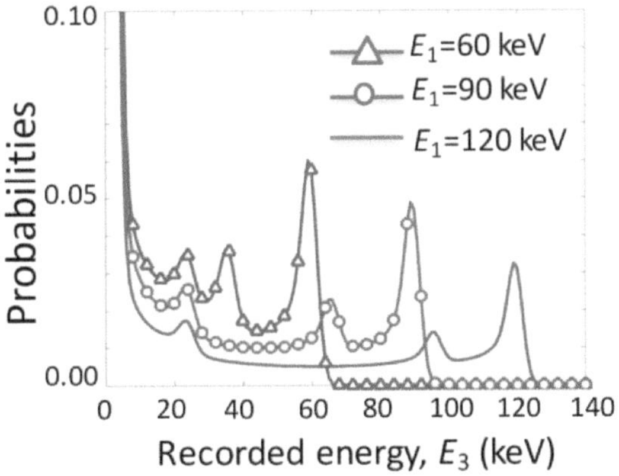

FIGURE 18.5 The spectral response of the CdTe detector with incident energy E_1 = 60, 90, and 120 keV, with flat field irradiation. The figure is from Ref. (3).

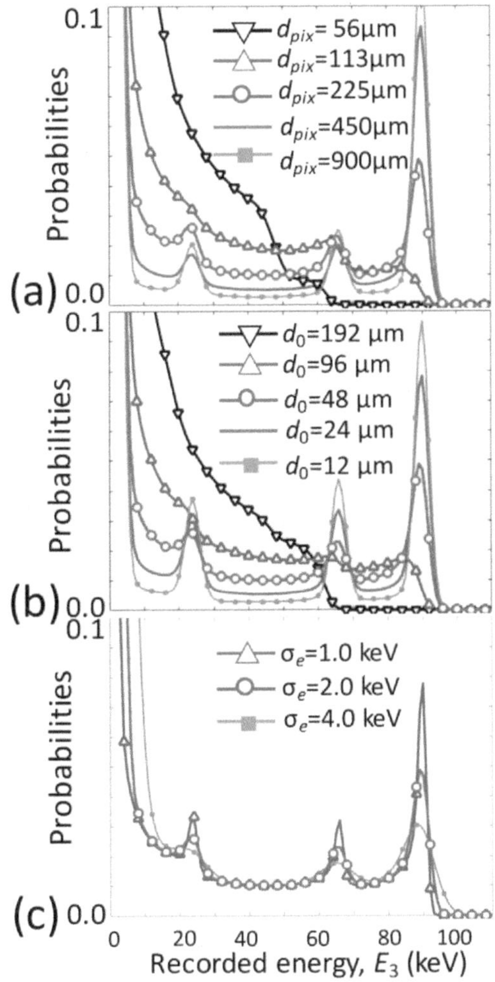

FIGURE 18.6 The spectral response to the incident energy E_1 = 90 keV with one of the following parameters changed one at a time, while the others were fixed at the standard setting: (a) the PCD pixel size d_{pix}, (b) the reference electronic charge cloud diameter d_0, and (c) electronic noise σ_e. The figures are from Ref. (3).

18.3.2 Use Case 2 (Imaging Performance with PCD Pixel Binning and Anti-Scatter Grids)

Use case 2 is to study the effect of PCD pixel binning and anti-scatter grids (6). Both signals and correlated noise of adjacent PCD pixels through different water thicknesses can be computed from the normalized covariance matrix. The effect of anti-scatter grids in terms of blocking x-rays and eliminating spill-in and spill-out cross-talks between PCD pixels can be taken into account by moving the "central pixel" that receives the x-rays and accumulating the signals and noise. The effect of $N \times N$ pixel binning can be taken into account by summing the outputs of multiple pixels into one output datum.

Figure 18.7 shows spectra obtained with no anti-scatter grids, 1-dimensional (1-D) anti-scatter grids (or blades), and 2-dimensional (2-D) anti-scatter grids. With each setting, the output pixel area of (900 μm)^2 was obtained by three different binning schemes: one (900 μm)^2 PCD pixel with no binning, binning 2 × 2 (450 μm)^2 PCD pixels, and binning 4×4 (225 μm)^2 PCD pixels. A sensitivity index (or generalized signal-to-noise ratio) for soft tissue contrast was computed and normalized against that of the ideal PCD (which had the detection rate of 100% with no spectral distortion). It can be seen that sensitivity index is affected by threshold energies, the PCD pixel sizes, anti-scatter grid designs, and binning schemes. One can also see that the maximum sensitivity index can be achieved at different threshold energies with different anti-scatter grid designs. Note that the spatial resolution in a vertical direction with 1-D anti-scatter grids and in both vertical and horizontal directions with no anti-scatter grids is worse than that with the ideal PCD due to spill-in cross-talk from neighboring pixels, and the increased photons resulted in the sensitivity index values being higher than those with 2-D anti-scatter grids in some cases.

18.3.3 Use Case 3 (PCD-CT Scan)

Use case 3 is to simulate PCD-CT scans (i.e., synthesize PCD-CT projections of a user-defined object) (3). Users need to prepare their own material-specific sinograms (i.e., line integrals of density images of soft tissue, bone, and K-edge materials) and the other data A–B and D–E specified in Figure 18.8, including the normalized covariance matrix computed by PcTK (Figure 18.3b). Then, a MATLAB® script included in the PcTK package can be used to generate noisy PCD projection data with spatio-energetic correlation between neighboring PCD pixels. Generating correlated noisy data is a slow process; thus, we provided a more computationally efficient script to generate noisy PCD data with no correlation. In Figure 18.8, an image for each energy window was reconstructed independently which showed artifacts near the brain-skull boundary.

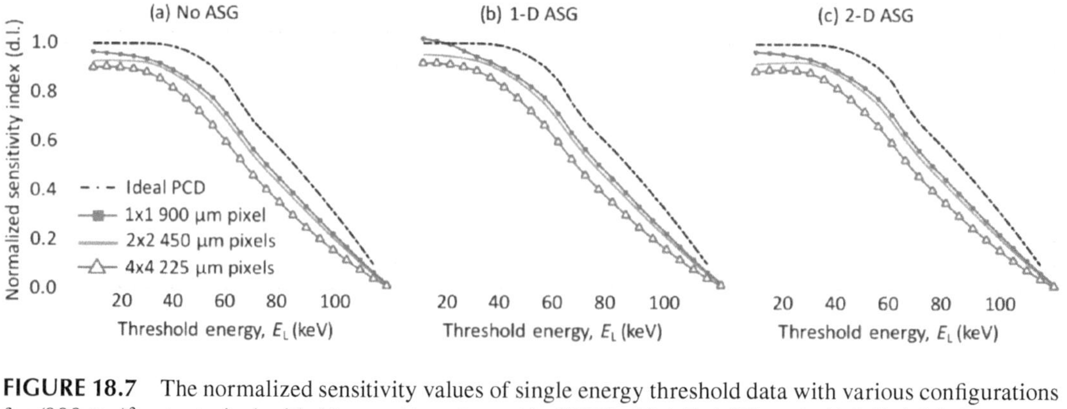

FIGURE 18.7 The normalized sensitivity values of single energy threshold data with various configurations for (900 μm)^2 output pixel with (a) no anti-scatter grids (ASG), (b) 1-D ASG, and, (c) 2-D ASG. The water thickness of 30 cm; 120 kVp; single energy threshold; CdTe detector. d.l. = dimension less. The figures are from Ref. (6).

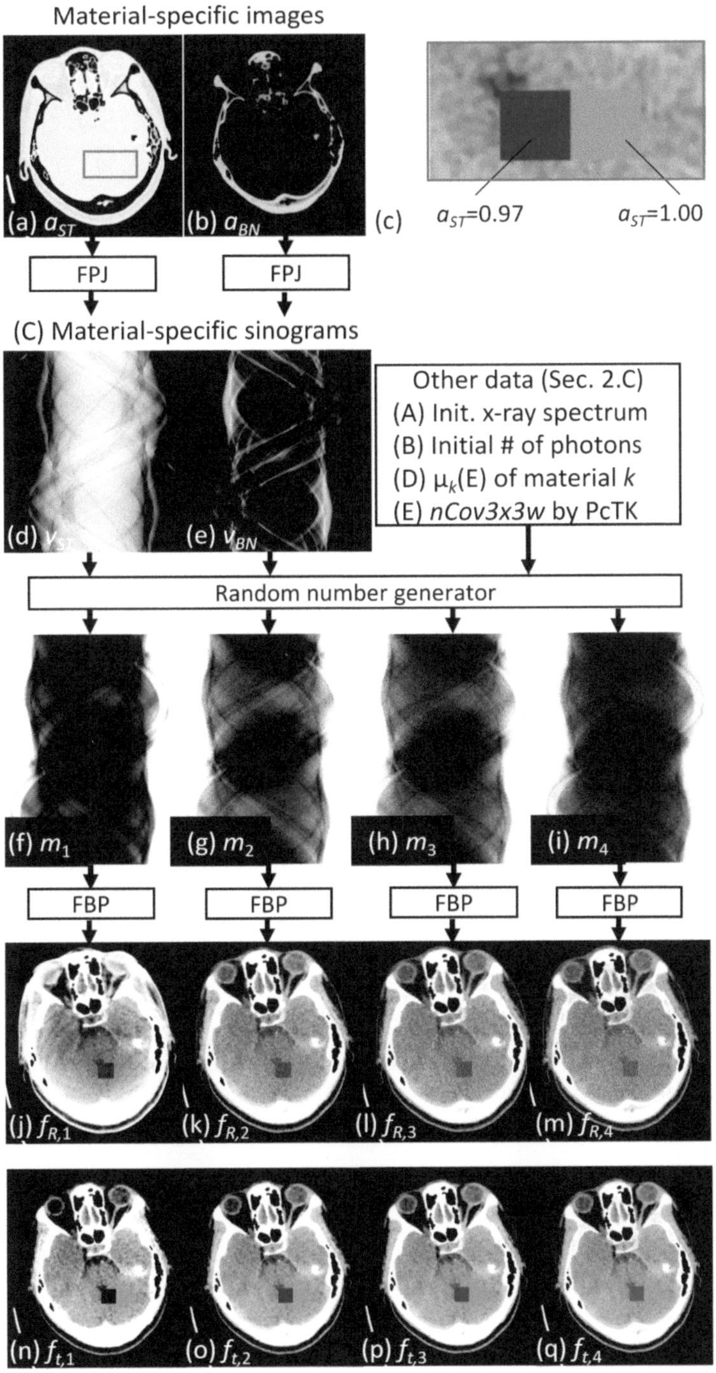

FIGURE 18.8 Materials prepared for and resulted from a simulated PCD-CT scan. (a–c) The density maps of soft tissue (a) and bone (b) with regions-of-interest with constant soft tissue density values (c). (d–e) Material-specific sinograms of soft tissue (h) and bone (i) generated from (a) and (b), respectively through forward projection (FPJ). (f–i) Noisy PCD projection data (counts) with cross-talk and spectral response effects of the four energy windows, generated using a random number generator and data (A)–(E) outlined in Section 2.C of Ref. (3). (j–m) CT images reconstructed from each of the PCD data (f)–(i) independently using filtered backprojection (FBP). (n–q) Monochromatic x-ray CT images synthesized from (a) and (b) at the center of the four energy windows used, 35 keV (n), 57 keV (o), 72 keV (p), and 100 keV (q). CT images are presented with the window width of 0.04 cm^{-1} and the window center at the value of a_{ST} = 1.0 region-of-interest (c). The figure is from Ref. (3).

The simulated PCD data can be used for many different purposes. One can reconstruct CT images of energy windows and assess the effect of spectral distortion. One can develop image reconstruction algorithms for, for example, spectral distortion compensation, noise reduction, signal enhancement, and material decomposition. Or one can optimize low-dose PCD-CT protocols.

18.4 CONCLUSION

We outlined PcTK with three use cases. We wish to promote PCD research in CT community and hope PcTK will be a valuable tool. Interested readers are encouraged to visit pctk.jhu.edu for more information and use PcTK package for their research.

ACKNOWLEDGMENTS

This work was supported by research agreements with Siemens Healthcare (JHU-2016-CT-1-01-Taguchi_C0022 and JHU-2018-CT-1-02-Taguchi_C00229096). We thank Drs. Steffen Kappler, Christoph Polster, Karl Stierstorfer, Okkyun Lee, Jingyan Xu, Matthew K. Fuld, Thomas G. Flohr, and George S. K. Fung for their contribution to the project. The authors have no relevant conflicts of interests.

REFERENCES

The author to whom correspondence should be addressed – Electronic addresses: ktaguchi@jhmi.edu, Telephone: +1 443 287 2425; Fax: +1 410 6141 1060.

1. Taguchi K, Iwanczyk JS. Vision 20/20: Single photon counting x-ray detectors in medical imaging. *Medical Physics*. 2013;40(10):100901.
2. Taguchi K, Stierstorfer K, Polster C, Lee O, Kappler S. Spatio-energetic cross talk in photon counting detectors: Numerical detector model (PcTK) and workflow for CT image quality assessment. *SPIE Medical Imaging 2018: Physics of Medical Imaging*. 2018;10573:10573–10535.
3. Taguchi K, Stierstorfer K, Polster C, Lee O, Kappler S. Spatio-energetic cross-talk in photon counting detectors: Numerical detector model (PcTK) and workflow for CT image quality assessment. *Medical Physics*. 2018;45(5):1985–1998.
4. Taguchi K, Polster C, Lee O, Stierstorfer K, Kappler S. Spatio-energetic cross talk in photon counting detectors: Detector model and correlated Poisson data generator. *Medical Physics*. 2016;43(12):6386–6404.
5. Taguchi K. Photon Counting Toolkit (PcTK) 2018. Available from: pctk.jhu.edu
6. Taguchi K, Stierstorfer K, Polster C, Lee O, Kappler S. Spatio-energetic cross-talk in photon counting detectors: N × N binning and sub-pixel masking. *Medical Physics*. 2018;45(11):4822–4843.

Part IV

Image Reconstruction for Spectral CT

19 Image Formation in Spectral Computed Tomography

Simon Rit[1], Cyril Mory[1], and Peter B. Noël[2]
[1]Univ Lyon, INSA-Lyon, Université Claude Bernard Lyon 1, UJM-Saint Etienne, CNRS, INSERM, CREATIS, Centre Léon Bérard, Lyon, France
[2]Department of Radiology, Perelman School of Medicine, University of Pennsylvania, Philadelphia, Pennsylvania, USA

CONTENTS

Spectral Computed Tomography (CT) can perform "color" x-ray detection; for example, photon-counting detectors can discriminate the energy of individual x-ray photons and divide them into several predefined energy bins, thereby providing a spectral analysis of the transmitted x-ray beam. By measuring the x-ray attenuation in two or more distinct energy bins, one can gain information about the elemental composition of an object, making it possible via material decomposition to distinguish between different materials, such as contrast agents and different types of tissues, in a single CT scan. This concept of spectral CT is based on the x-ray attenuation differences of various materials when simultaneously exposed by a spectrum of x-ray photons (which are emitted in a wide spectral range by a standard x-ray tube). Attenuation differences reflect the differences in material interactions with low- and high-energy photons, mainly Compton scatter and photoelectric effects in the diagnostic energy range. Interaction of x-rays with matter is described by the linear attenuation coefficient μ of an object, which depends on the three-dimensional (3D) position $\boldsymbol{x}$ in space and the one-dimensional (1D) energy ϵ of incident photons. The photon fluence Φ after the object of a monoenergetic pencil beam is described by the Beer-Lambert law:

$$\Phi = \Phi_0 \exp\left(-\int_{\mathcal{L}} \mu(\boldsymbol{x}, \epsilon) \mathrm{d}\ell \right) \tag{19.1}$$

with ϵ the beam energy, Φ_0 the initial beam fluence, and $\mathcal{L}$ the line corresponding to the beam.

Conventional CT scanners acquire a single sinogram, mixing all photons regardless of their energy. Reconstruction algorithms for single-energy CT either neglect the energy dependency of the incident beam or use corrections for multi-energy effects known as beam hardening [8], for example by assuming that a single material composes the object in the field-of-view [7]. Spectral CT scanners employ a variety of strategies to acquire multiple sinograms representative of different energy segments of the incoming spectra [38]. The purpose of this chapter is to present specific algorithmic solutions required to utilize this additional energy dimension in combination with conventional and advanced tomographic reconstruction algorithms.

The central goal of spectral processing steps is to reconstruct not only a 3D μ map at a given (effective) energy, but a four-dimensional (4D) μ for the energy range measured with two to five energy discrimination measurements provided by a spectral CT scanner. A simplified model becomes necessary and many contributions (also presented in this chapter) are based on a model proposed by Alvarez and Macovski [4]. This paradigm describes μ as a linear combination of a few energy-independent and space-independent functions, which they note:

$$\mu(\boldsymbol{x},\epsilon) \approx \sum_{m=1}^{\mathrm{M}} a_m(\boldsymbol{x}) f_m(\epsilon) \tag{19.2}$$

with $\boldsymbol{x}$ the 3D position in the object, M the number of basis functions, a_m the 3D space-dependent (but energy-independent) functions, and f_m the energy-dependent (but space-independent) functions. Two approaches have been proposed for the f_m functions and a_m volumes in human tissue. Both methods only require $\mathrm{M} = 2$ basis functions. One is to assume that the object attenuates x-rays as if it was composed of two materials, for example, water and bone [23]. The function f_m is then the mass-attenuation coefficient of material m, which solely depends on the energy, and the volume a_m is a map of the concentration of material m. The other approach proposes that image contrast is based on an x-ray particle model describing the physical interaction of photoelectric absorption and Compton scattering. The function f_m then approximates the energy dependence of the phenomenon m, and the volume a_m is a map of the cross-section for that type of interaction. In addition to the two functions to represent human materials, there can be additional components in the basis to represent non-human elements ($\mathrm{M} > 2$), for example, contrast materials having a K-absorption edge in the diagnostic energy range [57, 82]. Without loss of generality, we will refer to f_m as material-specific CT maps in the following sections.

The x-ray source of a CT scanner is polychromatic and characterized by an energy spectrum. Similarly, the signal measured by the detector is a function of the energies of impinging photons. The impinging spectrum is not equivalent to the measured one because the measurements can be distorted while the signal is picked up from the detector and processed by complex electronics. The ratio of the spectrum collected with a detector over the impinging spectrum is called a detector response function or pulse height distribution. These two energy functions can be merged into an *effective spectrum*, which is the product of the source spectrum and the detector response function. The concept of an effective spectrum can describe any spectral system, whether several effective spectra are acquired by using different source spectra, for example, with different source voltages, by using two detectors with different responses, for example, with different sensitive materials, or by using different energy thresholds for photon-counting detectors. Figure 19.1 illustrates the effective spectra of different systems.

Plugging the model of the linear attenuation coefficient (Equation 19.2) into the Beer-Lambert law (Equation 19.1) and accounting for the polychromatism of the effective spectra leads to the forward model of the inverse problem studied in this chapter

$$\hat{y}_{ib} = \int_{\mathbb{R}^+} s_b(\epsilon) \exp\left(-\int_{\mathcal{L}_i} \sum_{m=1}^{\mathrm{M}} a_m(\boldsymbol{x}) f_m(\epsilon) \mathrm{d}\ell \right) \mathrm{d}\epsilon \tag{19.3}$$

with $\hat{y}_{ib}$ the expectation of the measures for the i-th detector pixel and the b-th effective spectrum s_b (b stands for energy bin in photon counting systems). The goal of this inverse problem is to estimate

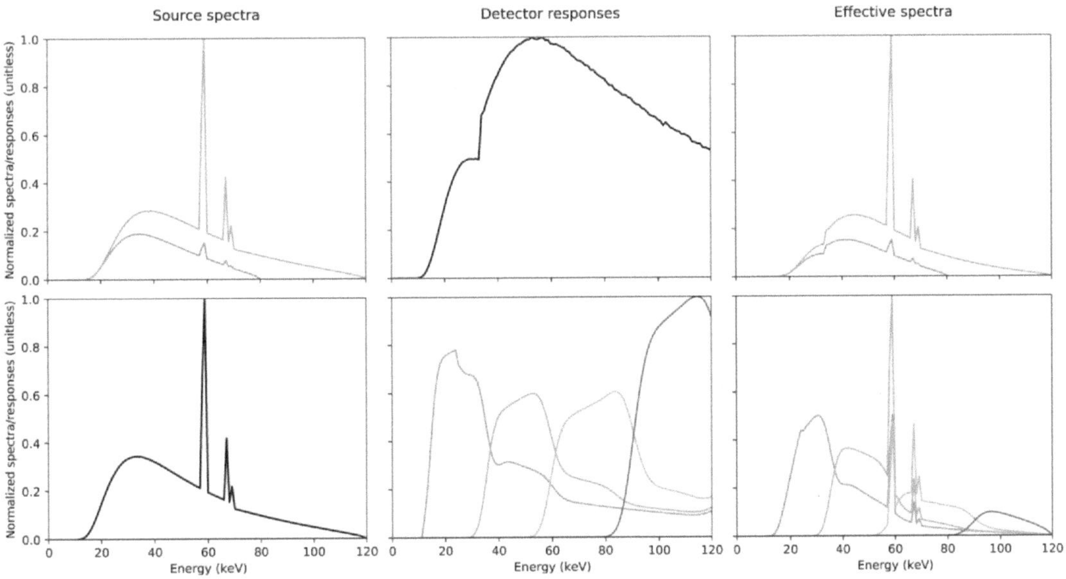

FIGURE 19.1 Examples of source spectra (left), detector responses (middle), and effective spectra (right), for a fast-switching x-ray source with an energy-integrating detector with a CsI scintillator (top, data from system #2 in [81]) and a photon-counting system with four energy bins (bottom, data from [16]).

the unknown material images $\boldsymbol{a}$ from measures $\boldsymbol{y}$. The effective spectra s can be estimated independently, before using the algorithms presented in this chapter [17, 40, 67]. The energy functions f are chosen based on the model in Equation 19.2. This forward model only accounts for the attenuation of primary rays and neglects scatter, pile-up, charge sharing, and other complex effects, unless those can be taken into account in the effective spectrum.

The following three sections introduce the main classes of spectral CT reconstruction algorithms (Figure 19.2): image-based and projection-based, which perform decomposition into

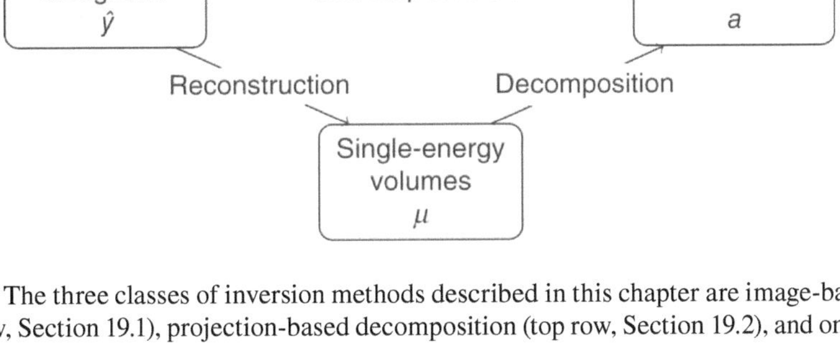

FIGURE 19.2 The three classes of inversion methods described in this chapter are image-based decomposition (bottom row, Section 19.1), projection-based decomposition (top row, Section 19.2), and one-step inversion (Section 19.3).

materials and tomographic reconstruction separately, and are therefore referred to as "two-step" methods, and one-step inversion, which merges both decomposition and reconstruction into a single inverse problem. The final sections describe possible regularizers for these ill-posed inverse problems and potential image quality issues specific to spectral CT decomposition and reconstruction.

19.1 IMAGE-BASED DECOMPOSITION

Image-based decomposition was initially developed for exploiting two (or more) CT acquisitions obtained at different tube-voltages on a conventional CT scanner [6]. With distinct spectra at different voltages, the resulting CT slices display energy dependent differences. Image-based decomposition assumes that the b-th single-energy CT represents the attenuation coefficient at a given (effective) energy e_b, which is true with monoenergetic CT acquisitions at a synchrotron [79], by reconstructing from the log-transformed projections $\ln(s_b(e_b)/y_{ib})$, or with the use of an efficient beam hardening correction. Under this assumption, the CT image $\mu(\cdot, e_b)$ of the b-th effective spectrum is, according to Equation 19.2, a linear combination of the sought space-dependent functions a_m and the energy-dependent functions f_m. Combining the measurements, one obtains at each spatial position $\boldsymbol{x}$ a small linear system of equations with as many equations as CT images:

$$\mu(\boldsymbol{x}) = \boldsymbol{F}\boldsymbol{a}(\boldsymbol{x}) \tag{19.4}$$

with

$$\mu(\boldsymbol{x}) = \begin{bmatrix} \mu(\boldsymbol{x}, e_1) \\ \mu(\boldsymbol{x}, e_2) \\ \vdots \\ \mu(\boldsymbol{x}, e_B)) \end{bmatrix}, \quad \boldsymbol{F} = \begin{bmatrix} f_1(e_1) & f_2(e_1) & \dots & f_M(e_1) \\ f_1(e_2) & f_2(e_2) & \dots & f_M(e_2) \\ \vdots & \vdots & \ddots & \vdots \\ f_1(e_B) & f_2(e_B) & \dots & f_M(e_B) \end{bmatrix} \quad \text{and} \quad \boldsymbol{a}(\boldsymbol{x}) = \begin{bmatrix} a_1(\boldsymbol{x}) \\ a_2(\boldsymbol{x}) \\ \vdots \\ a_M(\boldsymbol{x}) \end{bmatrix}. \tag{19.5}$$

Given its small size, this system can easily be solved, for example, with the Moore-Penrose pseudoinverse (which is the inverse of $\boldsymbol{F}$ if $\boldsymbol{F}$ is invertible). Moreover, since there is no spatial dependence of $\boldsymbol{F}$, this (pseudo-)inverse can be computed once for all voxels if the effective energy of the input CT images is known. Otherwise, it can be directly calibrated using materials with known linear attenuation properties. Image-based decomposition can be combined with regularization, for example to reduce noise [14, 15, 49, 76]. A simulated example using monochromatic spectra is provided in Figure 19.3.

The simplicity of image-based decomposition makes it an attractive solution. It is also extensively used in applications where access to raw data/sinograms is not available, as demonstrated in radiotherapy applications [80]. Another advantage compared to projection-based inversions is that there is no need to have projections acquired with the same geometry (source and detector positions and orientations) for all effective spectra, as is, for example, the case when two different x-ray sources are used for the acquisition of different spectra. The input CT images must still be perfectly registered, and this is true for all algorithms presented here. Even if two (or more) CT acquisitions could easily be acquired on any clinical CT scanner with different voltages, patient motion, for example, through breathing, reduces significantly the quality of spectral results. Another significant drawback of image-based decomposition is the impact of beam hardening when using conventional x-ray sources. Inaccuracies of beam hardening correction will have a direct influence on the result [71]. Advanced beam hardening correction

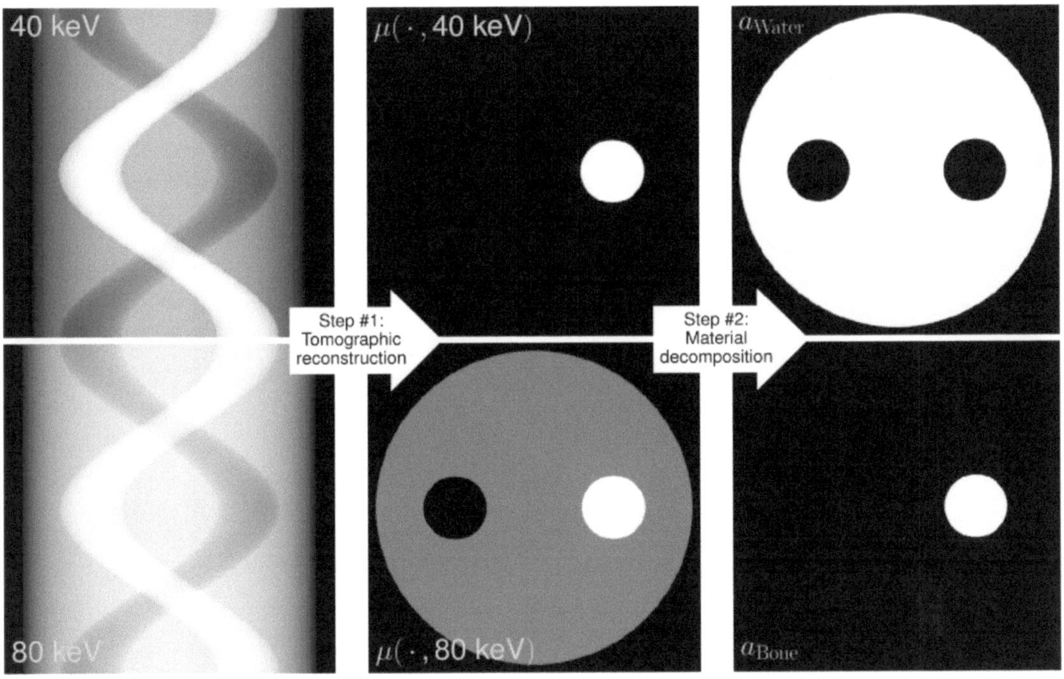

FIGURE 19.3 Left: noiseless simulated dual-energy log-transformed sinograms using monochromatic irradiations at 40 keV (top) and 80 keV (bottom). Middle: corresponding single-energy volumes g_b. Right: decomposed volumes a_m. The object is made of a liquid water component (top right) and cortical bone (bottom right). The linear attenuation coefficients used for the simulation are those of ICRP retrieved from x-ray lib [64], that is, $\mu_{\text{water}}(40\text{ keV}) = 0.27\,\text{cm}^{-1}$, $\mu_{\text{water}}(80\text{ keV}) = 0.18\,\text{cm}^{-1}$, $\mu_{\text{water}}(40\text{ keV}) = 1.19\,\text{cm}^{-1}$ and $\mu_{\text{bone}}(80\text{ keV}) = 0.41\,\text{cm}^{-1}$.

algorithms require the knowledge of the linear attenuation coefficients of the materials in the field-of-view, for example, by relying on the same model as Equation 19.2 [8]. Image-based decomposition is therefore simple because it forwards the complexity of Equation 19.3 from the decomposition to the beam hardening correction. The difficulty therefore lies in the latter and has lead to the development of algorithms, which correct for beam hardening in the image domain while decomposing by using a different model than Equation 19.2 [34]. Another approach, intermediate with one-step inversion (section 19.3), projects the current estimate to iteratively correct for beam hardening [35].

19.2 PROJECTION-BASED DECOMPOSITION

Projection-based methods perform first the decomposition in projection space before reconstructing material-specific CT maps (Figure 19.2).

19.2.1 Decomposition into Material Projections

Decomposition into material-specific projections aims to determine, for each pixel of the multi-energy sinogram, the corresponding line integral through the spatial maps a_m. For example, if the object consists of two materials as in Figure 19.3 and the basis functions f_m are the corresponding linear attenuation coefficients of the materials, the aimed decomposed data will be the sinogram

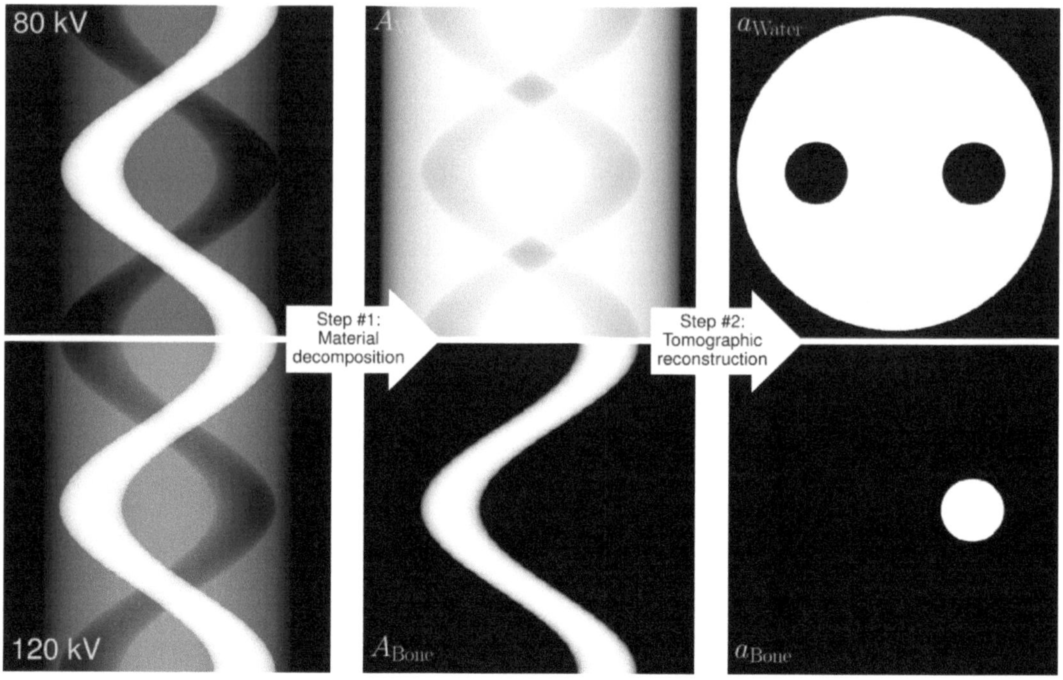

FIGURE 19.4 Left: noiseless simulated dual-energy sinograms of the object in Figure 19.3 using the 80 kV (top) and 120 kV (bottom) spectra and the detector response shown on top of Figure 19.1. Middle: decomposed sinograms A_m using projection-based decomposition with μ_{water} and μ_{bone} as basis functions f_m. Right: decomposed volumes a_m. The object is the same as in Figure 19.3.

of each material, as illustrated in Figure 19.4. Formally, Equation 19.3 is modified by inverting the order of the integral over the line $\mathcal{L}_i$ and the discrete sum over the M basis functions. Projection-based decomposition then utilizes the forward model:

$$\hat{y}_{ib} = \int_{\mathbb{R}^+} s_b(\epsilon)\exp\left(-\sum_{m=1}^{M} A_{im} f_m(\epsilon)\right) \mathrm{d}\epsilon \tag{19.6}$$

with the unknowns $A_{im} = \int_{\mathcal{L}_i} a_m(\boldsymbol{x})\mathrm{d}\ell$ corresponding to the i-th line integral through a_m. This decomposition yields a set $\boldsymbol{A}$ of M sinograms (one per basis function), which can each be reconstructed to obtain one volume per material. Similarly to the image-based problem, decomposing the acquired sinograms $\boldsymbol{y}$ into material-specific sinograms $\boldsymbol{A}$ is a small problem when processed pixel-by-pixel, with M unknowns to find from B measurements. However, the exponential function causes the problem to be non-linear and the (weighted) least squares data fidelity term is non-convex [1].

In their seminal paper [4], Alvarez and Macovski proposed to approximate the logarithm of the expectation of the measures $\hat{\boldsymbol{y}}$ by a P-th order polynomial of the A_{im}:

$$\ln \hat{y}_{ib} \simeq \sum_{p_1+p_2+\ldots+p_M \leq P} \alpha_{p_1 p_2 \ldots p_M} A_{i1}^{p_1} A_{i2}^{p_2} \ldots A_{iM}^{p_M} \tag{19.7}$$

with $\{p_1,\ldots,p_M\}$ the exponents and $\alpha_{p_0 p_1 \ldots p_M}$ the coefficients of the polynomial. Another solution is to directly approximate the inversion by a polynomial [28]:

$$A_{im} \simeq \sum_{q_1+q_2+\ldots+q_B \leq P} \beta_{q_1 q_2 \ldots q_B} \left(\ln \hat{y}_{i1}\right)^{q_1} \left(\ln \hat{y}_{i2}\right)^{q_2} \ldots \left(\ln \hat{y}_{iB}\right)^{q_B} \tag{19.8}$$

with $\{q_1,\ldots,q_B\}$ the exponents and $\beta_{q_0 q_1 \ldots q_B}$ the coefficients of this other polynomial. Both methods are very efficient solutions, probably best suited to dual-energy decomposition with two basis functions (B = M = 2). In any case, they are only approximations of Equation 19.6 or its inverse. The accuracy of this approximation can be improved by increasing the polynomial order P, but it also degrades the stability of the decomposition. Already in [4], the authors did not use all nine possible monomials and later studies suggested a rationale for adequately selecting a subset of monomials [29]. If the effective spectra s are known, the coefficients of the polynomials can be computed to best approximate the forward model, as $\boldsymbol{F}$ in image-based decomposition (Equation 19.4). Otherwise, one can directly calibrate the polynomial coefficients without estimating s by taking projections through multiple combinations of basis material layers with known thicknesses as, for example, in the calibration phantom of [2].

In 2008, in order to deal with three materials and four energy bins, Roessl *et al.* proposed to solve the problem in the maximum likelihood sense [57, 62], that is, to determine which are the most likely A_{im} given the measured y_{ib}. To maximize the log-likelihood, they used the Nelder-Mead downhill simplex method [47], which is a zero order optimization algorithm for convex problems, that is, which does not need the gradient of the cost function with respect to the optimized variables. Under standard clinical x-ray exposure, the statistical noise on y_{ib} results in very noisy decomposed sinograms, which must be filtered to become usable, as illustrated in Figure 19.5.

Brendel *et al.* [5] proposed to improve Roessl's optimization using the iterative coordinate descent. They also introduced spatial regularization in their minimization problem to limit noise in decomposed sinograms: in addition to being in agreement with the measured photon counts, the decomposed material line integrals in a pixel i must be similar to those in the neighboring pixels. However, regularizing in the projection domain is unusual and it can negatively impact the reconstructed images if it is inadequately chosen or weighted. Similar approaches based on solving an inverse problem include the work of Ducros *et al.* [16] and Abascal *et al.* [1] solving a weighted least-squares problems using a Gauss-Newton algorithm and an iterative Bregman scheme. The latter authors also used the Kullbac-Leibler divergence [21], which is more adapted to Poisson noise distributions and should lead to a result similar to the maximum likelihood approach of [57, 62].

Intermediate solutions between the polynomial models (Equations 19.7 and 19.8) and the full non-linear model (Equation 19.6) have been tailored for the case of more measurements than basis functions [2, 3, 26, 27, 41, 94]. Another approach is to use machine learning to solve this complex but small problem, for example, by using a neural network [93].

A significant advantage of projection-based decomposition over image-based decomposition (section 19.1) is that it does not suffer from beam hardening because the material maps $\boldsymbol{f}$ are energy-independent. However, it can only be applied if the measurements for different spectra are acquired with the same geometry, which is the case for dual-layer detectors and spectral photon-counting detectors but not for dual-source systems or fast-switching x-ray sources. For dual-source or fast-switching systems, one solution is to interpolate the sinograms to have corresponding measurements, but this step could limit the accuracy. Performing several successive acquisitions with different spectra on a standard CT is in theory feasible, but just like with image-based methods, patient motion is then a concern.

19.2.2 Tomographic Reconstruction

None of the methods presented in subsection 19.2.1 makes any assumption on how the material sinograms are reconstructed once they have been decomposed. In fact, any tomographic reconstruction

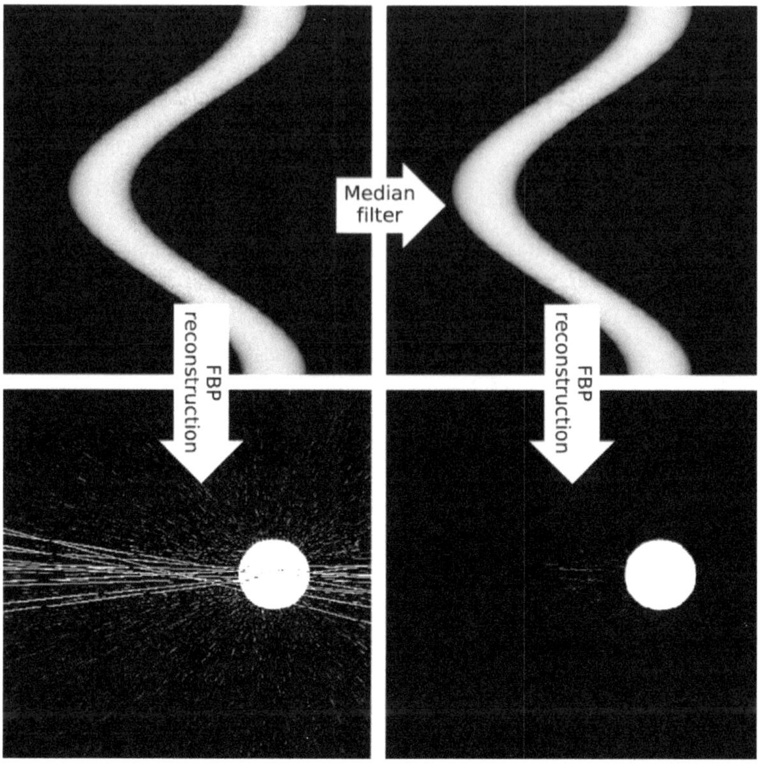

FIGURE 19.5 Sinogram of the bone (top) and its reconstruction (bottom) for the same object as Figure 19.4 with an additional solution of 1 mg/mL gadolinium filling the left hole of the water component. Data simulated using the 5-bin spectral model of the Philips small animal prototype in Lyon [65] corrupted with Poisson noise. The projection-based decomposition is the algorithm of Roessl *et al.* [57, 62] with the three-material basis $f = \{\mu_{\text{Water}}, \mu_{\text{Bone}}, \mu_{\text{Gadolinium}}\}$. Images reconstructed with a filtered backprojection reconstruction. The right sinogram resulted from a median filter to remove outliers. Outliers are in the low-count area, for rays that traverse both the bone and the gadolinium (see other reconstructions in Figure 19.6).

method can be used, including filtered backprojection algorithms. However, the decomposition is sensitive to noise and it is natural to account for this noise in an iterative reconstruction algorithm. A first solution is to use an estimate of the variance of the decomposed sinograms in a weighted least squares algorithm [61]. The material decomposition process also induces anti-correlated noise between the different materials [22], which suggests the use of reconstruction techniques that also account for covariances [60]. Variances and covariances can be estimated using the Cramér-Rao lower bound [56]. Sawatzky *et al.* [59] and Mory *et al.* [43] proposed such an approach. The core idea of these methods is that minimizing the usual least-squares data-attachment term yields the best linear unbiased estimator (BLUE) only when all data samples are uncorrelated and have equal variance. In all other cases, the BLUE is obtained by minimizing a generalized least squares (GLS) term, which involves the inverse of the covariance matrix of the noise. Although GLS is formally simple, it is computationally much more demanding since all material-specific CT maps f_m must be reconstructed simultaneously. It is not clear yet whether the improvement in image quality is worth the increased computational complexity [43].

19.3 ONE-STEP INVERSION

One-step methods generate material maps $\boldsymbol{a}$ straight from recorded photon counts $\boldsymbol{y}$. Similar to projection-based decomposition (section 19.2), these methods can rely, for example, on the forward model in Equation 19.3, but with the advantage of not requiring matching projections (similar to image-based decomposition section 19.1). It also circumvents the fundamental drawback of all two-step approaches: the first step may introduce errors, which cannot be compensated for in the second step. An excellent illustration of this latter problem is the presence of outliers in sinograms decomposed with non-regularized projection-based methods [57, 62]: as the decomposition process is non-linear, it may strongly amplify the statistical noise on the photon counts, resulting in some pixels with entirely incorrect values for the line integral. Reconstructing without first removing these outliers yields material-specific CT maps dominated by powerful streak artifacts (Figure 19.5).

19.3.1 Forward Problem and Cost Function

Most one-step reconstruction methods apply an identical forward model, which is the equivalent to Equation 19.3 except that the two integrals (over the energies ϵ and the line positions ℓ) are discretized. Note, there is no analytical solution to this problem. Discretizing the line integral is the basis of most iterative single-energy CT reconstruction algorithms and despite being posed as a linear inverse problem, single-energy iterative CT is computationally expensive, which partly explains why manufacturers have only recently started implementing it in commercial CT scanners [50]. One-step spectral CT is even more computationally expensive: with the same number of pixels and voxels, the number of measurements is multiplied by the number B of effective spectra (second index of $\boldsymbol{y}$) and the number of unknowns is multiplied by the number M of basis energy functions (second index of $\boldsymbol{a}$), plus the inverse problem is non-linear.

In the literature, the cost functions are constructed from different terms to solve this problem. For the data-attachment, the most widespread approach is to maximize the likelihood of observing the measurements $\boldsymbol{y}$, given the material-specific CT volumes $\boldsymbol{a}$ under the assumption that the measurements are corrupted by Poisson noise [18, 33, 40, 75, 83]. Other methods minimize a weighted-least squares data-attachment term, computed either on the photon counts [77] or on the ratio between photon counts and photon counts if there had been no attenuation [9, 12]. For the regularization, various conventional options have been considered: positivity [12, 33], total-variation [9, 18], or a similar measure based on the spatial gradient [33, 40, 77, 83].

19.3.2 Minimization

Given the size and non-linearity of the one-step inversion problem, the primary challenge is to minimize the cost function. Almost every method uses a different algorithm to solve its cost function and the landscape of solutions strongly resembles that of single-energy CT.

Several works attempt to adapt methods developed for single-energy CT, which assume a linear problem. Zhao *et al.* [92] linearize the cost function and use an algebraic reconstruction technique (ART) [19]. Li *et al.* [30] do the same using filtered backprojection reconstruction. Cai *et al.* [9] used a non-linear conjugate gradient. Chen *et al.* [12] used a heuristic non-convex adaptation of ASD-POCS [66]. Rodesch *et al.* [54] adapted the maximum likelihood polychromatic algorithm of De Man *et al.* [36].

Several works [33, 40, 83] used separable quadratic surrogates (SQS). The surrogate is a tool for *optimization transfer* [25], which aims at accelerating the minimization of the cost function. Formally, the function $\Phi_{\boldsymbol{x}_0} : \mathbb{R}^N \to \mathbb{R}$ is a surrogate of the cost function $\Psi : \mathbb{R}^N \to \mathbb{R}$ at $\boldsymbol{x}_0 \in \mathbb{R}^N$ if and only if $\Phi_{\boldsymbol{x}_0}$ is above Ψ on $\mathbb{R}^N$, and tangent to Ψ at $\boldsymbol{x}_0$, that is,

$$\begin{cases} \Phi_{\boldsymbol{x}_0}(\boldsymbol{x}) & \geq \Psi(\boldsymbol{x}) \quad \forall \boldsymbol{x} \in \mathbb{R}^N, \\ \Phi_{\boldsymbol{x}_0}(\boldsymbol{x}_0) & = \Psi(\boldsymbol{x}_0) \quad \text{and} \\ \Phi'_{\boldsymbol{x}_0}(\boldsymbol{x}_0) & = \Psi'(\boldsymbol{x}_0). \end{cases} \tag{19.9}$$

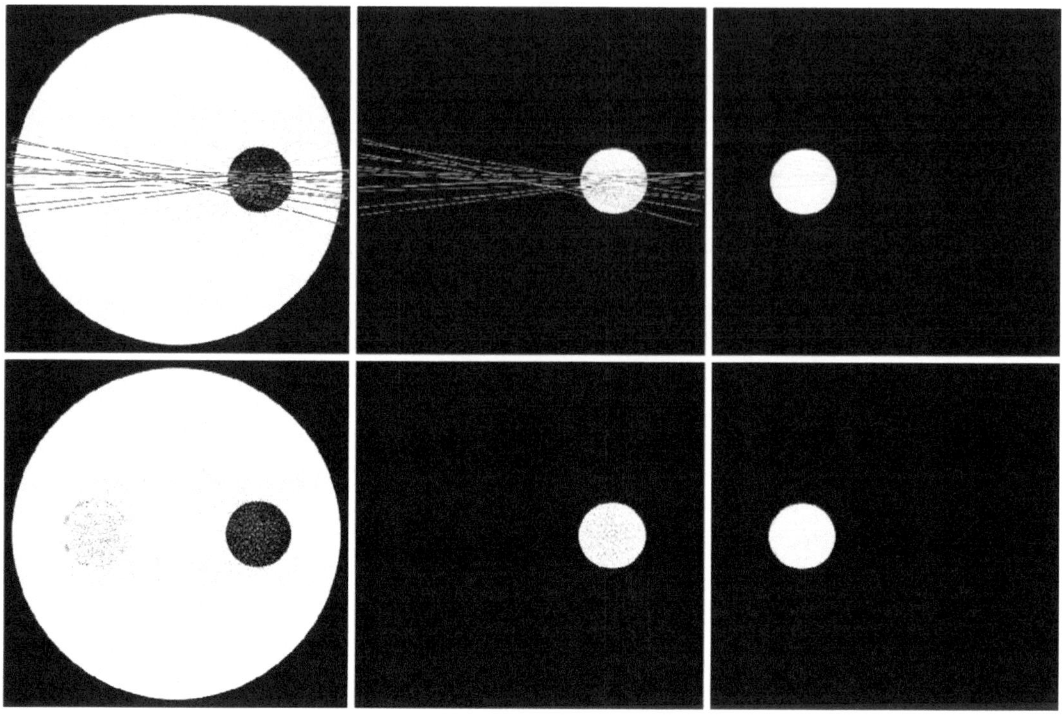

FIGURE 19.6 Projection-based (top, algorithm of [57, 62] combined with filtered-backprojection reconstruction) and one-step reconstruction (bottom, 500 iterations of the algorithm of [40] without subsets and without regularization) using the spectral model and the object described in Figure 19.5. From left to right: water, bone, and gadolinium maps. The grayscale is ±10% around the target concentration of each material.

It is separable if the contribution to Φ of one or a few unknowns can be separated from the ones of the other unknowns. The advantage is that the minimization can be split into many subproblems, each with one or a few unknowns, which can be solved in one iteration of Newton's algorithm, if these subproblems are quadratic. For spectral CT reconstruction, the existing SQS allows solving a subproblem with M unknowns per pixel [33, 40, 83]. Two SQS have been derived in the literature for one-step reconstruction [33, 83], but the inequality in Equation 19.9 is only demonstrated for the one in [33]. Since the problem is non-convex, SQS minimization would retrieve a local minimum if the initialization is not adequately chosen [33].

Some algorithms address the non-convexity using a primal-dual metric algorithm. Foygel Barber *et al.* developed the *Mirrored Convex/Concave Optimization for Nonconvex Composite Functions* (MOCCA) [18, 63], a primal-dual scheme derived from the Chambolle-Pock algorithm [11]. Tairi *et al.* [75] used a variable-metric primal algorithm [13].

Several of these algorithms have been compared in [44] on a simulated test case (three-material decomposition from a 5-bin photon-counting detector). All the algorithms converged to a visually similar solution, but there were substantial differences in convergence speed. Figure 19.6 demonstrates the potential benefit of one-step reconstruction, but it is clear that further research is required before one-step reconstruction can be routinely applied in a spectral CT scanner.

19.4 REGULARIZATION

The problem of decomposition and reconstruction for spectral CT is an ill-posed inverse problem, as is tomographic reconstruction alone [46]. Regularization is therefore required to obtain satisfying results.

In two-step decomposition algorithms, the regularization may be applied to each of the two steps, as pointed out in sections 19.1 and 19.2. Regularizing the first step is probably mandatory in both cases: this is well-known for tomographic CT reconstruction, the first step of image-based methods, and it empirically seems to be the case in projection-based decomposition (Figure 19.5), although this may depend on the number M of basis functions and the number B of effective spectra. The choice of the regularization and its strength is sensitive because it will impact the inputs of the second step. Inverting the decomposition in one step alleviates this difficulty.

There are many options for the regularization of spectral CT. As pointed out in section 19.2, only a small number of studies have suggested to regularize the decomposition of projections [1, 5, 16]. In general, the regularization is rather applied to the CT maps, that is, in the image domain. Any regularization used in tomographic reconstruction may be applied to each volume independently, for example, total variation (TV) [18, 63] or a differentiable approximation of TV [33, 40, 78, 83] (Figure 19.7), the $\ell 1$-norm of wavelets coefficients [87] or the $\ell 0$-norm of dictionaries [91]. Several such regularizers have been compared for spectral CT in [58].

Some authors have suggested to assume that the material-specific CT maps share the same structures and developed regularizations to take advantage of this similarity to improve the results. Similar strategies have been developed for dual-modality imaging such as anatomical priors from CT used in positron emission tomography (PET) reconstruction [52]. Total nuclear variation is a generalization of TV to multi-channel images, which was proposed for this specific goal [53]. Like TV, it favors a piecewise constant volume for each material, but it also favors volumes where edges have the same location and orientation. Several other multi-channel regularizers have been applied to spectral CT data [24, 48, 86].

A final class of regularization is the use of constraints to overcome a larger number of material-specific CT maps than energy measurements ($M > B$) [31–33, 42, 89]. Additional constraints are

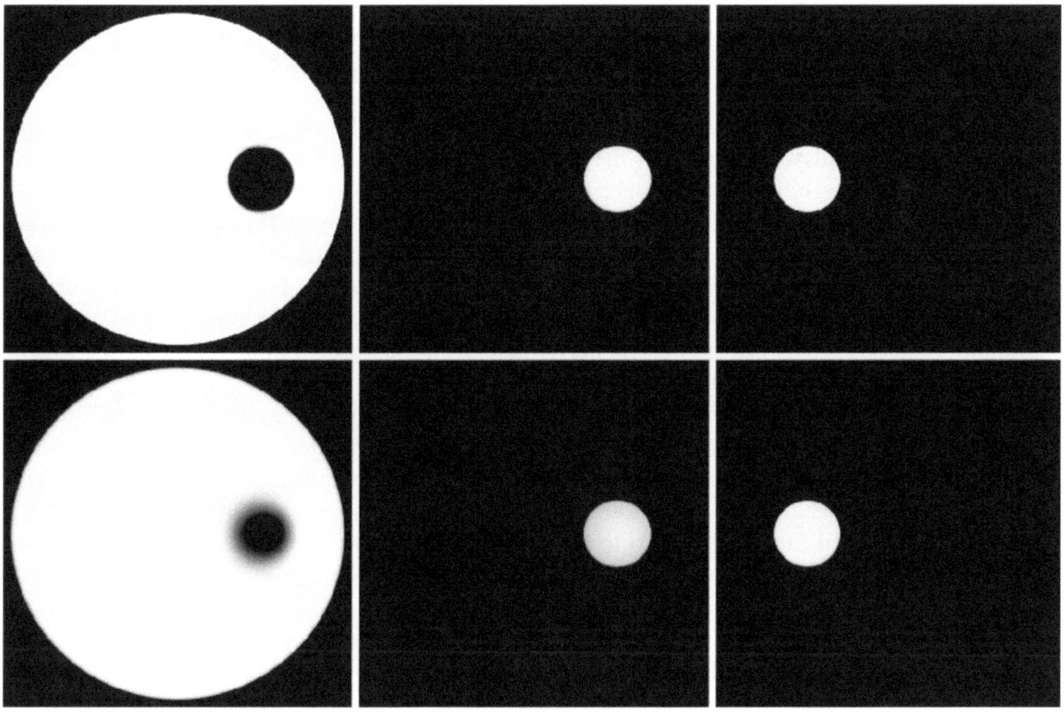

FIGURE 19.7 Effect of regularization on one-step reconstruction [40] from the same data as in Figure 19.6. The regularizer is Green's approximation of TV [20] on each material-specific CT map. The number of iterations was increased to 1000 to reach (visual) convergence. The regularization weights (one per material-specific CT map) have been first chosen to be maximum without visible cross-talk (top) and 100 times larger each (bottom). The grayscale is the same as in Figure 19.6.

added to those in Equation 19.4 or Equation 19.6 by assuming some predefined properties of the scanned materials based on volume and/or mass preservation between the sum of each material-specific CT maps and the mixture. These techniques have been applied in all types of inversions, image-based [31, 32, 42], projection-based [89], and one-step [33].

19.5 IMAGE QUALITY ISSUES SPECIFIC TO SPECTRAL CT

Spectral CT scanners can reconstruct regular CT-like volumes: the photon counts obtained from a spectral CT acquisition can be either fed to one of the spectral CT reconstruction methods described above, yielding material-specific maps, or merged back together into a single sinogram and reconstructed, generating a regular-CT volume (e.g., in Hounsfield Units, HU). Although they are reconstructed from identical input data, it turns out that material-specific CT volumes are typically much noisier than their HU counterpart. The two fundamental reasons for this phenomenon are: reconstructing several volumes instead of a single one reduces the amount of measured photons used per voxel, which results in higher noise (which can be compensated for by increasing the radiation exposure), and the non-linear decomposition process amplifies the noise.

With the introduction of photon-counting detectors into clinical routine, one can expect to see a reduction in detector pixel sizes [69, 84]. The increase in spatial resolution will extend the diagnostic range of CT imaging, for example, in the visualization of fine structures in the lung or along coronary arteries with stents [37, 65, 68]. In those cases, the high-resolution acquisition enables an improved sampling of high-frequency features and reduces noise aliasing [51]. However, for sections without fine details, a high-frequency noise will significantly reduce the image quality. In the future, it will be essential to incorporate these new circumstances into the image reconstruction and to optimize it through algorithmic solutions still to be developed. On this note, the additional energy dimension provides an increased amount of information, which can be utilized to denoise spectral images. The data can be utilized following strategies like prior image constraints [90] or dictionaries [39, 85] (section 19.4).

Additionally, material volumes are subject to decomposition errors, commonly referred to as "cross-talk": materials can appear in the wrong material-specific CT volumes. The severity of cross-talk depends on how much the materials' attenuation profiles differ from each other (the more similar they are, the stronger the cross-talk) and on how much noise is present in the photon counts (the noisier the data, the stronger the cross-talk). In one-step inversion methods, regularization can also cause cross-talk: regularizing one material creates discrepancies between the estimated photon counts and the measured ones, which are compensated by adding or removing some amount of another material. This effect is particularly intense on the borders of structures when a strong spatial regularization is applied, as illustrated in Figure 19.7.

Ring artifacts are a very common artifact in any type of CT imaging and can have a variety of sources. In conventional CT, if one detector element is out of calibration, the reading of this element may consistently be incorrect. As a consequence, the later reconstructed CT slice will be affected by rings. As photon-counting detectors are highly complex and sensitive compared to conventional detectors, a dedicated calibration needs to be performed. While this spectral technology, as well as calibration methods, are still under development, rings that may appear after reconstruction can be removed to a large degree by classical ring removal algorithms [45, 88]. Regarding rings or other artifacts, it is essential to understand that the current hardware does not represent an ideal detector. Novel sensor material (imperative for photon-counting CT), along the lines of cadmium telluride and cadmium zinc telluride, come with technical challenges which can be addressed by hardware as well as software solutions. Pile-up and spectral distortions are two of the main effects, which reduce the quality of spectral data from photon-counting detectors. Several investigators have developed techniques to model those shortcomings with different software-based techniques [10, 55, 70, 72–74]. These achievements represent an ideal opportunity to overcome some of those hardware shortcomings but they still need to be integrated in the image formation algorithms described in this chapter.

19.6 CONCLUSION

Spectral CT systems, especially systems equipped with a spectral photon-counting detector, are a promising development for the clinical routine. Many benefits concerning the diagnostic range have been discussed, which include low-dose, high-resolution, quantitative, and K-edge imaging. First prototype systems [69, 84] have been installed and have demonstrated benefits along the same lines. At the same time, one has to realize that this development comes with challenges, which translate into non-ideal imaging performances. The harmonization between hardware and software will significantly aid the process of overcoming those current shortcomings. In this chapter, we presented algorithmic solutions, which address a wide range of possible spectral CT implementations and the challenges that come along with each of them. In three sections, we introduced the main classes of spectral CT reconstruction algorithms: image-based and projection-based, which perform decomposition into materials and tomographic reconstruction separately and are therefore referred to as "two-step" methods, and one-step inversion, which merges both decomposition and reconstruction into a single inverse problem. For the coming years, while spectral CT will fully translate into the clinical routine, further algorithmic developments will be necessary to improve, for example, the sensitivity, to constantly extend the diagnostic range of CT imaging.

REFERENCES

1. J.F.P.J. Abascal, N. Ducros, and F. Peyrin. Nonlinear material decomposition using a regularized iterative scheme based on the Bregman distance. *Inverse Probl*, 34:124003, October 2018.
2. R.E. Alvarez. Estimator for photon counting energy selective x-ray imaging with multibin pulse height analysis. *Med Phys*, 38(5):2324–2334, May 2011.
3. R.E. Alvarez. Efficient, non-iterative estimator for imaging contrast agents with spectral x-ray detectors. *IEEE Trans Med Imaging*, 35(4):1138–1146, April 2016.
4. R.E. Alvarez and A. Macovski. Energy-selective reconstructions in x-ray computerized tomography. *Phys Med Biol*, 21(5):733–744, September 1976.
5. B. Brendel, F. Bergner, K. Brown, and T. Koehler. Penalized likelihood decomposition for dual layer spectral CT. In *Fourth international conference on image formation in X-ray computed tomography*, pages 41–44, Bamberg, Germany, 2016.
6. R.A. Brooks. A quantitative theory of the Hounsfield unit and its application to dual energy scanning. *J Comput Assist Tomogr*, 1(4):487–493, October 1977.
7. R.A. Brooks and G. Di Chiro. Beam hardening in x-ray reconstructive tomography. *Phys Med Biol*, 21(3):390–398, May 1976.
8. T.M. Buzug. *Computed Tomography: From Photon Statistics to Modern Cone-Beam CT.* Springer Science & Business Media, 2008.
9. C. Cai, T. Rodet, S. Legoupil, and A. Mohammad-Djafari. A full-spectral bayesian reconstruction approach based on the material decomposition model applied in dual-energy computed tomography. *Med Phys*, 40:111916, November 2013.
10. J. Cammin, J. Xu, W.C. Barber, J.S. Iwanczyk, N.E. Hartsough, and K. Taguchi. A cascaded model of spectral distortions due to spectral response effects and pulse pileup effects in a photon-counting x-ray detector for CT. *Med Phys*, 41(4):041905, March 2014.
11. A. Chambolle and T. Pock. A first-order primal-dual algorithm for convex problems with applications to imaging. *J Math Imaging Vis*, 40(1):120–145, May 2011.
12. B. Chen, Z. Zhang, E.Y. Sidky, D. Xia, and X. Pan. Image reconstruction and scan configurations enabled by optimization-based algorithms in multispectral CT. *Phys Med Biol*, 62:8763–8793, November 2017.
13. E. Chouzenoux, J.-C. Pesquet, and A. Repetti. Variable metric forward–backward algorithm for minimizing the sum of a differentiable function and a convex function. *J Optimiz Theory App*, 162(1):107–132, July 2014.
14. Q. Ding, T. Niu, X. Zhang, and Y. Long. Image-domain multi-material decomposition for dual-energy CT based on prior information of material images. *Med Phys*, 45(8):3614–3626, May 2018.
15. X. Dong, T. Niu, and L. Zhu. Combined iterative reconstruction and image-domain decomposition for dual energy CT using total-variation regularization. *Med Phys*, 41(5):051909, April 2014.

16. N. Ducros, J.F.P.-J. Abascal, B. Sixou, S. Rit, and F. Peyrin. Regularization of nonlinear decomposition of spectral x-ray projection images. *Med Phys*, 44:e174–e187, September 2017.
17. S. Ehn, T. Sellerer, K. Mechlem, A. Fehringer, M. Epple, J. Herzen, F. Pfeiffer, and P.B. Noël. Basis material decomposition in spectral CT using a semi-empirical, polychromatic adaption of the Beer-Lambert model. *Phys Med Biol*, 62:N1–N17, January 2017.
18. R. Foygel Barber, E.Y. Sidky, T. Gilat Schmidt, and X. Pan. An algorithm for constrained one-step inversion of spectral CT data. *Phys Med Biol*, 61(10):3784–3818, May 2016.
19. R. Gordon, R. Bender, and G.T. Herman. Algebraic reconstruction techniques (ART) for three-dimensional electron microscopy and x-ray photography. *J Theor Biol*, 29(3):471–481, December 1970.
20. P.J. Green. Bayesian reconstructions from emission tomography data using a modified EM algorithm. *IEEE Trans Med Imaging*, 9(1):84–93, March 1990.
21. T. Hohweiller, N. Ducros, F. Peyrin, and B. Sixou. Spectral CT material decomposition in the presence of Poisson noise: A Kullback–Leibler approach. *IRBM*, 38(4):214–218, 2017. Research in Imaging and Health TechnologieS 2017 (RITS 2017).
22. W.A. Kalender, E. Klotz, and L. Kostaridou. An algorithm for noise suppression in dual energy CT material density images. *IEEE Trans Med Imaging*, 7(3):218–224, September 1988.
23. W.A. Kalender, W.H. Perman, J.R. Vetter, and E. Klotz. Evaluation of a prototype dual-energy computed tomographic apparatus. I. Phantom studies. *Med Phys*, 13:334–339, May 1986.
24. D. Kazantsev, J.S. Jørgensen, M.S. Andersen, W.R.B. Lionheart, P.D. Lee, and P.J. Withers. Joint image reconstruction method with correlative multi-channel prior for x-ray spectral computed tomography. *Inverse Probl*, 34(6):064001, April 2018.
25. K. Lange, D.R. Hunter, and I. Yang. Optimization transfer using surrogate objective functions. *J Comput Graph Stat*, 9(1):1–20, March 2000.
26. O. Lee, S. Kappler, C. Polster, and K. Taguchi. Estimation of basis line-integrals in a spectral distortion-modeled photon counting detector using low-order polynomial approximation of x-ray transmittance. *IEEE Trans Med Imaging*, 36(2):560–573, February 2017.
27. O. Lee, S. Kappler, C. Polster, and K. Taguchi. Estimation of basis line-integrals in a spectral distortion-modeled photon counting detector using low-rank approximation-based x-ray transmittance modeling: K-edge imaging application. *IEEE Trans Med Imaging*, 36(11):2389–2403, November 2017.
28. L.A. Lehmann, R.E. Alvarez, A. Macovski, W.R. Brody, N.J. Pelc, S.J. Riederer, and A.L. Hall. Generalized image combinations in dual KVP digital radiography. *Med Phys*, 8(5):659–667, September 1981.
29. J.-M. Letang, N. Freud, and G. Peix. Signal-to-noise ratio criterion for the optimization of dual-energy acquisition using virtual x-ray imaging: Application to glass wool. *J Electron Imaging*, 13(3):436–449, July 2004.
30. M. Li, Y. Zhao, and P. Zhang. Accurate iterative FBP reconstruction method for material decomposition of dual energy CT. *IEEE Trans Med Imaging*, 38(3):802–812, March 2019.
31. Z. Li, S. Leng, L. Yu, Z. Yu, and C.H. McCollough. Image-based material decomposition with a general volume constraint for photon-counting CT. *Proceedings of SPIE–the International Society for Optical Engineering*, 9412, 2015.
32. X. Liu, L. Yu, A.N. Primak, and C.H. McCollough. Quantitative imaging of element composition and mass fraction using dual-energy CT: Three-material decomposition. *Med Phys*, 36:1602–1609, May 2009.
33. Y. Long and J.A. Fessler. Multi-material decomposition using statistical image reconstruction for spectral CT. *IEEE Trans Med Imaging*, 33(8):1614–1626, August 2014.
34. C. Maass, M. Baer, and M. Kachelriess. Image-based dual energy CT using optimized precorrection functions: A practical new approach of material decomposition in image domain. *Med Phys*, 36:3818–3829, August 2009.
35. C. Maass, E. Meyer, and M. Kachelriess. Exact dual energy material decomposition from inconsistent rays (MDIR). *Med Phys*, 38:691–700, February 2011.
36. B. De Man, J. Nuyts, P. Dupont, G. Marchal, and P. Suetens. An iterative maximum-likelihood polychromatic algorithm for CT. *IEEE Trans Med Imaging*, 20:999–1008, October 2001.
37. M. Mannil, T. Hickethier, J. von Spiczak, M. Baer, A. Henning, M. Hertel, B. Schmidt, T. Flohr, D. Maintz, and H. Alkadhi. Photon-counting CT: High-resolution imaging of coronary stents. *Invest Radiol*, 53:143–149, March 2018.
38. C.H. McCollough, S. Leng, L. Yu, and J.G. Fletcher. Dual- and multi-energy CT: Principles, technical approaches, and clinical applications. *Radiology*, 276(3):637–653, September 2015.

39. K. Mechlem, S. Allner, S. Ehn, K. Mei, E. Braig, D. Münzel, F. Pfeiffer, and P.B. Noël. A post-processing algorithm for spectral CT material selective images using learned dictionaries. *Biomed Phys Eng Express*, 3(2):025009, February 2017.
40. K. Mechlem, S. Ehn, T. Sellerer, E. Braig, D. Münzel, F. Pfeiffer, and P.B. Noël. Joint statistical iterative material image reconstruction for spectral computed tomography using a semi-empirical forward model. *IEEE Trans Med Imaging*, 37(1):68–80, January 2018.
41. K. Mechlem, T. Sellerer, S. Ehn, D. Münzel, E. Braig, J. Herzen, P.B. Noël, and F. Pfeiffer. Spectral angiography material decomposition using an empirical forward model and a dictionary-based regularization. *IEEE Trans Med Imaging*, 37(10):2298–2309, October 2018.
42. P. Mendonca, P. Lamb, and D. Sahani. A flexible method for multi-material decomposition of dual-energy CT images. *IEEE Trans Med Imaging*, 33(1):99–116, January 2014.
43. C. Mory, B. Brendel, K. Erhard, and S. Rit. Generalized least squares for spectral and dual energy CT: a simulation study. In *Sixth international conference on image formation in X-ray computed tomography*, pages 98–101, Salt Lake City, USA, 2018.
44. C. Mory, B. Sixou, S. Si-Mohamed, L. Boussel, and S. Rit. Comparison of five one-step reconstruction algorithms for spectral CT. *Phys Med Biol*, 63:235001, November 2018.
45. B. Münch, P. Trtik, F. Marone, and M. Stampanoni. Stripe and ring artifact removal with combined Wavelet–Fourier filtering. *Optics Express*, 17:8567–8591, May 2009.
46. F. Natterer. *The Mathematics of Computerized Tomography*. John Wiley & Sons, 1986.
47. J.A. Nelder and R. Mead. A simplex method for function minimization. *The Computer Journal*, 7(4):308–313, January 1965.
48. S. Niu, G. Yu, J. Ma, and J. Wang. Nonlocal low-rank and sparse matrix decomposition for spectral CT reconstruction. *Inverse Probl*, 34, February 2018.
49. T. Niu, X. Dong, M. Petrongolo, and L. Zhu. Iterative image-domain decomposition for dual-energy CT. *Med Phys*, 41(4):041901, April 2014.
50. X. Pan, E.Y. Sidky, and M. Vannier. Why do commercial CT scanners still employ traditional, filtered back-projection for image reconstruction? *Inverse Probl*, 25:1230009, January 2009.
51. A. Pourmorteza, R. Symons, A. Henning, S. Ulzheimer, and D.A. Bluemke. Dose efficiency of quarter-millimeter photon-counting computed tomography: First-in-human results. *Invest Radiol*, 53:365–372, June 2018.
52. J. Qi and R.M. Leahy. Iterative reconstruction techniques in emission computed tomography. *Phys Med Biol*, 51:R541–R578, August 2006.
53. D.S. Rigie and P.J. La Rivière. Joint reconstruction of multi-channel, spectral CT data via constrained total nuclear variation minimization. *Phys Med Biol*, 60(5):1741–1762, February 2015.
54. P.-A. Rodesch, V. Rebuffel, C. Fournier, F. Forbes, and L. Verger. Spectral CT reconstruction with an explicit photon-counting detector model: A one-step approach. *Medical Imaging 2018: Physics of Medical Imaging*, 10573: 1057353. International Society for Optics and Photonics, 2018.
55. E. Roessl, H. Daerr, and R. Proksa. A fourier approach to pulse pile-up in photon-counting x-ray detectors. *Med Phys*, 43:1295–1298, March 2016.
56. E. Roessl and C. Herrmann. Cramér-Rao lower bound of basis image noise in multiple-energy x-ray imaging. *Phys Med Biol*, 54:1307–1318, March 2009.
57. E. Roessl and R. Proksa. K-edge imaging in x-ray computed tomography using multi-bin photon counting detectors. *Phys Med Biol*, 52(15):4679–4696, August 2007.
58. M. Salehjahromi, Y. Zhang, and H. Yu. Comparison study of regularizations in spectral computed tomography reconstruction. *Sens Imaging*, 19, March 2018.
59. A. Sawatzky, Q. Xu, C.O. Schirra, and M.A. Anastasio. Proximal ADMM for multi-channel image reconstruction in spectral x-ray CT. *IEEE Tran Med Imaging,* 33(8):1657–1668, August 2014.
60. C.O. Schirra, B. Brendel, M.A. Anastasio, and E. Roessl. Spectral CT: A technology primer for contrast agent development. *Contrast Media Mol Imaging*, 9(1):62–70, January 2014.
61. C.O. Schirra, E. Roessl, T. Koehler, B. Brendel, A. Thran, D. Pan, M.A. Anastasio, and R. Proksa. Statistical reconstruction of material decomposed data in spectral CT. *IEEE Tran Med Imaging,* 32(7):1249–1257, July 2013.
62. J.P. Schlomka, E. Roessl, R. Dorscheid, S. Dill, G. Martens, T. Istel, C. Bäumer, C. Herrmann, R. Steadman, G. Zeitler, A. Livne, and R. Proksa. Experimental feasibility of multi-energy photon-counting K-edge imaging in pre-clinical computed tomography. *Phys Med Biol*, 53(15):4031–4047, August 2008.
63. T. Schmidt, R. Foygel Barber, and E. Sidky. A spectral CT method to directly estimate basis material maps from experimental photon-counting data. *IEEE Tran Med Imaging*, 36(9):1808–1819, April 2017.

64. T. Schoonjans, A. Brunetti, B. Golosio, M. Sanchez del Rio, V.A. Solé, C. Ferrero, and L. Vincze. The xraylib library for x-ray–matter interactions. Recent developments. *Spectrochim Acta B*, 66(11-12):776–784, November 2011.
65. S. Si-Mohamed, D. Bar-Ness, M. Sigovan, D.P. Cormode, P. Coulon, E. Coche, A. Vlassenbroek, G. Normand, L. Boussel, and P. Douek. Review of an initial experience with an experimental spectral photon-counting computed tomography system. *Nucl Instrum Meth A*, 873:27–35, November 2017.
66. E.Y. Sidky and X. Pan. Image reconstruction in circular cone-beam computed tomography by constrained, total-variation minimization. *Phys Med Biol*, 53(17):4777–4807, September 2008.
67. E.Y. Sidky, L. Yu, X. Pan, Y. Zou, and M. Vannier. A robust method of x-ray source spectrum estimation from transmission measurements: Demonstrated on computer simulated, scatter-free transmission data. *J Appl Phys*, 97(12):124701, June 2005.
68. R. Symons, Y. De Bruecker, J. Roosen, L. Van Camp, T.E. Cork, S. Kappler, S. Ulzheimer, V. Sandfort, D.A. Bluemke, and A. Pourmorteza. Quarter-millimeter spectral coronary stent imaging with photon-counting CT: Initial experience. *J Cardiovasc Comput*, 12(6):509–515, November 2018.
69. K. Taguchi. Energy-sensitive photon counting detector-based x-ray computed tomography. *Radiol Phys Technol*, 10:8–22, March 2017.
70. K. Taguchi, E.C. Frey, X. Wang, J.S. Iwanczyk, and W.C. Barber. An analytical model of the effects of pulse pileup on the energy spectrum recorded by energy resolved photon counting x-ray detectors. *Med Phys*, 37:3957–3969, August 2010.
71. K. Taguchi, T. Itoh, M.K. Fuld, E. Fournie, O. Lee, and K. Noguchi. "X-Map 2.0" for edema signal enhancement for acute ischemic stroke using non-contrast-enhanced dual-energy computed tomography. *Invest Radiol*, 53:432–439, July 2018.
72. K. Taguchi, C. Polster, O. Lee, K. Stierstorfer, and S. Kappler. Spatio-energetic cross talk in photon counting detectors: Detector model and correlated Poisson data generator. *Med Phys,* 43:6386, December 2016.
73. K. Taguchi, K. Stierstorfer, C. Polster, O. Lee, and S. Kappler. Spatio-energetic cross-talk in photon counting detectors: Numerical detector model (PcTK) and workflow for CT image quality assessment. *Med Phys*, 45:1985–1998, May 2018.
74. K. Taguchi, M. Zhang, E.C. Frey, X. Wang, J.S. Iwanczyk, E. Nygard, N.E. Hartsough, B.M.W. Tsui, and W.C. Barber. Modeling the performance of a photon counting x-ray detector for CT: Energy response and pulse pileup effects. *Med Phys*, 38:1089–1102, February 2011.
75. S. Tairi, S. Anthoine, C. Morel, and Y. Boursier. Simultaneous reconstruction and separation in a spectral CT framework with a proximal variable metric algorithm. In *Sixth international conference on image formation in X-ray computed tomography*, pages 32–35, Salt Lake City, USA, 2018.
76. S. Tao, K. Rajendran, C.H. McCollough, and S. Leng. Material decomposition with prior knowledge aware iterative denoising (MD-PKAID). *Phys Med Biol*, 63:195003, September 2018.
77. S. Tilley II, M. Jacobson, Q. Cao, M. Brehler, A. Sisniega, W. Zbijewski, and J.W. Stayman. Penalized-likelihood reconstruction with high-fidelity measurement models for high-resolution cone-beam imaging. *IEEE Trans Med Imaging*, 37(4):988–999, April 2018.
78. S. Tilley II, W. Zbijewski, J.H. Siewerdsen, and J.W. Stayman. A general CT reconstruction algorithm for model-based material decomposition. *Proceedings of SPIE–The International Society for Optical Engineering*, 10573, March 2018.
79. M. Torikoshi, T. Tsunoo, M. Sasaki, M. Endo, Y. Noda, Y. Ohno, T. Kohno, K. Hyodo, K. Uesugi, and N. Yagi. Electron density measurement with dual-energy x-ray CT using synchrotron radiation. *Phys Med Biol*, 48(5):673–685, March 2003.
80. W. van Elmpt, G. Landry, M. Das, and F. Verhaegen. Dual energy CT in radiotherapy: Current applications and future outlook. *Radiother Oncol*, 119(1):137–144, April 2016.
81. G. Vilches-Freixas, J.M. Létang, S. Brousmiche, E. Romero, M. Vila Oliva, D. Kellner, H. Deutschmann, P. Keuschnigg, P. Steininger, and S. Rit. Technical note: Procedure for the calibration and validation of kilo-voltage cone-beam CT models. *Med Phys*, 43(9):5199–5204, 2016.
82. X. Wang, D. Meier, K. Taguchi, D.J. Wagenaar, B.E. Patt, and E.C. Frey. Material separation in x-ray CT with energy resolved photon-counting detectors. *Med Phys*, 38:1534–1546, March 2011.
83. T. Weidinger, T.M. Buzug, T. Flohr, S. Kappler, and K. Stierstorfer. Polychromatic iterative statistical material image reconstruction for photon-counting computed tomography. *Int J Biomed Imaging*, 2016:5871604, 2016.
84. M.J. Willemink, M. Persson, A. Pourmorteza, N.J. Pelc, and D. Fleischmann. Photon-counting CT: Technical principles and clinical prospects. *Radiology*, 289:293–312, November 2018.

85. W. Wu, Y. Zhang, Q. Wang, F. Liu, P. Chen, and H. Yu. Low-dose spectral CT reconstruction using image gradient $\ell 0$–norm and tensor dictionary. *Appl Math Model*, 63:538–557, 2018.
86. W. Wu, Y. Zhang, Q. Wang, F. Liu, F. Luo, and H. Yu. Spatial-spectral cube matching frame for spectral CT reconstruction. *Inverse Probl*, 34(10):104003, 2018.
87. Q. Xu, A. Sawatzky, M.A. Anastasio, and C.O. Schirra. Sparsity-regularized image reconstruction of decomposed K-edge data in spectral CT. *Phys Med Biol*, 59(10):N65–N79, May 2014.
88. L. Yan, T. Wu, S. Zhong, and Q. Zhang. A variation-based ring artifact correction method with sparse constraint for flat-detector CT. *Phys Med Biol*, 61(3):1278–1292, February 2016.
89. L. Yu, X. Liu, and C.H. McCollough. Pre-reconstruction three-material decomposition in dual-energy CT. *Medical Imaging 2009: Physics of Medical Imaging*, 7258: 72583V. International Society for Optics and Photonics, 2009.
90. Z. Yu, S. Leng, Z. Li, and C.H. McCollough. Spectral prior image constrained compressed sensing (spectral PICCS) for photon-counting computed tomography. *Phys Med Biol*, 61:6707–6732, September 2016.
91. B. Zhao, H. Ding, Y. Lu, G. Wang, J. Zhao, and S. Molloi. Dual-dictionary learning-based iterative image reconstruction for spectral computed tomography application. *Phys Med Biol*, 57:8217–8229, December 2012.
92. Y. Zhao, X. Zhao, and P. Zhang. An extended algebraic reconstruction technique (E-ART) for dual spectral CT. *IEEE Trans Med Imaging*, 34(3):761–768, March 2015.
93. K.C. Zimmerman and T.G. Schmidt. Experimental comparison of empirical material decomposition methods for spectral CT. *Phys Med Biol*, 60(8):3175–3191, April 2015.
94. Y. Zou and M.D. Silver. Analysis of fast kV-switching in dual energy CT using a pre-reconstruction decomposition technique. *Medical Imaging 2008: Physics of Medical Imaging*, 6913: 691313. International Society for Optics and Photonics, 2008.

20 Spectral Distortion Compensation for Spectral CT

Okkyun Lee[1] *and Katsuyuki Taguchi*[2]

[1]Department of Robotics Engineering, Daegu Gyeongbuk Institute of Science and Technology, Daegu, Republic of Korea

[2]Russell H. Morgan Department of Radiology and Radiological Science, Johns Hopkins University School of Medicine, Baltimore, Maryland, USA

CONTENTS

20.1 INTRODUCTION

Photon counting detector (PCD)-based computed tomography (CT) exploits energy-dependent measurements from each of the PCD pixels to estimate basis line-integrals and has a great potential in many clinical applications such as more accurate material decomposition including K-edge imaging, reducing beam-hardening artifacts, and simultaneous multi-agent imaging [1, 2]. However, one of the challenges in the PCD-CT is the spectral distortion caused by physical effects such as charge sharing and K-escape fluorescence [1]. Conventional approaches

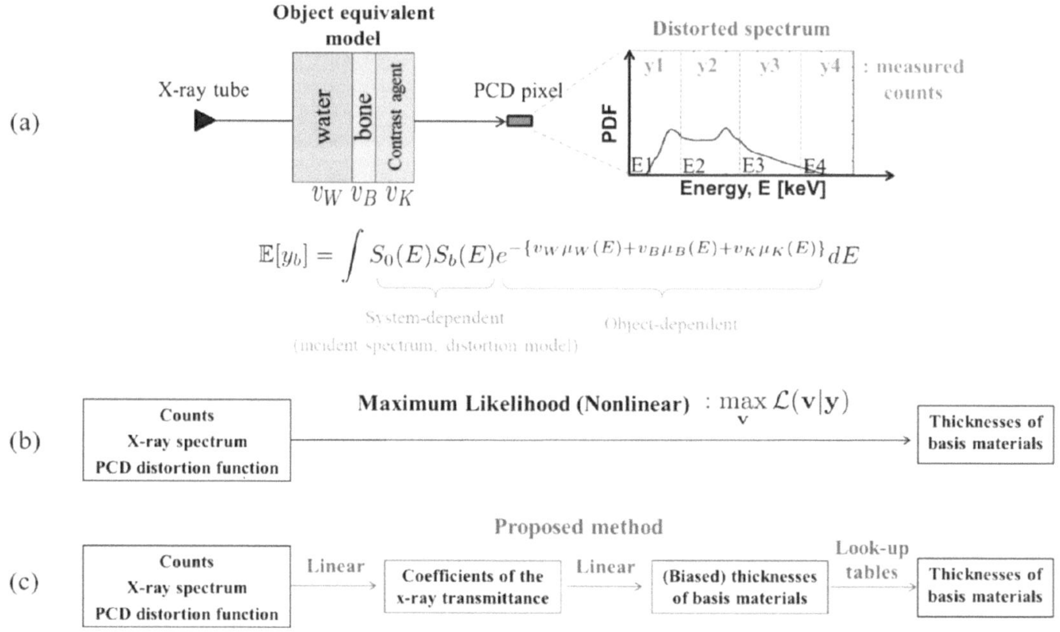

FIGURE 20.1 (a) Forward imaging chain that relates the basis line-integrals to the measured counts by the system-dependent model (x-ray incident spectrum and spectral distortion function in the PCD) and flowcharts for (b) the ML-based estimator and (c) the x-ray transmittance-based estimator.

to compensate for the spectral distortion include model-based methods and calibration-based methods. Model-based methods incorporate both the spectral distortion model and the x-ray incident spectrum in the PCD counts model and exploit the noise statistics in measured counts in the estimation (see Figure 20.1(a)). Maximum likelihood (ML)-based estimator belongs to this category [3, 4]: One can expect asymptotic optimal performance, but it requires accurate models for the incident spectrum and the spectral distortion in PCD, and it is computationally involved as it needs to solve a nonlinear optimization problem (see Figure 20.1(b)). On the other hand, calibration-based methods rely on calibration process without knowledge of the x-ray incident spectrum and the spectral distortion model [5–10]. It generates an estimator as a function of PCD measurements during the calibration process and use the estimator at the actual scan; thus, it is computationally efficient (note that all the time-consuming parts are shifted to the calibration process), but the performance depends on the heuristic calibration process. Recently, x-ray transmittance modeling-based three-step algorithm has been developed as a fast alternative to the ML-based estimator in the model-based methods [11, 12] (see Figure 20.1(c)). It decomposes the non-linear estimation process into two-linearized processes followed by an iterative bias correction step using look-up tables. It has been demonstrated by extensive studies that the three-step algorithm is as accurate as the ML-based estimators with additional benefit of computational efficiency; and also that the look-up tables used in the bias correction step may be numerically generated as long as the system models, that is, x-ray incident spectrum and spectral distortion, used in the algorithm are accurate [11–13]. Moreover, it was more robust than the ML-based estimator with low counts due to an implicit regularization in one of the linearized processes in the algorithm [11, 12] (see Figure 20.2); thus, this chapter will focus on the three-step algorithm as the spectral distortion compensation scheme on PCD-CT with a summary on other conventional schemes.

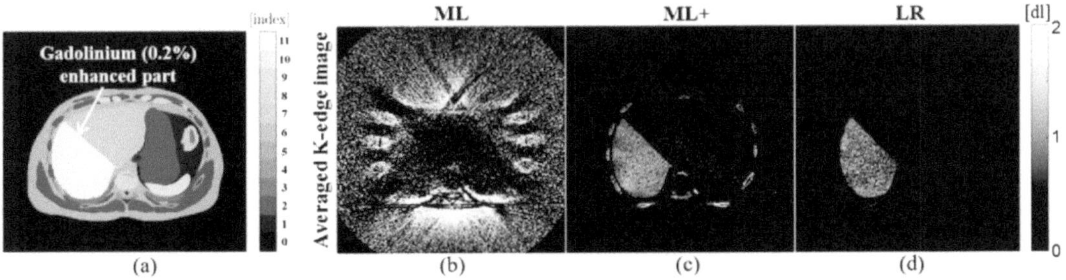

FIGURE 20.2 (a) An abdominal slice of modified X-CAT phantom [14] with gadolinium-enhanced part of liver for K-edge imaging (this figure corresponds to Figure 5(b) in [12]) and averaged K-edge images using (b) ML-based estimator (ML), (c) ML-based estimator with non-negativity constraint (ML+), and (d) the proposed three-step algorithm using low-rank (LR) approximation-based x-ray transmittance modeling ((b)-(d) correspond to Figure 13 in [12]). For more details including computational efficiency see [12]. Adapted from O. Lee, et al., "Estimation of basis line-integrals in a spectral distortion-modeled photon counting detector using low-rank approximation-based x-ray transmittance modeling: K-edge imaging application," *IEEE Trans. on Medical Imaging*, vol. 36, no. 11, pp. 2389–2403, 2017. Copyright 2017 by IEEE. Adapted with permission.

Outline of the chapter is as follows: Spectral distortions in PCD are described in Section 20.2. Conventional compensation schemes are summarized in Section 20.3, and the x-ray transmittance modeling-based three-step algorithm is described in Section 20.4. Section 20.5 is dedicated for practical implementation of the algorithm in the case of two-material decomposition as an example, and; followed by discussions in Section 20.6.

20.1.1 Notations

We define $\{E_m\}_{m=1}^{N_m}$ as a set of N_m points of the x-ray energy in the range of $E \in [E_{\min}, E_{\max}]$ with a sampling interval of 1keV. Let $X(E)$ be an arbitrary function over $[E_{min}, E_{max}]$, then we define $X \in \mathbb{R}^{N_m \times 1}$ as a discretized version of $X(E)$ such that the m-th component of X is equivalent to $X(E_m)$. We also define the unit [dl] as a dimensionless (or unitless).

20.1.2 Material Decomposition

The basic principle of material decomposition is that the linear attenuation coefficient $\mu_a(\boldsymbol{r}, E)$ [cm^{-1}] at position **r** and energy E can be modeled by a linear combination of energy-dependent basis functions such as linear attenuation coefficients of water ($\mu_W(E)$ [cm^{-1}]) and bone ($\mu_B(E)$ [cm^{-1}]):[1]

$$\mu_a(\mathbf{r}, E) = c_W(\mathbf{r})\mu_W(E) + c_B(\mathbf{r})\mu_B(E), \tag{20.1}$$

where $c_W(\boldsymbol{r})$ [dl] and $c_B(\boldsymbol{r})$ [dl] are basis coefficients of water and bone, respectively. The line-integral of (Eq. 20.1) can then be formulated as follows:

$$\begin{aligned}\int \mu_a(\mathbf{r}, E)d\mathbf{r} &= \int c_W(\mathbf{r})d\mathbf{r}\mu_W(E) + \int c_B(\mathbf{r})d\mathbf{r}\mu_B(E) \\ &= v_W\mu_W(E) + v_B\mu_B(E) \\ &= \mathbf{\Phi}(E)\mathbf{v},\end{aligned} \tag{20.2}$$

[1] One can also model it with linear attenuation coefficients of soft and hard tissues other than those of water and bone or physical phenomena such as photoelectric effect and Compton scattering. We consider here two-material decomposition for the sake of simplicity; however, one can extend it by additional basis functions for the K-edge imaging [3, 4, 9, 12].

where v_W [cm] and v_B [cm] are basis line-integrals (or thicknesses) of their corresponding basis coefficients (or materials), and $\mathbf{v} = [v_W, v_B]^T$ and $\mathbf{\Phi}(E) = [\mu_W(E), \mu_B(E)]$; thus, $\mathbf{\Phi} = [\mu_W, \mu_B] \in \mathbb{R}^{N_m \times 2}$.

20.2 SPECTRAL DISTORTIONS IN PHOTON COUNTING DETECTOR (PCD)

Measured energy spectrum at PCD is distorted due to count-rate independent spectral response effect (SRE) and count-rate dependent pulse pileup effect (PPE) [1, 4, 15–18]. The SRE is caused by various physical phenomena in the detector such as charge sharing, K-escape x-rays, and Compton scattering, and; the distortion due to the SRE becomes severe as the detector pixel size decreases, and it occurs regardless of the count rates. On the other hand, the PPE is caused by quasi-coincident photons incident to the PCDs, and it becomes severe as the count rate increases. While one eventually needs to address both the SRE and PPE, the PPE may be critical only when x-rays go through thin parts of the object (e.g., < 5 mm from skins) under clinical settings [1]. In contrast, the SRE is problematic for the entire scope of PCD application; thus, we will focus on compensating for the SRE.

The forward model for the expected measured counts with the SRE can be described as follows using (Eq. 20.2):[2]

$$\begin{aligned} \bar{y}_b(\mathbf{v}) &= \int_{E_b}^{E_{b+1}} \int_0^{\infty} S_0(E) \exp(-\mathbf{\Phi}(E)\mathbf{v}) \mathcal{S}_{SRE}(E, E') dE dE', \quad \text{for } b = 1, 2, \cdots, N_b, \\ &= \int_0^{\infty} S_0(E) \mathcal{S}_b(E) \exp(-\mathbf{\Phi}(E)\mathbf{v}) dE, \end{aligned} \tag{20.3}$$

where $\mathcal{S}_b(E) = \int_{E_b}^{E_{b+1}} \mathcal{S}_{SRE}(E, E') dE'$, N_b is the number of energy bins, E_b is the lower energy threshold for the b-th energy bin ($E_{N_b+1} = \infty$). $S_0(E)$ is the x-ray incident spectrum, and $\mathcal{S}_{SRE}(E, E')$ is a distribution function of a photon measured at energy E' when a photon is incident on the PCD pixel at energy E.[3] Using (Eq. 20.3), the measured counts including quantum noise is given as follows:

$$\mathbf{y} = \bar{\mathbf{y}}(\mathbf{v}) + \epsilon, \tag{20.4}$$

where $\mathbf{y} = [y_1, y_2, \cdots, y_{N_b}]^T$ is the vector of the measured counts, $\bar{\mathbf{y}}(\mathbf{v}) = [\bar{y}(\mathbf{v})_1, \bar{y}(\mathbf{v})_2, \cdots, \bar{y}(\mathbf{v})_{N_b}]^T$ is the expectation of $\mathbf{y}$, and $\epsilon = [\epsilon_1, \epsilon_1, \cdots, \epsilon_{N_b}]^T$ is the vector of the quantum noise.

Figure 20.3(a) shows examples of the normalized x-ray incident spectrum $S_0(E') / \int S_0(E) dE$ (140 kVp, 10 mm aluminum filtration [20]) and the normalized distorted spectrum measured at PCD due to the SRE ($\int S_0(E) \mathcal{S}_{SRE}(E, E') dE / \int\int S_0(E) \mathcal{S}_{SRE}(E, E') dE dE'$) with various detector pixel sizes (113, 225, 450, and 900 μm; generated by PcTK toolkit [19]). Note that the amount of distortion is substantial for all detector pixel sizes and it becomes severe as the pixel size decreases. Figure 20.3(b) shows examples of $\mathcal{S}_{SRE}(E, E')$ (with detector pixel size 450 μm) along the energy E' for several selected energies $E = 40$, 80, and 120 keV.

---

[2] We omitted a dependency on the direction of the line-integral in this model for the sake of simplicity; however, one can easily modify the model to include it.

[3] Note that $\int \mathcal{S}_{SRE}(E, E') dE'$ can be larger than one in practice due to cross-talks between PCD pixels [19].

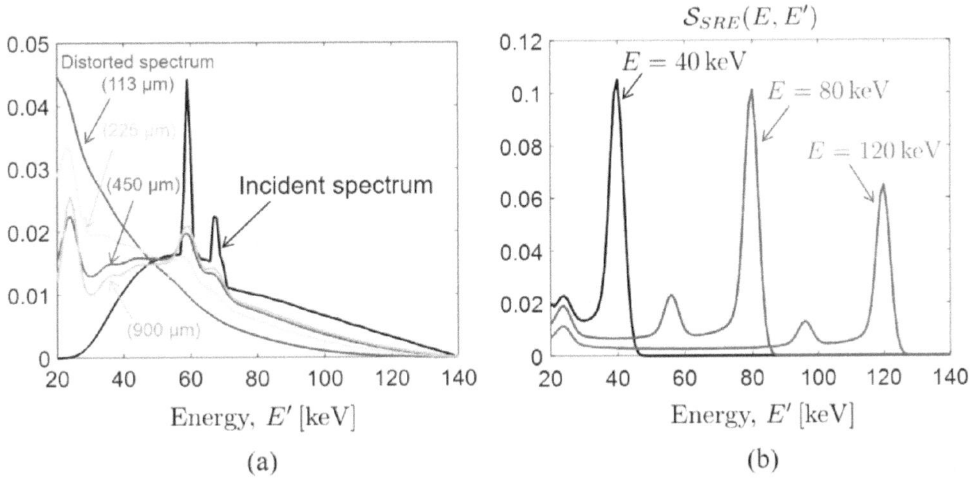

FIGURE 20.3 (a) Examples of (normalized) distorted x-ray incident spectrums due to the SRE for various detector pixel sizes (113, 225, 450, and 900 μm) and (b) spectral distortion functions, $\mathcal{S}_{SRE}(E,E')$, when $E = 40, 80,$ and 120 keV and the detector pixel size is 450 μm.

20.3 CONVENTIONAL COMPENSATION SCHEMES FOR PCD-CT

20.3.1 Maximum Likelihood (ML)-Based Estimator

The measured photon counts can be considered as independent random variables following Poisson distributions; thus, the likelihood function of the basis line-integrals can be formulated as follows:

$$f(\mathbf{v} \mid \mathbf{y}) = \prod_{b=1}^{N_b} \frac{\overline{y}_b(\mathbf{v})^{y_b}}{y_b\,!} \exp(-\overline{y}_b(\mathbf{v})). \tag{20.5}$$

The ML estimator can then be described as [3, 4],

$$\hat{\mathbf{v}} = \arg\min_{\mathbf{v}} \mathcal{L}(\mathbf{v} \mid \mathbf{y}), \tag{20.6}$$

where $\mathcal{L}(\mathbf{v} \mid \mathbf{y})$ is the negative log-likelihood as follows:

$$\mathcal{L}(\mathbf{v} \mid \mathbf{y}) = \sum_{b=1}^{N_b} [\overline{y}_b(\mathbf{v}) - y_b \ln(\overline{y}_b(\mathbf{v}))]. \tag{20.7}$$

We can also impose a boundary constraint on the basis line-integrals in (Eq. 20.7) [12, 21]. The goal of the ML estimator is to estimate $\mathbf{v}$ from the measured counts $\mathbf{y}$ given the incident spectrum $S_0(E)$ and the spectral distortion model $\mathcal{S}_{SRE}(E,E')$.

20.3.2 A-Table Estimator

A-table estimator exploits a first order Taylor expansion of the log-normalized counts:

$$\text{-}\ln(\mathbf{y}/\overline{\mathbf{y}}(\mathbf{0})) = M\mathbf{v} + \mathbf{n}, \tag{20.8}$$

where M is a sensing matrix and $\mathbf{n}$ is a residual of the expansion. It first calculates the sensing matrix and noise covariance[4] using calibration data, and; applies them on the actual scan data to estimate $\mathbf{v}$ as follows:

$$\hat{\mathbf{v}} = (M^T CM)^{-1} M^T [-\ln(\mathbf{y}/\overline{\mathbf{y}}(\mathbf{0}))], \tag{20.9}$$

where C is the noise covariance matrix. It also calculates the bias correction table (BCT) in the calibration process to correct for a bias in the estimated $\mathbf{v}$ due to the linearization:

$$\hat{\mathbf{v}}_{corrected} = \hat{\mathbf{v}} - BCT(\hat{\mathbf{v}}). \tag{20.10}$$

20.3.3 Polynomial Fitting-Based Estimator

Polynomial fitting-based estimator exploits a polynomial expansion of the log-normalized counts to estimate the basis line-integrals [5–7], and it can be described as follows:

$$\hat{v}_W (\text{or } \hat{v}_B) = c_0 + \sum_{b=1}^{N_b} c_{(1,b)} \ln(y_b / \overline{y}_b(\mathbf{0})) + \sum_{b=1}^{N_b} \sum_{b' \geq b}^{N_b} c_{(2,bb')} \ln(y_b / \overline{y}_b(\mathbf{0})) \ln(y_{b'} / \overline{y}_{b'}(\mathbf{0})) + \cdots.$$

It first calculates all the polynomial coefficients using the calibration data,[5] and; applies them to the actual scan data to estimate $\hat{\mathbf{v}}$. Note that the calibration process becomes unstable due to the substantially increased number of coefficients as the number of energy bins and the degree of the polynomial increases. Recently, a weighting scheme using subsets of energy bins [10] was developed so that the instability due to a large number of energy bins ($N_b \geq 2$) can be reduced; however, an additional calibration process using the polynomial expansion is required for the weighting scheme.

20.4 X-RAY TRANSMITTANCE MODELING-BASED THREE-STEP ESTIMATOR

In this section, we describe the x-ray transmittance modeling-based three-step estimator as the following order: (1) x-ray transmittance modeling, (2) linearized PCD forward counts model, (3) the three-step estimator, and (4) theoretical analysis.

20.4.1 X-Ray Transmittance Modeling

We define the exponentially attenuated energy-dependent line-integrals as the x-ray transmittance, $X(E)$:

$$X(E) = \exp\left(-\int \mu_a(\mathbf{r}, E) d\mathbf{r}\right) = \exp(-\boldsymbol{\Phi}(E)\mathbf{v}). \tag{20.11}$$

The x-ray transmittance modeling is to design a few energy-dependent bases $\{D_k(E)\}_{k=1}^{N_k}$ and then approximate the x-ray transmittance by a linear combination of those bases as follows:

$$X(E) = \sum_{k=1}^{N_k} D_k(E)\theta_k + \delta X(E), \text{ for } E_{min} \leq E \leq E_{max}, \tag{20.12}$$

[4] One can design the noise covariance either as independent or dependent of v [8, 9, 21].
[5] Various combinations of basis line-integrals and corresponding log normalized measurements.

where $\delta X(E)$ is the approximation error and θ_k is the coefficient for the $D_k(E)$. Note that the x-ray energy E is limited between E_{min} and E_{max}, and in practice, these values can be determined from the x-ray incident spectrum (see (Eq. 20.3) and Figure 20.3(a)). Once we design the bases $\{D_k(E)\}_{k=1}^{N_k}$, we can use them to linearize the PCD forward counts model and then derive the three-step estimator as will be described later. Key observations on the x-ray transmittance modeling are that the number of bases N_k should be less than or equal to the number of energy bins N_b (the reason will be given in Section 20.4.2) and that the bases need to be designed as accurate as possible with the limited number of energy bins; thus, we focus on how to design the bases, $\{D_k(E)\}_{k=1}^{N_k}$.

One possible solution is to use low-order polynomials as the bases to model the x-ray transmittance without K-edge materials; we showed that four polynomial curves (0–3 degrees) are sufficient to model the smooth x-ray transmittances accurately [11]. However, the smooth low-order polynomials are not adequate to model an x-ray transmittance with K-edge material such as iodine (K-edge in 33.2 keV) or gadolinium (K-edge in 50.2 keV), and the low-order polynomials are not the optimal bases but heuristically selected ones. To address these issues, we recently developed a low-rank approximation-based x-ray transmittance modeling as a generalized approach to model an arbitrarily shaped x-ray transmittance regardless of the presence or absence of K-edge materials. The main idea of this approach is, instead of using fixed bases such as the low-order polynomials, to design bases that best describes a set of x-ray transmittances with various shapes. The set of x-ray transmittances can be generated by multiple combinations of materials depending on specific aims, for example, mixtures of various thicknesses of water and bone for two-material decomposition or those of water, bone, and a K-edge material for three-material decomposition including the K-edge imaging. An example of a set of normalized x-ray transmittances generated from various thicknesses of water (10 cm to 30 cm with 1 cm interval) is shown in Figure 20.4(a). A mathematical description for designing the bases is given as follows: Let $X_t(E)$ be the x-ray transmittance from the t-th combination of line-integrals and its discretized version X_t constitute the t-th column of the x-ray transmittance matrix, then the design of the bases can be formulated by the following optimization problem:

$$(\hat{D},\hat{\Theta}) = \arg\min_{D,\Theta} \|XW - D\Theta\|_F, \tag{20.13}$$

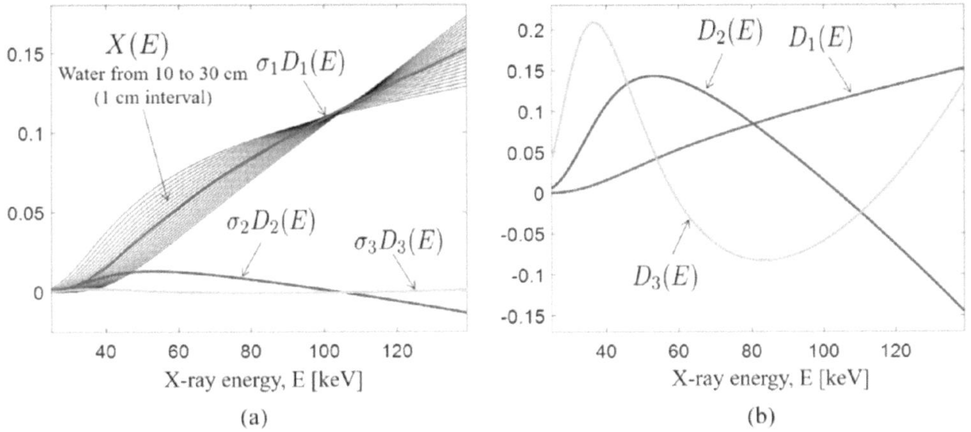

FIGURE 20.4 (a) Various (normalized to have a unit ℓ_2 norm) x-ray transmittances $X(E)$ generated from water 10 cm to 30 cm with 1 cm interval and three left singular vectors $\{D_k(E)\}_{k=1}^{3}$ calculated from these transmittances using the low-rank approximation (scaled by their associated singular values $\{\sigma_k\}_{k=1}^{3}$, and; the largest singular value has been normalized to one) and (b) the three left singular vectors without the scaling.

where $\|\cdot\|_F$ denotes the Frobenius norm, $X = [X_1, X_2, \cdots, X_{N_t}] \in \mathbb{R}^{N_m \times N_t}$ is the x-ray transmittance matrix with N_t different shapes of x-ray transmittances, $D = [D_1, D_2, \cdots, D_{N_k}] \in \mathbb{R}^{N_m \times N_k}$ is the discretized version of the bases set, $\Theta = [\theta_1, \theta_2, \cdots, \theta_{N_t}] \in \mathbb{R}^{N_k \times N_t}$ is the corresponding coefficients matrix, and the dimension satisfies $N_k << N_m << N_t$. $W \in \mathbb{R}^{N_t \times N_t}$ is a diagonal matrix whose i-th diagonal component is $W_{ii} = \| X_i \|_2^{-1}$ to normalize the matrix X so that each x-ray transmittance has a unit ℓ_2 norm. The role of this normalization is to prevent the design biased on modeling x-ray transmittances having large norm.[6] Note that $\text{rank}(D\Theta) \leq N_k$; thus, (Eq. 20.13) is equivalent to the following low-rank approximation problem:

$$\hat{X} = \arg\min_{\tilde{X}} \left\| XW - \tilde{X} \right\|_F, \quad \text{s.t. } \text{rank}(\tilde{X}) \leq N_k, \tag{20.14}$$

where N_k is the given rank. The unique solution of (Eq. 20.14) is given by Eckart and Young [22]: First N_k left singular vectors of the normalized x-ray transmittance matrix. For example, the first three left singular vectors calculated from the set of x-ray transmittance in Figure 20.4(a) are shown in Figure 20.4(b). We also plot the scaled left singular vectors by their corresponding singular values in Figure 20.4(a). The first singular vector delineates the global tendency of the set of x-ray transmittance, and the remaining singular vectors adjust the details of the shape, but; the effect substantially declines as the singular values decrease. It demonstrates the effectiveness of the low-rank approximation-based x-ray transmittance modeling with a limited number of energy-dependent bases. Section 20.5 provides numerical analysis on $\delta X(E)$ from the low-rank approximation-based x-ray transmittance modeling in a broad range of attenuations of water and bone.[7]

20.4.2 Linearized PCD Forward Counts Model

Substituting (Eq. 20.12) into (Eq. 20.3), the forward counts model (Eq. 20.4) can be linearized with the basis coefficients θ as follows:

$$\begin{aligned} \mathbf{y} &= B\theta + \eta + \epsilon \\ &\approx B\theta + \epsilon, \end{aligned} \tag{20.15}$$

where b-th row and k-th column of the sensing matrix $B \in \mathbb{R}^{N_b \times N_k}$ is given by

$$B_{(b,k)} = \int_{E_{min}}^{E_{max}} S_0(E) S_b(E) D_k(E) dE. \tag{20.16}$$

The modeling error η comes from the approximation error $\delta X(E)$ in (Eq. 20.12), and it is given by

$$\eta_b = \int_{E_{min}}^{E_{max}} S_0(E) S_b(E) \delta X(E) dE. \tag{20.17}$$

Section 20.5 provides numerical analysis on η for a broad range of attenuations of water and bone.[8]

---

[6] The x-ray transmittance with the largest norm is $X(E) = 1$ (without object).

[7] $N_k = 3$ was sufficient to have less than 2% of the relative approximation error on average in a broad range of attenuations of water, bone, and gadolinium (see [12]).

[8] The relative ratio of the norm of the modeling error η to that of the quantum noise was about 50% when $N_k = 3$ (25% when $N_k = 4$) on average in a broad range of attenuations of water, bone, and gadolinium (the number of incident photons was 275,000; see the supplementary material of [12]).

Note that the number of bases should be less than or equal to the number of energy bins ($N_k \leq N_b$) to avoid (Eq. 20.15) to be an under-determined problem. Note also that the original nonlinear counts model is linearized with the coefficients θ.

20.4.3 Three-Step Estimator

Using the linearized forward counts model in (Eq. 20.15), we can derive the three-step estimator as presented in this section. Practical implementations with an example of two-material decomposition will be given in Section 20.5.

20.4.3.1 1st Step: Estimation of the X-Ray Transmittance

The first step is to estimate the x-ray transmittance using the linearized model (Eq. 20.15). We first calculate the coefficients θ from the measured counts $\mathbf{y}$ by solving the following penalized least squares fitting:

$$\begin{aligned}\hat{\theta} &= \arg\min_{\theta} \|\mathbf{y} - B\theta\|^2 + \lambda\|C\theta\|^2 \\ &= (B^T B + \lambda C^T C)^{-1} B^T \mathbf{y},\end{aligned} \tag{20.18}$$

where $C \in \mathbb{R}^{N_k \times N_k}$ is a regularization matrix. The x-ray transmittance can then be calculated as follows:

$$\hat{X} = \sum_{k=1}^{N_k} D_k \hat{\theta}_k. \tag{20.19}$$

20.4.3.2 2nd Step: Estimation of the Basis Line-integrals

The second step is to estimate the basis line-integrals from the result of the first step (Eq. 20.19) using the least squares fitting as follows:

$$\begin{aligned}\hat{\mathbf{v}} &= \arg\min_{\mathbf{v}} \left\|\ln(\hat{X}) + \mathbf{\Phi}\mathbf{v}\right\|_2^2 \\ &= \mathbf{\Phi}^{\dagger}[-\ln(\hat{X})].\end{aligned} \tag{20.20}$$

In practice, the following two issues need to be addressed before taking the log-transform to the estimated x-ray transmittance: (1) negative values in the estimated x-ray transmittance and (2) noise boosting from the log-transform. More specifically, the second issue comes from the observation that the x-ray transmittance decreases toward zero at each of the x-ray energies as the amount of attenuation increases, and it happens rather quickly in the lower energy part where the attenuation coefficients have large values. Therefore, the lower energy part is the most error-prone part of the logarithm operation, since the log-transform can boost even a small error in the small value of the estimated x-ray transmittance. To address these issues, we implement two safeguard schemes: the first scheme is to discard $R(\hat{X})$ points in the lowest energies of the estimated $\hat{X}$ and the second one is to clip the values of $\hat{X}$ under a predefined threshold value. We call these a pruning process and the detailed implementation is described in Section 20.5.

20.4.3.3 3rd Step: Iterative Bias Correction

Note that the linearization processes in the previous steps make the estimation computationally efficient and also that the regularization in the first step and the safeguard schemes in the second step stabilize possible noise boosting during the estimation. However, these linearization and stabilization processes can cause a bias in the estimated $\hat{\mathbf{v}}$; thus, the third step is necessary to correct for the bias. The conventional method is to use a bias look-up table ($BCT(\mathbf{v})$) generated before the actual scans using calibration data of various thicknesses of objects [8, 9]. More specifically, $BCT(\mathbf{v}) = [BCT_W(\mathbf{v}), BCT_B(\mathbf{v})]^T$, where $BCT_W(\mathbf{v})$ and $BCT_B(\mathbf{v})$ are the bias of water and bone, respectively, when the ground truth of basis line-integral is $\mathbf{v}$; thus, each $BCT_{\{W\ or\ B\}}(\mathbf{v})$ is a two-dimensional look-up table.[9] The bias of $\hat{\mathbf{v}}$ then can be corrected as follows:

$$\hat{\mathbf{v}}_{corrected} \leftarrow \hat{\mathbf{v}} - BCT(\hat{\mathbf{v}}). \tag{20.21}$$

In order to substantially reduce the bias in $\hat{\mathbf{v}}$, the argument of the generated $BCT(\cdot)$ must be close enough to the ground truth, which is a challenge in practice; however, the difference between the two variables can be decreased (and so does the residual bias) by repeating (Eq. 20.21) and updating $\hat{\mathbf{v}}$ iteratively as follows:

$$\hat{\mathbf{v}}^{(q)} = \hat{\mathbf{v}}^{(q-1)} - BCT^{(q)}(\hat{\mathbf{v}}^{(q-1)}), \text{ for } q = 1, 2, \cdots, \text{Iter}_{\max}, \tag{20.22}$$

where the superscript q denotes the index of iterations; thus, $\hat{\mathbf{v}}^{(0)}$ is the initial estimation without bias correction, and $\hat{\mathbf{v}}^{(q)}$ indicates the bias-corrected result with q iterations. Note that the benefit of using the iterative approach is apparent as described in the following section.

20.4.4 Theoretical Analysis

We provide theoretical analysis for the stability and convergence in the first and third steps of the algorithm, respectively.

20.4.4.1 Stability Analysis for the Estimation of the Basis Coefficients

The role of the cost function in (Eq. 20.18) can be separated into the data fidelity term and the regularization term, and each of the terms needs the following assumptions $\mathcal{A}1$ and $\mathcal{A}2$, respectively, for the analysis:

$$\mathcal{A}1: \lambda \to 0,\ \eta \to \mathbf{0},\ \det(B) \neq 0,\ \mathbf{y} > \mathbf{0},$$
$$\mathcal{A}2: \lambda \to 0,\ \|\eta\|_2 < \|\bar{\mathbf{y}}(\mathbf{v})\|_2.$$

Both assumptions require $\lambda \to 0$, so the analysis will be done without the regularization term. The meanings of the second to the fourth assumptions in $\mathcal{A}1$ are the x-ray transmittance modeling is precise, the square ($N_k = N_b$) sensing matrix B is invertible, and at least one photon is measured in each energy bin, respectively.[10] The second assumption in $\mathcal{A}2$ means that the amount of modeling error is less than that of the original signal in the model.[11] Using the above assumptions, we can prove the following two analyses:

1. Data fidelity term: It becomes a simple least squares fitting in general (when $N_k \leq N_b$), but it provides a unique ML solution when $N_k = N_b$ under the assumption $\mathcal{A}1$ (see Proposition 1 in [11]).

---

[9] The dimension of the table increases as the number of basis materials increases. For example, if one considers the additional third basis for the sake of K-edge imaging, then three-dimensional bias correction tables for water, bone, and the K-edge material will be needed [12].

[10] Note that the third and fourth assumptions in $\mathcal{A}1$ are trivial.

[11] The second assumption in $\mathcal{A}2$ is reasonable in practice and much less restrictive than that of the $\mathcal{A}1$.

2. Regularization term: Under the assumption $\mathcal{A}2$, the relative mean squared error of the estimated coefficients in (Eq. 20.18) can be upper-bounded as follows when $N_k = N_b$:

$$\mathbb{E}\left[\frac{\|\hat{\theta}-\theta\|_2^2}{\|\theta\|_2^2}\right]^{\frac{1}{2}} \le \kappa(B)\frac{\sqrt{\sqrt{N_b}\|\bar{\mathbf{y}}\|_2 + \|\eta\|_2^2}}{\|\bar{\mathbf{y}}\|_2 - \|\eta\|_2}, \tag{20.23}$$

where $\kappa(B)$ is the condition number of the sensing matrix B. Note that (Eq. 20.23) is a generalized sensitivity analysis compared to those of Proposition 2 and corollary 3 in [12], where the sensitivity analysis was performed with additional assumption of $\bar{y}_1 = \bar{y}_2 = \cdots = \bar{y}_{N_b}$. The proof of (Eq. 20.23) is the same with those provided in [12] with the additional property of $\|\bar{\mathbf{y}}\|_1 \le \sqrt{N_b}\,\|\bar{\mathbf{y}}\|_2$.[12] Note that the positivity of the denominator of the upper-bound is guaranteed from the second assumption in $\mathcal{A}2$ and that the error bound is a strictly increasing function of the amount of attenuation,[13] the number of energy bins (N_b), the modeling error ($\|\eta\|_2$), and the condition number $\kappa(B)$; thus, the sensitivity analysis in (Eq. 20.23) demonstrates the necessity of the regularization in the first step. One may be confused that the number of energy bins can make the error bound increase, but note that there is a trade-off between N_b and $\|\eta\|_2$: $\|\eta\|_2$ increases as N_b decreases, and *vice versa* (see [12] for the numerical assessments). It is worth to mention that the sensitivity analysis in (Eq. 20.23) also shows the benefit of using the low-rank approximation-based x-ray transmittance modeling in the stability point of view since it guarantees the least amount of modeling error with the fewest bases possible. We have also found that having equal weight on the coefficients vector θ (i.e., $C = I$, where I is an identity matrix) is not effective as the regularization matrix due to a large variation on the magnitude of the coefficients θ. For example, the magnitude of each coefficient is proportional to the associated singular value of the basis after the low-rank approximation; thus, we set the regularization matrix as $C = \hat{\Sigma}^{-1}$, where $\hat{\Sigma} \in \mathbb{R}^{N_k \times N_k}$ is the singular value matrix from the low-rank approximation,[14] to provide the equal penalty on the coefficients normalized by the singular values (see [12] for the numerical assessments for the comparison of different regularization matrices).

20.4.4.2 Convergence Analysis for the Iterative Bias Correction Method

Under the assumption $\mathcal{A}3$ (shown below), a sufficient condition for the conventional correction method to be unbiased is the condition $\mathcal{A}4$ with $L = 0$ and $q = 1$ (see Proposition 3 in [11]), and a sufficient condition for the proposed iterative method converges to the unbiased solution is the condition $\mathcal{A}4$ with $L < 1$ and $q = 1,2,\cdots$ (see Proposition 4 in [11]).

$$\mathcal{A}3: \mathbb{E}[BCT^{(q)}(\hat{\mathbf{v}}^{(q-1)})] = BCT^{(q)}(\mathbb{E}[\hat{\mathbf{v}}^{(q-1)}]) \tag{20.24}$$

$$\mathcal{A}4: \left\|BCT^{(q)}(v_1) - BCT^{(q)}(v_2)\right\|_2 \le L\|v_1 - v_2\|_2, \tag{20.25}$$

[12] Due to the inequality of $\|\bar{\mathbf{y}}\|_1 \le \sqrt{N_b}\,\|\bar{\mathbf{y}}\|_2$, the upper-bound in (Eq. 20.23) is less tight than those in Proposition 2 and corollary 3 in [12].

[13] The upper-bound in (Eq. 20.23) is a strictly decreasing function of $\|\bar{\mathbf{y}}\|_2$, which is inversely proportional to the amount of attenuation.

[14] We use the normalized singular value matrix so that the least non-zero element becomes 1.

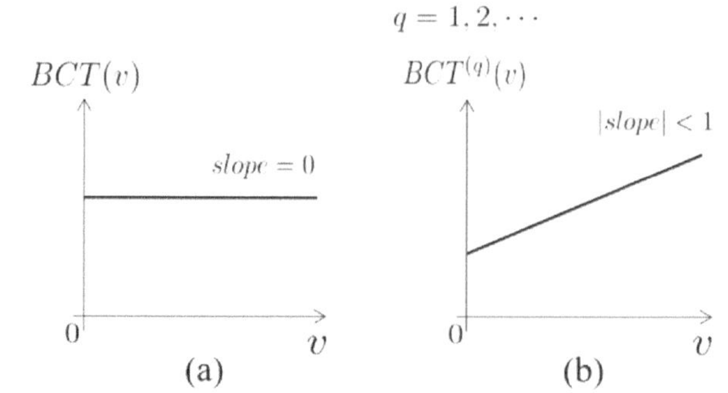

FIGURE 20.5 Example of bias correction tables for the (a) conventional non-iterative and (b) proposed iterative bias correction method to be unbiased. The problem is simplified to the one-material decomposition; thus, the x-axis denotes the thickness of the material and y-axis denotes the corresponding bias.

where $\mathbf{v}_1$ and $\mathbf{v}_2$ are arbitrary basis line-integrals. The assumption $\mathcal{A}3$ describes that $BCT^{(q)}(\mathbf{v})$ satisfies the equality of Jensen's inequality [23], and it is well known that an affine function is guaranteed to satisfy it.[15] The condition $\mathcal{A}4$ describes that $BCT^{(q)}(\mathbf{v})$ satisfies the Lipschitz continuity with the Lipschitz constant L with the usual metric (Euclidean distance). In other words, between any two points, the difference in their biases is smaller than the difference in their values (line integrals). Thus, it is a reasonable condition unless the BCTs have an abrupt change in their values. Figures 20.5(a) and (b) show examples of $BCT^{(q)}(\mathbf{v})$ for the conventional and iterative bias correction methods to be unbiased, respectively. The problem is simplified to the one-dimensional case, that is, one basis material, and $BCT^{(q)}(\mathbf{v})$ is assumed to be affine, that is, $\mathcal{A}3$ is guaranteed. Note that the condition to be unbiased for the proposed iterative bias correction method is less restrictive compared to that of the conventional (non-iterative) correction method, and it clearly shows the benefit of using the iterative approach.

20.5 PRACTICAL IMPLEMENTATIONS: EXAMPLE OF TWO-MATERIAL DECOMPOSITION

This section describes details of practical implementations of the three-step algorithm to the case of two-material decomposition: The following subsections correspond to the first, second, and third step of the algorithm, respectively, followed by results for the estimation of thicknesses of water and bone in slab-geometry with a comparison to those of the ML-based estimator. We set the energy thresholds as 20, 40, 60, and 80 keV and set $N_b = N_k = 4$. We used the spectral distortion function for the detector size of 450 μm and the incident x-ray spectrum shown in Figure 20.3. We then set $E_{min} = 25$ keV and $E_{max} = 139$ keV, and also set the number of incident photons as $\int S_0(E)dE = 3\times 10^5$.

20.5.1 X-Ray Transmittance Modeling

The first thing to do is to generate the x-ray transmittance matrix for the low-rank approximation. We use various combination of water (0–35 cm with 0.5 cm interval) and bone (0–5 cm with 0.2 cm interval) to generate the various shape of x-ray transmittances, that is, x-ray transmittance matrix. We also use multiple combination of water (0.25–35 cm with 0.5 cm interval) and bone (0.1–5 cm with 0.2 cm interval) to generate various x-ray transmittances as a test data set so that they can be

[15] Note that being an affine function is a sufficient condition for $\mathcal{A}3$. In [11], $\mathcal{A}3$ was demonstrated by numerical assessment for a broad range of basis line-integrals of the photoelectric effect and Compton scattering.

used for validating the model using quantitative analysis. Once the x-ray transmittance matrix is prepared, one can apply the low-rank approximation to get the energy-dependent bases. Figures 20.6(a) and (b) show a normalized singular value distribution and first four left singular vectors of the x-ray transmittance matrix (i.e., four energy-dependent bases), respectively. Note that all the singular values except the first four are less than 1% of the first singular value. Figures 20.6(c) and (d) show examples of x-ray transmittance modeling as a linear combination of the four bases shown in Figure 20.6(b) when the object is pure water 10 cm, and a mixture of water 25 cm and bone 2 cm, respectively. Figure 20.6(e) illustrates a two-dimensional map of the relative approximation error, $\frac{\|X-\delta X\|_2}{\|X\|_2} \times 100\%$, and Figure 20.6(f) the ratio of the magnitude of the modeling error to that of

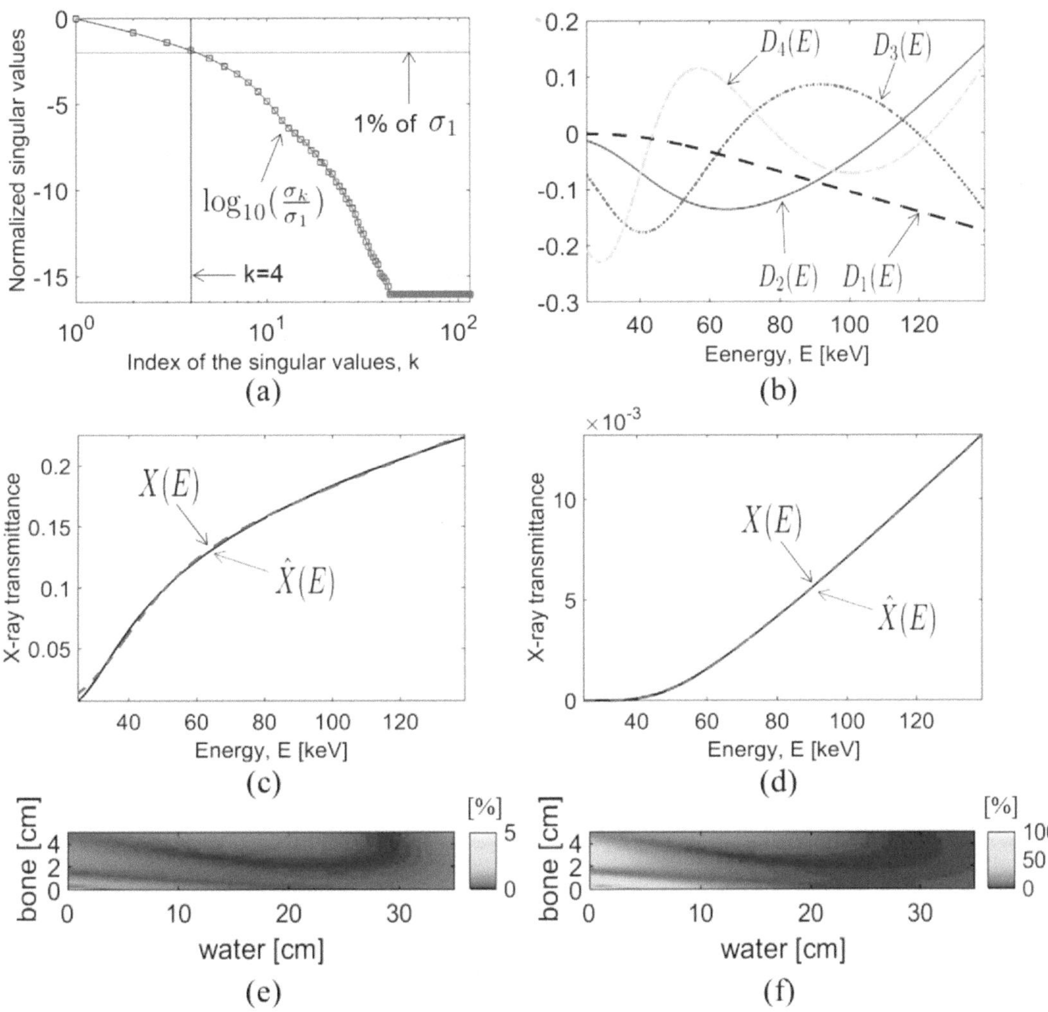

FIGURE 20.6 (a) Distribution of singular values for the x-ray transmittance matrix (the first four singular values are 42.44, 6.42, 1.76, and 0.6; these values will be used in the regularization matrix as described in Section 20.4.4.1), (b) four left singular vectors, (c) examples of x-ray transmittance modeling when water 10 cm and bone 0 cm and (d) when water 25 cm and bone 2 cm, (e) two-dimensional map for the relative approximation error, and (f) two-dimensional map of the ratio of the magnitude of the modeling error to that of the quantum noise on average (for each of the coordinates, that is, the corresponding combination of water and bone, the test data of the x-ray transmittance is generated).

the quantum noise on average, $\frac{\|\eta\|_2}{\sqrt{\mathbb{E}\|\epsilon\|^2}} \times 100\%$, using the test data set as the ground truth X. Note that the relative approximation error is much less than 5% throughout the whole attenuation range and also that the modeling error is relatively smaller than that of the quantum noise in general.

20.5.2 Pruning Process

Figure 20.7(a) shows two safeguard schemes to stabilize the second step of the algorithm (see Section 20.4.3.2). First, one should determine the number of neglecting points, $R(\hat{X})$, in the estimated x-ray transmittance $\hat{X}$ and discard it (see the appendix C in [12] for a detailed description of how to calculate $R(\hat{X})$); and crop the values in the $\hat{X}$ below the threshold, $0.02 \times \max(\hat{X})$. Figure 20.7(b) illustrates two-dimensional map of $R(X)$ where X is the ground truth of the x-ray transmittance.

20.5.3 Bias Correction Tables

BCTs need to be generated *a priori* to the actual scan, and detailed procedure is given as follows:

1. Determine the attenuation range for basis materials, that is, thicknesses of water and bone in this case, that sufficiently cover the amount of attenuation for a target object. Here, we set the water from 0 cm to 35 cm with 1 cm of interval and bone from 0 cm to 5 cm with 0.5 cm of interval.
2. Generate multiple noise realizations (10,000 in this example) for measured counts using the forward model in (Eq. 20.3) and (Eq. 20.4) for each of the combinations of the materials.

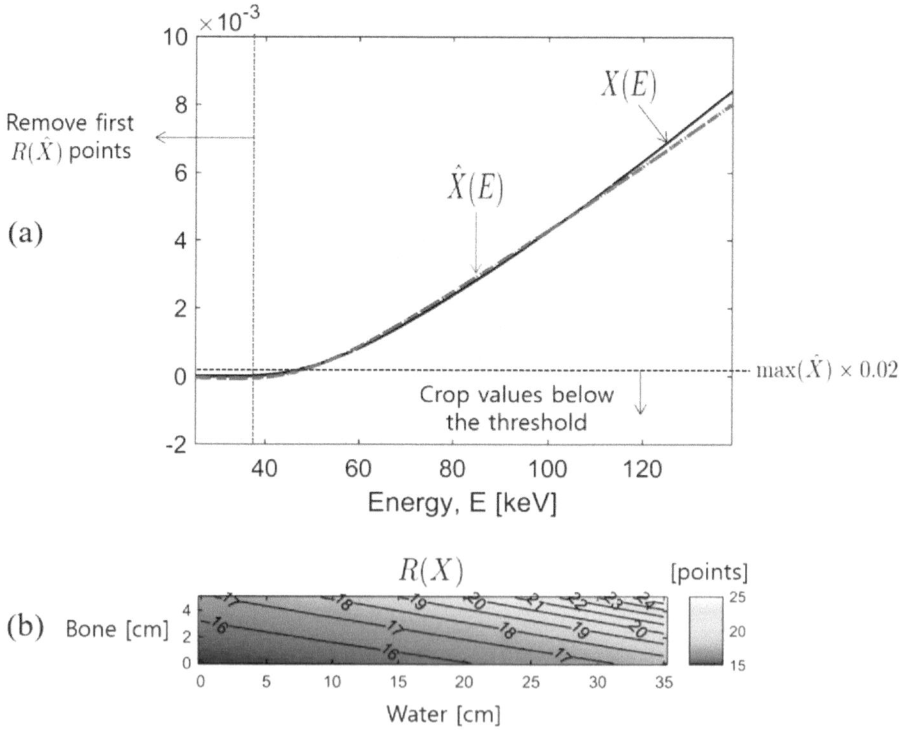

FIGURE 20.7 (a) Two safe-guard schemes applied in the estimated x-ray transmittance (water 28 cm and bone 2 cm) to stabilize the second step and (b) two-dimensional map of the $R(\hat{X})$ when X is a ground truth. Specific values used to calculate $R(\hat{X})$ are $E_b = 70$ keV, $R_{\min} = 15$, $R_{\max} = 25$, $c_1 = 1$, and $c_2 = 33.36$ (see [12] for the role of these values).

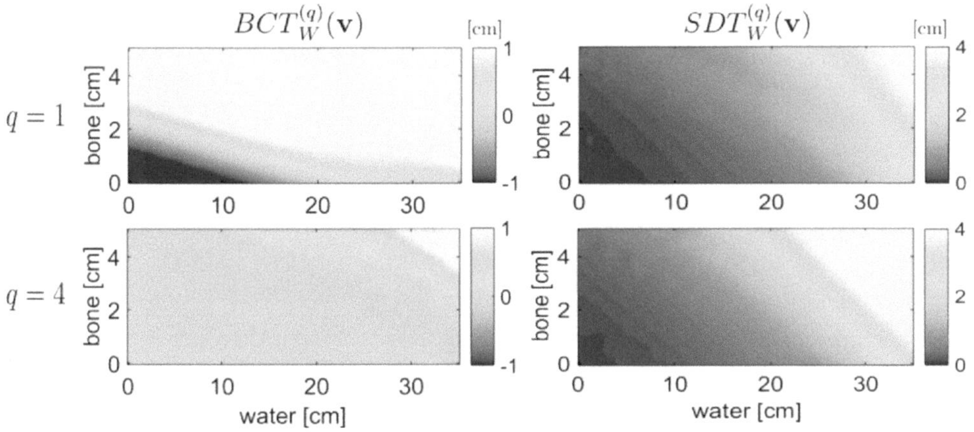

FIGURE 20.8 Bias correction tables (first column) and standard deviation tables (second column) of water when $q = 1$ (first row) and $q = 4$ (second row) for the selected parameters of $\lambda = 4$ and $\text{Iter}_{\text{max}} = 3$.

3. Set various values of the regularization parameter (λ in (Eq. 20.18))[16] and, for each of the values, apply the first and second steps of the algorithm to the synthesized noisy counts to calculate the bias for water and bone, and then generate BCTs for each of the materials.
4. Using (Eq. 20.22), generate following BCTs for a sufficiently large number of iterations (Iter_{max}). For each iteration, interpolate the BCTs so that the discretization error can be minimized. Here, we interpolated it with 0.2 cm of interval for water and 0.1 cm for bone.
5. Throughout the processes 3 and 4, one can also generate the standard deviation tables and use them to determine the regularization parameter and number of iterations.
6. Calculate the average amount of bias and standard deviation for the entire table for each of the iterations and candidate values for the λ.
7. Find the minimum iteration number that satisfies below the given average bias (1 mm for water in this example) for each of the λ, and; then find the λ that shows the minimum average standard deviation at the iteration found before. Use that λ, iteration number, and the corresponding BCTs for the actual scan (here, $\lambda = 4$ and $\text{Iter}_{\text{max}} = 3$).[17]

Figure 20.8 illustrates the two-dimensional BCTs ($BCT_W^{(q)}(\mathbf{v})$) and standard deviation tables ($SDT_W^{(q)}(\mathbf{v})$) for water. Note that the bias of water in the table is substantially reduced after applying the proposed correction method three times. On the other hand, the standard deviation increased after the three iterations; but, the results in the next section will show that the standard deviation satisfies the Cramer-Rao lower bound (CRLB), numerically demonstrating that the proposed method is nearly the minimum variance and unbiased (MVU) estimator.

20.5.4 Numerical Results

We have done all the necessary preprocessing for the three-step algorithm, that is, low-rank approximation-based x-ray transmittance modeling and determining the regularization parameters and the number of iterations for the bias correction step. We apply the three-step algorithm with these preprocessed results for estimating the basis line-integrals (i.e., thicknesses of water and bone) of

[16] For computational efficiency, one can set several candidates for regularization parameter and then iteratively refine the candidate values.
[17] See [12] for another suggestion for selecting the regularization parameter and the number of iterations.

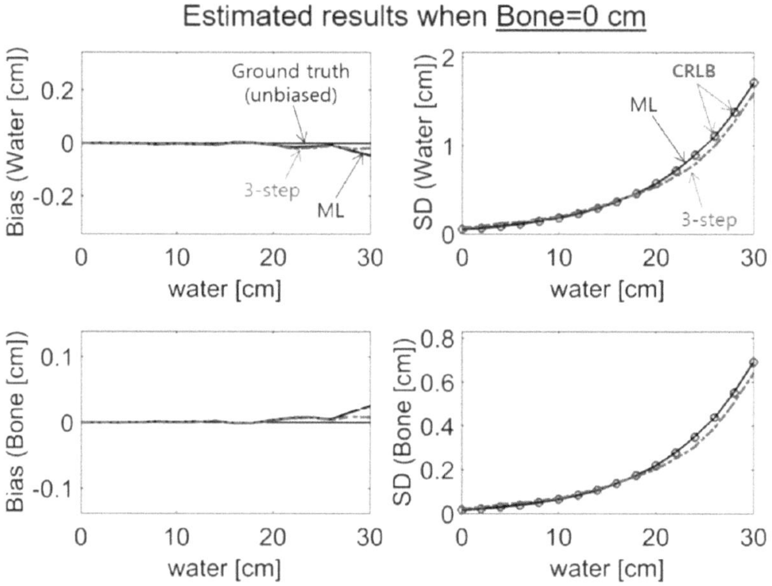

FIGURE 20.9 Bias and SD of the estimated results (thicknesses of water and bone) using the three-step algorithm and the ML-based estimator. The object consists of water, 0–30 cm with 2 cm interval, without a bone.

simple slab-geometry consisting of water (0 cm to 30 cm with 2 cm interval) and bone (0 cm or 3 cm); and, compare the results to those of the ML-based estimator. For the ML-based estimator, we used the derivative-free Nelder-Mead algorithm [24] using a software package (*fminsearch*: MATLAB® R2013a, The MathWorks Inc., Natick, MA) to solve (Eq. 20.6).

Figure 20.9 shows the bias (first column) and standard deviation (SD; second column) for the estimated thicknesses of water (first row) and bone (second row) using the three-step algorithm and the ML-based estimator when the bone is absent in the object. We also plot the ideal results (0 for the bias and the CRLB for the SD [25, 26]) to compare the estimate to the ground truth. As we can see in this figure, the results of the three-step algorithm are comparable to those of the ML-based estimator, almost unbiased and achieve the CRLB.

Figure 20.10 also shows the same results with those of Figure 20.9 but when the 3 cm of bone is present in the object. The tendency is similar to that of without bone (Figure 20.9): the results of the three-step algorithm are comparable to those of the ML-based estimator. However, the bias of the ML-based estimator increases as the amount of water increases from 20 cm to 30 cm due to the lack of sufficient statistics from a large amount of attenuation [27]. On the other hand, the three-step algorithm shows a consistent tendency regardless of the amount of attenuation due to that the implicit regularization in the first step stabilizes the estimation and also that the iterative bias correction method effectively reduces the bias [11, 12].

20.6 DISCUSSIONS

The three-step algorithm has been developed for spectral compensation in PCD-CT as a fast alternative to the conventional ML-based estimator. It requires the x-ray incident spectrum and spectral distortion model as an input to the algorithm, and estimates the x-ray transmittance in the first step, estimates basis line-integrals in the second step, and corrects for the bias in the third step. The algorithm is computationally efficient due to the linearized estimation steps and demonstrated by extensive simulation studies that it achieves almost the MVU estimator and also that the estimation

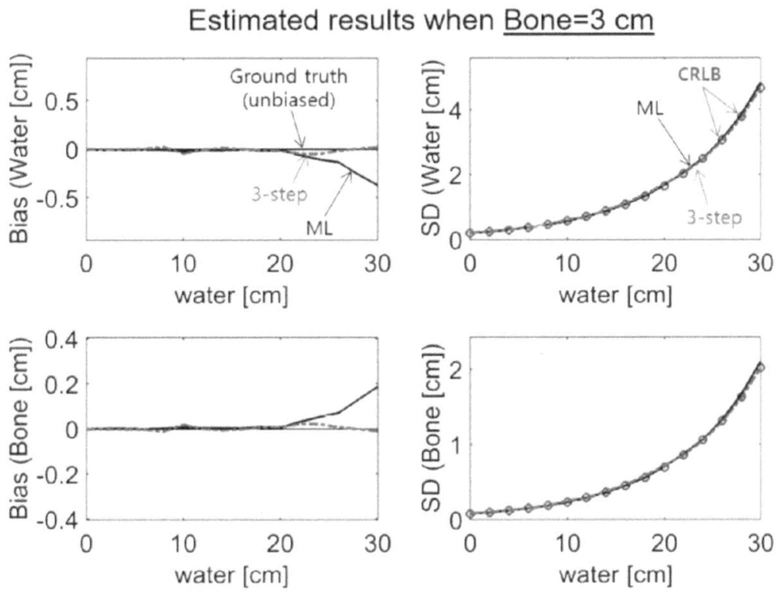

FIGURE 20.10 Bias and SD of the estimated results (thicknesses of water and bone) using the three-step algorithm and the ML-based estimator. The object consists of water, 0–30 cm with 2 cm interval, and bone, 3 cm.

results are robust to the x-ray dose level compared to those of the ML-based estimator [11, 12]. Recently, a preliminary study has been shown that the three-step algorithm also works in the prototype PCD-CT system using a simple water-equivalent phantom with bone and iodine inserts [13], but more rigorous validation and analysis are necessary for applying the algorithm to clinical cases.

We acknowledge that the computational efficiency of the ML-based estimator depends on how to implement it. Nonetheless, it is evident that all the linearization steps with closed-form solutions in the three-step algorithm are a benefit in the computational efficiency compared to that of solving a non-linear optimization problem as in the ML-based estimator. Detailed computation time for the three-step algorithm and the ML-based estimator can be found in [11] and in the supplementary material of [12].

All the compensation schemes described in this chapter are performed on the sinogram domain, that is, both model-based and calibration-based methods estimate line-integrals of the basis materials from the PCD outputs. It is also worth to mention that there are calibration-based compensation schemes performed on the image reconstructed from the PCD outputs to estimate basis images for the corresponding materials [28, 29]. Recently, various iterative schemes have also been developed to directly estimate basis images from the PCD outputs [30, 31]. Pros and cons as well as a comparison of those various approaches are of interest and should be found elsewhere.

REFERENCES

1. K. Taguchi and J. S. Iwanczyk, "Vision 20/20: Single photon counting x-ray detectors in medical imaging," *Med. Phys.*, vol. 40, no. 10, pp. 100901, Oct. 2013.
2. D. P. Cormode, S. Si-Mohamed, D. Bar-Ness, M. Sigovan, P. C. Naha, J. Balegamire, F. Lavenne, P. Coulon, E. Roessl, M. Bartels, M. Rokni, I. Blevis, L. Boussel, and P. Douek, "Multicolor spectral photon-counting computed tomography: *In vivo* dual contrast imaging with a high count rate scanner," *Sci. Rep.*, vol. 7, no. 4784, pp. 1–11, 2017.
3. E. Roessl and R. Proksa, "K-edge imaging in x-ray computed tomography using multi-bin photon counting detectors," *Phys. Med. Biol.*, vol. 52, pp. 4679–4696, 2007.

4. J. P. Schlomka, E. Roessl, R. Dorscheid, S. Dill, G. Martens, T. Istel, C. Bäumer, C. Herrmann, R. Steadman, G. Zeitler, A. Livne, and R. Proksa, "Experimental feasibility of multi-energy photon-counting K-edge imaging in pre-clinical computed tomography," *Phys. Med. Biol.*, vol. 53, pp. 4031–4047, 2008.
5. W. R. Brody, G. Butt, A. Hall, and A. Macovski, "A method for selective tissue and bone visualization using dual energy scanned projection radiography," *Med. Phys.*, vol. 8, no. 3, pp. 353–357, May 1981.
6. L. A. Lehmann, R. E. Alvarez, A. Macovski, and W. R. Brody, "Generalized image combinations in dual KVP digital radiography," *Med. Phys.*, vol. 8, no. 5, pp. 659–667, Sept. 1981.
7. H. N. Cardinal and A. Fenster, "An accurate method for direct dual-energy calibration and decomposition," *Med. Phys.*, vol. 17, no. 3, pp. 327–341, May 1990.
8. R. E. Alvarez, "Estimator for photon counting energy selective x-ray imaging with multibin pulse height analysis," *Med. Phys.*, vol. 38, no. 5, pp. 2324–2334, May 2011.
9. R. E. Alvarez, "Efficient, non-iterative estimator for imaging contrast agents with spectral x-ray detectors," *IEEE Trans. on Medical Imaging*, vol. 35, no. 4, pp. 1138–1146, Apr. 2016.
10. D. Wu, L. Zhang, X. Zhu, X. Xu, and S. Wang, "A weighted polynomial based material decomposition method for spectral x-ray CT imaging," *Phys. Med. Biol.*, vol. 61, pp. 3749–3783, 2016.
11. O. Lee, S. Kappler, C. Polster, and K. Taguchi, "Estimation of basis line-integrals in a spectral distortion-modeled photon counting detector using low-order polynomial approximation of x-ray transmittance," *IEEE Trans. on Medical Imaging*, vol. 36, no. 2, pp. 560–573, Feb. 2017.
12. O. Lee, S. Kappler, C. Polster, and K. Taguchi, "Estimation of basis line-integrals in a spectral distortion-modeled photon counting detector using low-rank approximation-based x-ray transmittance modeling: K-edge imaging application," *IEEE Trans. on Medical Imaging*, vol. 36, no. 11, pp. 2389–2403, Nov. 2017.
13. O. Lee, C. Polster, S. Kappler, K. Rajendran, C. H. McCollough, S. Leng, and K. Taguchi, "Application of the x-ray transmittance modeling-based three-step algorithm to experimental data from a prototype PCD-CT system," *Proceedings of 5th International Conference on Image Formation in X-Ray Computed Tomography (CT meeting)*, May 20-23 2018.
14. W. P. Segars, M. Mahesh, T. J. Beck, E. C. Frey, and B. M. W. Tsui, "Realistic CT simulation using the 4D XCAT phantom," *Med. Phys.*, vol. 35, no. 8, pp. 3800–3808, Aug. 2008.
15. K. Taguchi, E. C. Frey, X. Wang, J. S. Iwanczyk, and W. C. Barber, "An analytical model of the effects of pulse pileup on the energy spectrum recorded by energy reolved photon counting x-ray detectors," *Med. Phys.*, vol. 37, no. 8, pp. 3957–3969, Aug. 2010.
16. K. Taguchi, M. Zhang, E. C. Frey, X. Wang, J. S. Iwanczyk, E. Nygard, N. E. Hartsough, B. M. W. Tsui, and W. C. Barber, "Modeling the performance of a photon counting x-ray detector for CT: Energy response and pulse pileup effects," *Med. Phys.*, vol. 38, no. 2, pp. 1089–1102, Feb. 2011.
17. J. Xu, W. Zbijewski, G. Gang, J. W. Stayman, K. Taguchi, M. Lundqvist, E. Fredenberg, J. A. Carrino, and J. H. Siewerdsen, "Cascaded systems analysis of photon counting detectors," *Med. Phys.*, vol. 41, no. 10, pp. 101907 (1–15), Oct. 2014.
18. J. Cammin, J. Xu, W. C. Barber, J. S. Iwanczyk, N. E. Hartsough, and K. Taguchi, "A cascaded model of spectral distortions due to spectral response effects and pulse pileup effects in a photon-counting x-ray detector for CT," *Med. Phys.*, vol. 41, no. 4, pp. 041905 (1–15), Apr. 2014.
19. K. Taguchi, K. Stierstorfer, C. Polster, O. Lee, and S. Kappler, "Spatio-energetic cross-talk in photon counting detectors: Numerical detector model (PcTK) and workflow for CT image quality assessment," *Med. Phys.*, vol. 45, no. 5, pp. 1985–1998, May 2018.
20. J. Punnoose, J. Xu, A. Sisniega, W. Zbijewski, and J. H. Siewerdsen, "Technical Note: Spektr 3.0-a computational tool for x-ray spectrum modeling and analysis," *Med. Phys.*, vol. 43, no. 8, pp. 4711–4717, Aug. 2016.
21. P. L. Rajbhandary, S. S. Hsieh, and N. J. Pelc, "Segmented targeted least squares estimator for material decomposition in multibin photon-counting detectors," *J Med Imaging (Bellingham)*, vol. 4, no. 2, pp. 023503 (1–8), 2017.
22. C. Eckart and G. Young, "The approximation of one matrix by another of lower rank," *Psychometrika*, vol. 1, no. 3, pp. 211–218, Sept. 1936.
23. J. L. W. V. Jensen, "Sur les fonctions convexes et les inégalités entre les valeurs moyennes," *Acta Mathematica*, vol. 30, no. 1, pp. 175–193, 1906.
24. J. C. Lagarias, J. A. Reeds, M. H. Wright, and P. E. Wright, "Convergence properties of the Nelder-Mead simplex method in low dimensions," *SIAM J. Optim.*, vol. 9, no. 1, pp. 112–147, 1998.
25. S. M. Kay, *Fundamentals of Statistical Signal Processing, Volume I: Estimation Theory*, Prentice-Hall, Upper Saddle River, NJ, 1993.

26. E. Roessl and C. Herrmann, "Cramér-Rao lower bound of basis image noise in multiple-energy x-ray imaging," *Phys. Med. Biol.*, vol. 54, pp. 1307–1318, 2009.
27. C. Cloquet and Michel Defrise, "MLEM and OSEM deviate from the Cramer-Rao bound at low counts," *IEEE Trans. on Nuclear Science*, vol. 60, no. 1, pp. 134–143, Feb. 2013.
28. S. Kappler, A. Henning, B. Krauss, F. Schoeck, K. Stierstorfer, T. Weidinger, and T. Flohr, "Multi-energy performance of a research prototype CT scanner with small-pixel counting detector," *Proc. of SPIE*, vol. 8668, pp. 86680O, 2013.
29. S. Faby, S. Kuchenbecker, S. Sawall, D. Simons, H. P. Schlemmer, M. Lell, and M. Kachelriess, "Performance of today's dual energy CT and future multi energy CT in virtual non-contrast imaging and in iodine quantification: A simulation study," *Med. Phys.*, vol. 42, no. 7, pp. 4349–4366, July 2015.
30. T. G. Schmidt, R. F. Barber, and E. Y. Sidky, "A spectral CT method to directly estimate basis material maps from experimental photon-counting data," *IEEE Trans. on Medical Imaging*, vol. 36, no. 9, pp. 1808–1819, Sept. 2017.
31. K. Mechlem, S. Ehn, T. Sellerer, E. Braig, D. Münzel, F. Pfeiffer, and P. B. Noël, "Joint statistical iterative material image reconstruction for spectral computed tomography using a semi-empirical forward model," *IEEE Trans. on Medical Imaging*, vol. 37, no. 1, pp. 68–80, Jan. 2018.

21 Novel Regularization Method with Knowledge of Region Types and Boundaries

Kenji Amaya[1] *and Katsuyuki Taguchi*[2]
[1]Tokyo Institute of Technology, Tokyo, Japan
[2]Johns Hopkins University, Baltimore, Maryland, USA

CONTENTS

21.1 INTRODUCTION

Photon counting detector-based x-ray computed tomography (PCD-CT) is now recognized as the future of CT. As outlined in Chapters 5–9 PCD-CT not only improves the CT images for existing clinical applications, but also enables new applications such as probing into material properties. However, the linear attenuation coefficients of some soft tissues are closed to each other; thus, the material decomposition problem is often ill-conditioned. In order to overcome this problem, it is effective to use the *a priori* information. One of the effective *a priori* information often used in many inverse problems including image restoration and image reconstruction is the geometrical information. For example, the values of neighboring pixels are not expected to be significantly different to each other in most cases, while pixel values are expected to change discontinuously across the boundary of each material region as shown in Figure 21.1. A different class of *a priori* information is available for PCD-CT: Material

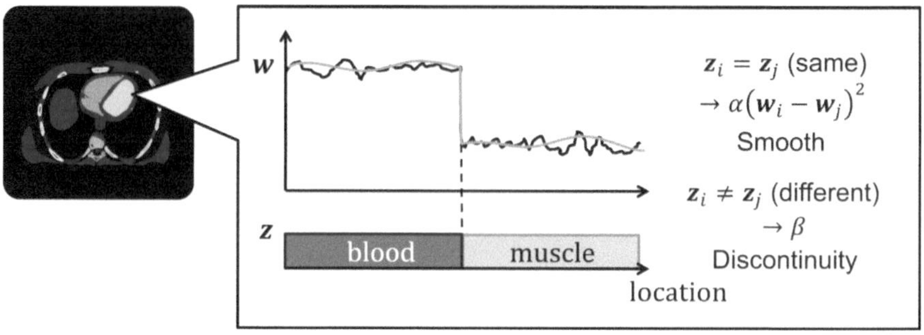

FIGURE 21.1 Attenuation coefficients change continuously within the same tissue region; however, they change abruptly and discontinuously across region boundaries.

properties. The objects are not arbitrary but human bodies in medical imaging, and there is *a priori* information on the materials of organs such as bone, heart, liver, and fat. There are international and national databases for densities and fractions-by-weight of elements (or chemical compositions) of biological composite materials [1] and for energy-dependent mass attenuation coefficients of various elements [2]. We propose to use such statistical information effectively during the image reconstruction process.

In this chapter, we introduce a novel-image reconstruction method called "Joint Estimation Maximum *A Posteriori*" (JE-MAP), which jointly estimates images of the energy-dependent linear attenuation coefficients *and* maps of tissue types, both from PCD data using material decomposition as shown in Figure 21.2. [3] The method implements image reconstruction using prior information about tissue types as well as tissue type identification using information of the noise distribution during CT projection. The JE-MAP algorithm employs maximum *a posteriori* (MAP) estimation based on voxel-based latent variables for the tissue types [4], incorporates the geometrical and statistical prior information about human organs using a voxel-based coupled Markov random field (MRF) model [5] and a Gaussian mixture model [6], respectively, and approximates photon quantum noise using a Gaussian distribution.

In the following subsections, we outline JE-MAP algorithm in detail and demonstrate how JE-MAP works using a 1-dimensional (1D) deburring as an example. We then apply JE-MAP to PCD-CT and present computer simulations results comparing with filtered backprojection (FBP) and penalized maximum likelihood (PML) with a quadratic penalty.

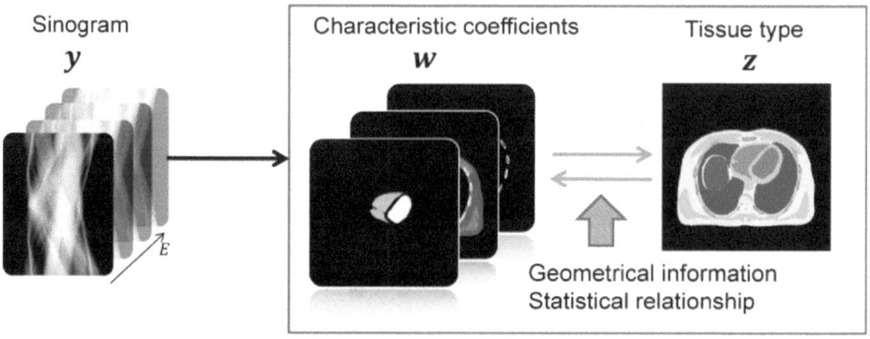

FIGURE 21.2 Diagram of "Joint Estimation Maximum *A Posteriori*" (JE-MAP) method.

21.2 METHODS

21.2.1 1D Deburring Problem Setting

We outline the JE-MAP method and demonstrate how it works using a simple example, a 1D deburring problem. The goal in this case is to estimate a set of the true pixel values and a set of tissue types for each of 1D discrete pixels from noisy and blurred 1D observed data. Let w_i be the true value on pixel $i = 1,...,I$ and a 1D vector $\mathbf{W} = \{w_i \mid i = 1,...,I\}$ be a set of the true pixel values on the 1D image.

We introduce another unknowns, latent variables z_i, to express the tissue type at each image pixel i. We employ Potts model with the 1-of-K scheme [7] to represent the tissue type. [8]

$$z_i \in \left\{(1,0,...,0)^T,...,(0,0,...,1)^T\right\}, z_i \in \{0,1\}^K. \tag{21.1}$$

Thus, each image pixel is labeled by one of K tissue types and $\mathbf{Z} = \{z_i \mid i = 1,...,I\}$ is a set of the latent variables for the 1D image.

Figure 21.3 shows the 1D problem we tackle in this section, with the vertical axis representing the true pixel values and the colors of the line indicating the tissue types. The number of pixels of this example is $I = 100$ and the number of tissue types is $K = 3$.

The quantity we observe is a blurred and noisy version of the image pixel values. Let $j = 1,...,J$ represents a set of indices of an observed data and let $\hat{V} = \{\hat{v}_j \mid j = 1,...,J\}$ be a set of blurred and noisy measured data (see, e.g., Figure 21.4) with $\hat{v}_j$ being the observed value for pixel j. The Gaussian noise parameters were $\mu_\varepsilon = 0$ and $\sigma_\varepsilon = 0.01$.

Again, our goal is to estimate the 1D image vector **W** and the tissue type vector **Z** shown in Figure 21.3 from a blurred noisy image $\hat{\mathbf{V}}$ shown in Figure 21.4.

21.2.2 Forward System Modeling

The relationship among the true pixel value w_i, the true but blurred image to be observed v_j, and the observed noisy and blurred data $\hat{v}$ can be expressed as:

$$v_j = \sum_i^I d_{ji} w_i, \tag{21.2}$$

$$\hat{v}_j = v_j + \varepsilon_j, \tag{21.3}$$

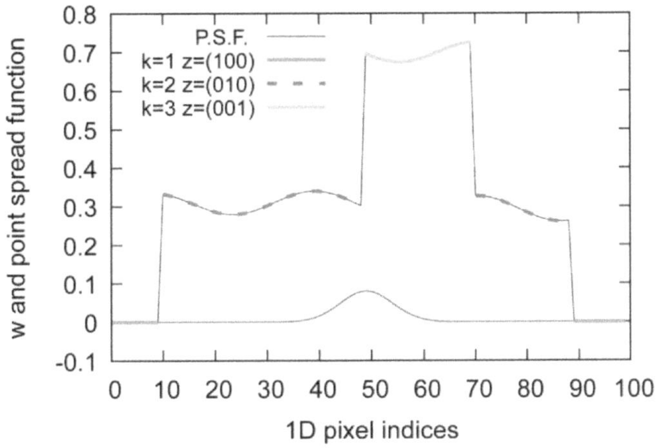

FIGURE 21.3 The true pixel values and tissue types of the 1D deburring problem.

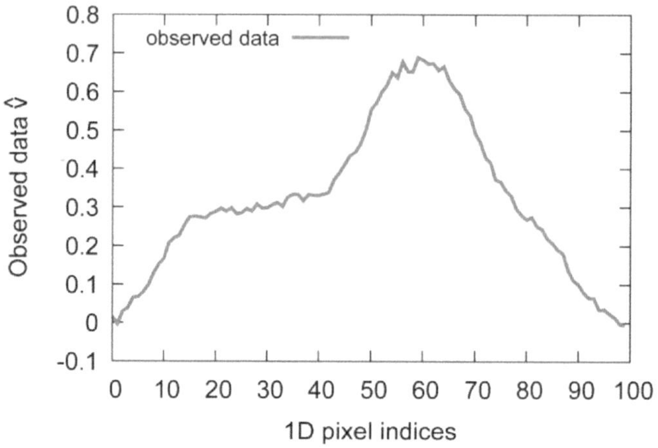

FIGURE 21.4 An example of blurry and noisy observed/measured image.

where d_{ji} and ε_j represents the blurring process and added noise, respectively, and the elements d_{ji} are given by

$$d_{ji} = \frac{1}{\sqrt{2\pi}} \exp\left(-\frac{(i-j)^2}{2\zeta^2} \right) \tag{21.4}$$

with the parameter ζ defining the degree of blurring (a smaller *zeta* resulting in a narrower Gaussian peak in Eq. (21.4), and thus, less blurry images). The point spread function with $\zeta = 5.0$ is shown in Figure 21.3. The noise ε_j is Gaussian distributed:

$$\varepsilon_j \sim \mathcal{N}(\mu_\varepsilon, \sigma_\varepsilon). \tag{21.5}$$

21.2.3 Cost Function

The 1D problem can be formulated as a joint estimation of the two unknown quantities, **W** and **Z**, which can be performed by maximizing the posterior probability. The solution can be found by

$$\begin{gathered}(\boldsymbol{W}^*, \boldsymbol{Z}^*) = \underset{w,z}{\arg\min}\{-\ln p(\hat{\boldsymbol{V}} \mid \boldsymbol{W}) - \ln p(\boldsymbol{W}, \boldsymbol{Z})\}, \\ \text{subjectto } \boldsymbol{w}_i \geq \boldsymbol{0} \ (i = 1, \ldots, I),\end{gathered} \tag{21.6}$$

where $p(\hat{\boldsymbol{V}} \mid \boldsymbol{W})$ is the likelihood distribution and $p(\boldsymbol{W}, \boldsymbol{Z})$ is the prior distribution.

21.2.4 Likelihood Modeling

Noisy and blurred measured data $\hat{\boldsymbol{V}}$ given the true object **W**, thus, the true blurred image v_j, are expressed by a Gaussian distribution:

$$-\ln p(\hat{\boldsymbol{V}} \mid \boldsymbol{W}) = \frac{1}{2} \sum_{j=1}^{J} (\hat{v}_j - v_j)^T \sigma_{\varepsilon,j}^{-1} (\hat{v}_j - v_j). \tag{21.7}$$

21.2.5 Prior Distribution Modeling

We define the prior distribution as a combination of a region-based coupled MRF model [5] and a statistical relationship between $\boldsymbol{W}$ and $\boldsymbol{Z}$, both of which are outlined in the following subsections.

$$\ln p(\boldsymbol{W},\boldsymbol{Z}) := \ln p_{\mathrm{MRF}}(\boldsymbol{W},\boldsymbol{Z}) + \ln p_{\mathrm{sta}}(\boldsymbol{W},\boldsymbol{Z}). \tag{21.8}$$

21.2.5.1 Region-Based Coupled MRF Model

We adopt a region-based coupled MRF model to express geometrical continuity within a region and discontinuity across a region boundary, both of characteristic coefficients as observable variables and region types as latent variables. Let $ne(i)$ be a set of index of neighboring voxels around image pixel i. Considering Potts model of region types, we design the region-based coupled MRF model as follows:

$$-\ln p_{\mathrm{MRF}}(\boldsymbol{W},\boldsymbol{Z}) = \mathcal{E}(\boldsymbol{W},\boldsymbol{Z}) + \ln B_{\mathrm{MRF}}, \tag{21.9}$$

$$\begin{aligned}\mathcal{E}(\boldsymbol{W},\boldsymbol{Z}) = \frac{1}{2}\sum_{i=1}^{I}\sum_{i'\in ne(i)} &\{\beta_1(z_i \cdot z_{i'})(\boldsymbol{w}_i \boldsymbol{w}_{i'})^2 \\ &+\beta_2(1 - z_i \cdot z_{i'})\left\{(\boldsymbol{w}_i - \boldsymbol{w}_{i'}) - \left(\mu(z_i) - \mu(z_{i'})\right)\right\}^2\right\},\end{aligned} \tag{21.10}$$

where $\mathcal{E}(\boldsymbol{W},\boldsymbol{Z})$ represents the energy function of Gibbs distribution and C_{MRF} is the normalization constant. $\mu(z_i)$ represents the statistical expected value of characteristic coefficients for z_i. When two region types z_i and $z_{i'}$ for neighboring pixels i and i', respectively, are the same, the first term of Eq. (21.10) encourages the smoothness while the second term vanishes. In contrast, when the region types are different, the second term encourages the difference in pixel values at the boundary of organs to be close to the expected difference, while the first term vanishes. Two parameters, β_1 and β_2, balance the effect of the corresponding term.

21.2.5.2 Gaussian Mixture Model

We model the statistical relationship between characteristic coefficients $\boldsymbol{w}$ and a region type z using a multivariate Gaussian distribution, and therefore, model the relationship between $\boldsymbol{w}$'s and all of the possible region types z's for an image pixel using a multivariate Gaussian mixture model.

$$\begin{aligned}-\ln p_{\mathrm{sta}}(\boldsymbol{W},\boldsymbol{Z}) &= -\beta_3\sum_{i=1}^{I}\{\ln p(z_i) + \ln p(\boldsymbol{w}_i \mid z_i)\} \\ &= \beta_3\sum_{i=1}^{I}\left\{\ln K + \sum_{k=1}^{K} z_i^{(k)}\left\{\frac{1}{2}(\boldsymbol{w}_i - \mu_k)^T \Sigma_k^{-1}(\boldsymbol{w}_i - \mu_k) + \ln C_k\right\}\right\},\end{aligned} \tag{21.11}$$

where β_3 is a weighting parameter, $z_i^{(k)}$ means the kth element of z_i, and μ_k, Σ_k, and C_k are the expected value, the covariance matrix, and the normalization constant of the multivariate Gaussian distribution for kth region type, respectively. We assume that a probability of tissue type z at pixel i, $p(z_i)$, is uniformly distributed; however, one can use prior knowledge to make it more accurate.

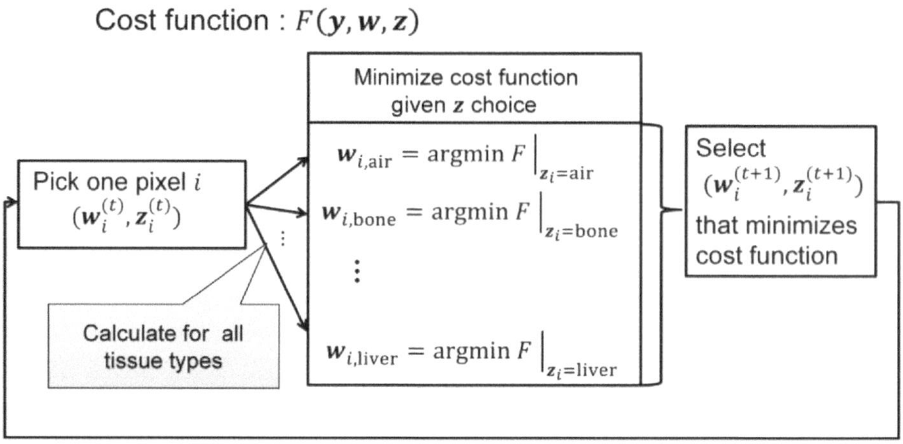

FIGURE 21.5 The flow of Iterated Conditional Modes (ICM) algorithm for the joint estimation.

21.2.6 Iterative Estimation Algorithm

Unlike usual image reconstruction problems, there are two unknowns for each pixel, and one set of unknowns, the tissue type z, is a discrete variable, while the other unknowns, the pixel value $\boldsymbol{w}$, is a continuous variable. If one performs an exhaustive search for all of the possible discrete variables z_i for all of the pixels is, it would result in a combinatorial explosion. We adopt Iterated Conditional Modes (ICM) algorithm [9] to find the minimum of the cost function. The flow of the algorithm is shown in Figure 21.5. ICM is an algorithm designed for a joint estimation problem like ours, which, at each sub-iteration, minimizes the cost function for one pixel i by first finding a sub-minimizer $\boldsymbol{w}_i$ with a discrete variable z_i being fixed at one of K tissue types using iterative coordinate descent for the continuous variable $\boldsymbol{w}_i$, performing the sub-minimization for all of the possible tissue types K, and then selecting the combination of $\boldsymbol{w}_i$ and z_i that minimizes the cost for i and using the selected combination in the next sub-iteration. The cost is minimized for a different pixel in the next sub-iteration, and repeat the process. One (global) iteration is completed once all of the pixels are swept by sub-iterations, and ICM starts the next (global) iteration. The cost function is convex with respect to $\boldsymbol{w}_i$ in each update; therefore, its constrained minimization can be computed analytically and efficiently with the Karush-Kuhn-Tucker conditions. [10]

21.2.7 Reconstruction of 1D Blurred Image with JE-MAP

We first compare the performances of JE-MAP and a conventional PML method using the reconstruction of the 1D image (Figure 21.3) from noisy blurred data (Figure 21.4), and then demonstrate the mechanism of JE-MAP. The PML method used a quadratic penalty term; thus, its cost function consisted of the likelihood term (Eq. (21.7)) and a simple MRF model, which is the first term of Eq. (21.10) with a constant tissue type z. The iterative coordinate descent algorithm was used to minimize the cost function. The parameter to control the strength of the penalty, $beta_1$, was set at the same value as JE-MAP such that the difference between the two methods was attributed to the other terms. The 1D image reconstructed by PML is shown in Figure 21.6. It can be seen that region boundaries/edges are blurred and there are some deviations from the truth at non-edge regions. In contrast, the 1D image reconstructed by JE-MAP (Figure 21.7) demonstrates that the region boundaries are sharp, that heterogeneous profiles at non-edge regions are accurate, and that tissue types (indicated by colors) are accurately estimated.

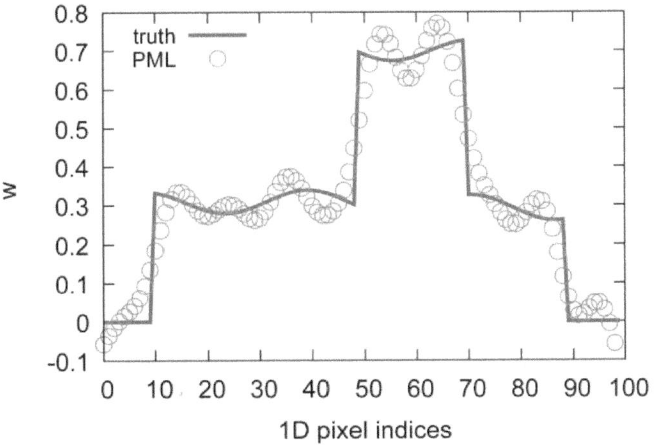

FIGURE 21.6 The 1D image reconstructed by PML.

Figure 21.8 shows the changes of the cost function values by one sub-iteration. In each global iteration step, 100 sub-iterations were performed to update all of the pixels in a randomized order. There are 100 color dots between whole numbers (i.e., in one global iteration) in Figure 21.8, which represents a chosen tissue type z_i for pixel i in a sub-iteration.

Figure 21.9 presents the updated tissue types at pixels $\mathbf{z}$ after one sub-iteration is performed on a pixel indicated by an open white circle. Green, blue, and red indicates the tissue type of 1, 2, and 3, respectively. The initial tissue type was set at $z_i = 1$ for all of the pixels. It can be seen that the correct tissue types were getting chosen as the iteration progressed as pixels at the region boundaries switch to correct tissue types.

Figure 21.10 shows the corresponding pixel values of the 1D image $\mathbf{W}$ at each sub-iteration. The initial values were the measured, blurred, and noisy image. The blurred edges (see, e.g., the edges at pixel indices of 50 and 70) gradually became sharp as iteration progresses and under/overshoot near the edges were suppressed as the tissue type boundaries grew to the exact locations. Pixel values (thus, colors) of the pixel-of-interest change after a sub-iteration is performed on the pixel.

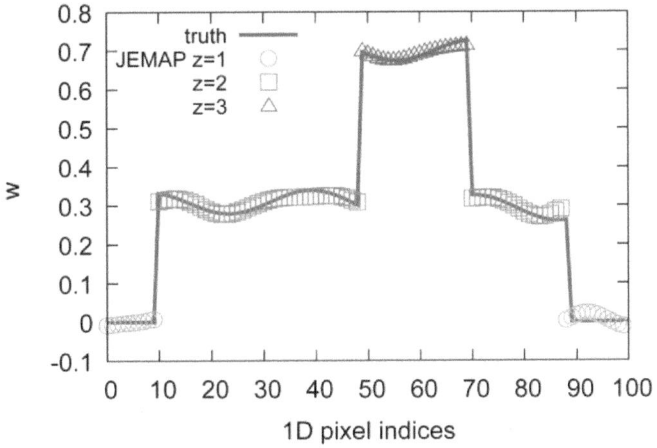

FIGURE 21.7 The 1D image reconstructed by JE-MAP. The color of each plot indicates the estimated tissue type z.

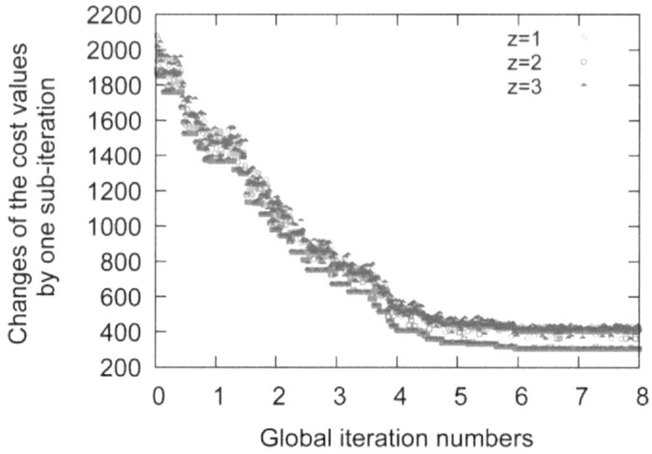

FIGURE 21.8 The change of the cost function values after each iteration.

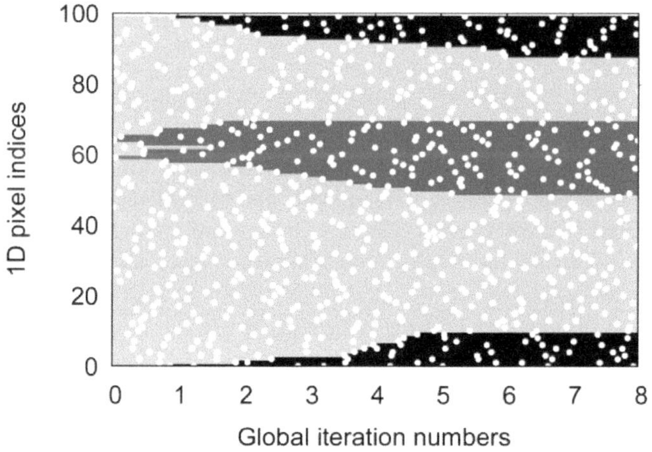

FIGURE 21.9 The chosen tissue types **Z** at each iteration.

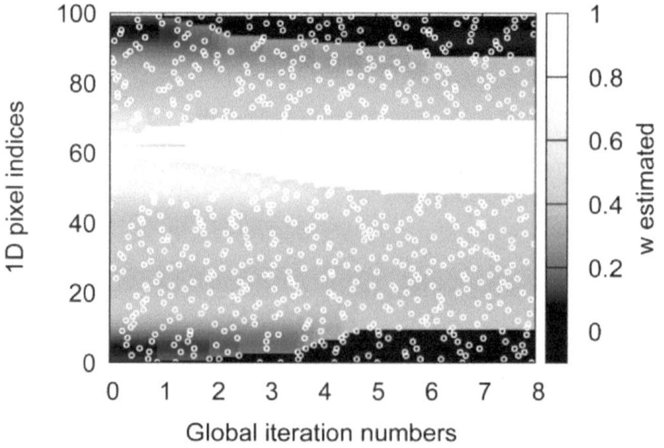

FIGURE 21.10 The change of the intensity of 1D image **W** during the iteration process.

21.3 EXTENTION TO PCD-CT

In the previous section, we described the JE-MAP method and demonstrated 1D blurred noisy image as an example. In this section, we apply the JE-MAP method to PCD-CT and our goal is to estimate both the characteristic coefficients and the material type for each image pixel from the sinogram data measured by PCD-CT.

Let $w = \{w_i \mid i = 1,...,I\}$ be a set of characteristic coefficients for the tomographic image and $z = \{z_i \mid i = 1,...,I\}$ be a set of the latent variable. For each pixel, a pair of characteristics coefficients are defined as $w = (w_{pe}, w_{CS})^T$, which correspond to the two phenomena of x-ray interactions, the photoelectric effect and Compton scattering. The energy-dependent linear attenuation coefficients at energy E at an image pixel can then be described as a linear combination of the product of energy-dependent basis functions and the corresponding characteristic coefficients. This latent variable is given to each image pixel as a label that represents one of K tissue types.

Furthermore, let $j = 1,...,J$ be a sinogram pixel index, with J the total number of sinogram pixels and let $V = \{v_j \mid j = 1,...,J\}$ be a set of line integrals of the characteristic coefficients in the sinogram, which can be calculated by forward projection of W as:

$$v_j = \sum_{i \in \text{ray}(j)} d_{ij} w_i, \tag{21.12}$$

where ray(j) is a set of image voxels through which a ray goes to sinogram pixel j in the forward projection process, and d_{ij} is an element of the forward projection matrix from image to sinogram.

The Poisson likelihood of the sinogram V given the PCD-CT measurement $\hat{Y}$ is approximated by multivariate Gaussian distributions of v_j given the parameters v_j^* and P_j^*:

$$L(V \mid \hat{Y}) \approx \prod_{j=1}^{J} \mathcal{N}(v_j \mid v_j^*, P_j^*). \tag{21.13}$$

The details of calculation of the Gaussian parameters v_j^* and P_j^* are discussed in the reference [3].

21.3.1 Evaluation Methods

In this section, we demonstrate the performance of the JE-MAP method using the results and figures presented in [3].

21.3.1.1 Phantom and Scan

We performed a computer phantom simulation to evaluate our algorithm. We used a modified thorax image of the XCAT phantom [11] with the nine tissue types shown in Figure 21.11. The phantom image covered $40 \times 40\ \text{cm}^2$ by 512×512 pixels, and heterogeneous geometrical textures were added to make the image pixel values inside organs not uniform. For contrast agent, we assumed that a dual-phase injector were used in clinics and set its concentration in heart blood as 0.4% and 0.8%, which provides enhancements similar to clinical images. There was no information available on the distribution of characteristic coefficient values for human organ; thus, the textures were added in a following way: we randomly generated high- or low-density pixels corresponding to the tissue type each pixel belong to and blurred the image by Gaussian filter. Each organ was processed separately such that the organ boundaries remained sharp.

We simulated parallel beam projections with Poisson noise and the following parameters: tube voltage 140 kV, 10^5 x-ray photons incident per projection ray, 360 projections over 180°, 728 detectors with 0.78125 mm width, same as the width of the phantom image pixel, and four energy thresholds at 10, 40, 70, and 100 keV. A hundred noise realizations were performed.

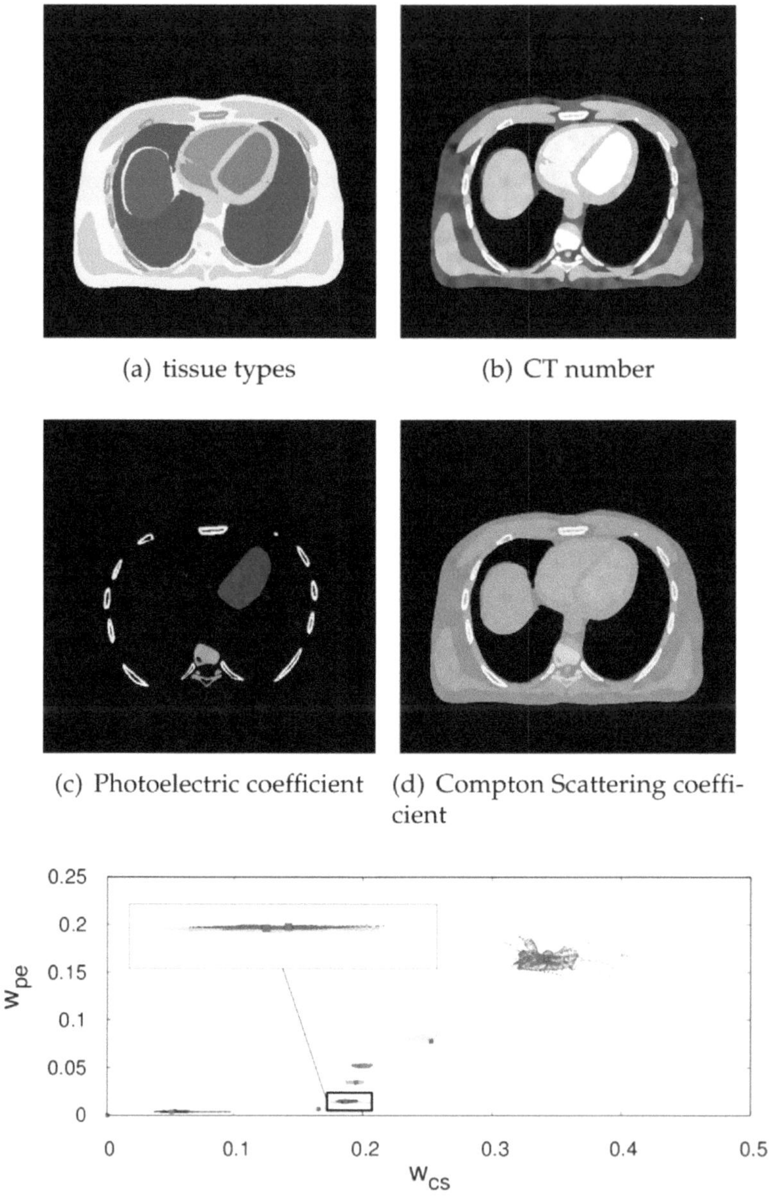

(a) tissue types (b) CT number

(c) Photoelectric coefficient (d) Compton Scattering coefficient

(e) characteristic coefficients

FIGURE 21.11 Thorax of the modified XCAT phantom. Geometrical textures were added to each tissue such that the pixel values inside an organ are not homogeneous. (a) The nine tissue types including air indicated by different colors. (b) The monochromatic CT image at 70 keV. WW 600 HU and WL 0 HU. (c, d) The images of two characteristic coefficients, photoelectric effect (c) and Compton scattering (d). (e) The scatter plot of characteristic coefficients in the phantom. (Figures are from Ref. [3])

21.3.2 Reconstruction and Tissue Type Classification

First, material decomposition was performed to obtain two sinograms of the characteristic coefficients from the PCD data. Then, images of the characteristic coefficients were reconstructed using the following three methods: FBP, PML, and JE-MAP. The FBP images were used as an initial estimate for both PML and JE-MAP. For tissue type identification for FBP and PML, we employed pixel-based identification, that is, for each image pixel a tissue type is chosen which gives the minimum L2-norm distance from the statistically expected values to the image pixel value.

FBP with a Shepp-Logan filter was performed on each of the two sinograms of the characteristic coefficients independently to obtain the corresponding image.

PML minimizes the negative Gaussian log-likelihood of the data in Eq. (21.13) with a quadratic regularizer $R(\boldsymbol{W})$ weighted by $\beta_1 = 5\times 10^4$:

$$\boldsymbol{W}^* = \arg\min_{\boldsymbol{W}}\{-\ln\ L(\boldsymbol{W} \mid \hat{\boldsymbol{Y}}) + \ln\ R(\boldsymbol{W})\},$$
$$R(\boldsymbol{W}) = \frac{1}{2}\sum_{i=1}^{N}\sum_{i'\in ne(i)} \beta_1 (w_i - w_{i'})^2 \tag{21.14}$$

JE-MAP was performed with $\beta_1 = 6.0\times 10^4$, $\beta_2 = 1.5$, and $\beta_3 = 1.0$. We preset the expected values and covariance matrices of characteristic coefficients used in JE-MAP with the number of tissue types $K = 9$ and each latent variable corresponds to tissue type shown in Table 21.1. The covariance matrix Σ_k was sampled from the phantom and scaled by $\beta_4 = 1.0\times 10^{-2}$.

$$\Sigma_k = \beta_4 \Sigma_{\text{sample},k}\,. \tag{21.15}$$

Monochromatic CT images at 70 keV were synthesized from the characteristic coefficient images. For better understanding of the role of the four terms in JE-MAP, we reconstructed the images with only one of the four parameters $\beta_1, \beta_2, \beta_3$, and β_4 being changed at a time and the image quality was qualitatively evaluated.

21.3.3 Quantitative Evaluation

The standard deviation, σ, of pixel values over 100 noise realizations was measured. The averaged value over adipose regions shown in Figure 21.12(a) was used to measure the image noise.

The spatial resolution was quantified by fitting an error function to each horizontal edge profile in the region shown in Figure 21.12(b).

$$\text{Edge}(x) = \frac{\delta_1}{2}\left(1 + \text{erf}\left(\frac{x - \delta_2}{\sqrt{2}\delta_3}\right)\right) + \delta_4, \tag{21.16}$$

TABLE 21.1
Color Table for Tissue Types in the Phantom (Table is from Ref. [3])

Tissue Type	Color Name	Color
Air	black	
Muscle	green	
Lung	brown	
Spine	light gray	
Rib	dark gray	
Adipose	yellow	
Liver	blue	
Blood w/0.4% Iodine	light magenta	
Blood w/0.8% Iodine	dark magenta	

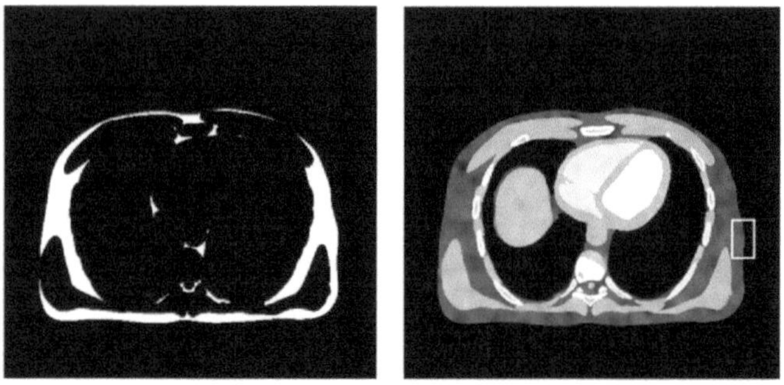

(a) ROI of adipose (b) Horizontal profile region for FWHM

FIGURE 21.12 The mean of the standard deviation values was obtained in the inner region of adipose (a), and the FWHMs were calculated from horizontal edges inside the region indicated by the white box in (b). (Figures are from Ref. [3])

In Eq. (21.16), δ_3 indicates the sharpness of the edge, from which the full-width-at-half-maximum (FWHM) was calculated as $\text{FWHM} = 2\sqrt{2\ln 2}\delta_3$. The FWHM was averaged over all profiles to obtain a measure for the spatial resolution.

The accuracy of the CT images was quantified by calculating the bias of the monochromatic CT images for each pixel, and the mean bias was calculated over the entire region inside the phantom. The accuracy of the tissue types was assessed in a binary fashion on a pixel basis. When the chosen tissue type for the image pixel was the correct tissue type, it was considered an accurate outcome; if it was not the correct tissue type, it was considered an inaccurate outcome. The ratio of the number of accurate outcomes to the number of image pixels is the accuracy of the tissue types.

21.3.4 Evaluation Results

Figure 21.13 presents the estimated tissue types and monochromatic CT images at 70 keV from one noise realization, and Figure 21.14 shows profiles along the line shown in Figure 21.13(f) for each reconstruction method. A strong salt and pepper noise can be seen in the FBP image (st.dev. = 46.8 HU in entire phantom), which resulted in a salt and pepper pattern in the tissue type image as well. PML provided CT images with less noise (st.dev. = 38.5 HU); however, it blurred the organ boundaries as seen in Figure 21.14, which, in turn, resulted in wrong tissue type identification near the organ boundaries. For example, it can be seen that there are pixels mis-identified as adipose tissue at the boundaries between the heart muscle and the lung. JE-MAP reconstructed CT images with much less noise (st.dev. = 27.4 HU), while the boundaries of organs remained sharp (Figure 21.14) resulting in more accurate tissue type identification at the boundaries. There are some regions in the tissue images of PML and JE-MAP where muscle and liver tissues were mislabeled because the characteristic coefficients of muscle and liver are too close to each other to be separated (see Figure 21.11(e)).

The calculation of JE-MAP took 942.59 sec for 33 iterations while PML took 867.35 sec for 33 iterations, using single Intel(R) Xeon(R) CPU E5-2643 v3 @ 3.40 GHz. The difference is small, which demonstrates that computing the additional terms for JE-MAP and performing ICM were not computationally significant compared to performing forward projection. Note that the present program codes have not been optimized in any way in this simulation.

Figure 21.15 presents JE-MAP images when one of the four parameters was smaller than the default setting used in Figure 21.13, and Figure 21.16 shows the images with larger parameters. The use of a smaller β_1 made the images heterogeneous but noisy (Figure 21.15(a, d)), while the use of

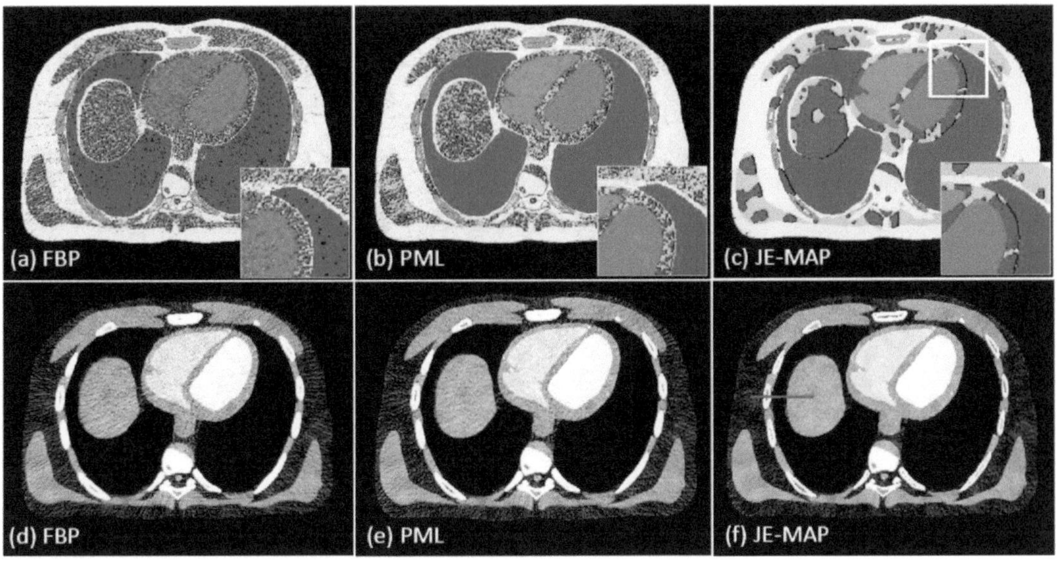

FIGURE 21.13 Images of the estimated tissue types (a-c) and monochromatic CT images at 70 keV (d-f). WW 600 HU, WL 0 HU. (Figures are from Ref. [3])

a larger β_1 resulted in a camouflage pattern caused by mislabeled tissue types (Figure 21.16(a, d)). Decreasing β_2 resulted in salt and pepper noise (Figure 21.16(b, e)), while increasing β_2 made the shape of the organs smoother (Figure 21.16(b, e)). Both β_3 and β_4 had the same effect on the images, and decreasing either β_3 or β_4 weakened the relationship between the characteristic coefficients so that the pixels were identified as either tissue type. Increasing either β_3 or β_4 made the characteristic coefficients (thus, CT pixel values) to be closer to the statistically expected values, suppressing the geometrical heterogeneous textures inside the organs.

Figure 21.17 shows the bias and standard deviation of the CT images at 70 keV and the accuracy of the tissue type identification. The mean values were measured for each organ excluding pixels near the boundaries of organs and are presented together with the mean values of the entire phantom

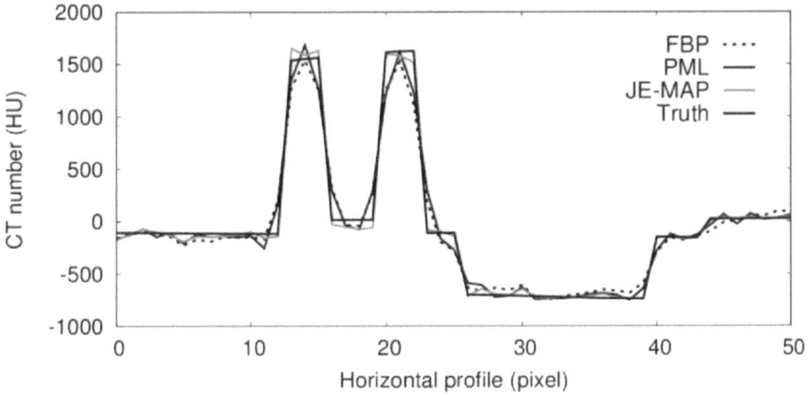

FIGURE 21.14 Profiles of CT images at 70 keV along the line in Figure 21.2(f) through adipose, rib, lung, a thin layer of adipose, and the liver. (Figures are from Ref. [3])

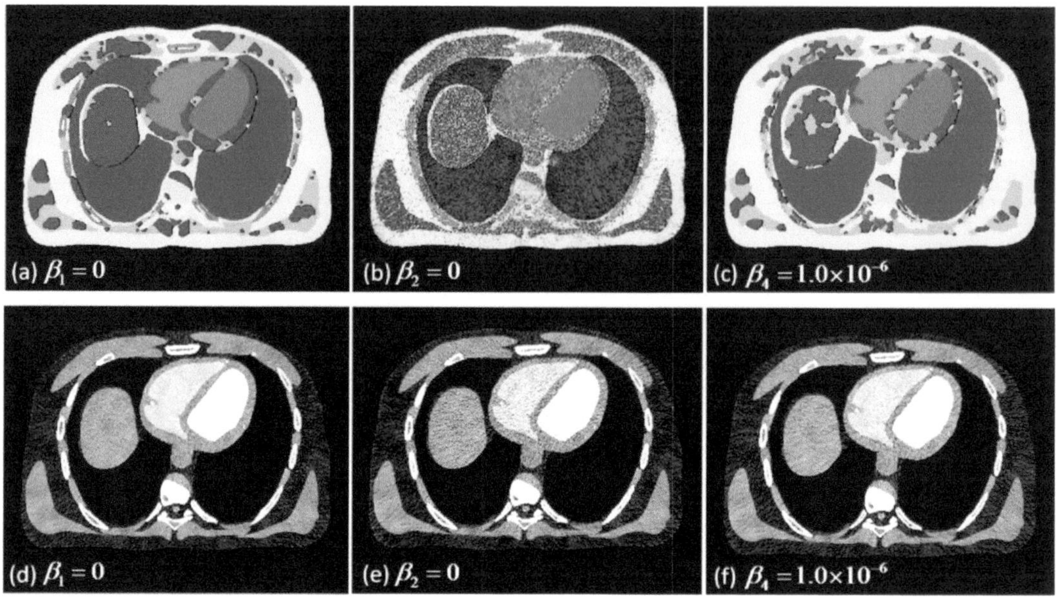

FIGURE 21.15 Images of the estimated tissue types (a-c) and monochromatic CT images at 70 keV (WW 600 HU, WL 0 HU) (d-f) obtained by JE-MAP using one of parameters smaller than those used for Figure 21.13: (a, d) smaller β_1, (b, e) smaller β_2, and (c, f) smaller β_4. (Figures are from Ref. [3])

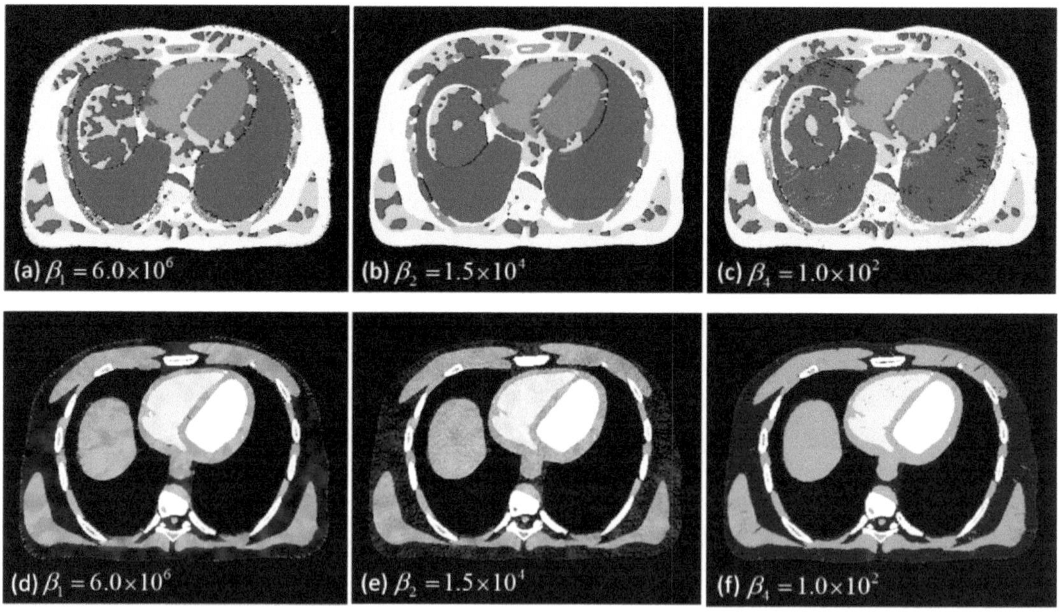

FIGURE 21.16 Images of the estimated tissue types (a-c) and monochromatic CT images at 70 keV (WW 600 HU, WL 0 HU) (d-f) obtained by JE-MAP using one of parameters larger than those used for Figure 21.13: (a, d) smaller β_1, (b, e) smaller β_2, and (c, f) smaller β_4. (Figures are from Ref. [3])

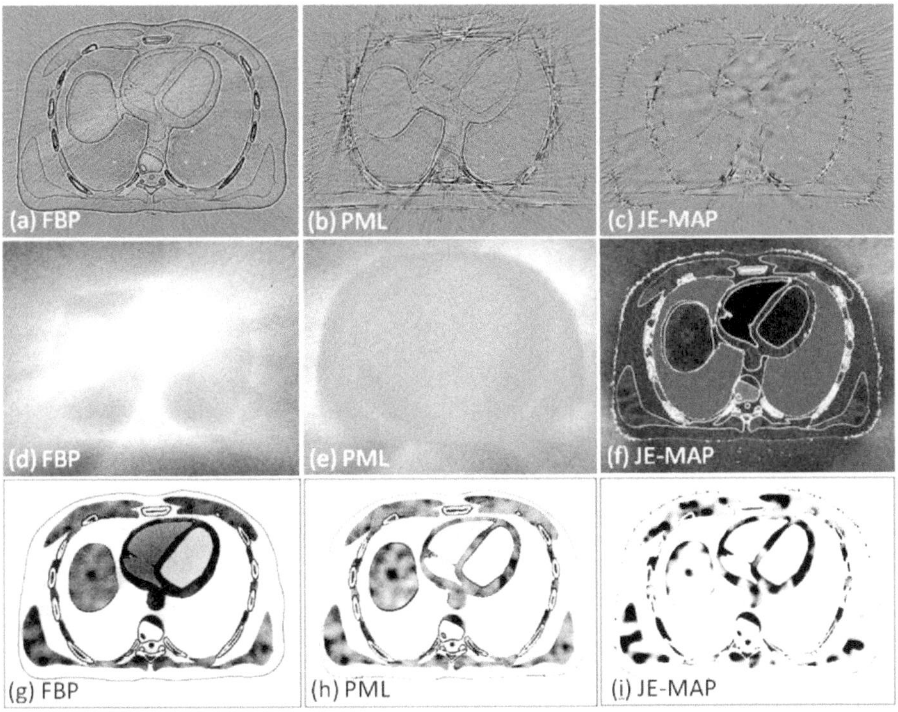

FIGURE 21.17 Results of 100 noise realizations: (a-c) bias and (d-f) noise of CT images and (g-i) the accuracy of tissue type identification. Display window width and level are: (a-c) 100 HU, 0 HU, (d) 100 HU, 100 HU, (e, f) 30 HU, 60 HU, (d) 100 HU, 100 HU, and (g-i) 50%, 100%. (Figures are from Ref. [3])

in Tables 21.2, 21.3, and 21.4. It can be seen that JE-MAP provided the best values in most indexes. The bias was as small as 0.1 HU with JE-MAP. The image noise of the entire phantom (Table 21.3) was 46.8 HU for FBP, 38.5 HU for PML and 27.4 HU for JE-MAP. The accuracy of tissue types improved from 71.7% for FBP and 80.1% for PML to 86.9% for JE-MAP. The accuracy of muscle with JE-MAP was lower than other organs, which are attributed to the mislabeling as liver.

TABLE 21.2
Mean Bias in Homogeneous Tissue Regions (Table is from Ref. [3])

	Bias (HU)		
Tissue Type	**FBP**	**PML**	**JE-MAP**
Air	0.1	0.0	0.0
Muscle	1.0	0.3	0.3
Lung	−1.0	−0.1	0.0
Spine	6.2	−0.6	−0.4
Rib	−1.0	46.8	3.4
Adipose	0.0	0.2	0.0
Liver	2.6	0.5	0.0
Blood w/ 0.4% Iodine	3.5	0.6	0.4
Blood w/ 0.8% Iodine	4.4	0.6	−0.3
Entire Phantom	−1.8	−0.9	−0.1

TABLE 21.3
Mean Standard Deviation in Homogeneous Tissue Regions (Table is from Ref. [3])

	Standard Deviation (HU)		
Tissue type	**FBP**	**PML**	**JE-MAP**
Air	28.0	34.9	23.6
Muscle	46.2	38.4	21.6
Lung	43.1	37.8	24.3
Spine	56.5	39.9	26.8
Rib	49.1	39.4	38.8
Adipose	39.9	37.9	21.2
Liver	59.1	39.0	20.4
Blood w/ 0.4% Iodine	63.5	39.9	16.5
Blood w/ 0.8% Iodine	64.0	39.9	18.8
Entire Phantom	46.8	38.5	27.4

TABLE 21.4
Mean Accuracy in Homogeneous Tissue Regions (Table is from Ref. [6])

	Accuracy (%)		
Tissue type	**FBP**	**PML**	**JE-MAP**
Air	99.9	100.0	100.0
Muscle	34.3	49.7	54.6
Lung	98.1	100.0	100.0
Spine	99.6	100.0	100.0
Rib	100.0	100.0	99.8
Adipose	94.1	94.0	100.0
Liver	41.9	52.8	91.6
Blood w/ 0.4% Iodine	41.4	90.5	100.0
Blood w/ 0.8% Iodine	68.4	95.0	100.0
Entire Phantom	71.7	80.1	86.9

The resolution-noise tradeoff curves were shown in Figure 21.18, where the top-left end-point of the curves was obtained from the images reconstructed by the corresponding method. JE-MAP provided the best tradeoff performance.

21.4 CONCLUSION

In this chapter, we have introduced a new joint estimation framework employing MAP estimation based on pixel-based latent variables for tissue types. The JE-MAP method makes the continuous Baysian estimation from detected noisy photon counts possible by integrating the geometrical information described by latent MRF, statistical relationship between tissue types and the characteristic coefficients, and Poisson noise models of PCD data. A simple example

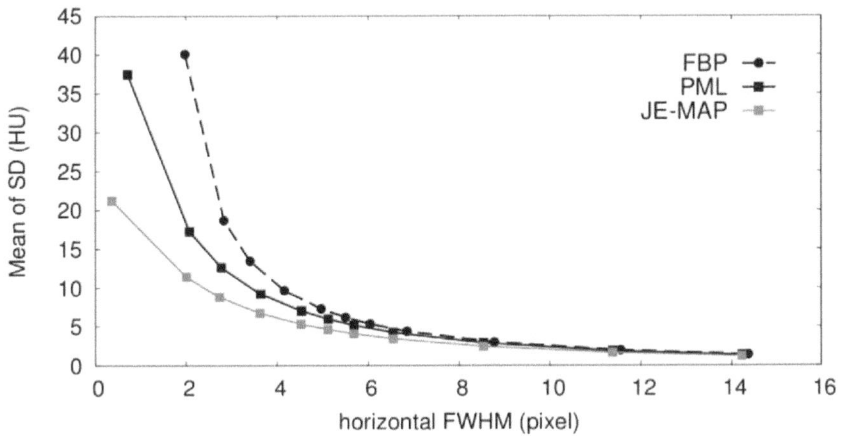

FIGURE 21.18 Noise-resolution tradeoff curves. The top-left point of each method is the values from the estimated images, and the curves are obtained by blurring each image with a Gaussian filter with various parameters. (Figures are from Ref. [3])

of 1D image reconstruction was provided to help readers understand how JE-MAP works visually and clearly.

The use of the additional information on tissue types improves the resolution-noise tradeoff of the images, and the use of improved images improves the accuracy of the tissue type identification. The JE-MAP method provided more accurate tissue type identification, decreased image noise, sharper edges, while maintaining heterogeneous tissue textures. The joint estimation framework has a potential for an even further improvement by introducing more prior information about tissues in human body, for example, the location, size, and number of tissues, or limited variation of neighboring tissues, which will be easily formulated by pixel-based latent variables.

ACKNOWLEDGMENTS

The work was supported in part by research agreements with Siemens Healthineers (JHU-2013-CT-125-01-Taguchi-C00212554 and JHU-2018-CT-1-02-Taguchi-C00229096). We are grateful for Mr. Kento Nakada and Dr. George S. K. Fung for their contribution to JE-MAP algorithm development and Drs. Matthew K. Fuld, Thomas G. Flohr, Steffen Kappler, Karl Stierstorfer, and Christopher Polster for their support.

REFERENCES

1. Yongyue Zhang, Michael Brady, and Stephen Smith. Segmentation of brain MR images through a hidden Markov random field model and the expectation-maximization algorithm. *IEEE Transactions on Medical Imaging*, 20(1):45–57, 2001.
2. Stan Z Li. *Markov Random Field Modeling in Image Analysis*, Vol. 26. Springer, London, 2009.
3. Christopher M Bishop et al. *Pattern Recognition and Machine Learning*, Vol. 4. Springer New York, 2006.
4. D. R. White, I. J. Wilson, J. Booz, J. J. Spokas, and R. V. Griffith. ICRU report 44, tissue substitutes in radiation dosimetry and measurement. *Journal of the International Commission on Radiation Units and Measurements*, 1989.
5. James H. Hubbell and Stephen M. Seltzer. X-ray mass attenuation coefficients. *NIST Standard Reference Database*, 126, 1996.

6. Kento Nakada, Katsuyuki Taguchi, George S. K. Fung, and Kenji Amaya. Joint estimation of tissue types and linear attenuation coefficients for photon counting CT. *Medical Physics*, 42(9):5329–5341, 2015.
7. Ryota Hasegawa, Masato Okada, and Seiji Miyoshi. Image segmentation using region-based latent variables and belief propagation. *Journal of the Physical Society of Japan*, 80(9):3802, 2011.
8. Ryota Hasegawa, Masato Okada, and Seiji Miyoshi. Image segmentation using region-based latent variables and belief propagation. *Journal of the Physical Society of Japan*, 80(9):3802, 2011.
9. Julian Besag. On the statistical analysis of dirty pictures. *Journal of the Royal Statistical Society. Series B (Methodological)*, 259–302, 1986.
10. Rangarajan K. Sundaram. *A First Course in Optimization Theory*. Cambridge University Press, 1996.
11. W. P. Segars, G. Sturgeon, S. Mendonca, Jason Grimes, and B. M. W. Tsui. 4d xcat phantom for multi-modality imaging research. *Medical Physics*, 37(9):4902–4915, 2010.

Index

NOTE: Page numbers in **bold** and *italics* refer to tables and figures, respectively.

C

D

Q

R

S

T

Y

Z